New Frontiers in Head and Face Medicine

New Frontiers in Head and Face Medicine

Editor: Edward Clark

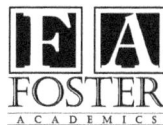

FA
FOSTER
ACADEMICS

www.fosteracademics.com

www.fosteracademics.com

FA **FOSTER**
ACADEMICS

Cataloging-in-Publication Data

New frontiers in head and face medicine / edited by Edward Clark.
     p. cm.
Includes bibliographical references and index.
ISBN 978-1-63242-771-7
     1. Head--Diseases. 2. Face--Diseases. 3. Head--Diseases--Treatment. 4. Face--Diseases--Treatment.
5. Head--Diseases--Diagnosis. 6. Face--Diseases--Diagnosis. 7. Otolaryngology. I. Clark, Edward.
RC936 .N49 2019
617.51--dc23

Foster Academics,
118-35 Queens Blvd., Suite 400,
Forest Hills, NY 11375, USA

ISBN 978-1-63242-771-7 (Hardback)

Contents

Preface

Head and face medicine deals with the conditions of the structures of the head, face and neck. It encompasses a number of sub-disciplines specializing in different aspects of injuries, diseases and trauma, such as facial plastic and reconstructive surgery, head and neck oncologic surgery and otology, among others. Plastic surgery is a specialization in medicine, which involves the reconstruction, restoration and alteration of a body part. Reconstructive surgery which aims to reconstruct a body part, and cosmetic surgery that is performed for aesthetic reasons are encompassed under plastic surgery. Abdominoplasty, blepharoplasty, lip enhancement, rhinoplasty, cheek augmentation, etc. are some of the facial augmentation procedures under plastic surgery. Craniofacial surgery is a form of reconstructive surgery, in which congenital and acquired deformities of the head, face, skull, neck and jaws are addressed. Cleft lip and palate, rare craniofacial clefts, isolated and syndromic craniosynostosis, Crouzon's syndrome, craniofacial microsomia, etc. are treated in this domain. This book provides significant information of this discipline to help develop a good understanding of head and neck medicine and associated specializations. The extensive content herein provides the readers with a thorough understanding of the subject. This book aims to equip students and experts with the advanced topics and upcoming concepts in this area.

The information contained in this book is the result of intensive hard work done by researchers in this field. All due efforts have been made to make this book serve as a complete guiding source for students and researchers. The topics in this book have been comprehensively explained to help readers understand the growing trends in the field.

I would like to thank the entire group of writers who made sincere efforts in this book and my family who supported me in my efforts of working on this book. I take this opportunity to thank all those who have been a guiding force throughout my life.

Editor

Quantitative relations between the eyeball, the optic nerve, and the optic canal important for intracranial pressure monitoring

Michael Vaiman[1,3*], Paul Gottlieb[2] and Inessa Bekerman[2]

Abstract

Objective: To find correlations between diameters of the optic nerve sheath (ONSD), the eyeball, and the optic canal that might be important for intracranial pressure monitoring.

Methods: In a prospective cohort study, the CT data of consecutive 400 adults (18+) with healthy eyes and optic nerves and absence of neurological diseases were collected and analyzed. When the CT scans were obtained, the diameters of the optic nerve sheath, the eyeball, and the optic canal were measured and statistically analyzed. The data obtained from the left and from the right eyeballs and optic nerves were compared. The correlation analysis was performed within these variables, with the gender, and the age.

Results: In healthy persons, the ONSD varies from 3.65 mm to 5.17 mm in different locations within the intraorbital space with no significant difference between sexes and age groups. There is a strong correlation between the eyeball transverse diameter (ETD) and ONSD that can be presented as ONSD/ETD index. In healthy subjects, the ONSD/ETD index equals 0.19.

Conclusion: The calculation of an index when ONSD is divided by the ETD of the eyeball presents precise normative database for ONSD intracranial pressure measurement technique. When the ONSD is measured for intracranial pressure monitoring, the most stable results can be obtained if the diameter is measured 10 mm from the globe. These data might serve as a normative database at emergency departments and in general neurological practice.

Keywords: Optic nerve sheath diameter, Computed tomography

Introduction

Intracranial pressure monitoring by means of measuring changes in the optic nerve sheath' diameter (ONSD) became practical in the 1990s. It was postulated that the presence of enlarged optic nerve sheaths suggests that raised intracranial pressure is transmitted intraorbitally [1-3]. While this fact is already well established and its importance is understood, some disagreement remains in its quantitative part. The ONSD is measured by sonography, CT, and MRI but no generally accepted protocol was designed. Different authors indicated normal/abnormal threshold (a cutoff value) of the ONSD from 5 mm to 5.9 mm with numerous variations between these numbers [4,5]. The recent review on methods of intracranial pressure monitoring estimated the accuracy of the ONSD method as low [6].

Numerous publications on the topic [1-5,7,8], actually all of them, report measurements of the ONSD only and do not take into account variations of forms and sizes of the eyeball and the optic canal as like the intraorbital part of the optic nerve is located not between these two anatomical structures but in the open space. There is a possibility that dimensions of these two structures might correlate with the ONSD influencing the accuracy of the ONSD method of intracranial pressure monitoring. If the ONSD is used as a technique for intracranial pressure monitoring, various additional factors are to be taken into account.

* Correspondence: vaimed@yahoo.com
[1]Department of Otolaryngology, Head and Neck Surgery, Assaf Harofe Medical Center, Affiliated to Sackler Faculty of Medicine, Tel Aviv University, Zerifin, Israel
[3]33 Shapiro Street, Bat Yam 59561, Israel
Full list of author information is available at the end of the article

First, the eyeball is a constantly voluntary and involuntary moving object even when at rest and the head of the optic nerve moves with it [9]. For example, if at the moment of the image taking a patient will gaze 3 mm above the horizontal line, the distal part of the optic nerve will move 3 mm below the horizontal line; and if fixational eye movements will turn the eye 3 mm to the left, the optic nerve head will move 3 mm to the right. All that movements might change the ONSD close to the globe. The researches ignore this possibility and they usually measure the ONSD only 3 mm behind the globe [1-5,7,8]. The authors have chosen this location because the sheath is wide in this area (bulging dura mater region).

Second, the axial length of the eyeball (anterior-to-posterior diameter) is different in cases with myopia, emmetropia, and hypermetropia [10]. Third, myopia, congenital and acquired glaucoma, retinoblastoma and some other disorders can change the size of the eyeball [11]. Forth, the optic canal of the sphenoid bone can be wide, normal, or narrow and specifically its orbital opening can be wide or narrow that can influence the ONSD because the sheath acts as periosteum of the sphenoid bone inside the canal [12]. All these variations might influence the accuracy of the ONSD method of intracranial pressure monitoring.

The purpose of the current research was to establish normative data of the ONSD in various locations within its intraorbital part with the help of data obtained by computer tomography (CT) technique and to analyze their possible correlations with the eyeball transverse diameter (ETD) and the optic canal diameters. We planned to measure the ONSD in several distances from the globe together with the diameters of the optic canal and the eyeball, analyze possible correlations, and recommend the most convenient approach to be used in practice in cases when ONSD is measured for the purpose of detection of elevated intracranial pressure.

Materials and methods
Study design and setting
In a prospective cohort study, we collected and analyzed the CT data of consecutive 400 adult patients (18+) that were admitted to the Department of Radiology at our Medical Center from Jan 2011 to February 2014. The study protocol conformed to the ethical guidelines of the 1975 Declaration of Helsinki as reflected a *priori* after approval by the institution's Helsinki committee. We examined the patients who were admitted to the Emergency Department, were referred to the CT investigation that included the head and neck region, and appeared to be neurologically and ophthalmologically healthy.

Exclusion procedure was organized in two steps. First, the patients with documented ophthalmologic, cerebral, or neurophthalmologic disorders were excluded as well as patients with injuries around the orbits. At this stage, we also checked the data of the blood tests to exclude intoxications that might affect CNS. Second, the selected patients were examined by an ophthalmologist and by a neurologist in order to exclude overlooked eye disorders or cerebral pathology. Special attention was paid in order to exclude cases with ischemic, toxic, hereditary, nutritional, or compressive neuropathies, glaucoma, cataract, etc. Therefore, four criteria were used to include a case into our study: 1) a neurologist did not find any CNS-specific pathology; 2) an ophthalmologist did find any eye/optic nerve-specific pathology; 3) CT investigation did not detect any cranial pathology or existing pathology of the optic nerve; 4) blood tests did not indicate any toxic elements that might affect the CNS.

The patient flow was as follows: from the 587 consecutive patients, 122 were excluded at the first step, 65 were excluded at the second step. The data collection was stopped when we obtained 400 healthy cases.

Variables analyzed
1. ETD (retina to retina), 2. ONSD at 3 mm behind the globe, 3. ONSD at 10 mm behind the globe, 4. ONSD at 3 mm from the anterior lumen of the optic canal, and 5. area of the anterior lumen of the optic canal.

Data sources and measurements
All the CT scans were obtained by the 256-slice CT scanner (Brilliance iCT, Philips Healthcare). We implemented the standard Philips protocols for head and neck imaging in all cases, single slice section 3 mm [13-15]. When the CT scans were obtained, the left and right ETD and the ONSD were measured by the computer program (Figures 1 and 2). The transverse diameter of the eyeball was chosen because the ONSD is usually measured in the transverse plain. The optic canal is rarely round in its orbital orifice; usually it is oval. That is why we measured two diameters for its orbital opening. Window parameters were: spine window, middle third; WW 60, WL 360, (sometimes abbreviated as C:60,0. W:360,0 spine), accuracy 1 pixel. All measurements were made using the same window, contrast and brightness. The error margin was expressed by means of the technical error of measurement (TEM) to calculate the intra-evaluator variability and inter-evaluator variability between two evaluators. The same equipment and methodological procedures for measurements were adopted by both evaluators.

Analysis
Measurements of five above mentioned variables were analyzed. A within-group repeated measures experimental statistical analysis was used to test the variables. To verify the normality of the data, normal probability plots

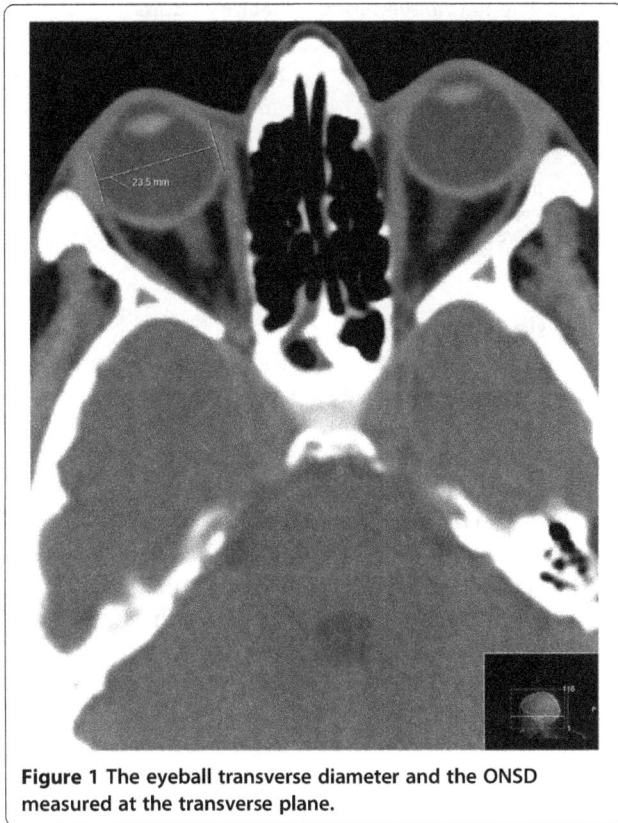

Figure 1 The eyeball transverse diameter and the ONSD measured at the transverse plane.

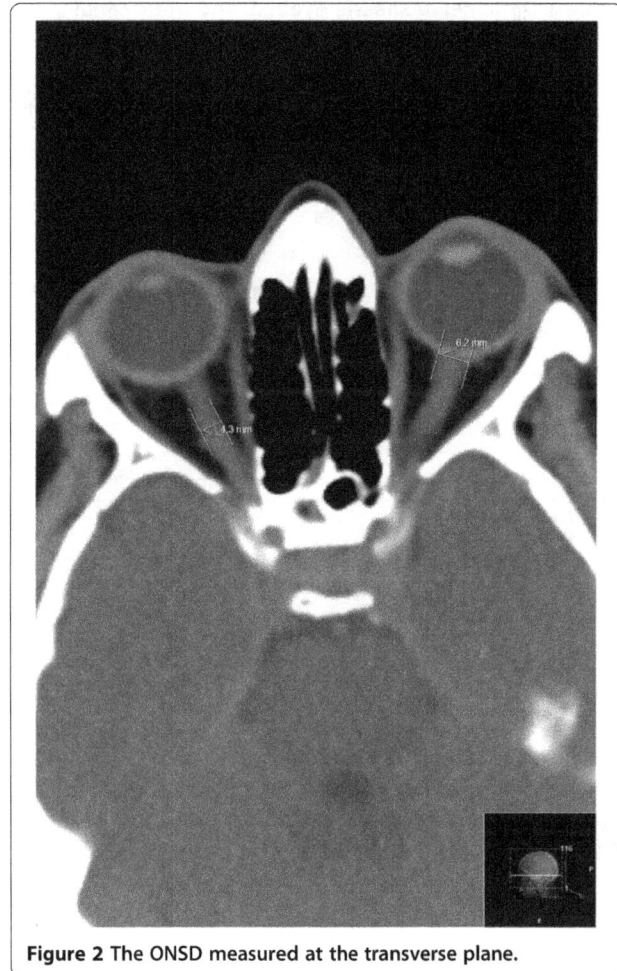

Figure 2 The ONSD measured at the transverse plane.

and basic descriptive statistics (mean, standard deviation (SD), min, and max) were calculated for every variable (the diameters). The data obtained from the left eyeball and the optic nerve and from the right eyeball and the nerve was compared. The correlation analysis was performed with gender and age groups (group I: 18-30; group II: 30-65; group III: 65+).

The correlation analysis was performed between the following pairs of variables: ETD to ONSD at 3 and 10 mm from the globe; ONSD converted to area at 3 mm from the lumen of the optic canal to the area of the lumen. The correlation analysis between the optic canal measurements and the proximal ONSD were performed not between their diameters but between their areas because the nerve is round and the optic canal is oval. The data were statistically evaluated by three-dimensional analysis of variance, SPSS, Standard version 17.0 (SPSS, Chicago, IL, 2007), and χ [2] criterion using 95% confidence interval. The level of significance for all analyses was set at $p < 0.05$.

Results

In our cohort, there were 214 females and 186 males, age range was from 18 to 94 (mean 46). Distribution among age groups was as follows: group I (18-30) - 89; group II (30-65) - 156; group III (65+) - 155.

Altogether, 800 eyeballs, ONSD, and optic canals were measured. For the TEM calculation, two measurements were obtained from each location (n = 1600 measurements for each of three variables). The difference between the first and second measurements were then determined and the relative TEM (technical error of measurement expressed in %) was calculated to be 3.77 acceptable. For inter-evaluator TEM, it varied from 3.18 to 3.58 for different locations (acceptable).

Tables 1 and 2 present the results of the measurements. Analyzing these data it was detected that standard deviation of the mean ONSD, minimal, and maximal variations of the ONSD are the highest at 3 mm position while at 10 mm position they are the lowest. Variations of the proximal part of the ONSD that is close to the anterior opening of the optic canal are also less significant if compared with the 3 mm position. For this location, however, strong positive correlation exists between the ONS area (calculated from ONSD data) and the area of the orbital orifice of the optic canal. At the orifice itself the correlation is almost

Table 1 Optic nerve sheath, eyeball, and optic canal anterior (orbital) opening CT measurements (in mm)

Distance/position	Right eye			Left eye		
	Mean ± SD	Max	Min	Mean ± SD	Max	Min
Distal ONSD*	4.94 ± 1.51	7.5	3.5	5.17 ± 1.34	7.9	3.8
Middle ONSD**	4.35 ± 0.76	7.6	3.3	4.45 ± 0.62	5.9	3.3
Proximal ONSD***	3.84 ± 0.82	5.2	2.7	3.65 ± 0.70	4.8	2.9
Proximal ONS area	11.58 ± 1.8	21.23	5.7	10.46 ± 1.5	18	6.6
Transverse	22.822 ± 1.7	25.5	20.0	22.936 ± 1.8	25.8	19.4
Eyeball diameter						
Optic canal anterior opening						
Longer diameter	4.8 ± 1.8	5.8	3.5	5.0 ± 1.8	5.8	3.6
Shorter diameter	4.2 ± 1.6	4.8	2.9	4.2 ± 1.7	4.8	2.8
Area (mm²)	15.83 ± 2.3	19	7.2	16.49 ± 2.7	21.86	7.9

*3 mm behind the globe.
**10 mm behind the globe.
***3 mm before entering the anterior opening of the optic canal.

100% (r = 0.96), and at 3 mm from the orifice it remains 0.82. In comparison, at 10 mm from the globe location r = 0.44 only.

Analyzing further the obtained results, we paid attention that ONSD taken from the middle section of the intraorbital part of the optic nerve correlates with the ETD of the eyeball and that this correlation can be presented as an index. This index is calculated as ONSD divided by the transverse diameter of the eyeball (ONSD/ETD) and is presented in the Table 3 as 0.19 with standard deviation of 0.01-0.02.

We did not find statistically significant differences correlated with gender of the patients (p = 0.15), and their age (I vs. II, p = 0.25; I vs. III, p = 0.09; II vs. III, p = 0.36). In our cases, measurements taken from the right eyeball and optic nerve were slightly smaller than the left side measurements but this difference is also statistically insignificant (p = 0.44).

Table 2 Correlation between the optic nerve sheath, eyeball, and optic canal anterior (orbital) opening measurements (in mm)

Correlation between	Right eye	Left eye
	r	r
Distal ONSD*/ETD	0.74	0.69
Middle ONSD**/ETD	0.79	0.77
Proximal ONS area***/OC lumen area	0.82	0.84
ONS area at lumen/OC area at the lumen	0.96	0.95

*3 mm behind the globe.
**10 mm behind the globe.
***3 mm before entering the anterior lumen of the optic canal.
ETD – eyeball transverse diameter.
OC – optic canal.

Table 3 The nerve/eye index in healthy adults

ONSD/ETD index	Right eye	Left eye
Average	0.19 ± 0.01	0.19 ± 0.02
Max	0.26	0.26
Min	0.15	0.15

The index is calculated as ONSD taken from the middle part of the intraorbital path of the optic nerve divided by the transverse diameter of the eyeball (ONSD/ETD).

Discussion

The pathophysiology of optic nerve sheath enlargement as a result of intracranial hypertension has been established well already [6,7,16]. The ONSD technique itself is not perfected yet and some improvements might be suggested. Analyzing the obtained data, we believe that the 3 mm distance from the globe is not the ideal location to measure ONSD for intracranial pressure monitoring. We cannot ignore constant physiological tremor, slow drifts, flicking movements, tracking movements, smooth pursuits, saccades, and other eye movements [17,18]. Whatever method is used for the ONSD measurement – CT, MRI, or ultrasound – images are taken from a constantly moving object even when a patient is given instruction to look straight forward, and even when the eyes are closed. Currently, the quantitative estimate of how the movements of the eyeball change shape and size of the bulging dura mater region is lacking. We cannot recommend measuring the ONSD close to the globe until this question is clarified. In addition to that, the enlargement of ONSD behind the globe was also found in papilledema, optic nerve lesions, optic atrophy, and endocrine orbitopathy [19,20].

We did not find statistically significant differences in ONSD correlated with age. The optic nerves experience the age-dependent nerve fiber loss as any other nerve in the human body. However, while total axon count in the optic nerve decreases with age, mean axon diameter increases with age [21]. At the same time, the thickness of dura mater increases with age [22]. While all these processes take place simultaneously, we might suggest that the ONSD remains approximately the same during a lifetime.

The size of the eyeball correlates with the ONSD. This fact can be used to our advantage. The optic nerve/eyeball diameter index is much less variable variance than ONSD and could be used for intracranial pressure monitoring with more precise results.

Movements of the eyeball can change ONSD close to the globe therefore 3 mm distance from the globe is not an ideal location to measure ONSD to monitor intracranial pressure. If ONSD is measured close to the orbital orifice of the optic canal, the measurements can be influences by the correlation between dimensions of the

ONS and the optic canal. If the canal itself and especially if its anterior opening is wide or narrow, the ONSD measurement will correlate with it. Therefore, the proximal location is also not ideal for measuring the ONSD for intracranial pressure purposes. The middle part of the intraorbital optic nerve route experience less variations in size in normal healthy people. We do not dictate that ONSD should be measured at 10 mm from the globe sharp; the intraorbital part of the optic nerve varies in length (usually from 1.5 to 2.4 cm) and the ONSD can be measured at 8 mm or 12 mm from the globe but definitely not at 3 mm location. In any case, for the most precise detecting of the elevated intracranial pressure, we recommend to use the optic nerve/ eyeball diameter index. This index is calculated as ONSD taken from the middle part of the intraorbital path of the optic nerve divided by the transverse diameter of the eyeball (ONSD/ETD). While standard deviation of the ONSD measurements varies from 0.62 to 1.51 at various locations, the standard deviation of the ONSD/ETD index is 0.01-0.02 that insures very precise normative data. From three eyeball diameters, we selected the ETD because the majority of the authors writing on ONSD technique for intracranial pressure monitoring measure ONSD in the transverse plain and because anterior-to-posterior eyeball diameter varies in cases of myopia, emmetropia, and hypermetropia significantly.

Limitations of the research

All the CT scans were obtained by the 256-slice CT Philips scanner. It might be possible that scanners of different trademarks could provide slightly different results of measurements as well as MRI or sonography evaluation.

Generalisability

External validity of the study results is based on recent efforts in standardization of CT nomenclature and protocols for various CT scanner manufacturers (GE, Philips, Toshiba, Hitachi, Siemens). All these scanner manufacturers provide features to automatically initiate a prescribed axial, helical or dynamic scan when a threshold level of contrast enhancement is reached at a specified region of interest (in our case, the orbit and the optic canal) [23].

Conclusion

In healthy persons, the ONSD varies from 3.65 mm to 5.17 mm in different locations within the intraorbital space with no significant difference between sexes and age groups. More precise results can be obtained through the calculation of an index when ONSD is divided by the ETD of the eyeball. In healthy subjects, the ONSD/ETD index equals 0.19. When the ONSD is measured for intracranial pressure monitoring, the most stable results can be obtained if the diameter is measured 10 mm from the globe. These data might serve as a normative database when ONSD technique is used for intracranial pressure monitoring at emergency departments and in general neurological practice.

Competing interests

The authors declare that they have no financial and non-financial conflict of interest.

Authors' contributions

MV – study concept, study design, analysis of the data, manuscript draft, manuscript final version; PG and IB – collection of the data, data analysis. All authors read and approved the final manuscript.

Author details

[1]Department of Otolaryngology, Head and Neck Surgery, Assaf Harofe Medical Center, Affiliated to Sackler Faculty of Medicine, Tel Aviv University, Zerifin, Israel. [2]Department of Radiology, Assaf Harofe Medical Center, Affiliated to Sackler Faculty of Medicine, Tel Aviv University, Zerifin, Israel. [3]33 Shapiro Street, Bat Yam 59561, Israel.

References

1. Hansen HC, Helmke K: The subarachnoid space surrounding the optic nerves. An ultrasound study of the optic nerve sheath. *Surg Radiol Anat* 1996, **18**(4):323–8.
2. Helmke K, Hansen HC: Fundamentals of transorbital sonographic evaluation of optic nerve sheath expansion under intracranial hypertension. I. Experimental study. *Pediatr Radiol* 1996, **26**(10):701–5.
3. Helmke K, Hansen HC: Fundamentals of transorbital sonographic evaluation of optic nerve sheath expansion under intracranial hypertension II. Patient study. *Pediatr Radiol* 1996, **26**(10):706–10.
4. Kimberly HH, Shah S, Marill K, Noble V: Correlation of optic nerve sheath diameter with direct measurement of intracranial pressure. *Acad Emerg Med* 2008, **15**(2):201–4.
5. Geeraerts T, Launey Y, Martin L, Pottecher J, Vigué B, Duranteau J, Benhamou D: Ultrasonography of the optic nerve sheath may be useful for detecting raised intracranial pressure after severe brain injury. *Intensive Care Med* 2007, **33**(10):1704–11.
6. Raboel PH, Bartek J Jr, Andresen M, Bellander BM, Romner B: Intracranial pressure monitoring: invasive versus non-invasive methods-a review. *Crit Care Res Pract* 2012, **2012**:950393. doi: 10.1155/2012/950393. Epub 2012 Jun 8.
7. Moretti R, Pizzi B: Optic nerve ultrasound for detection of intracranial hypertension in intracranial hemorrhage patients: confirmation of previous findings in a different patient population. *J Neurosurg Anesthesiol* 2009, **21**:16–20.
8. Tayal VS, Neulander M, Norton HJ, Foster T, Saunders T, Blaivas M: Emergency department sonographic measurement of optic nerve sheath diameter to detect findings of increased intracranial pressure in adult head injury patients. *Ann Emerg Med* 2007, **49**(4):508–14.
9. Martinez-Conde S, Macknik SL: Fixation eye movements across vertebrates: comparative dynamics, physiology, and perception. *J Vis* 2008, **8**(14):28.1–16.
10. Tomlinson A, Phillips CI: Applanation tension and axial length of the eyeball. *Brit J Ophthal* 1970, **54**:548–553.
11. Charman WN: Optics of the Human Eye. In *Visual Optics and Instrumentation*. Edited by Cronly Dillon J. Boca Raton: CRC Press; 1991:1–26.
12. Prado PA, Ribeiro EC, De Angelis MA, Smith RL: Biometric study of the optic canal during cranial development. *Orbit* 2007, **26**(2):107–11.
13. Wintermark M, Maeder P, Verdun FR, Thiran JP, Valley JF, Schnyder P, Meuli R: Using 80 kVp versus 120 kVp In Perfusion CT Measurement Of Regional Cerebral Blood Flow. *AJNR Am J Neuroradiol* 2000, **21**(10):1881–1884.
14. Smith WS, Roberts HC, Chuang NA, Ong KC, Lee TJ, Johnston SC, Dillon WP: Safety and feasibility of a CT protocol for acute stroke: combined CT, CT

angiography, and CT perfusion imaging in 53 consecutive patients. *AJNR Am J Neuroradiol* 2003, **24**(4):688–90.

15. Wintermark M, Fischbein NJ, Smith WS, Ko NU, Quist M, Dillon WP: **Accuracy of dynamic perfusion CT with deconvolution in detecting acute hemispheric stroke.** *AJNR Am J Neuroradiol* 2005, **26**(1):104–12.

16. Hayreh SS: **The sheath of the optic nerve.** *Ophthalmologica* 1984, **189**(1–2):54–63.

17. Schütz AC, Trommershäuser J, Gegenfurtner KR: **Dynamic integration of information about salience and value for saccadic eye movements.** *Proc Natl Acad Sci U S A* 2012, **109**(19):7547–52.

18. Richard A, Churan J, Guitton DE, Pack CC: **Perceptual compression of visual space during eye-head gaze shifts.** *J Vis* 2011, **11**(12). doi:10.1167/11.12.1.

19. Mashima Y, Oshitari K, Imamura Y, Momoshima S, Shiga H, Oguchi Y: **High-resolution magnetic resonance imaging of the intraorbital optic nerve and subarachnoid space in patients with papilledema and optic atrophy.** *Arch Ophthalmol* 1996, **114**(10):1197–203.

20. Skalka HW: **Neural and dural optic nerve measurements with A-scan ultrasonography.** *South Med J* 1978, **71**(4):399–400.

21. Mikelberg FS, Yidegiligne HM, White VA, Schulzer M: **Relation between optic nerve axon number and axon diameter to scleral canal area.** *Ophthalmology* 1991, **98**(1):60–3.

22. Jimenez-Hamman MC, Sacks MS, Malinin TI: **Quantification of the collagen fiber architecture of human cranial dura mater.** *J Anat* 1998, **192**:99–106.

23. Kalra MK, Saini S: **Standardized nomenclature and description of CT scanning techniques.** *Radiology* 2006, **241**:657–660.

2

Efficacy of platelet rich fibrin in the reduction of the pain and swelling after impacted third molar surgery

Ozkan Ozgul[1*], Fatma Senses[2], Nilay Er[3], Umut Tekin[2], Hakan Hıfzı Tuz[4], Alper Alkan[5], Ismail Doruk Kocyigit[2] and Fethi Atil[2]

Abstract

Background: Impacted third molar removal is a routine procedure in oral and maxillofacial surgery. Platelet-rich fibrin (PRF) is a second generation platelet concentration which is produced by simplified protocol. The aim of this study was to assess the effectiveness of PRF in the healing process by evaluating the changes in pain and swelling after third molar surgery.

Methods: Fifty-six patients (23 male, 33 female) who provide the inclusion criteria were selected to participate in this study. The evaluation of the facial swelling was performed by using a horizontal and vertical guide. The pain was evaluated in the postoperative period using a visual analog scale (VAS) of 100 mm.

Results: Horizontal and vertical measurements showed more swelling at the control side (without PRF) in 3th day postoperatively ($p < 0.05$). There were no statistically significant differences regarding pain among the groups.

Conclusion: As a conclusion, PRF seems to be effectiveness on postoperative horizontal swelling after third molar surgery. PRF could be used on a routine basis after third molar extraction surgery.

Keywords: PRF, Third molar surgery, Pain, Swelling

Background

The removal of impacted third molars is common oral surgical procedure. Surgical extraction of third molars is often accompanied by pain, swelling, trismus, and general oral dysfunction during the healing period [1–5]. Careful surgical technique and scrupulous perioperative care can minimize the frequency of complications and limit their severity [2].

Various pharmacological and/or extraction methods have been used for maintaining patients social activities. These include non-steroid anti-inflammatory drugs (NSAIDs), laser treatment, steroids and ultrasound [6–9]. However, the amount and intensity of edema, pain and trismus occurring after surgical extraction cannot be eliminated completely.

Platelet-rich fibrin (PRF) is a second generation platelet concentration which is produced by simplified protocol. PRF consists of a fibrin matrix polymerized in a tetramolecular structure, the incorporation of platelets, leukocyte, and cytokines, and the presence of circulating stem cells [10–12]. There are many studies showing accelerating wound healing of PRF in periodontal defects, cyst cavities and sinus floor augmentation in the literature [13–15]. There are limited studies on the effects of PRF on postoperative pain and swelling [16, 17].

The aim of this study is to evaluate the incidence and severity of postoperative swelling and pain following mandibular third molar surgery using PRF as a healing material in the extraction sockets. The null hypothesis tested was that PRF would effect the postoperative swelling and pain positively.

* Correspondence: ozkanozgul@yahoo.com
[1]Department of Oral and Maxillofacial Surgery, Faculty of Medicine, Ufuk University, Ankara, Turkey
Full list of author information is available at the end of the article

Method

This study was carried in two different Oral and Max-illofacial Surgery Departments. Institutional ethics com-mittee's approval was obtained for the protocol of the study. [Kırıkkale University, Faculty of dentistry local ethic committee 09/03 (15.04.2013)]. Based on previ-ously treated trial cases we conducted a power analysis (Power and Precision software, Biostat, Englewood, NJ, USA). The findings indicated a minimum sample size of $n = 50$, based on an α of 5 % and a power of 80 %. Con-sidering a possible loss of about 10 % of patients, we used 56 participants.

After preoperative evaluation and obtaining written in-formed consent, total of 56 patients (23 male, 33 female) ranging from 18-28 years who could follow postopera-tive instructions were selected for the study.

Clinical inclusion criteria were as follows:

1) Bilateral fully impacted third molars which have the same degree of surgical difficulty comparing one side with the other (Fig. 1).
2) No preexisting medical conditions or no use of medication that would influence or alter wound healing
3) No active pathology associated with the third molars
4) No temporomandibular joint disorder history that would affect the pain sensation after surgery.

Fifty-six patients (23 male-, 33 female) who met the inclusion criteria were selected to participate in this study. Pell and Gregory [18] classification was used to determine the difficulties of the patients included in the study. Of these 56 patients distribution of the classifica-tion was as: 20 horizontal, 15 mezioangular, 21 vertical. PRF and the technique were explained to patient and in-formed consent was taken from all patients.

Patients underwent surgical treatment in accordance with the rules of antisepsis and asepsis. All bilateral third molars surgeries were performed by a single experienced operator in each centers. Prior to the extractions, 10 ml of venous blood was collected from each patient by a surgical nurse and was placed in glass-coated plastic tubes. Tubes were transferred to a centrifuge device and centrifuged for 10 min at 3000 rpm according to Chouk-roun et al [14].

Following centrifugation, PRF was dissected approxi-mately 2 mm below its connection to the red corpuscle beneath to include remaining platelets, which have been proposed to localize below the junction between PRF and the red corpuscle. Then PRF was squeezed between gauzes to transform into a membrane (Fig. 2).

All patients underwent bilateral removal of 3rd molar in single appointment that were the same degree of surgical difficulty. Mandibular and buccal blocks were adminis-tered using articaine containing 1:200,000 epinephrine (Ultracain DS; Aventis, Istanbul, Turkey). Horizontal and vertical incisions were performed and a full-thickness mucoperiosteal flap was raised and the tooth was removed with elevators. Following the extraction, the socket was thoroughly irrigated so that pathologic tissue (eg, granula-tion tissue), follicular remnants, and bony spicules were removed from the cavity (Fig. 3). Following that PRF was placed in the socket on one side which was chosen ran-domly by coin toss and other side was taken as control group (Fig. 4). Both extraction cavities were primarily closed with 3-4 interrupted sutures using 3.0 silk sutures. Postoperatively, amoxicillin 1000 mg (Alfoxil 1gr; Fako, Istanbul, Turkey) twice daily, paracetamol 500 mg (Vermi-don 500 mg; Sandoz, Istanbul, Turkey) thrice daily and chlorhexidine mouthwash thrice daily were administered to all patients for a week.

Patients were blind to the knowledge of PRF placed side in order not to affect visual analog scale (VAS) scores. The pain was evaluated in the postoperative period using a VAS of 100 mm. After the surgery, the patients were instructed to note their postoperative dis-comfort and/or pain on the scale, which was designed as 0 indicating no pain whereas 100 indicating the worst ever experienced . The evaluation of the postoperative

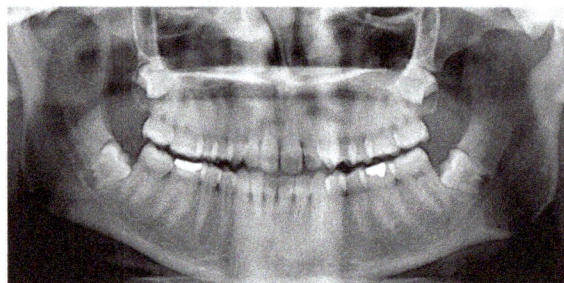

Fig. 1 PRF was prepared to place into extraction socket

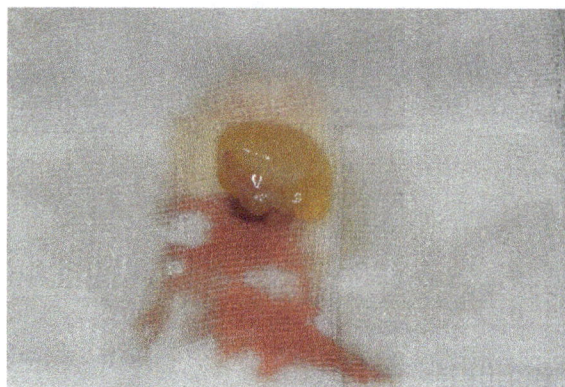

Fig. 2 Bilateral impacted third molars which have the same degree of surgical difficulty comparing one side with the other

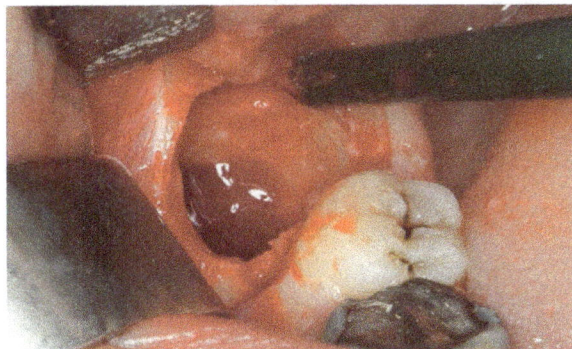

Fig. 3 Extraction socket

pain was carried out at 24 h, 72 h and seven days after the procedure.

The evaluation of the facial swelling was done by using a horizontal and vertical guide with a flexible ruler. For horizontal guide two points marked at the ear tragus and buccal comissura, and the distance between them was measured and recorded. The same procedure was performed for vertical guide at lateral chantus of the eye and gonion. The evaluation of the postoperative facial swelling was carried out at 24 th hours, 72th hours and seventh day after the procedure. The postoperative evaluations were performed by surgeons that were blinded to the operative procedures, in order to eliminate unwanted bias. The evolution of swelling was evaluated by subtracting the value obtained at each postoperative period by the obtained at baseline [19].

Statistical analysis was performed using the software program SPSS 20.0 (SPSS 20.0 for Windows; SPSS Inc., Chicago, IL, USA), at a significance level of $\alpha = 0.05$. For analysis of swelling the Shapiro–Wilk test was used to evaluate the distribution of the data (normal or non-normal), the Wilcoxon test for paired samples was used since the data were not normally distributed. Regarding the pain statistical analysis were performed by using one–way analysis of variance (ANOVA). If there were

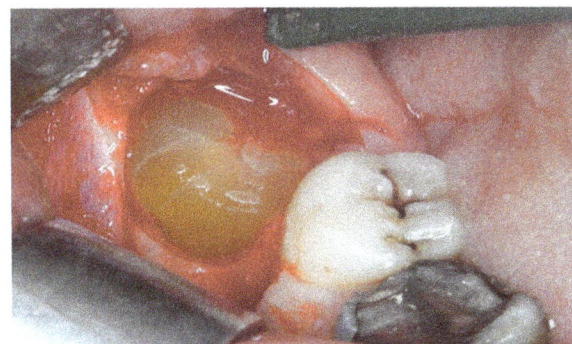

Fig. 4 PRF placed into extraction socket on one side

difference between the measurements, the data were analyzed by the Paired Sample test.

Results
Statistically significant differences were observed in first and third days horizontal measurements between PRF and control side ($p < 0.05$). And more swelling was seen at the control side. The pain scores were measured by using VAS. There were no statistically significant differences observed between groups (Tables 1, 2 and 3).

Discussion
The surgical removal of impacted third molars cause trauma of the soft tissue and bony structures in the oral cavity. The postoperative signs and symptoms of pain, edema and limited mouth opening due to muscle spasm might occur [20, 21].

Fibrin glue [also known as fibrin sealant or fibrin adhesive (platelet rich plasma, PRF)] is a protein based product developed for tissue hemostasis and sealing. Platelet–based materials combine plasma proteins and platelets [22].

PRF described by Choukrouns is prepared naturally without addition of thrombin, and it is hypothesized that PRF has a natural fibrin framework and can protect growth factors from proteolysis [13]. PRF releases high quantities of three main growth factors transforming growth factor β-1 (TGF beta-1), platelet-derived growth factor AB (PDGF-AB), vascular endothelial growth factor (VEGF), and an important coagulation matricellular glycoprotein (thrombospondin-1, TSP-1) during 7 days. Apart from these PRF also secrete EGF, FGF, and three important proinflammatory cytokines- IL-1b, IL-6, and TNF-α which obtained with a simple centrifugation procedure, to stimulate several biological functions such as chemotaxis, angiogenesis, proliferation, differentiation, modulation, thereby representing a possible therapeutic device for a more rapid and effective regeneration of hard and soft tissues [14, 16, 17]. Platelets also play a role in host defense mechanisms at the wound site, by delivering signaling peptides which attract macrophage cells. Platelet concentrates may contain small amounts of leukocytes that synthesize interleukins involved in the non-specific immune reaction [22].

Recently the use of PRF has been proposed as an aid for enhancing regeneration of osseous and epithelial tissues in oral surgery. Several in vitro studies, animal experiments and clinical trials suggested that platelet concentrates may effectively trigger stimulation of osseous and soft tissue regeneration, and reduce inflammation, pain and side effects. The clinical efficacy of PRF in oral surgical procedures is debated as contrasting results have been reported in different clinical procedures [22–25].

Table 1 Results of Postoperative Swelling (horizontal measurements)

Horizontal swelling			
Postoperative evaluation times	Control side Mean(SD)	PRF side Mean (SD)	P-value
1st day	4.64 (4.27)	3.28 (3.02)	0.041*
3rd day	3.62(3.51)	1.83(2.52)	0.001*
7th day	0.73 (1.89)	0.57 (1.87)	0.634

*statistically significant differences amongs groups

Use of PRF in oral cavity has been implicated in different procedures such as extraction socket preservation, intrabony defects, sinus augmentation, and sinus lift procedures for implant placement, bone augmentation, root coverage procedures, and healing in donor site with successful results [22].

Recently some studies evaluated the effect of platelet rich plasma (PRP) to the extraction sockets healing and postoperative complications [26, 27]. Several studies showing animal experiments and clinical trials showed that PRF might affect the regeneration of soft and hard tissue, healing and reduce the side effects [22, 24].

Zhang et al [25] evaluate the influence of PRF on bone regeneration in sinus augmentation. After a healing period of 6 months no statistical differences found between PRF and the control groups.

According to a study by Choukroun et al. a cystic cavity filled with PRF would be totally healed in 2 months instead of the 6 to 12 months required for physiologic healing [22].

There are some controversies in the literature. A study evaluating the effectiveness of PRF in the treatment of intrabony defects of chronic periodontitis patients, thirty-two defects were treated with PRF or a conventional open flap debridement alone. They showed that PRF can be used in the treatment of intrabony defects of chronic periodontitis patients [28]. Lee et al [24] used the PRF for restoration of peri-implant defects in rabbit. Their results showed the possibility of PRF use in bone regeneration.

Contradictory, Aroca et al [15] evaluated that the claimed benefits for soft tissue wound healing induced by PRF membranes and they reported that their results failed to show any beneficial effect of PRF membrane in

Table 2 Results of Postoperative Swelling (vertical measurements)

Vertical swelling			
Postoperative evaluation times	Control side Mean(SD)	PRF side Mean (SD)	P-value
1st day	5.92 (7.42)	5.19 (8.12)	0.306
3rd day	4.00 (6.42)	3.42 (6.55)	0.589
7th day	1.28 (3.95)	0.82 (3.81)	0.061

Table 3 Results of Postoperative pain

VAS scores			
Postoperative evaluation times	Control side Mean(SD)	PRF side Mean (SD)	P-value
1st day	42.84 (29.77)	47.16 (30.59)	0.413
3rd day	26.48 (30.36)	25.50 (29.95)	0.296
7th day	9.41 (16.57)	10.21 (19.75)	0.503

terms of root coverage or short-term wound healing for the treatment of multiple gingival recessions.

Mozatti et al [26] evaluated that the effects of PRP on inflammation process, wound healing, pain and swelling after third molar extraction. They reported that PRP was more effective on wound healing in the extraction socket. Our results supported that PRF was more effective on the swelling in the third day after third molar surgery.

Alissa et al [27] evaluated the influence of PRP on healing of extraction sockets. They reported that PRP may have some benefits in reducing complications such as alveolar osteitis, swelling, pain and improving healing of soft tissue.

Kumar et al [17] investigated the effect of platelet-rich fibrin (PRF) on postoperative pain, swelling, trismus, periodontal healing they concluded that case group had less pain, swelling, and trismus on the first postoperative day compared with the control group. Their results also showed increased and faster periodontal healing in the case group.

In another study by Singh et al [16] they concluded that use of PRF after bilaterally third molar surgeries resulted in less pain compared to control side.

In the present study, PRF was used after third molar extraction, swelling and pain were evaluated. Statistically significant difference was found concerning first and third day horizontal measurements of PRF and control sides with more swelling at the control side ($p < 0.05$). These results are in accordance with Kumar et al [17].

The present study found no significant difference between PRF and control sides in terms of pain which is similar to Singh et al [16], but different from Kumar et al [17] study where the control and PRF groups consisted of different patients. As the results of the study the null hypothesis was partially rejected since there was no positive effect of PRF seen on the pain.

There are some limits to our study; the present study was conducted on bilaterally removed third molars at the same session the results of pain might have been influenced by the control side. Also the use of 3-D optical scanner for the measurements of facial swelling might have given more precise recordings however the funding of the study did not support such expenses. We recommend that further studies investigating this manner should consider the mentioned limitations of the present study.

Conclusion

As a conclusion, PRF seems to be efficient on postoperative horizontal swelling after third molar surgery. PRF could be used for control swelling after third molar extraction surgery. Studies with a larger sample that will need a bilateral third molar removal that will be extracted in different sessions with a longer follow-up is warranted to obtain a more statistically meaningful results with respect to bone regeneration.

Abbreviations
NSAID: Non-steroid anti-inflammatory drugs; PRF: Platelet-rich fibrin; PRP: Platelet-rich plasma; VAS: Visual analog scale.

Competing interest
All authors declare that they have no competing interests.

Authors' contributions
All authors contributed extensively to the work presented in this paper. OO searched the articles for the review, drafted the manuscript and wrote the manuscript. FS and NE have performed the surgeries. IDK and AA performed the postoperative measurements. IDK and FA designed the study and helped in wrote the manuscript. AA and HHT drafted the manuscript and reviewed it critically. UT revised the final version of the manuscript. All authors read and approved the final version of the manuscript.

Author details
[1]Department of Oral and Maxillofacial Surgery, Faculty of Medicine, Ufuk University, Ankara, Turkey. [2]Department of Oral and Maxillofacial Surgery, Faculty of Dentistry, Kırıkkale University, Kırıkkale, Turkey. [3]Department of Oral and Maxillofacial Surgery, Faculty of Dentistry, Trakya University, Edirne, Turkey. [4]Department of Oral and Maxillofacial Surgery, Faculty of Dentistry, Hacettepe University, Ankara, Turkey. [5]Department of Oral and Maxillofacial Surgery, Faculty of Dentistry, Erciyes University, Kayseri,, Turkey.

References
1. Koerner KR, Medlin KE. Clinical procedures for third molar surgery. 2nd ed. South Sheridan: PennWell; 1995.
2. Szmyd L. Impacted teeth. Dent Clin North Am. 1971;15:299–318.
3. Nageshwar. Comma incision for impacted third molars. J Oral Maxillofac Surg. 2002;60(12):1506–9.
4. Fonseca RJ, Frost DE, Hersh EV, Levin LM. Oral and maxillofacial surgery: anaesthesia/dentoalveolar surgery/office management. 1st ed. Philadelphia: Saunders; 2001.
5. Kirk DG, Liston PN, Tong DC, Love RM. Influence of two different flap designs on incidence of pain, swelling, trismus, and alveolar osteitis in the week following third molar surgery. Oral Surg Oral Med Oral Pathol Oral Radiol Endod. 2007;104:e1–6.
6. Bagan JV, Lopez JS, Valencia E. Clinical comparison of dexketoprofen trometamol and dipyrone in postoperative dental pain. J Clin pharmacol. 1998;38:55–64.
7. Björnsson GA, Haanaes HR, Skoglund LA. Naproxen 500 mg bid versus acetaminophen 1000 mg qid: effect on swelling and other acute postoperative events after bilateral third molar surgery. J Clin Pharmacol. 2003;43:849–58.
8. Spilka CJ. The placebo of corticosteroids and antihistamines in oral surgery. Oral Surg Oral Med Oral Pathol. 1961;14:1034–42.
9. Skjelbred P, Løkken P. Post-operative pain and inflammatory reaction reduced by injection of a corticosteroid. A controlled trial in bilateral oral surgery. Eur J Clin Pharmacol. 1982;21(5):391–6.
10. Dohan DM, Choukroun J, Diss A, Dohan SL, Dohan AJ, Mouhyi J, et al. Platelet-rich fibrin (PRF): A second-generation platelet concentrate.Part III: Leucocyte activation: A new feature for platelet concentrates? Oral Surg Oral Med Oral Pathol Oral Radiol Endod. 2006;101:E51–5.
11. Gaultier F, Navarro G, Donsimoni JM, Dohan D. Platelet concentrates. Part 3: Clinical applications. Implantodontie. 2004;13:3–11. French.
12. Simonpieri A, Choukroun J, Girard MO, Ouaknine T, Dohan D. Immediate post-extraction implantation: interest of the PRF. Implantodontie. 2004;13: 177–89. French.
13. Simonpieri A, Del Corso M, Sammartino G, Dohan Ehrenfest DM. The Relevance of Choukroun's Platelet-Rich Fibrin and Metronidazole During Complex Maxillary Rehabilitations Using Bone Allograft. Part I: A New Grafting Protocol. Implant Dent. 2009;18:102–11.
14. Choukroun J, Adda F, Schoeffler C, Vervelle A. Une opportunité en paro-implantologie: le PRF. Implantodontie. 2001;42:55–62.
15. Aroca S, Keglevich T, Barbieri B, Gera I, Etienne D. Clinical evaluation of a Modified Coronally Advanced Flap Alone or in Combination With a Platelet-Rich Fibrin Membrane for the Treatment of Adjacent Multiple Gingival Recessions: A 6-Month Study. J Periodontol. 2009;80:244–52.
16. Singh A, Kohli M, Gupta N. Platelet rich fibrin: a novel approach for osseous regeneration. J Maxillofac Oral Surg. 2012;11(4):430–4.
17. Kumar N, Prasad K, Ramanujam L, K R, Dexith J, Chauhan A. Evaluation of Treatment Outcome After Impacted Mandibular Third Molar Surgery With the Use of Autologous Platelet-Rich Fibrin: A Randomized Controlled Clinical Study. J Oral Maxillofac Surg. 2014 Dec 13. doi: 10.1016/j.joms.2014. 11.013. [Epub ahead of print]
18. Pell GJ, Gregory BT. Impacted mandibular third molars: classification and modified techniques for removal. Dent Digest. 1933;39:330–8.
19. Alcântara CE, Falci SG, Oliveira-Ferreira F, Santos CR, Pinheiro ML. Pre-emptive effect of dexamethasone and methylprednisolone on pain, swelling, and trismus after third molar surgery: a split-mouth randomized triple-blind clinical trial. Int J Oral Maxillofac Surg. 2014;43:93–8.
20. Grossi GB, Maiorana C, Garramone RA, Borgonovo A, Creminelli L, Santoro F. Assesing postoperative discomfort after third molar surgery:A prospective study. J Oral Maxillofac Surg. 2007;65:901–17.
21. Baqain Z, Karaky AA, Sawair F, Khraisat A, Duaibis R, Rajab LD. Frequency estimates and risk factors for post operative morbidity after third molar removal:A prospective cohort study. J Oral Maxillofac Surg. 2008;66(11): 2276–83.
22. Choukroun J, Diss A, Simonpieri A, Girard MO, Schoeffler C, Dohan SL, et al. Platelet-rich fibrin (PRF): A second-generation platelet concentrate.Part IV: Clinical effects on tissue healing. Oral Surg Oral Med Oral Pathol Oral Radiol Endod. 2006;101:E56–60.
23. Su CY, Kuo YP, Tseng YH, Su CH, Burnouf T. In vitro release of growth factors from platelet-rich fibrin (PRF): a proposal to optimize the clinical applications of PRF. Oral Surg Oral Med Oral Pathol Oral Radiol Endod. 2009; 108(1):56–61.
24. Lee JW, Kim SG, Kim JY, Lee YC, Choi JY, Dragos R, et al. Restoration of a peri-implant defect by platelet- rich fibrin. Oral Surg Oral Med Oral Pathol Oral Radiol Endod. 2012;113(4):459–63.
25. Zhang Y, Tangl S, Huber CD, Lin Y, Qiu L, Rausch-Fan X. Effects of Choukroun's platelet-rich fibrin on bone regeneration in combination with deproteinized bovine bone mineral in maxillary sinus augmentation:A histological and histomorphometric study. J Cranio-Maxillofac Surg. 2012; 40(4):321–8.
26. Mozzatti M, Martinasso G, Pol R, Polastri C, Cristiano A, Muzio G, et al. The impact of plasma rich in growth factors on clinical and biological factors involved in healing processes after third molar extraction. J Biomed Mater Res. 2010;95(3):741–6.
27. Alissa R, Esposito M, Horner K, Oliver R. The influence of platelet-rich plasma on the healing of extraction sockets: an explorative randomised clinical trial. Eur J Oral Implantol. 2010;3(2):121–34.
28. Thorat MK, Pradeep AR, Pallavi B. Clinical effect of autulogous platelet-rich fibrin in the treatment of intra-bony defects : a controlled clinical trial. J Clin Periodontol. 2011;38:925–32.

3

Evaluation of the anesthetic effect of epinephrine-free articaine and mepivacaine through quantitative sensory testing

Sareh Said Yekta-Michael[1,2*†], Jamal M Stein[1†] and Ernst Marioth-Wirtz[2]

Abstract

Introduction: Long lasting anesthesia of the soft tissue beyond the dental treatment affects patients in daily routine. Therefore a sophisticated local anesthesia is needed. The purpose of this study was an evaluation of the clinical use of epinephrine-free local anesthetic solutions in routine short-time dental treatments.

Materials and methods: In a prospective, single-blind, non-randomized and controlled clinical trial, 31 patients (16 male, 15 female patients) undergoing short-time dental treatment under local anesthesia (plain solutions of articaine 4% and mepivacaine 3%) in area of maxillary canine were tested with quantitative sensory testing QST. Paired-Wilcoxon-testing (signed-rank-test) and Mc Nemar tests have been used for statistical results.

Results: Significant differences in all tested parameters to the time of measurements were found. Mepivacaine showed a significantly stronger impact for the whole period of measurement (128 min) on thermal and mechanical test parameters and to the associated nerve fibers.

Conclusion: Plain articaine shows a faster onset of action associated with a shorter time of activity in comparison to plain mepivacaine. In addition to this articaine shows a significant low-graded effect on the tested nerve-fibers and therefore a least affected anesthesia to the patient. The clinical use of an epinephrine-free anesthetic solution can be stated as possible option in short dental routine treatments to the frequently used vasoconstrictor containing local anesthetics. Patients may benefit from shorter numbness.

Keywords: Articaine, Mepivacaine, Local anesthesia, Maxillary infiltration, Trigeminal region, Epinephrine-free

Introduction

In dental treatment, the management of pain is an important factor for patient comfort and a critical element of patient care [1,2]. A huge amount of local anesthetic agents are used nowadays, but only a few of these available agents have been exposed to be more beneficial in dental routine. These few compounds, which mostly contain a vasoconstrictor e.g. epinephrine, are widely used [3]. The clinical benefit of local anesthetics combined with vasoconstrictors is obvious: local ischemia is provided by the supplement in the region of attention,

which extends the duration activity and reduces the systemic toxicity of the anesthetic agent [4,5].

However, there are also clinical situations, which do not allow the use of agents containing vasoconstrictors, particularly epinephrine. Clinical findings and contraindication in anamnesis are e.g. hypertension, hyperthyreosis, diabetes mellitus and all advice of vasoconstrictions [6-11]. In order to avoid systemic adverse reactions, local anesthetic solutions should always contain the minimum concentration of epinephrine [4]. It is very important for the clinician to be acquainted with the characteristics of the agent. Especially pharmacological action, toxicity and maximal dose are important parameters to know.

In addition attention has to be payed to the onset, the depth of anesthesia and the duration of activity related to the planned dental procedure. Unfortunately the compounds, which are commonly used and contain a

---

* Correspondence: ssaidyekta@ukaachen.de
†Equal contributors
[1]Department of Conservative Dentistry, Periodontology and Preventive Dentistry, Aachen University, Aachen, North Rhine-Westphalia, Germany
[2]Interdisciplinary Center for Clinical Research, RWTH Aachen University, Aachen, North Rhine-Westphalia, Germany

vasoconstrictor, have a disadvantage, especially concerning routine nonsurgical short-time dental treatments. There is a discrepancy between the time for dental procedures and the time of agent's activity, especially on patient's soft tissue [4]. Several studies have proved that soft tissue anesthesia can last for 3 – 4 hours beyond the treatment when an agent with vasoconstrictor was used [12,13]. In particular the long-lasting anesthesia of soft tissue, causing unpleasant numbness beyond the dental treatment, affects the patient in daily routine. Eminently because of this negative effect on patient's comfort, local anesthesia has to be justified for routine short-time dental treatments.

A situation-related compound, which approaches the possibility of a safe and adequate dental care and the need of the patient, meaning a least affecting anesthesia, has to be chosen [4,14]. Studies have confirmed that plain solutions of local anesthesia provide an alternative option to the commonly used compounds [14]. Although a variety of plain local anesthetic solutions are available, they are rarely used in daily routine. The plain solutions Mepivacaine shows the typical structure of an amino-amide local anesthetic and was object of different studies [15]. In contrast to other local anesthetics of the amino-amid type, plain mepivacaine shows vasoconstrictor-properties at its disposal [15,16].

Articaine is also a local anesthetic of an amide type. But since it possesses vasodilatation-properties [16], it is mostly used in association with a vasoconstrictor increasing the local anesthetic efficacy. The characteristic property of articaine is its chemical structure: a thiophene-ring in addition to an ester linkage. This chemical structure represents an exception in the line of local anesthetics in clinical use [1]. Several studies have exposed that articaine is the local anesthetic agent with the best properties of diffusion within soft and hard tissue [4].

In order to test the effect of soft tissue-anesthesia and in particular the effect of the compound being used on sensory modalities of large and small fibers (Aβ-, C- and Aδ- fibers), a reliable noninvasive psychophysical test-method can be performed; the quantitative sensory testing (QST). This QST procedure has become an integrable diagnostic tool in clinical routine with a standardized battery of thermal and mechanical parameters [17,18]. It has already been used successfully in the trigeminal region of face [17-21]. In the present study QST was adapted to the hairy skin of the infraorbital region (V2) during small dental interventions in maxillary premolares.

The aim of the current study is to elevate the clinical use of vasoconstrictor-free local anesthetics in routine short-time dental treatments and especially to discover the effect of the local anesthetic agents (articaine/mepivacaine) on sensory modalities of large and small fibers (Aβ-, C- and Aδ- fibers) and the differences of

the resulting soft-tissue anesthesia. The purpose is to discover a situation-justifying agent, which can be used by the clinician for routine short-time dental treatments and also improves the situation of the patient due to the limited duration of soft-tissue anesthesia.

Materials and methods
Patients
Thirty-one patients (15 female, male 16) covering an age between 20 and 40 years (27.4 ± 4.0 years, mean ± SD) in need of small nonsurgical dental treatment in region of maxillary premolares were included in this prospective, controlled non-randomized, single blind study. Only patients, who fulfilled the inclusion criteria and none of the exclusion criteria, were tested.

The inclusion criteria involved the necessity of a dental filling therapy in maxillary premolar region, filling-free maxillary canines, the wish of the patient and the medical indication for a dental local anesthesia in the region of the dental treatment and furthermore the age of the patients (20 – 40 years). The exclusion criteria were all kinds of cardiovascular-, metabolic-, CNS-, immune system- disease; furthermore coagulopathy, circulatory disorder, recent operations, contagious diseases, sulfite sensitivity or allergy to any part of the solution, psychiatric illness, drug consumption and pregnancy. All patients have been without any medication for 48 hours.

All participants gave their informed consent prior to the inclusion in this study according to the 1964 declaration of Helsinki. The study took place at the department of conservative dentistry, periodontology and preventive dentistry of RWTH University Aachen. The protocol passed the local ethics committee (number of the acceptance by the ethic committee EK 076/11).

Thermal and mechanical detection and pain thresholds were determined by the quantitative sensory testing protocol (QST) [17,18,22]. In several studies it was recommended to reduce the originally QST protocol of 13 parameters to less parameters without affecting the informative value of the measurement in order to ensure an integration into clinical practice. With thermal and mechanical stimuli of QST it is possible to show distinct neuroanatomic pathways with Aβ, Aδ, and C fiber populations [21,23,24].

Because of the limited time of clinical routine it was necessary to design a test-protocol obtaining the sensory profiles within dental treatment. Therefore in the present study 7 of the 13 possible test parameters of QST were included into the test protocol; containing CDT, cold detection threshold; WDT, warm detection threshold; CPT, cold pain threshold; HPT, heat pain threshold; MDT, mechanical detection threshold; MPT, mechanical pain threshold and VDT, vibration detection threshold. In addition to that the pulp sensory of the canine was tested in a circle of 5 minutes for the whole test period by using a cold test, which seeks a response to the thermal stimulus (Figure 1).

Clinical examination- treatment protocol

At the beginning of every test period a control test was implemented in order to demonstrate the test method to the patient and to collect normative data. For realizing a painless small dental treatment (fissure-filling-therapy in premolares on both sides of maxilla) a maxillary local infiltration anesthesia in canine region was performed. For that, plain solutions of articaine 4% (Ultracain D®, Sanofi-Aventis, Paris, France) and mepivacaine 3% (Meaverin®, Actavis, New Jersey, USA) were applied. The local anesthetics were given to all patients, alternately on the right and left side of maxilla; in conclusion every agent was nearly administered equal times on every side. Thereby an amount of 1.00 ml solution was given in 30 sec per dental syringe (Uniject k®, Fa. Sanofi-Aventis, Paris, France) always performed by the same dentist. Immediately after the injection the first test of the test-interval was performed; each test, containing QST and the test of pulp sensibility, took 9 min. During the five-minute breaks between every single test-interval, the dental treatment was performed. Patients were lying on a dental chair and kept their eyes closed throughout the QST procedure. Half of the group was tested on the right side first, the other half on the left side. All tests were performed by the same trained examiner.

Quantitative sensory testing

The test protocol containing thermal and mechanical detection, as well as pain thresholds, was always applied in the same order. Thereby the patients were tested thermal before mechanical testing occured.

All thermal stimuli were assigned by a special computer-controlled peltier type thermode with a stimulation area of 16×16 mm^2 (TSA-II, Medoc Ltd., Israel). Starting at a temperature-baseline of 32°C, the temperature of the thermode decreased or increased by 1°C/sec to determine thermal detection and pain thresholds (CDT, WDT, CPT, and HPT). The patients were asked to press a

computer mouse button as soon as they observed the corresponding cold, warm, cold pain, or heat pain sensation. After receiving measurement results, the temperature of the thermode returned to baseline-temperature for each thermal threshold. In order to protect the patient's skin, the range of stimulation temperatures was controlled between 0 – 50°C. The test-procedure for cold and warm detection thresholds (CDT, WDT) was performed firstly. Afterwards cold pain- and heat pain thresholds (CPT, HPT) were determined.

The mechanical test procedure contained the thresholds for MDT, MPT and VDT.

MDT was rated with modified von Frey filaments featuring forces of 0.08, 0.2, 0.4, 0.7, 1.6, 4, 6, 10, 14, 20, 40, 60, 80, 100, 150, 260, 600, 1.000, 1.800, 3.000 mN (Touch-Test Sensory Evaluators; North Coast Medical, Morgan Hill, CA, USA).

For performing the measurement of MPT, custom-made weighted pinprick stimulators with forces of 8, 16, 32, 64, 128, and 256 mN and a contact area of ca. 0.2 mm diameter were applied to hairy skin of the infra-orbital region.

MDT and MPT were set by the method of limits starting with a clearly noticeable filament of 16 mN and a non-painful pinprick stimulator of 8 mN.

Both thresholds were defined as the geometric mean of 5 series of descending and ascending stimulus intensities [25,26].

The vibration stimuli were applied by a 64-Hz Rydel-Seifer tuning fork (OF033N; Aesculap, Tuttlingen, Germany) that was placed over the maxilla (infraorbital nerve area). Threshold measurement was performed 3 times starting with maximum vibration amplitude. As soon as the subject indicated disappearance of vibratory sensation, the threshold was read on a scale ranging from 0/8 to 8/8 (steps of 1/8). VDT was defined as the arithmetic mean of 3 runs [25,26].

Statistical analysis

All statistics were done in an explorative manner; no adjustment of significance level for multiple testing was performed. The function of statistic was to investigate

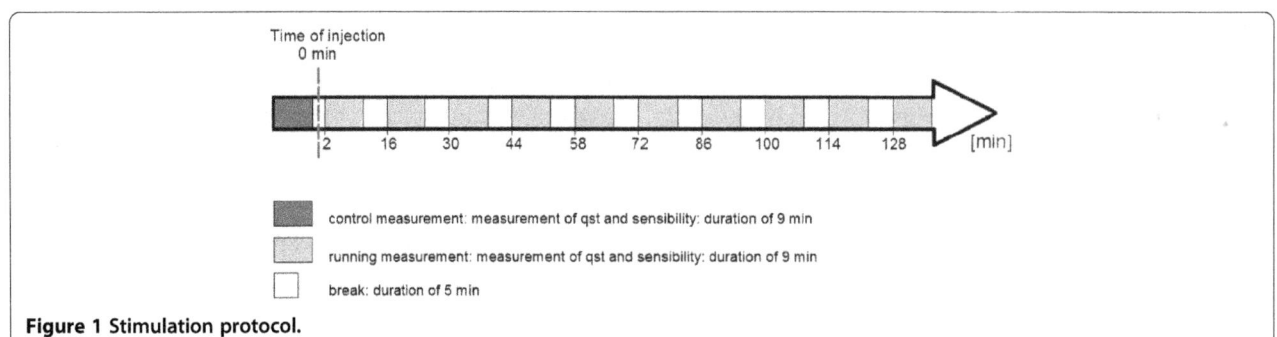

Figure 1 Stimulation protocol.

differences between the anesthesia-tread of both agents at testing time; furthermore to discover the differences between the measurement of control tests and continuing measurement tests. For all QST parameters differences between the agents were performed using the Wilcoxon-signed rank test. Testing the pulp sensibility the Mc Nemar Test was performed. Significance level was accepted at $p < 0.05$. Statistical analysis was done with SigmaStat 11.0 (SPSS Inc., USA) and SAS (SAS Institute Inc., USA).

Results

Altogether, thirty-one patients, sixteen male and fifteen female, with a mean age of $27.4 \pm 4,0$ years (mean ± SD), a mean size of 173.6 ± 6.3 cm (mean ± SD) and a mean weight of $69,3 \pm 10,6$ kg (mean ± SD) could be included.

Thermal testing

The effect of both anesthetic agents showed significant differences at each time of measurement for CDT as well as for WDT (Table 1, Figure 2). Equivalent amounts of the two local anesthetics exerted a different effect on the intense temperature-detection thresholds. Mepivacaine showed a stronger influence ($p < 0.05$) on the temperature sensitivity across all points of measuring, as well as higher detection thresholds ($p < 0.05$) in CDT and WDT than articaine. For both, CDT ($p < 0.001$) and WDT ($p < 0.01$), the values of control measurement were not achieved until the end of measurement progress. Until the last point of measurement (128th minute) a significant difference between the control measurement and the course measurements existed. Moreover, significant differences in anesthesia profiles occured in CPT as well as in HPT. By comparing the analysis of the control value and the course measurements an end of significant differences for cold pain threshold (CPT) was reached within the measurement period in both preparations. Articaine reached the value of control measurement earlier ($t = 72$ min, $p > 0.05$) than mepivacaine ($t = 100$ min, $p > 0.05$). Only at heat pain threshold (HPT) no significant differences were registered for articaine from the point of mensuration ($t = 100$ min, $p > 0.05$) to the received value of the control measurement. Even CPT and HPT showed that mepivacaine had a greater effect on thermal pain thresholds ($p < 0.05$) and maintained this throughout the measuring time.

Mechanical testing

For MDT as well as MPT, significant differences between the measured sensitivity thresholds were recorded at each time of testing (Table 2, Figure 3). At the tactile detection threshold MDT the measurement values of the control measurement were not reached in mepivacain over the entire measurement time course ($p < 0.05$). At the local anesthetic articaine a comparison with the course of measurements shows that the biggest interference of MDT was directly after the injection. In following development sensitivity of the skin returned steadily. Up to 100th Minute, a significant discrepancy between the control measurement and course measurements were demonstrated ($p < 0.05$). From the 114th minute no significant difference with the control measurement consisted ($p > 0.05$).

On MPT, articaine abolished the difference to the control test result from the point of the 72 min ($p > 0.05$). The significant difference between control measurement and results of process of mepivacaine existed until the end of measurement ($p < 0.05$). Mepivacaine had a stronger influence ($p > 0.05$) over the entire time of measurement on MDT as well as on MPT; in direct comparison to articaine, relevant thresholds were increased significantly during the whole period of time. Almost over the entire measurement in VDT, mepivacaine had a stronger effect than articaine, whereas only two measurements showed a significant discrepancy between the two agents. Again, both pharmaceutical values of the control measurement were achieved for the measurement progress, whereas that proceeded faster for articaine ($t = 58$ min, $p > 0.05$) than for mepivacaine ($t = 114$ min, $p > 0.05$; Figure 3).

Testing the pulp sensibility

The measurements of testing pulp sensitivity of the anesthetized tooth showed significant differences between the two local anesthetics at three points of measurement. The success rate for maxillary buccal infiltration in canine area to produce pulpal anesthesia using articaine was 74.19%, while the success rate was 90.32% using mepivacaine solution. By using mepivacaine it was possible to anesthetize more patients at the treated teeth region for a longer time. For both agents returning to baseline pulp sensibility was obtained within the testing period, while this point was reached earlier using articaine as agent ($t = 44$ min, $p > 0.05$) than using mepivacaine as agent ($t = 58$ min, $p > 0.05$; Figure 4).

The results of duration of pulp sensitivity testing showed a similar course. A period in which a positive sensitivity testing was considerably increased was 16 to 58 minutes for mepivacaine. At this period the two drugs showed differences, whereas the minutes 30 and 44 were significant ($p < 0.05$). In both preparations no significant differences between the measurement of control and the course measurements, starting at 86th minute, were observed ($p > 0.05$).

Discussion

Method and external parameter

In this prospective study, a non-randomized controlled clinical trial, 31 patients (16 male, 15 female patients)

Table 1 Measurement results of the QST thermal testing (CDT, CPT, WDT, HPT)

Time of measurement [min]	CDT					CPT				
	Articaine 4%		Mepivacaine 3%			Articaine 4%		Mepivacaine 3%		
	median [°C]	p-value control vs. course	median [°C]	p-value control vs. course	p-value articaine vs. mepivacaine	median [°C]	p-value control vs. course	median [°C]	p-value control vs. course	p-value articaine vs. mepivacaine
Control- measurement	29,90	-	30,30	-	-	14,30	-	15,50	-	-
2	7,90	<0,001	0,00	<0,001	0,346	0,00	<0,001	0,00	<0,001	0,85
16	16,60	<0,001	0,00	<0,001	0,036	0,00	<0,001	0,00	<0,001	0,129
30	25,20	<0,001	1,10	<0,001	<0,001	9,60	0,005	0,00	<0,001	<0,001
44	26,80	<0,001	14,50	<0,001	<0,001	12,40	0,070	0,00	<0,001	0,022
58	26,10	<0,001	23,30	<0,001	0,004	10,50	0,029	0,00	<0,001	0,047
72	26,80	<0,001	26,30	<0,001	0,018	13,70	0,139	3,10	<0,001	0,02
86	28,00	0,003	27,50	<0,001	0,034	15,00	0,631	10,80	0,006	0,013
100	28,20	0,012	27,30	<0,001	0,011	15,50	0,822	12,50	0,094	0,011
114	28,30	0,004	28,10	<0,001	0,245	16,30	0,524	14,30	0,411	0,053
128	28,40	<0,001	28,40	<0,001	0,36	17,30	0,123	15,40	0,493	0,037

Table 1 Measurement results of the QST thermal testing (CDT, CPT, WDT, HPT) (Continued)

Time of measurement [min]	WDT					HPT				
	Articaine 4%		Mepivacaine 3%		p-value articaine vs. mepivacaine	Articaine 4%		Mepivacaine 3%		p-value articaine vs. mepivacaine
	Median [°C]	p-value control vs. course	Median [°C]	p-value control vs. course		Median [°C]	p-value control vs. course	Median [°C]	p-value control vs. course	
Control- measurement	34,30	-	34,30	-	-	42,40	-	43,50	-	-
2	50,00	<0,001	50,00	<0,001	0,042	50,00	<0,001	50,00	<0,001	0,156
16	48,60	<0,001	50,00	<0,001	0,021	50,00	<0,001	50,00	<0,001	0,074
30	41,00	<0,001	50,00	<0,001	<0,001	48,30	<0,001	50,00	<0,001	<0,001
44	38,70	<0,001	50,00	<0,001	<0,001	48,00	<0,001	50,00	<0,001	<0,001
58	37,20	<0,001	46,20	<0,001	<0,001	47,30	<0,001	50,00	<0,001	0,007
72	36,50	<0,001	42,80	<0,001	<0,001	45,50	<0,001	49,60	<0,001	0,006
86	36,20	<0,001	40,10	<0,001	0,002	44,30	0,007	47,30	<0,001	0,008
100	36,50	<0,001	37,70	<0,001	0,016	45,00	0,052	47,50	0,002	0,008
114	35,60	0,003	36,80	<0,001	0,041	42,80	0,376	47,40	<0,001	<0,001
128	35,90	0,006	36,50	0,002	0,024	44,10	0,102	46,20	0,003	0,013

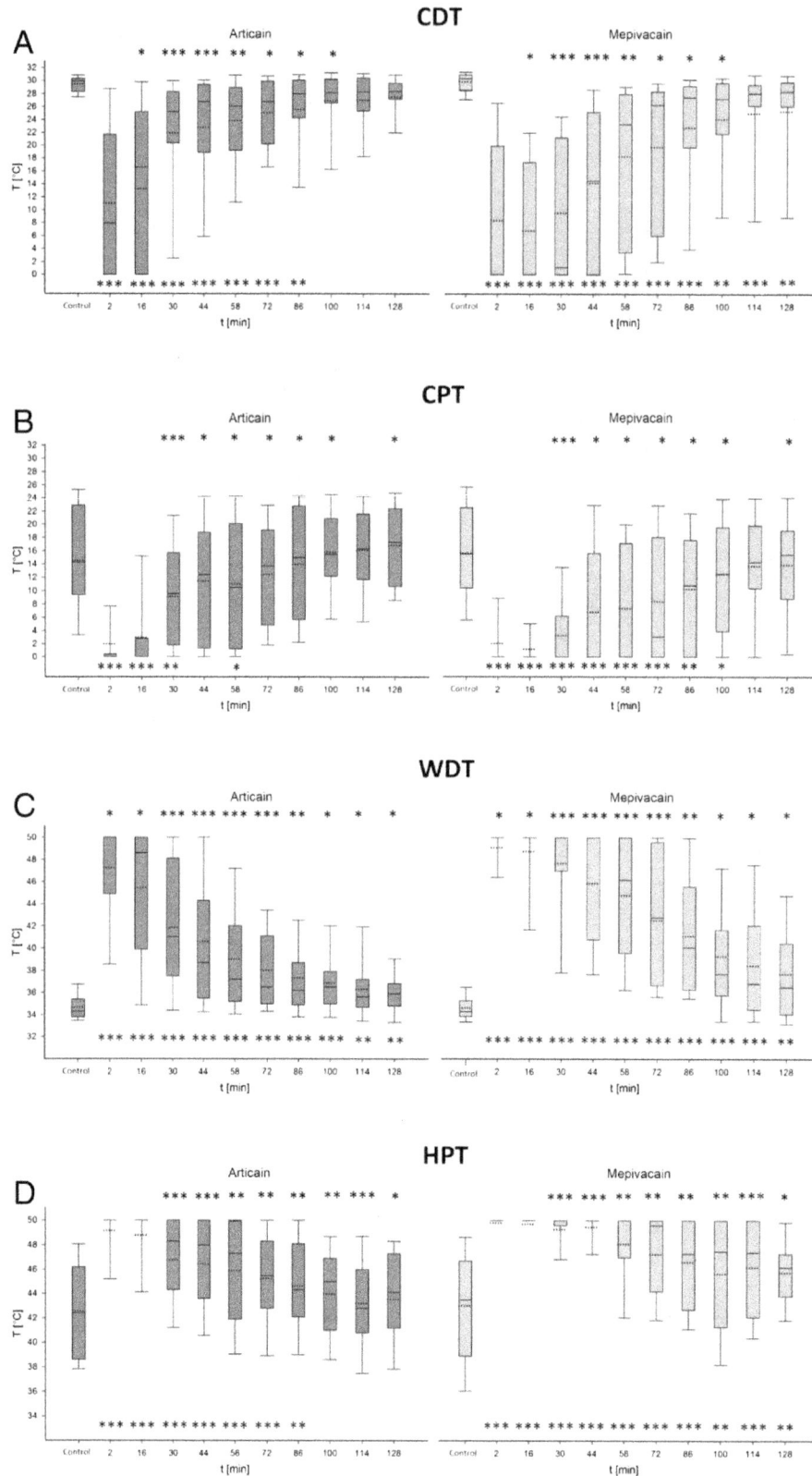

Figure 2 (See legend on next page.)

(See figure on previous page.)
Figure 2 Presentation of the results of the thermal QST parameters (A: CDT Articain, CDT Mepivacain; B: CPT Articain, CPT Mepivacain; C: WDT Articain, WDT Mepivacain D: HPT Articain, HPT Mepivacain) and the results of the statistical analysis for the individual measurement points (inclusive standard deviation). Significant differences are indicated by asterisks (paired Wilcoxon test: p *** ≤ 0.001; ** p ≤ 0.01, p ≤ 0.05 *, ns = not significant). The upper asterisks indicate significant differences between the measured values of articaine and mepivacaine to the respective measurement time. The lower asterisks indicate significant differences between the control measurement value and the running values of each anesthetic. Median value (solid line) and mean value (dotted line) are shown within the boxplots.

were tested with QST while undergoing a short-time dental treatment under local anesthesia in area of maxillary canine.

As previous studies proved that a difference in the perception of sensitive stimuli between healthy men and women does exist in this study, attention was paid to a homogeneous distribution of gender in order to avoid prejudicing the results. Furthermore, the age lowers the pain threshold (higher sensitivity) and leads to a slightly different reception of hot and cold stimuli [20,24,27,28]. In this study, the age of patients was limited in order to avoid any influences on the measurement results.

In previous studies QST was used successfully in the infraorbital region as detection method [20,24]. This study discovered the investigation area for the examination as a suitable method. This is attributable to the fact that on the one hand the region of canine represents an extremely sensitive area of innervation (N.trigeminus, N.infraorbitalis V2) and on the other hand the requirement of reproducibility is satisfied since the canine-region is used, despite individual anatomical differences, as a reference point for the repeated application of the measuring instruments. A difference in perception between the left and right sides of the examined QST parameters could not be determined [24,29].

In this study attention was particularly paid to the side distribution using local anesthetics. Both preparations were used on both sides for equal times. Thereby side distribution did not have an impact on the results.

In dentistry, choosing the right local anesthetics is of huge importance, the aspects of biocompatibility, tolerability and allergic potential should be considered [25,30]. The effect of local anesthetics on sensitivity can be evaluated in different ways. Commonly used methods examine the sensitivity of the anesthetized tooth, i.e. by checking the sensibility of the nerve fibers within the pulp. In order to check them, physical methods which involve thermal- (cold or heat application), electrical- and electro-optical measurement are used [26]. But those methods do not offer a review of the sensitivity of soft tissue, since it is also numbed by the used agent. Nevertheless the anesthesia of soft tissue, which most often affects the patient beyond the dental treatment, is an inevitable side effect of local anesthesia in dentistry and should be limited temporally, if possible. Especially for minor procedures, such as a routine-small-non surgical dental treatment, a discrepancy

between the time of dental treatment implementation and the effect of anesthesia within the treated area as well as on the soft tissue does exist. Within currently available methods to study the function of sensory Aδ-, Aß- and C-fibers, QST is a reliable and repeatable method [20,24,31].

A comparison between different local anesthetics of equal amounts is restricted, since different anesthetic-agents have various relative efficacies and various intrinsic activities.

Local anesthetics with an approximately similar relative efficacy and intrinsic activity, but a different molecular weight, can only be compared theoretically in equimolar solutions. Studies working with equimolar solutions are only partially applied in practical clinical use. The applicability of data obtained in this study has priority for dental daily routine. In the present study, always the same volume (1.00 ml) of the different anesthetic-agent was applied, despite the fact that different doses were applied to each side. The used volume was taken to ensure both: first of all that local anesthesia of tooth for the short dental procedure was adequate and furthermore that the investigation of the anesthetic effect on soft tissue performing QST was in a realizing range (128 minutes) for the patient.

Action of local anesthetics on pulpal sensitivity/effect of the local anesthetic to the QST parameters and their associated nerve fibers

The investigation of the effect of anesthesia on pulp sensibility showed that there are significant differences between the compared preparations. Mepivacaine is the stronger preparation in the applied volume. It has both, a stronger effect in terms of absolute number of negative samples than articaine, as well as the time until positive samples of sensitivity are measured. Articaine, however, shows a faster onset of action associated with a short duration of action.

Articaine has a higher number of negative samples of detectable sensitivity immediately after the application. This observation is also consistent with results of other studies. Because of a good bone- and soft tissue penetration of the active agent articaine, a possible reason for the rapid onset of action can be proven in different studies [32-34]. Mepivacaine reaches the maximum effect at a later point of time (t = 16 min).

In vitro studies confirm a consistent finding that articaine seems to be superior in the anesthetic efficacy. In an *in vitro* study Potocnik et al. were able to show that

Table 2 Measurement results of the QST mechanical testing (MDT, MPT, VDT)

Time of measurement [min]	MDT Articaine 4%		MDT Mepivacaine 3%			MPT Articaine 4%		MPT Mepivacaine 3%			VDT Articaine 4%		VDT Mepivacaine 3%		
	Median [mN]	p-value control vs. course	Median [° mN]	p-value control vs. course	p-value articaine vs. mepivacaine	Median [mN]	p-value control vs. course	Median [mN]	p-value control vs. course	p-value articaine vs. mepivacaine	Median [x/8]	p-value control vs. course	Median [x/8]	p-value control vs. course	p-value articaine vs. mepivacaine
Control-measurement	0,06	-	0,06	-	-	5,66	-	5,66	-	-	7,00	-	7,00	-	-
2	122,47	<0,001	4242,64	<0,001	0,004	362,04	<0,001	362,04	<0,001	0,037	5,00	<0,001	5,00	<0,001	0,625
16	69,28	<0,001	2323,79	<0,001	<0,001	362,04	<0,001	362,04	<0,001	0,02	6,00	<0,001	5,00	<0,001	0,041
30	7,75	<0,001	197,48	<0,001	<0,001	90,51	<0,001	362,04	<0,001	<0,001	6,00	0,002	5,00	<0,001	<0,001
44	0,53	<0,001	28,28	<0,001	<0,001	22,63	<0,001	181,02	<0,001	<0,001	6,00	0,008	6,00	<0,001	0,104
58	0,53	<0,001	11,83	<0,001	<0,001	11,31	<0,001	90,51	<0,001	<0,001	6,00	0,063	6,00	<0,001	0,054
72	0,13	<0,001	1,06	<0,001	<0,001	5,66	0,016	22,63	<0,001	<0,001	7,00	0,25	6,00	0,078	0,129
86	0,06	<0,001	0,28	<0,001	<0,001	5,66	0,188	22,63	<0,001	<0,001	6,00	0,375	6,00	0,016	0,098
100	0,06	0,009	0,13	<0,001	<0,001	5,66	1	11,31	<0,001	<0,001	7,00	0,25	6,00	0,008	0,055
114	0,06	0,055	0,13	<0,001	<0,001	5,66	1	5,66	0,01	0,005	7,00	0,109	6,00	0,125	0,844
128	0,06	0,055	0,13	<0,001	<0,001	5,66	1	5,66	0,02	0,01	7,00	0,313	6,00	0,063	0,375

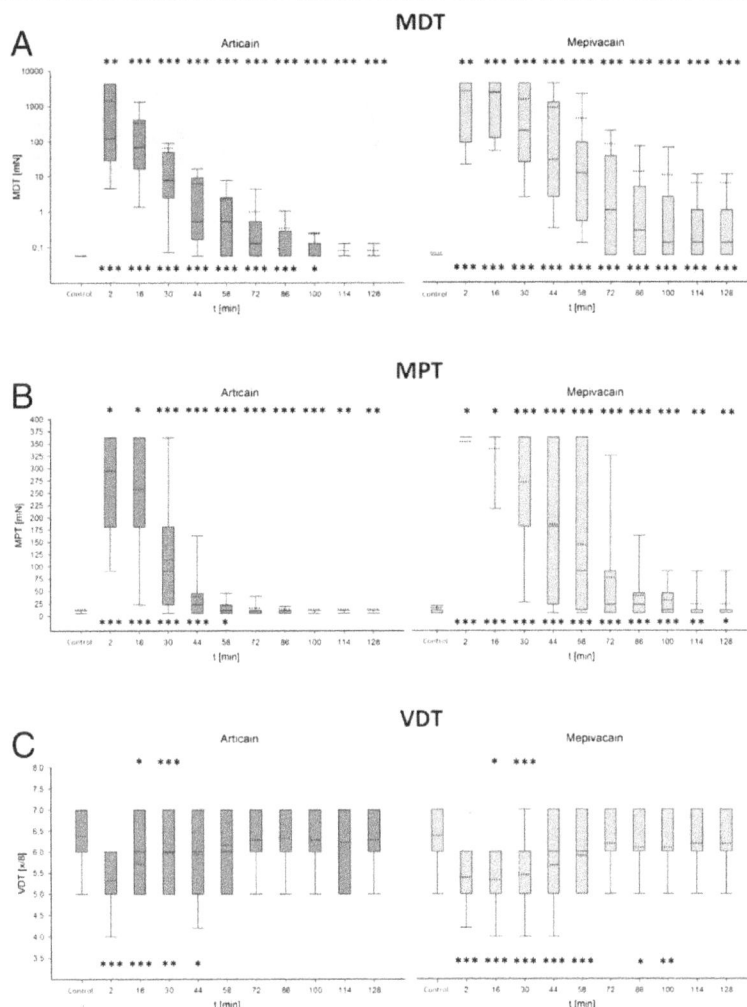

Figure 3 Presentation of the results of the mechanical QST parameters (A: MDT Articain, MDT Mepivacain; B: MPT Articain, MPT Mepivacain; C: VDT Articain, VDT Mepivacain) and the results of the statistical analysis for the individual measurement points (inclusive standard deviation). Control measurement and anesthesia course of the two local anesthetics in direct comparison. Significant differences are indicated by asterisks (paired Wilcoxon test: p *** ≤ 0.001; ** p ≤ 0.01, p ≤ 0.05 *, ns = not significant). The upper asterisks indicate significant differences between the measured values of articaine and mepivacaine to the respective measurement time. The lower asterisks indicate significant differences between the control measurement value and the running values of each anesthetic. Median value (solid line) and mean value (dotted line) are shown within the boxplots.

at sural nerve of a rat articaine 4% anesthetic solution was more effective than a lidocaine 4% or mepivacaine 3% solution [35]. This result has also been demonstrated in other *in vitro* studies on isolated nerves of frogs and rats [36].

In a comparative clinical trial Cowan could show that in a dental infiltration anesthesia with equal volumes (1.00 ml) of anesthetic agents the anesthetic effect of articaine without an added vasoconstrictor is less than the anesthetic effect of lidocaine 2% and mepivacaine 3% [15]. A similar result was also obtained by Winther and Nathalang in a comparative study. They discovered that the epinephrine-free solution could cause lack of adequate clinical analgesia in both, 2% and in 4% concentration, in contrast to epinephrine-containing articaine

solutions [37]. In a comparison of 1% solutions of both local anesthetics Sommer et al. showed that mepivacaine had almost the doubled action time as articaine [38]. A possible reason may be the low but existing vasoconstrictor effect of mepivacaine and the pronounced vasodilatory effect of articaine. These substance properties play only a minor role in the *in vitro* model of the isolated nerve, whereas they are quite detectable in clinical use because of the vascularized tissue [1]. In contrast to that, Rahn et al. demonstrated that a 2% articaine-epinephrine-free solution compared to standard articaine (4% articaine with epinephrine solution of 1/200.000) can be perfectly used in clinical routine and has even be proven in surgical intervention. This performance was also confirmed by Kämmerer et al. who successfully used

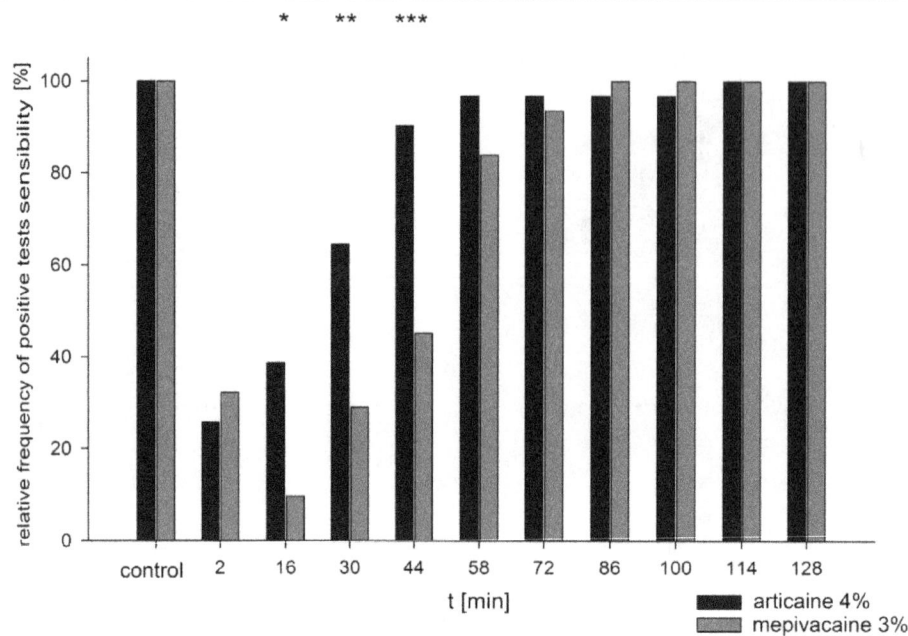

Figure 4 Representation of the relative frequency of positive samples to the sensitivity of the individual measuring time points for both local anesthetics in direct comparison.

a 4% articaine-epinephrine-free solution for tooth extraction in the mandible [14,39]. A comparison of dental anesthetic success of local anesthetics between this study and other studies shows that the observed anesthesia success in this study agrees with the values obtained in other studies. The anesthesia success for mepivacaine is assessed as high (t = 16 min, anesthesia success 90.32%) and for articaine as moderate (t = 2 min, anesthesia success 74.19%). Moore et al. were able to achieve a comparative success with articaine 4% anesthesia without epinephrine in a maxillary infiltration anesthesia (1.00 ml) of 75.8%. This almost agrees with the results of this study [40-43].

The study demonstrates that the applied amount of 1.00 ml of the anesthetic agent articaine is sufficiently high to achieve adequate success of anesthesia during small dental procedures.

The results of the QST parameters permit conclusions of certain nerve fibers [18,31]. Differences of the two preparations are obvious.

The two preparations show significant differences of the individual measuring times to each other and also of the control value compared to the values of each continuing measurements.

No significant difference between the control values and the measurement values of articaine in five of seven tests could be observed. This was only achieved at two of seven test parameters by mepivacaine. However, a differentiated end of the blockade and the regeneration of individual nerve fibers from the active ingredient of the local anesthetic are not evident. Accordingly, the sensitivity

to the local anesthetic does not only depend on the diameter of the individual nerve fibers, but notably on the choice of the active substance and its physicochemical properties [44]. In opposite to the conventional amide anesthetics mepivacaine, which is only degraded in the liver, articaine, being metabolized in the liver and in plasma by Pseudocholinesterasen, shows a short interference of the thresholds which were measured. Furthermore, plain articaine has its strongest effect just after the injection at the first measurement point (based on the sensitivity of the tooth anesthetized). Whereas this can firstly be registered a measurement point later in the case of mepivacaine. Thus, the excellent tissue penetration and rapid onset of action can be confirmed for the active agent articaine, which is awarded in various studies. Both factors are based on the physicochemical properties, in particular increased by the thiophene lipophilicity. This allows a more efficient diffusion of articaine through soft tissue than other local anesthetics [32-34].

Aβ- fibers (MDT, VDT)

The study of myelinated Aβ-fibers took place via QST parameters MDT and VDT. This demonstrates that there are significant differences at all measuring times between the two preparations at MDT. The active agent mepivacaine showed a stronger influence on MDT as articaine at all measuring times. A significant difference between the control value and the value of the course of the active agent mepivacaine was detectable on the entire range of measurement. In contrast to that, articaine

Evaluation of the anesthetic effect of epinephrine-free articaine and mepivacaine...

23

did not show any significant difference at the end of the measurement time (114 minutes). In various studies, which were already carried out on the face, MDT presented to be particularly sensitive test parameters [18].

The local anesthetic effect on these test parameters might be the reason for the long time influence.

The VDT test parameters show significant differences of the two preparations concerning the measuring times of 16 and 30 minutes. Again, mepivacaine was more effective than articaine.

The comparison between the control values and the progress values showed no significant difference at the end of measurement for both active substances, although the end of significant differences was reached earlier by articaine than by mepivacaine. The results show that the myelinated Aβ-fibers, which are associated with the test parameters, recover very fast from the local anesthetic action. This agrees with previous studies [45,46]. Especially articaine seems to affect Aβ-fibers less than mepivacaine. However, it should be noted that there can be a transmission of the vibration to the maxillary bone protrusion [24]. This may lead to stimulation of unanesthetized areas, a distortion of the measured values and that VDT loses informative value compared with MDT.

Aδ- fibers (CDT, MPT, HPT)

The test parameters associated with the Aδ-fiber activity show at almost all points of time significant differences between the two preparations. Thereby mepivacaine has a stronger effect on the test parameters than articaine.

The test parameters HPT and MPT do not show significant differences between the progress values and the control value for articaine within the study period of 128 minutes at the end of the measurements.

The results suggest that articaine has less influence on Aδ-fiber activity than mepivacaine. Also the regeneration of nerve fibers from the local anesthetic effect of articaine is faster than the regeneration from the effect of mepivacaine.

C-fibers (WDT, CPT, HPT)

The test parameters associated with the C-fiber activity showed at almost all points of measurement a significantly stronger effect of mepivacaine compared to articaine. During the test a significant difference of both agents remains at WDT parameters until the end of the measurement period. However, a stronger influence of the test parameter was recorded for mepivacaine. Surprisingly, it appears that at CPT the significant difference between the value of measurements and the control value was canceled for both agents. This occured faster in the case of articaine than in the case of mepivacaine.

As far as HPT is considered, only articaine achieved the end of significant difference during the measurement, whereas mepivacaine still showed significant discrepancy during the measurement range to the end of measurement.

Conclusion

The aim of the study was to investigate the analgesic effect of tooth as well as the anesthetic numbing effect of soft tissue which is caused by local anesthetics as 4% articaine and 3% mepivacaine which do not contain a vasoconstrictor. The results of this study show that mepivacaine causes a longer analgesia to the anesthetized tooth and has a stronger influence on the investigated thermal and mechanical test parameters at all measurement points of time. Plain articaine 4% shows an earlier onset of action associated with a shorter time of activity in comparison to plain mepivacaine 3%. This can result in more frequent injections of the local anesthetic agent, if articaine is used. In addition to this articaine shows a significant low-graded effect on the tested nerve-fibers and therefore a least affected anesthesia to the patient. Plain articaine 4% is very close to the demands of a differentiated anesthesia. The clinical use of an epinephrine-free anesthetic solution can be stated as possible option in short dental routine treatments to the frequently used vasoconstrictor containing local anesthetics.

Competing interests
The authors declare that they have no competing interests.

Authors' contributions
SYM and JMS contributed to the conception, design and coordination of the study as well as the acquisition of data. EMW performed the statistical calculations. SYM and EMW drafted and wrote the manuscript. SYM and JMS revised the manuscript. All authors read and approved the final manuscript.

References
1. Malamed SF, Sykes P, Kubota Y, Matsuura H, Lipp M. Local anesthesia: a review. Anesth Pain Control Dent. 1992;1(1):11–24.
2. Meechan JG. Pain control in local analgesia. Eur Arch Paediatr Dent. 2009;10(2):71–6.
3. Jeske AJ, Blanton PL. Selection of local anesthetics in dentistry: clinical impression versus scientific assessment. J Am Coll Dent. 2006;73(3):21–4.
4. Daubländer M, Kämmerer PW, Willershausen B, Leckel M, Lauer HC, Buff S, et al. Clinical use of an epinephrine-reduced (1/400,000) articaine solution in short-time dental routine treatments-a multicenter study. Clin Oral Investig. 2011;16(4):1289–95.
5. Davenport RE, Porcelli RJ, Iacono VJ, Bonura CF, Mallis GI, Baer PN. Effects of anesthetics containing epinephrine on catecholamine levels during periodontal surgery. J Periodontol. 1990;61(9):553–8.
6. Heavner JE. Local anesthetics. Curr Opin Anaesthesiol. 2007;20(4):336–42.
7. Hogan QH. Pathophysiology of peripheral nerve injury during regional anesthesia. Reg Anesth Pain Med. 2008;33(5):435–41.
8. Laragnoit AB, Neves RS, Neves IL, Vieira JE. Locoregional anesthesia for dental treatment in cardiac patients: a comparative study of 2% plain lidocaine and 2% lidocaine with epinephrine (1:100,000). Clinics (Sao Paulo). 2009;64(3):177–82.

9. Meechan JG. Local anaesthesia: risks and controversies. Dent Update. 2009;36(5):278–80.

10. O'Malley TP, Postma GN, Holtel M, Girod DA. Effect of local epinephrine on cutaneous bloodflow in the human neck. Laryngoscope. 1995;105(2):140–3.

11. Sader R. Lokalanästhesie, hämorrhagische Diathesen und medikamentöse Therapie. MKG-Chirurg. 2009;2:125–41.

12. Malamed SF, Gagnon S, Leblanc D. Efficacy of articaine: a new amide local anesthetic. J Am Dent Assoc. 2000;131(5):635–42.

13. Winther JE, Patirupanusara B. Evaluation of carticaine - a new local analgesic. Int J Oral Surg. 1974;3(6):422–7.

14. Kämmerer PW, Palarie V, Daubländer M, Bicer C, Shabazfar N, Brüllmann D, et al. Comparison of 4% articaine with epinephrine (1:100,000) and without epinephrine in inferior alveolar block for tooth extraction: double-blind randomized clinical trial of anesthetic efficacy. Oral Surg Oral Med Oral Pathol Oral Radiol Endod. 2011;113(4):495–9.

15. Cowan A. Clinical assessment of a new local anesthetic agent-carticaine. Oral Surg Oral Med Oral Pathol. 1977;43(2):174–80.

16. Willatts DG, Reynolds F. Comparison of the vasoactivity of amide and ester local anaesthetics. An intradermal study. Br J Anaesth. 1985;57(10):1006–11.

17. Mücke M, Cuhls H, Radbruch L, Baron R, Maier C, Tölle T, et al. Quantitative sensory testing. Schmerz. 2014;28(6):635–48.

18. Rolke R, Magerl W, Campbell KA, Schalber C, Caspari S, Birklein F, et al. Quantitative sensory testing: a comprehensive protocol for clinical trial. Eur J Pain. 2006;10(1):77–88.

19. Said-Yekta S, Smeets R, Esteves-Oliveira M, Stein JM, Riediger D, Lampert F. Verification of nerve integrity after surgical intervention using quantitative sensory testing. J Oral Maxillofac Surg. 2011;70(2):263–71.

20. Yekta SS, Koch F, Grosjean MB, Esteves-Oliveira M, Stein JM, Ghassemi A, Riediger D, Lampert F, Smeets R. Analysis of trigeminal nerve disorders after oral and maxillofacial intervention. Head Face Med. 2010 Oct 26;6:24. doi:10.1186/1746-160X-6-24.

21. Yekta SS, Lückhoff A, Ristić D, Lampert F, Ellrich J. Impaired somatosensation in tongue mucosa of smokers. Clin Oral Investig. 2012;16(1):39–44.

22. Ellrich J, Ristic D, Yekta SS. Impaired thermal perception in cluster headache. J Neurol. 2006;253(10):1292–9.

23. Svensson P, Baad-Hansen L, Thygesen T, Juhl GI, Jensen TS. Overview on tools and methods to assess neuropathic trigeminal pain. J Orofac Pain. 2004;18(4):332–8.

24. Yekta SS, Smeets R, Stein JM, Ellrich J. Assessment of trigeminal nerve functions by quantitative sensory testing in patients and healthy volunteers. J Oral Maxillofac Surg. 2010;68(10):2437–51.

25. Becker DE, Reed KL. Local anesthetics: review of pharmacological considerations. Anesth Prog. 2012;59(2):90–101.

26. Gopikrishna V, Pradeep G, Venkateshbabu N. Assessment of pulp vitality: a review. Int J Paediatr Dent. 2009;19(1):3–15.

27. Gibson S, Farrell M. A review of age differences in the neurophysiology of nociception and the perceptual experience of pain. Clinic J Pain. 2004;20(4) 227–39. Review

28. Heft M, Cooper B, O'Brian K, Hemp E, O'Brian R. Aging effects on the perception of noxious and non-noxious thermal stimuli applied to the face. Aging (Milano). 1996;8:35–41.

29. Matos R, Wang K, Jensen JD, Jensen T, Neuman B, Svensson P, et al. Quantitative sensory testing in the trigeminal region: site and gender differences. J Orofac Pain. 2011;25(2):161–9.

30. Becker DE, Reed KL. Essentials of local anesthetic pharmacology. Anesth Prog. 2006;53(3):98–108.

31. Chong PS, Cros DP. Technology literature review: quantitative sensory testing. Muscle Nerve. 2004;29(5):734–47.

32. Lima-Júnior JL, Dias-Ribeiro E, de Araújo TN, Ferreira-Rocha J, Honfi-Júnior ES, Sarmento CF, Seabra FR, de Sousa Mdo S. Evaluation of the buccal vestibule-palatal diffusion of 4% articaine hydrochloride in impacted maxillary third molar extractions, Med Oral Patol Oral Cir Bucal. 2009;1;14(3):E129-32.

33. Oertel R, Rahn R, Kirch W. Clinical pharmacokinetics of articaine. Clin Pharmacokinet. 1997;33(6):417–25.

34. Vree TB, Gielen MJ. Clinical pharmacology and the use of articaine for local and regional anaesthesia. Best Pract Res Clin Anaesthesiol. 2005;19(2):293–308.

35. Potocnik I, Tomsic M, Sketelj J, Bajrovic FF. Articaine is more effective than lidocaine or mepivacaine in rat sensory nerve conduction block in vitro. J Dent Res. 2006;85(2):162–6.

36. Muschaweck R, Rippel R. A new local anesthetic (carticaine) from the thiopene-series. Prakt Anaesth. 1974;9(3):135–46.

37. Winther JE, Nathalang B. Effectivity of a new local analgesic Hoe 40 045. Scand J Dent Res. 1972;80(4):272–8.

38. Sommer S, Fruhstorfer H, Nolte H. Comparative studies of the local anaesthetic action of carticaine 1% and mepivacaine 1%. Anaesthesist. 1978;27(7):65–8.

39. Rahn R, Hauzeneder W, Flanze L. Efficiency of a 2% epinephrine-free Articain solution (Ultracain 2%) for dental local anesthesia. Dtsch Stomatol. 1991;41(10):379–82.

40. Evans G, Nusstein J, Drum M, Reader A, Beck M. A prospective, randomized, double-blind comparison of articaine and lidocaine for maxillary infiltrations. J Endod. 2008;34(4):389–93.

41. Moore PA, Boynes SG, Hersh EV, DeRossi SS, Sollecito TP, Goodson JM, et al. The anesthetic efficacy of 4 percent articaine 1:200,000 epinephrine: two controlled clinical trials. J Am Dent Assoc. 2006;137(11):1572–81.

42. Srinivasan N, Kavitha M, Loganathan CS, Padmini G. Comparison of anesthetic efficacy of 4% articaine and 2% lidocaine for maxillary buccal infiltration in patients with irreversible pulpitis. Oral Surg Oral Med Oral Pathol Oral Radiol Endod. 2009;107(1):133–6.

43. Tortamano IP, Siviero M, Costa CG, Buscariolo IA, Armonia PL. A comparison of the anesthetic efficacy of articaine and lidocaine in patients with irreversible pulpitis. J Endod. 2009;35(2):165–8.

44. Gokin AP, Philip B, Strichartz GR. Preferential block of small myelinated sensory and motor fibers by lidocaine: in vivo electrophysiology in the rat sciatic nerve. Anesthesiology. 2001;95(6):1441–54.

45. Rosenberg PH, Heinonen E. Differential sensitivity of A and C nerve fibres to long-acting amide local anaesthetics. Br J Anaesth. 1983;55(2):163–7.

46. Sakai T, Tomiyasu S, Yamada H, Ono T, Sumikawa K. Quantitative and selective evaluation of differential sensory nerve block after transdermal lidocaine. Anesth Analg. 2004;98(1):248–51.

4

Shear bond strength of Biodentine, ProRoot MTA, glass ionomer cement and composite resin on human dentine *ex vivo*

Markus Kaup[1], Christoph Heinrich Dammann[1], Edgar Schäfer[2] and Till Dammaschke[1*]

Abstract

Introduction: The aim of this study was to compare the shear bond strength of Biodentine, ProRoot MTA (MTA), glass ionomer cement (GIC) and composite resin (CR) on dentine.

Methods: 120 extracted human third molars were embedded in cold-cured-resin and grinned down to the dentine. For each material 30 specimens were produced in standardised height and width and the materials were applied according to manufacturers' instructions on the dentine samples. Only in the CR group a self-etching dentine-adhesive was used. In all other groups the dentine was not pre-treated. All specimens were stored at 37.5 °C and 100% humidity for 2d, 7d and 14d. With a testing device the shear bond strength was determined (separation of the specimens from the dentine surface). The statistical evaluation was performed using ANOVA and Tukey-test ($p < 0.05$).

Results: At all observation periods the CR showed the significant highest shear bond strength ($p < 0.05$). After 2d significant differences in the shear bond strength were detectable between all tested materials, whereby CR had the highest and MTA the lowest values ($p < 0.05$). After 7d and 14d the shear bond strengths of MTA and Biodentine increased significantly compared to the 2d investigation period ($p < 0.05$). Biodentine showed a significantly higher shear bond strength than MTA ($p < 0.05$), while the difference between Biodentine and GIC was not significant ($p > 0.05$).

Conclusions: After 7d Biodentine showed comparable shear bond values than GIC, whereas the shear bond values for MTA were significantly lower even after 14d. The adhesion of Biodentine to dentine surface seams to be superior compared to that of MTA.

Keywords: Biodentine, Composite resin, Glass ionomer cement, ProRoot MTA, Shear bond strength

Introduction

In the early 1990s the development of mineral trioxide aggregate (MTA) introduced a new class of dental calcium silicate cements (CSCs) based on Portland cement, originally developed as a perforation repair material. Since then it has been widely used for repair-purposes of furcations and root canals, as a root-end filling material, for direct and indirect pulp-capping and the treatment of extern and intern resorptions with high success rates [1-3].

Beside a long setting time the major drawbacks of MTA are its relatively low compression and flexural strength, which are lower than those of dentine [4]. These factors are limiting the field of application to low stress-bearing areas [5]. Hence, MTA can not be used e.g. as base, base build-up, core material or as temporary restoration.

This triggered the development of new formulas of calcium silicate-based cements to overcome these drawbacks and keep the advantages. Biodentine (Septodont, St.-Maur-des-Fossés, France) can be considered as an outcome of this process. This calcium silicate based cement uses synthetically created pure raw materials in comparison to the impure base materials of MTA. Biodentine mainly consists of tri- and dicalcium silicate as the main

* Correspondence: tillda@uni-muenster.de
[1]Department of Operative Dentistry, Westphalian Wilhelms-University, Albert-Schweitzer-Campus 1, building W 30, 48149 Münster, Germany
Full list of author information is available at the end of the article

material, calcium carbonate as filler for enhancing mechanical properties and accelerating the hardening of the cement and zirconium dioxide as a radiopacifier [5-7]. In contrast to MTA, which uses only distilled water for setting, Biodentine uses a mix of distilled water, calcium chloride and a hydrosoluble polymer. Calcium chloride acts as an accelerator of the setting reaction [8]. The hydrosoluble polymer reduces the necessary water of the reaction [7]. With these improvements of the composition the initial setting time of Biodentine (12 min) is much lower than that of MTA (180 min) [6]. Biodentine is bioactive and biocompatible like MTA [6,9] and possesses the same good sealing abilities than other CSCs [7].

The microhardness, flexural and compressive strength of Biodentine are higher than those of other CSCs and more comparable to dentine [7,10]. Thus, Biodentine can also be used as an alternative to glass ionomer cements (GICs) in restorative dentistry [11].

Besides having a fast setting time and a high compressive strength any material used for posterior fillings must also have the ability to create a bond between the material and the dentine like GICs or dentine adhesives. A material used as a base or base build-up should provide an adequate seal, be able to prevent leakage and remain in place under dislodging forces, such as chewing pressure or the application of other restorative material, thus having adhesive properties to dentine. Hence, the bond strength of restorative materials is an important factor in clinical practice.

However, to the best of our knowledge there is no study available, which compares the shear bond strength of Biodentine, MTA, glass ionomer cement, and composite resin on a planar dentine surface in the same experimental setup. Thus, the aim of this *ex vivo* study was to determine the shear bond strength of Biodentine on dentine after 2, 7, and 14 days and to compare this values with another CSC (ProRoot MTA; Dentsply-Maillefer, Ballaigues, Switzerland), a glass ionomer cement (ChemFil rock; Dentsply, Konstanz, Germany) and a composite resin for bulk filling (X-tra base universal; VOCO, Cuxhaven, Germany). All these different materials are recommended to replace missing dentine in restorations or endodontic therapies.

The null-hypotheses of this study were that (i) the shear bond strengths to dentine of Biodentine and MTA are equal and that (ii) Biodentine and MTA possess lower shear bond strengths GIC and composite resin in combination with a dentine adhesive.

Methods

120 human third molar teeth were stored in sterile saline solution directly after extraction and refrigerated at 5 °C for less than two weeks. The handling of all human samples followed strictly the "Declaration of Helsinki". To produce plane-parallel samples the molar teeth were embedded in a cold-curing resin (Technovit 4071; Kulzer, Wehrheim, Germany) and ground with sandpaper (1200 grain) down to the dentine surface.

An impression of a columnar metal blank with a diameter of 3.28 mm and height of 4 mm was taken with polyether rubber impression material (Dimension Penta H and Impregum Garant L DuoSoft; 3 M ESPE, Seefeld, Germany). This negative form was used to ensure standardisation of samples. The mould made of polyether rubber was placed on the dentine samples and was completely filled with the particular test material avoiding any air entrapments, voids or gaps. The cross sectional area of the specimens was 8.5 mm^2 and the test material had complete contact to the dentine surface without touching the enamel. All plane-parallel dentine samples were rinsed with distilled water and air dried directly before the application of the test materials.

ProRoot MTA, Biodentine, ChemFil rock and X-tra base universal were strictly handled in accordance with the manufactures´ instructions. Thus, for ProRoot MTA, Biodentine, and the GIC ChemFil rock the dentine was not further treated before application. After placing the polyether rubber mould on the dentine surface it was completely filled with the appropriate material with the aid of a cement plugger.

Only in the composite resin group the dentine was pretreated with the recommended self-etching dentine adhesive (Futurabond DC Single Dose; VOCO, Cuxhaven, Germany). After light-curing (Elipar Highlight; 3 M ESPE, Seefeld, Germany) the X-tra base universal composite resin was put in the mould and light-cured by increment technique.

30 specimens were produced from every test material for shear bond testing after two, seven and 14 days (n = 10 per day) and stored in an incubator (U 29; Memmert, Schwabach, Germany) at 37.5 °C and 100% humidity. The polyether rubber moulds were removed from all specimens so that only the cylindrical test material adhered perpendicular to the dentine surface.

The shear bond strength was evaluated with the universal testing device LF Plus (Lloyd Instruments, Bognor Regis, Great Britain). All specimens were mounted in a metal mould which served as drive surface for a metal plunger. This plunger overlaid the specimen surface and touched the cylindrical test material at the contact with the dentine surface in a right angle (90°). The testing device moved with a defined feed speed of 1 mm/min towards the plunger. The shear bond strength needed to separate the test materials from the dentine surface was calculated with a special software program (Nexygen Version 4.5; Lloyd Instruments, Bognor Regis, Great Britain). The values were statistically analysed using analysis of variance (ANOVA) and post-hoc Tukey-test ($p < 0.05$).

Shear bond strength of Biodentine, ProRoot MTA, glass ionomer cement and composite resin...

27

The bonding failure modes of the restorative materials to the dentine surface were evaluated by using a laser scanning microscope (BZ 9000, Keyence, Osaka, Japan):

Mode 1. adhesive failure that occurred at the filling material and dentine interface
Mode 2. cohesive failure within the filling material
Mode 3. mixed failure mode

Results

Shear bond strength

The values of the shear bond strength and the statistical evaluation are given in Table 1. At all observation periods ProRoot MTA showed the lowest shear bond strength of all tested materials. After two days a slight touch with the metal plunger was effectual to detach all ProRoot MTA samples from the dentine surface. Thus, shear bond strength was not measurable and set to be "0". Although the dentine bonding of ProRoot MTA increased over time after 14 d still 20% of the specimens showed no measurable bonding to the dentine surface. The shear bond strength for Biodentine after 2 d was nearly 3 MPa and tripled within one week to more than 9 MPa. The GIC ChemFil rock reached a shear bond strength of about 10 MPa after two days which was comparable to the values determined after one and two weeks. Hence, an in- or decrease of the values did not occur over time. The composite resin X-trabase universal in combination with the dentine adhesive Futurabond DC showed mean shear bond strengths of about 30 MPa with no significant changes over time.

The statistical evaluation revealed that the composite resin in combination with a dentine adhesive had the significantly highest shear bond strength of all tested materials at all observation periods (p < 0.05). After two days significant differences between all materials were obtained, while the composite resin in combination with a dentine adhesive had the highest and ProRoot MTA the lowest values (p < 0.05). After one week Biodentine showed a significantly higher shear bond strength than ProRoot MTA (p < 0.05), while the difference between Biodentine and GIC was not significant (p > 0.05). The

shear bond strength of ProRoot MTA and Biodentine increased significantly compared to the 2 d observation period (p < 0.05). Comparable results were obtained after two weeks. The shear bond values for ProRoot MTA further increased as the values after 14 d they were significantly higher than those after 2 d and 7 d (p < 0.05), whiles no significant changes were detected in the Biodentine group between the 7 d and 14 d observation period (p > 0.05).

Failure mode

In the ProRoot MTA group 63.33% of the specimens showed an adhesive, 13.33% a cohesive and 23.33% a mixed failure mode (Figure 1), whereas in the Biodentine group a cohesive failure mode was noticed in 56.66% of the specimens and an adhesive failure mode occurred in 43.33% of the cases (Figure 2). In GIC samples the failure modes was mainly cohesive (93.33%) and in a minor part a mixture between an adhesive and cohesive failure (6.66%) (Figure 3). The composite resin and dentine adhesive showed an adhesive failure mode in 66.66% and a mixture between an adhesive and cohesive failure mode in 33.33% of the samples (Figure 4). Detailed results are given in Table 2.

Discussion

Shear bond strength measurements

Theoretically, bond strength is defined as the interfacial adhesion between substrate and the bonded material, mediated by an adhesive layer. In practice, this is often not the case, and instead, fractures may take place in the bond material, the substrate, or both and may extend beyond the initial bonded area. What is actually being measured is the fracture force of a bonded system for a particular method of load application and should only cautiously be interpreted as bond strength [12]. Hence, the failure modes of e.g. GIC [12,13] and Biodentine [14,15] to dentine were largely cohesive within the cement rather than at the interface. Therefore, the rigidity of the material has a significant influence on the interpretation of bond strength [12] and thus the true clinical bond to dentine is probably different from the data given here.

Table 1 Shear bond strength (mean and standard deviation) of the tested materials on dentine after 2 d, 7 d and 14 d

Material	2 d	7 d	14 d
ProRoot MTA	0.0[a]	0.85 (±1.42)[a*]	4.96 (±4.54)[a**]
Biodentine	3.14 (±1.09)[b]	9.75 (±2,19)[b*]	9.34 (±1.01)[b*]
ChemFil rock (GIC)	10.92 (±5.69)[c]	9.73 (±4.03)[b]	9.94 (±1.44)[b]
X-trabase (composite resin) + Futurabond DC (dentine adhesive)	32.74 (±4.66)[d]	32.75 (±4.61)[c]	30.48 (±4.43)[c]

Values with the same superscript letters were not statistically different at p = 0.05.
* = statistically significant difference of the shear bond strength values in comparison to the values at the 2 d observation period (p < 0.05).
** = statistically significant difference of the shear bond strength values in comparison to the values at the 7 d observation period (p < 0.05).
All values are given in MPa. The statistical evaluation was performed using ANOVA and Tukey-test (p < 0.05).

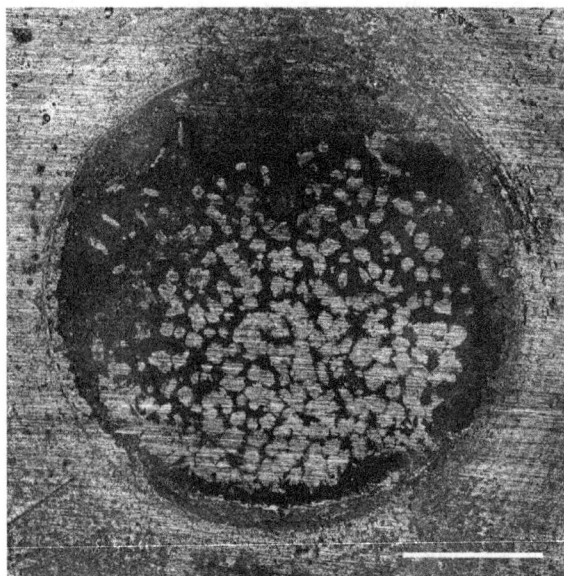

Figure 1 Example of a mixed failure mode of ProRoot MTA on dentine after 14 d. Original magnification x5. Bar represents 1 mm.

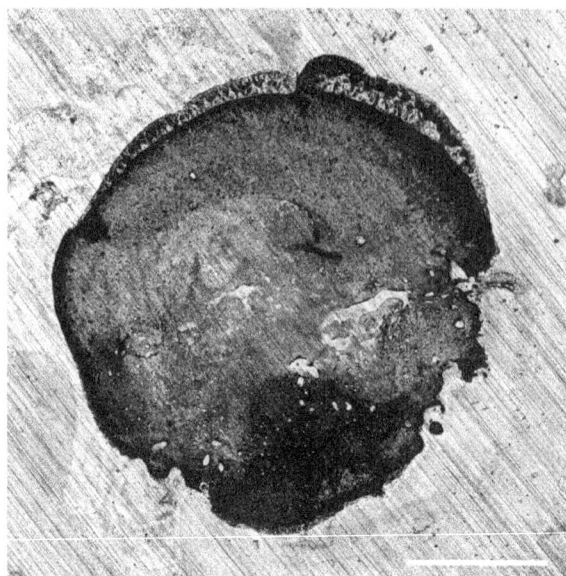

Figure 3 Example of a cohesive failure mode of ChemFil rock on dentine after 14 d. Original magnification x5. Bar represents 1 mm.

Another important point to be noted is that the materials were not tested immediately after their initial setting, which is the real clinical scenario where the restored teeth are immediately subjected to masticatory stress. Here the samples were stored without any load up to 14 d before loading, which may have influenced the results. It has also to be kept in mind that the present study was performed using sound and healthy dentine. Thus, in cariously affected dentine the shear bond strength may be lower.

Hence, laboratory-generated shear bond values should be interpreted and transferred to the clinical situation with some caution [12].

Bonding of CSCs to dentine

If the tricalcium silicate powder of a CSC is mixed with water a calcium-silicate-hydrate as well as calcium hydroxide is formed, which provides a high alkaline pH

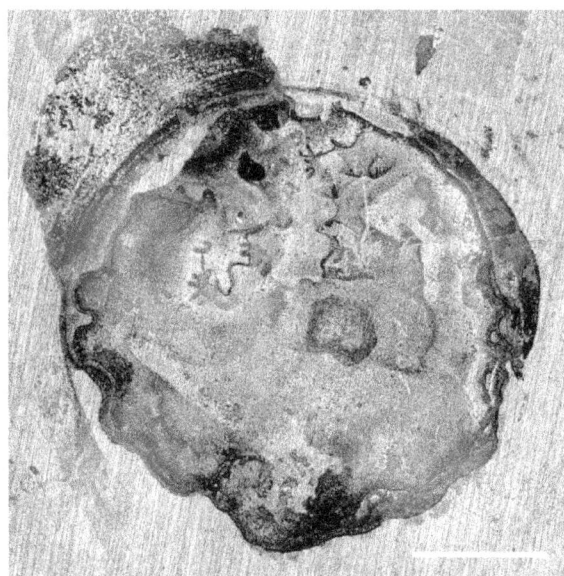

Figure 2 Example of a cohesive failure mode of Biodentine on dentine after 14 d. Original magnification x5. Bar represents 1 mm.

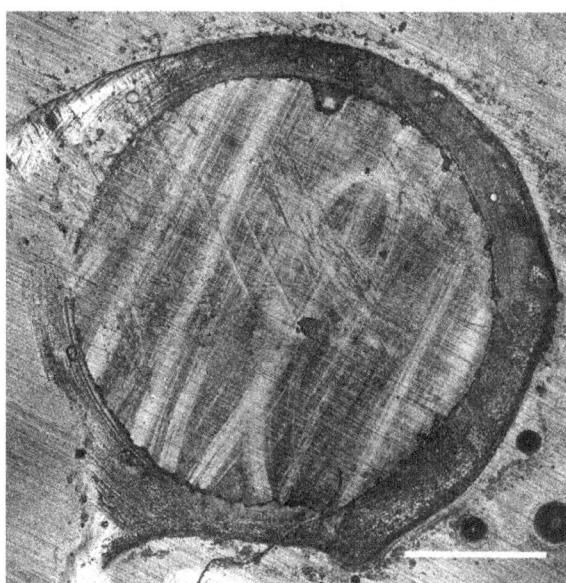

Figure 4 Example of an adhesive failure mode of X-trabase (composite resin) in combination with Futurabond DC (dentine adhesive) on dentine after 14 d. Original magnification x5. Bar represents 1 mm.

Table 2 Failure mode of ProRoot MTA (MTA), Biodentine (BD), ChemFil rock (GIC) and X-trabase (composite resin) in combination with Futurabond DC (CR) on dentine after 2 d, 7 d and 14 d

sample no.	MTA 2 d	MTA 7 d	MTA 14 d	BD 2 d	BD 7 d	BD 14	GIC 2 d	GIC 7 d	GIC 14 d	CR 2 d	CR 7 d	CR 14 d
1	1	1	1	1	1	1	2	2	2	1	1	1
2	1	1	1	1	1	1	2	2	2	1	1	1
3	1	1	2	1	1	1	2	2	2	1	1	1
4	1	1	2	1	2	2	2	2	2	1	1	1
5	1	1	2	1	2	2	2	2	2	1	1	1
6	1	1	2	1	2	2	2	2	2	3	1	3
7	1	1	3	1	2	2	2	2	2	3	1	3
8	1	3	3	2	2	2	2	2	2	3	1	3
9	1	3	3	2	2	2	2	3	2	3	1	3
10	1	3	3	2	2	2	2	3	2	3	1	3

1 = adhesive failure mode that occurred at the filling material and dentine interface.
2 = cohesive failure mode within the filling material.
3 = mixed failure mode.

[6]. This is in contrast to most other dental cements like GIC, which are highly acidic during the setting reaction [16]. The exact mechanism regarding the bonding of CSCs to dentine is still unclear. Discussed is a chemical bond as well as a micromechanical anchorage via cement tags in the dentinal tubules [16-19]. E.g. after placement of MTA on dentine, hydroxyapatite crystals nucleate and grow, filling the microscopic space between MTA and the dentine surface. Initially this seal is mechanical. Over time, the reaction between hydroxyapatite and dentine leads to a chemical bonding [19]. Hence, MTA appeared to bond chemically to dentine via diffusion-controlled reaction between its apatitic surface and dentine, forming an adherent interfacial layer that was firmly attached to the dentin wall [19]. It was shown that MTA trigger the precipitation of carbonated apatite, promoting a controlled mineral nucleation on dentine that was observed as the formation of an interfacial layer with tag-like structures [18]. This mechanism, theoretically, could initially lead also to the retention of the cement by the dentine through a micromechanical bonding system [20]. The alkaline Biodentine may induce a caustic denaturation and permeability of the organic collagen component of interfacial dentine [16]. Hence, for Biodentine a recent study showed the formation of intratubular tags in conjunction with an interfacial mineral interaction layer referred to as the "mineral infiltration zone" [16]. The interfacial layer formed between Biodentine and dentine may be comparable to that formed between dentine and MTA [21]. In contrast to Atmeh et al. [16] the migration of ions into dentine was not shown for Biodentine by Gjorgievska et al. [21] This leads to the conclusion that the adhesion of Biodentine is mainly micromechanical, and not ion-exchange based. Nevertheless, Biodentine showed excellent adaptability toward dentine [21].

Comparison to other Biodentine studies

To the best to our knowledge this is the first study that determined the shear bond strength values of Biodentine to a planar prepared coronal dentine surface. Nevertheless, the results of the present study are in the same range (6.2 MPa to 9.1 MPa) than push-out bond strength values [14,15,22-24]. However, the comparison of push-out bond strength of different CSCs with the results of the present study should be interpreted with some caution due to the different subject and methodology used in previous studies.

Interestingly the shear bond strength of Biodentine increased significantly from 2 d to one week. This may be explained by the fact that that the setting reaction of CSCs might continue for more than a month [25]. After 7 d and 14 d there was no significant difference in the shear bond strength of Biodentine and the GIC ChemFill rock. Thus, it may be concluded from this result that Biodentine may be used for replacement of missing dentine in comparable indications to GIC. In contrast the shear bond strength of ProRoot MTA was significant lower at all investigation periods which may be interpreted as a clinical disadvantage of MTA concerning tooth restoration.

Comparison to MTA

Identically to Biodentine to the best of our knowledge no data about shear bond strength of MTA to a planar prepared coronal dentine surface is available in literature. ProRoot MTA showed the lowest shear bond strength of all tested materials. A slight touch with the metal plunger was effectual to detach all ProRoot MTA samples from the dentine surface in the two days group. Nevertheless, the shear bond strength increased up to 5 MPa after two weeks. An increase of the shear bond strength values over time was also reported in push-out strength tests which range from 3.03 ± 1.28 MPa after 2 d [15] and between 4.75 ± 1.71 MPa [26] up to 9.0 ± 0.9 MPa [22] after 7 d, for example. Similar to the present study in general the push-out strength of Biodentine was higher compared to ProRoot MTA [22,23].

The different results of ProRoot MTA and Biodentine may be explained by the different particle size of these CSCs, which affects the penetration of cement into dentinal tubules in tag-like structures leading to a micromechanical anchor [17]. A smaller particle size and uniform components might have a role in better interlocking of Biodentine with dentine [15]. It was shown that calcium and silicon uptake into dentine leading the formation of tag-like structures in Biodentine was higher than in Pro-Root MTA [17]. In contrast to ProRoot MTA the Biodentine-liquid contains calcium chloride as setting accelerator. It was discussed if the addition of calcium chloride may enhance the resistance of CSCs to displacement from dentine and thus to improve shear bond strength [20].

Comparison to GIC

Since their introduction in 1972 [27], GICs have been widely used as dental restorative materials, luting cements and base materials [12,28]. One of their main advantages is the chemical bonding to tooth substrate by relative ease of use [29]. This is comparable to CSCs but there is a difference in the adhesive mechanism between acidic GIC and alkaline CSCs. The exact mechanism of GIC bonding to dentine is still unknown [12]. Several bonding mechanisms are discussed in literature: GIC bonds chemically directly to dentine by ionic bonding with hydroxyapatite to tooth substrate [30] even in presence of a smear layer [12]. Micromechanical bonding is also possible [12] and bonding to collagen has as well been suggested in a recent study [31]. The application of acidic GIC on dentine resulted in a demineralising effect on inorganic dentine components [16]. Polyalkenoic acids from the GIC is absorbed irreversibly onto hydroxyapatite from the dentine surface [32,33]. GIC forms an interaction zone by movement of ions from the cement into the surface layer of the tooth [21,34,35]. Hence, an ion exchange layer appears interfacial between dentine and GIC [36]. Whereas some authors reported about the formation of a hybrid layer and GIC tags in dentinal tubules after dentine conditioning and smear layer removal [37]. That could not be confirmed in other studies [38]. Hence, there was little evidence of tag-like structures when GIC is applied on dentine when the smear layer was not removed [16].

Bond strengths of GIC have been studied extensively using conventional shear testing methods but there is quite a bit of variation of the bond strengths of GIC on dentine surfaces that have not been conditioned [12,13,30,39]. For the GIC used in the present study (ChemFil rock) the

manufacturer specified the shear bond strength to be 11.75 ± 4.75 MPa [40], which is in the range of the values found here.

Comparison to X-trabase and Futurabond DC

The composite resin in combination with a dentine adhesive was included in this study as a positive control because it is well know that such materials possess the highest shear bond strength on dentine surfaces. Thus, the shear bond strength of X-trabase and Futurabond DC was about three times higher than that of GIC, Biodentine or ProRoot MTA. The present shear bond strength is in accordance with values found in literature for Futurabond DC ranging from 38.5 ± 14.8 MPa [41] to 39.30 ± 4.30 MPa [42] which confirms the accuracy of the method.

Failure mode

The analysis of the failure modes showed that for Biodentine the predominant failure type was cohesive, while for ProRoot MTA most of the failures were adhesive between the filling material and the dentine interface. This finding is in agreement with previous studies evaluating ProRoot MTA [43-45] or comparing Biodentine and ProRoot MTA [14,15] in push-out tests.

As already discussed for the shear bond strength these results could be attributed to the different particle size of Biodentine and MTA, which affects the penetration of filling materials into dentinal tubules. Biodentine has a smaller particle size and uniform components that may contribute to better adhesion and interlocking with the dentine, which consequently results in cohesive failures within the filling material [15]. In addition, the ability of Biodentine to form tag-like structures into dentinal tubules increased the micromechanical attachment [15,16].

The microscopically observation revealed a predominantly cohesive failure mode within the tested GIC. These findings correspond to results previously reported [46-48] and it is believed that this cohesive failure occurs in GIC is due to the porosity within the cement itself. This porosity will act as a stress concentration point where the fracture will initiate [47]. It may be speculated in how far this will apply for Biodentine.

For the used composite resin and the dentine adhesive (X-trabase + Futurabond DC) the failure mode was determined to be 2/3 adhesive and 1/3 a mixture between adhesive and cohesive. This is not in fully accordance with the recent literature where a predominantly cohesive [41] or all failure modes (adhesive, cohesive, mixture) [42] were described for Futurabond DC.

Conclusion

The null-hypotheses of this study could not be fully confirmed: Biodentine possess a shear bond strength to dentine comparable to a GIC, which was higher than that of ProRoot MTA but lower than that of composite resin in combination with a dentine adhesive. The shear bond strength of CSCs is increasing with time as the material cures.

Thus, under the aspect of dentine adhesion it may be concluded from the results of the present study that Biodentine may be used to replace missing dentine. Nevertheless, because the interaction of CSCs and the dentine surface is not fully understand yet further research concerning dentine-cement-interaction and dentine adhesion of CSCs is necessary.

Abbreviations
CR: Composite resin; CSC: Calcium silicate cement; GIC: Glass ionomer cement; MTA: Mineral Trioxide Aggregate.

Competing interests
The authors declare that they have no competing interests.

Authors' contributions
All authors have contributed significantly to this work and contributed to the paper in the equal parts: MK had the idea for the research and developed the concept, performed the in vitro experiments, participated in literature research and carried out proofreading. CHD performed the in vitro experiments, participated in literature research and carried out proofreading. ES participated in the design of the study, in literature research, writing of the manuscript, performed the statistical analysis and carried out proofreading. TD participated in study development, material testing, literature research, writing of the manuscript and carried out proofreading. All authors read and approved the final manuscript. All authors are in agreement with the content of the manuscript.

Author details
[1]Department of Operative Dentistry, Westphalian Wilhelms-University, Albert-Schweitzer-Campus 1, building W 30, 48149 Münster, Germany.
[2]Central Interdisciplinary Ambulance in the School of Dentistry, Albert-Schweitzer-Campus 1, building W 30, 48149 Münster, Germany.

References
1. Parirokh M, Torabinejad M. Mineral trioxide aggregate: a comprehensive literature review - Part I: chemical, physical, and antibacterial properties. J Endod. 2010;36:16–27.
2. Torabinejad M, Parirokh M. Mineral trioxide aggregate: a comprehensive literature review - Part II: leakage and biocompatibility investigations. J Endod. 2010;36:190–202.
3. Parirokh M, Torabinejad M. Mineral trioxide aggregate: a comprehensive literature review - Part III: Clinical applications, drawbacks, and mechanism of action. J Endod. 2010;36:400–13.
4. Camilleri J, Montesin FE, Curtis RV, Pitt Ford TR. Characterization of Portland cement for use as a dental restorative material. Dent Mater. 2006;22:569–75.
5. Camilleri J, Montesin FE, Juszczyk AS, Papaioannou S, Curtis RV, McDonald F, et al. The constitution, physical properties and biocompatibility of modified accelerated cement. Dent Mater. 2008;24:341–50.
6. Camilleri J, Sorrentino F, Damidot D. Investigation of the hydration and bioactivity of radiopacified tricalcium silicate cement, Biodentine and MTA Angelus. Dent Mater. 2013;29:580–93.
7. Pradelle-Plasse N, Tran XV, Colon P. Physico-chemical properties. In: Goldberg M, editor. Biocompatibility or cytotoxic effects of dental composites. Oxford: Coxmoor; 2009. p. 184–94.
8. Bortoluzzi EA, Broon NJ, Bramante CM, Felippe WT, Tanomaru Filho M, Esberard RM. The influence of calcium chloride on the setting time, solubility, disintegration, and pH of mineral trioxide aggregate and white Portland cement with a radiopacifier. J Endod. 2009;35:550–4.
9. Laurent P, Camps J, De Méo M, Déjou J, About I. Induction of specific cell responses to a Ca_3SiO_5-based posterior restorative material. Dent Mater. 2008;24:1486–94.
10. Laurent P, Aubut V, About I. Development of a bioactive Ca_3SiO_5 based posterior restorative material (Biodentine™). In: Goldberg M, editor. Biocompatibility or cytotoxic effects of dental composites. Oxford: Coxmoor; 2009. p. 195–200.
11. Koubi G, Colon P, Franquin JC, Hartmann A, Richard G, Faure MO, et al. Clinical evaluation of the performance and safety of a new dentine substitute, Biodentine, in the restoration of posterior teeth – a prospective study. Clin Oral Investig. 2013;17:243–9.
12. Erickson RL, Glasspoole EA. Bonding to tooth structure: a comparison of glass-ionomer and composite-resin systems. J Esthet Dent. 1994;6:227–44.
13. Ewoldsen N, Covey D, Lavin M. The physical and adhesive properties of dental cements used for atraumatic restorative treatment. Spec Care Dent. 1997;17:19–24.
14. Elnaghy AM. Influence of acidic environment on properties of Biodentine and white mineral trioxide aggregate: a comparative study. J Endod. 2014;40:953–7.
15. Guneser MB, Akbulut MB, Eldeniz AU. Effect of various endodontic irrigants on the push-out bond strength of Biodentine and conventional root perforation repair materials. J Endod. 2013;39:380–4.
16. Atmeh AR, Chong EZ, Richard G, Festy F, Watson TF. Dentin-cement interfacial interaction: calcium silicates and polyalkenoates. J Dent Res. 2012;91:454–9.
17. Han L, Okiji T. Uptake of calcium and silicon release from calcium silicate-based endodontic materials into root canal dentine. Int Endod J. 2011;44:1081–7.
18. Reyes-Carmona JF, Felippe MCS, Felippe WT. The biomineralization ability and interaction of Mineral Trioxide Aggregate and Portland cement with dentin in a phosphate-containing fluid. J Endod. 2009;35:731–6.
19. Sarkar NK, Caicedo R, Ritwik P, Moiseyeva R, Kawashima I. Physicochemical basis of the biologic properties of mineral trioxide aggregate. J Endod. 2005;31:97–100.
20. Reyes-Carmona JF, Felippe MS, Felippe WT. The biomineralization ability of mineral trioxide aggregate and Portland cement on dentine enhances the push-out strength. J Endod. 2010;36:286–91.
21. Gjorgievska ES, Nicholson JW, Apostolska SM, Coleman NJ, Booth SE, Slipper IJ, et al. Interfacial properties of three different bioactive dentine substitutes. Microsc Microanal. 2013;19:1450–7.
22. Aggarwal V, Singla M, Miglani S, Kohli S. Comparative evaluation of push-out bond strength of ProRoot MTA, Biodentine, and MTA Plus in furcation perforation repair. J Conserv Dent. 2013;16:462–5.
23. El-Ma'aita AM, Qualtrough AJE, Watts DC. The effect of smear layer on the push-out bond strength of root canal calcium silicate cements. Dent Mater. 2013;29:797–803.
24. Elnaghy AM. Influence of QMix irrigant on the micropush-out bond strength of Biodentine and white mineral trioxide aggregate. J Adhes Dent. 2014;16:277–83.
25. Chedella SCV, Berzins QW. A differential scanning calorimetry study of the setting reaction of MTA. Int Endod J. 2010;43:509–18.
26. Gancedo-Caravia L, Garcia-Barbero E. Influence of humidity and setting time on the push-out strength of mineral trioxide aggregate obturations. J Endod. 2006;32:894–6.
27. Wilson AD, Kent BE. A new translucent cement for dentistry. The glass ionomer cement. Br Dent J. 1972;132:133–5.
28. Smith DC. Development of glass-ionomer cement systems. Biomater. 1998;19:467–78.
29. Naasan MA, Watson TF. Conventional glass ionomers as posterior restorations. A status report for the American Journal of Dentistry. Am J Dent. 1998;11:36–45.
30. Wilson AD, McLean JW. Glass-ionomer cements. Chicago: Quintessence; 1988.
31. Akinmade A. The adhesion of glass polyalkenoate cements to collagen. J Dent Res. 1994;73(Spec Iss):181.
32. Ellis J, Jackson AM, Scott RP, Wilson AD. Adhesion of carboxylate cements to hydroxyapatite. III. Adsorption of poly(alkenoic acids). Biomater. 1990;11:379–84.
33. Misra DN. Adsorption of low molecular weight polyacrylic acid on hydroxyapatite: role of molecular association and apatite dissolution. Langmuir. 1991;7:2422–4.
34. Ngo HC, Mount G, Mc Intyre J, Tuisuva J, von Doussa RJ. Chemical exchange between glass-ionomer restorations and residual carious dentine in permanent molars: An in vivo study. J Dent. 2006;34:608–13.

35. ten Cate JM, van Duinen RNB. Hypermineralization of dentinal lesions adjacent to glass-ionomer cement restorations. J Dent Res. 1995;76:1266–71.

36. Wilson AD, Prosser HJ, Powis DM. Mechanism of adhesion of polyelectrolye cements to hydroxyapatite. J Dent Res. 1983;62:590–2.

37. Yip HK, Tay FR, Ngo HC, Smales RJ, Pashley DH. Bonding of contemporary glass ionomer cements to dentin. Dent Mater. 2001;17:456–70.

38. Hosoya Y, García-Godoy F. Bonding mechanism of Ketac-molar aplicap and Fuji IX GP to enamel and dentin. Am J Dent. 1998;11:235–9.

39. Hewlett ER, Caputo AA, Wrobet DC. Glass ionomer bond strength and treatment of dentin with polyacrylic acid. J Prosthet Dent. 1991;66:767–72.

40. Dentsply. ChemFil rock – advanced glass ionomer restorative. Scientific compendium. Milford: Dentsply Caulk; 2011. p. 25–6.

41. Wagner A, Wendler M, Petschelt A, Belli R, Lohbauer U. Bonding performance of universal adhesives in different etching modes. J Dent. 2014;42:800–7.

42. Abdalla AI. Bond strength of a total-etch and two self-etch adhesives to dentin with and without intermediate flowable liner. Am J Dent. 2010;23:157–60.

43. Hong ST, Bae KS, Baek SH, Kum KY, Shon WJ, Lee W. Effects of root canal irrigants on the push-out strength and hydration behaviour of accelerated mineral trioxide aggregate in its early setting phase. J Endod. 2010;36:1995–9.

44. Saghiri MA, Shokouhinejad N, Lotfi M, Aminsobhani M, Saghiri AM. Push-out bond strength mineral trioxide aggregate in the presence of alkaline pH. J Endod. 2010;36:1856–9.

45. Shokouhinejad N, Nekoofar MH, Iravani A, Kharrazifarad MJ, Dummer PMH. Effect of acidic environment on the push-out bond strength of mineral trioxide aggregate. J Endod. 2010;36:871–4.

46. McCarthy MF, Hondrum SO. Mechanical and bond strength properties of light-cured and chemically cured glass ionomer cements. Am J Orthod Dentofacial Orthop. 1994;105:135–41.

47. Tanumiharja M, Burrow MF, Tyas MJ. Microtensile bond strength of glass ionomer (polyalkenoate) cements to dentine using four conditioners. J Dent. 2000;28:361–6.

48. Triana R, Prado C, Garro J, García-Godoy F. Dentin bond strength of fluoride releasing materials. Am J Dent. 1994;7:252–4.

5

Epidermal growth factor enhances osteogenic differentiation of dental pulp stem cells *in vitro*

Casiano Del Angel-Mosqueda[1,2,4], Yolanda Gutiérrez-Puente[2,3], Ada Pricila López-Lozano[1,2,4], Ricardo Emmanuel Romero-Zavaleta[1], Andrés Mendiola-Jiménez[5], Carlos Eduardo Medina-De la Garza[1,5], Marcela Márquez-M[5,6] and Myriam Angélica De la Garza-Ramos[1,4*]

Abstract

Introduction: Epidermal growth factor (EGF) and basic fibroblast growth factor (bFGF) play an important role in extracellular matrix mineralization, a complex process required for proper bone regeneration, one of the biggest challenges in dentistry. The purpose of this study was to evaluate the osteogenic potential of EGF and bFGF on dental pulp stem cells (DPSCs).

Material and methods: Human DPSCs were isolated using CD105 magnetic microbeads and characterized by flow cytometry. To induce osteoblast differentiation, the cells were cultured in osteogenic medium supplemented with EGF or bFGF at a low concentration. Cell morphology and expression of CD146 and CD10 surface markers were analyzed using fluorescence microscopy. To measure mineralization, an alizarin red S assay was performed and typical markers of osteoblastic phenotype were evaluated by RT-PCR.

Results: EGF treatment induced morphological changes and suppression of CD146 and CD10 markers. Additionally, the cells were capable of producing calcium deposits and increasing the mRNA expression to alkaline phosphatase (ALP) and osteocalcin (OCN) in relation to control groups ($p < 0.001$). However, bFGF treatment showed an inhibitory effect.

Conclusion: These data suggests that DPSCs in combination with EGF could be an effective stem cell-based therapy for bone tissue engineering applications in periodontics and oral implantology.

Keywords: Dental pulp stem cells, Epidermal growth factor, Basic fibroblast growth factor, Osteogenic differentiation, Bone mineralization, Bone remodelling

Introduction

The multi-lineage differentiation capacity of mesenchymal stem cells (MSCs) has been amply studied in recent years because of its implication in tissue engineering and regenerative medicine [1, 2]; however, this field is currently faced with the critical challenge of developing novel approaches to regenerate large bone defects. Some years ago, Gronthos and colleagues isolated dental pulp stem cells (DPSCs) from human third molars confirming that these cells present the ability to differentiate into odontogenic/osteogenic cells [3–5]. Previous reports have shown that the osteogenic differentiation on DPSCs is successfully induced by chemical cues such as dexamethasone, ascorbic acid, and β-glycerophosphate [6–8]. Although these compounds have proven efficacy, analysis of the role of growth factors in osteogenesis has been the aim of several studies focused on improving extracellular matrix mineralization, a physiological process characterized by high expression of alkaline phosphatase (ALP) and osteocalcin (OCN), followed by calcium deposition [9, 10].

Epidermal growth factor (EGF) and basic fibroblast growth factor (bFGF) are powerful mitogens for many cell types including MSCs [11–13]. Ideally, it is expected that these factors maintain the self-renewal and multipotency capacities of these cells [14] but it is known that they can also promote differentiation towards specialized

* Correspondence: myriam.garzarm@uanl.edu.mx
[1]Unidad de Odontología Integral y Especialidades, Centro de Investigación y Desarrollo en Ciencias de la Salud, Universidad Autónoma de Nuevo León, Monterrey, Nuevo León, México
[4]Facultad de Odontología, Universidad Autónoma de Nuevo León, Monterrey, Nuevo León, México
Full list of author information is available at the end of the article

lineages such as osteoblasts, a process largely controlled by various growth factors [15, 16]. Certain studies show that bFGF affects osteogenic differentiation of DPSCs [17] through inhibition of ALP enzymatic activity and mineralization [18]. This effect has also been shown in stem cells from human exfoliated deciduous teeth (SHED) and periodontal ligament stem cells (PDLSCs) [19, 20]. On the other hand, it is well-known that an extensive variety of mesenchymal cells normally express the epidermal growth factor receptor (EGFR), a tyrosine kinase receptor that activates intracellular signalling pathways that determine their fate [21–23]. Emerging evidence suggests that EGF works as an enhancer of mineralization during differentiation of MSCs derived from bone marrow [24, 25]; however, the effect of EGF on osteogenic differentiation of DPSCs is unknown.

The purpose of this study was to evaluate the role of EGF and bFGF in order to identify crucial growth factors associated with enhancing osteogenic differentiation of DPSCs. We hypothesized that EGF supplementation may increase mineralization on the osteogenic differentiation of these cells. Our results provide evidence that EGF treatment, but not bFGF, is capable of increasing calcium deposit formation as well as ALP and OCN gene expression compared to traditional osteogenic medium. These observations indicate that EGF could be an effective adjuvant for improving bone regeneration in periodontics and oral implantology.

Material and methods

Subjects

Pulp samples were obtained from 12 human premolars extracted for orthodontic purposes from healthy patients; finally, the dental pulp tissues of the youngest patient (18 years of age) were used. The protocol was approved by the Ethics Committee, School of Dentistry of the Universidad Autónoma de Nuevo León (UANL) and performed in accordance with the ethical standards laid down in the 1964 Declaration of Helsinki. Informed consent was obtained from all donors.

Cell culture

Dental pulp explants were digested with 3 mg/ml collagenase type I and 4 mg/ml dispase (Sigma-Aldrich, St. Louis, MO, USA) at 37 °C for 1 h. The cell suspension was centrifuged at 300 g for 10 min, washed and then filtered through a 70 µm nylon filter (BD Biosciences, San Jose, CA, USA). Dental pulp cells were maintained in α-modified Eagle's medium (α-MEM) supplemented with 10 % fetal bovine serum (FBS) (Gibco-Invitrogen, Carlsbad, CA, USA), 2 mM L-glutamine, 100 U/ml penicillin, 100 µg/ml streptomycin and 0.25 µg/ml amphotericin B (Sigma-Aldrich) at 37 °C in a humidified

atmosphere with 5 % CO_2 for 3 weeks. The medium was renewed every 3 days.

Magnetic cell sorting

Cell isolation was performed following the manufacturer's protocol. Briefly, cultured cells were resuspended in PBS with 1 % bovine serum albumin (BSA) (Sigma-Aldrich) and then incubated with CD105 magnetic microbeads (Miltenyi Biotech, Bergish Gladbach, Germany) for 15 min at 4 °C. Cells were washed and loaded into a MS column placed in the magnetic field of a MiniMACS™ Separator (Miltenyi Biotech). Magnetically-labelled cells were collected and subcultured until passage 3 under the same growth conditions.

Flow cytometry analysis

To confirm the typical MSC immunophenotype, magnetic-isolated cells were incubated with the following monoclonal antibodies: CD105-FITC, CD73-PE, CD13-PE, CD45-FITC, CD34-PE, HLA-DR-PerCp, CD14-PE, CD11b-PE (BD Biosciences) and CD90-FITC (Miltenyi Biotech). Antibodies were added to ~1 x 10^5 cells per sample and then incubated for 30 min at 4 °C in dark. Stained cells were washed and then resuspended in PBS with 4 % paraformaldehyde. All samples were analyzed in a FACSCalibur™ flow cytometer system (BD Biosciences).

Formalin-induced fluorescence assay

DPSCs were plated onto 6-well plates (Corning-Costar, Corning, NY, USA) at a density of ~3 x 10^4 per well and cultured for 7 days in α-MEM as a negative control, and osteogenic medium (OM) as a positive control, composed of α-MEM, 10^{-7} M dexamethasone, 50 µg/ml ascorbic acid and 10 mM β-glycerophosphate (Sigma-Aldrich). At the same time, cells were incubated with OM containing 10 ng/ml of human EGF (OM + EGF) (Miltenyi Biotech) and OM containing 10 ng/ml of human bFGF (OM + bFGF) (Life Technologies, Rockville, MD, USA). Cultured cells were washed and then fixed with 10 % neutral-buffered formalin (BDH Chemicals, Ltd, UK) for 30 min. Fixed cells were incubated with 1 µg/ml DAPI (Thermo Scientific, Waltham, MA, USA) at room temperature for 5 min in dark. Cells were analyzed in a Zeiss Axiovert 200 M fluorescence microscope (Carl Zeiss, Göttingen, Germany).

Immunocytochemistry

DPSCs were plated onto 8-well chamber slides (Lab-Tek Chamber Slide, Nunc, Germany) at a density ~2.5 x 10^3 per well and maintained in α-MEM, OM, OM + EGF and OM + bFGF for 7 days. Cultured cells were fixed with cold methanol for 10 min and then incubated in PBS with 2 % BSA at room temperature for 30 min.

Fixed cells were incubated with mouse anti-human CD146-FITC (Miltenyi Biotech) and mouse anti-human CD10-FITC (BD Biosciences) monoclonal antibodies, counterstained with DAPI and then analyzed by fluorescence microscopy.

Osteogenic differentiation

DPSCs were plated onto 24-well plates (Corning-Costar) at a density of ~6 x 10^3 cells per well and cultivated in α-MEM for 24 h. The DPSCs were washed and then maintained in different culture media: α-MEM, OM, OM + EGF and OM + bFGF at 37 °C in a humidified atmosphere with 5 % CO_2 for 21 days. All media were renewed every 3 days.

Alizarin red S assay

After 21 days of osteogenic induction, the cells were fixed with 10 % neutral-buffered formalin for 30 min. Fixed cells were washed and then incubated with 2 % alizarin red S (ARS) (pH 4.2) (Sigma-Aldrich) at room temperature for 30 min in dark with gentle shaking. After staining, they were washed 4 times with PBS. The cells were analyzed by light microscopy and then incubated with cetylpyridinium chloride (CPC) 100 mM at 37 °C for 1 h to solubilize the extracellular calcium deposits attached to ARS. Two hundred microliters of each sample were transferred onto 96-well black plates (Corning-Costar). The ARS concentration was determined by absorbance at 495 nm in an iMark™ Absorbance Microplate Reader (Bio-Rad, Hercules, CA, USA) [26].

Reverse transcriptase polymerase chain reaction (RT-PCR)

Total RNA from DPSCs, cultured in α-MEM, OM, OM + EGF and OM + bFGF was isolated using the TRIzol method (Invitrogen Corp, Carlsbad, CA, USA). For the cDNA synthesis, the ImProm-II Reverse Transcription System kit (Promega, Madison, WI, USA) was used according to the manufacturer's instructions. PCR reactions to β-actin, alkaline phosphatase (ALP), bone sialoprotein (BSP), osteocalcin (OCN) and osteopontin (OPN) were performed in a MJ-Mini™ Staff Thermal cycler (Bio-Rad), following the protocol previously described [27]. PCR products were resolved on 1.5 % agarose gel electrophoresis, running at 100 V for 35 min. The gels were stained with 1 μg/ml ethidium bromide (Bio Basic Inc, Markham, ON, Canada) and displayed in a UV Transilluminator Doc™ Gel (Bio-Rad). All the reagents were used as a negative control for PCR except cDNA. In our study, all tests were performed three times (Table 1).

Statistical analysis

The ARS levels were analyzed using one-way analysis of variance (ANOVA) and Tukey's test for multiple

Table 1 Primer sequences for osteogenic differentiation analysis using reverse transcriptase-polymerase chain reaction (RT-PCR)

Gene	Sequence of oligonucleotides (5'- 3')	Tm °C
β-Actin	Forward: GGCATCCTGACCCTGAAGTA Reverse: GGGGTGTTGAAGGTCTCAAA	51
OCN	Forward: GAGCCCCAGTCCCCTACC Reverse: CCGATAGAGGTCCTGAAAG	58
BSP	Forward: CAGCGGAGGAGACAATGGAG Reverse: TTCAACGGTGGTGGTTTTCC	58
OPN	Forward: CAACGAAAGCCATGACCACA Reverse: CAGGTCCGTGGGAAAATCAG	54
ALP	Forward: GGTGAACCGCAACTGGTACT Reverse: CCCACCTTGGCTGTAGTCAT	54

comparisons among groups and p-values < 0.01 were considered statistically significant in all treatments. Data analysis was performed with SPSS software (SPSS Inc, Chicago, IL, USA).

Results

Isolation and phenotypic characterization of DPSCs

Adherent unsorted cells showed different sizes and morphologies after 3 weeks under cell growth conditions (Fig. 1a), in contrast, CD105+ magnetically-sorted cells showed a relatively homogeneous morphology characterized by spindle-shaped appearance with oval-central nuclei. Additionally, several colony-forming unit fibroblasts (CFU-F) were observed until passage 3 (Fig. 1b–d). Sorted cells had positive or negative expression by flow cytometry to the following surface markers: 99.47 % CD105-FITC, 97.89 % CD73-PE, 85.03 % CD90-FITC, 86.76 % CD13-PE, 0 % CD45-FITC, 0.11 % CD34-PE, 0.02 % HLA-DR-PerCp, 0.38 % CD14-PE and 0.39 % CD11b-PE (Fig. 1e). These results confirm that our cell culture presented the typical MSC immunophenotype: CD105+/CD73+/CD90+/CD13+/CD45−/CD34−/HLA-DR−/CD14−/CD11b−.

Morphological changes and expression of CD146 and CD10 surface markers

After 7 days in α-MEM incubation, DPSCs showed a fibroblastic-elongated morphology and tended to align themselves in parallel lines (Fig. 2a). Similar cell morphology was also observed in OM treated-cells (Fig. 2b). However, DPSCs in OM + EGF treatment showed clear morphological differences, characterized by polygonal-shaped appearance with spherical-peripheral nuclei and low cytoplasm content (Fig. 2c); moreover, these changes in OM + bFGF treatment were not observed (Fig. 2d). Additionally, the presence of EGF seems to induce a different organization pattern in cell culture, in comparison to the OM group. The highest cell confluence was observed in cells incubated with EGF or bFGF, in relation to α-MEM and OM control groups. Immunofluorescence

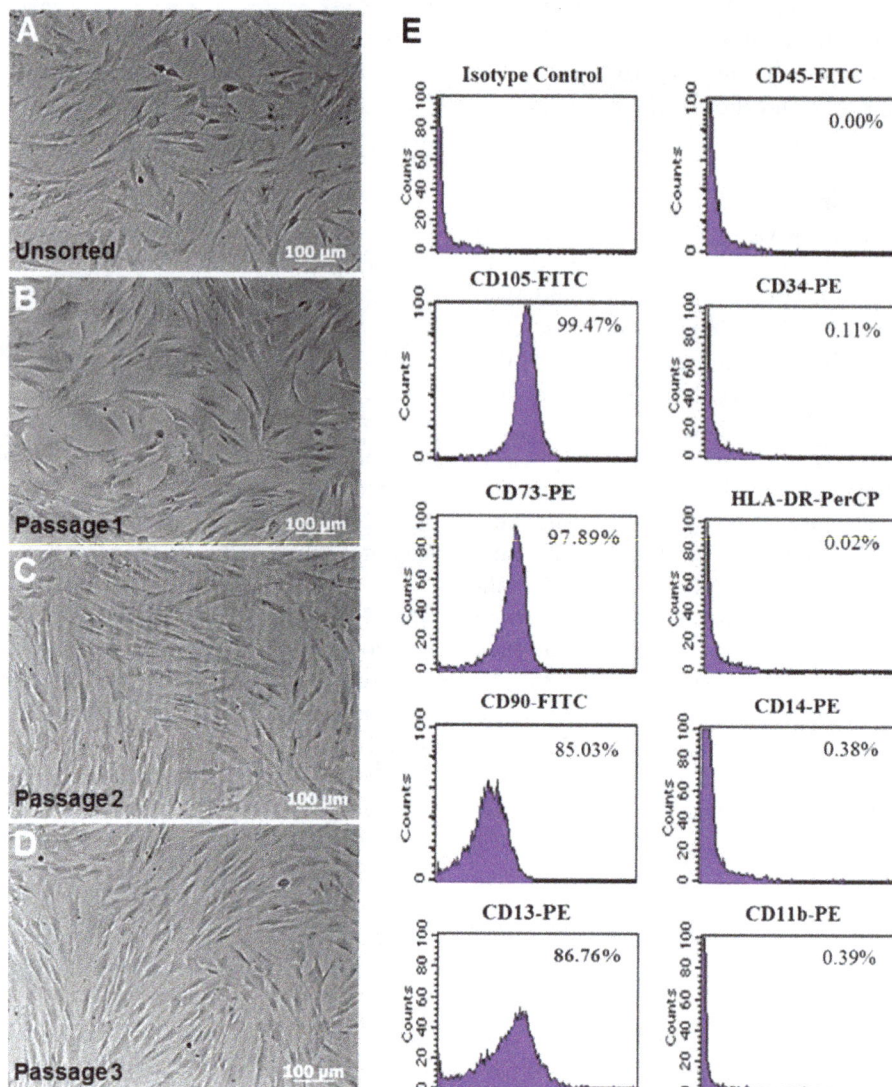

Fig. 1 Cell culture and flow cytometry analysis of isolated dental pulp stem cells (DPSCs). **a** Representative phase-contrast micrographs shows unsorted-cells derived from human dental pulp tissue after 14 days of cell culture. **b–d** CD105$^+$ magnetically-sorted DPSCs cultured in α-MEM without osteogenic induction. Morphologically, cells appear as typical fibroblastic and spindle shape during 3 passages. Original magnification 10x, scale bar =100 μm. **e** Flow cytometric analysis presented as histograms that show cell fluorescence intensity on the horizontal axis and cell frequency distribution on the vertical axis. Percentage results show positive expression to immunophenotype associated with mesenchymal stem cell (MSC) lineage as well as a lack of expression for hematopoietic markers

analysis confirmed that cells cultivated in α-MEM for 7 days were highly positive to CD146 and CD10 surface markers (Fig. 2e, i). Although, the OM group was capable of decreasing expression of both markers (Fig. 2f, j), EGF treated-cells showed the strongest inhibitory effect (Fig. 2g, k). In contrast, bFGF treated-cells seem to maintain expression levels in relation to α-MEM group (Fig. 2h, l).

Extracellular calcium deposition by ARS assay

After 21 days under osteogenic induction, a complete cell confluence in all treatments was observed. At this stage, the α-MEM group was negative to ARS (18.81 μg/ml);

however, in OM, OM + EGF, and OM + bFGF treatments, calcium deposition were observed (Fig. 3a). Microscopic analysis confirmed the absence of mineralized nodules in α-MEM (Fig. 3b). DPSCs treated only with OM showed high levels of ARS (792.64 μg/ml) and prominent mineralization nodules (Fig. 3c). Interestingly, OM supplemented with EGF induced a clear increase in abundance and size of calcium deposits (Fig. 3d), in addition to a significant increase in the mineralization levels evaluated by ARS (1686.31 μg/ml), in comparison to OM control group (Fig. 3f). In contrast, supplementation with bFGF showed a statistical

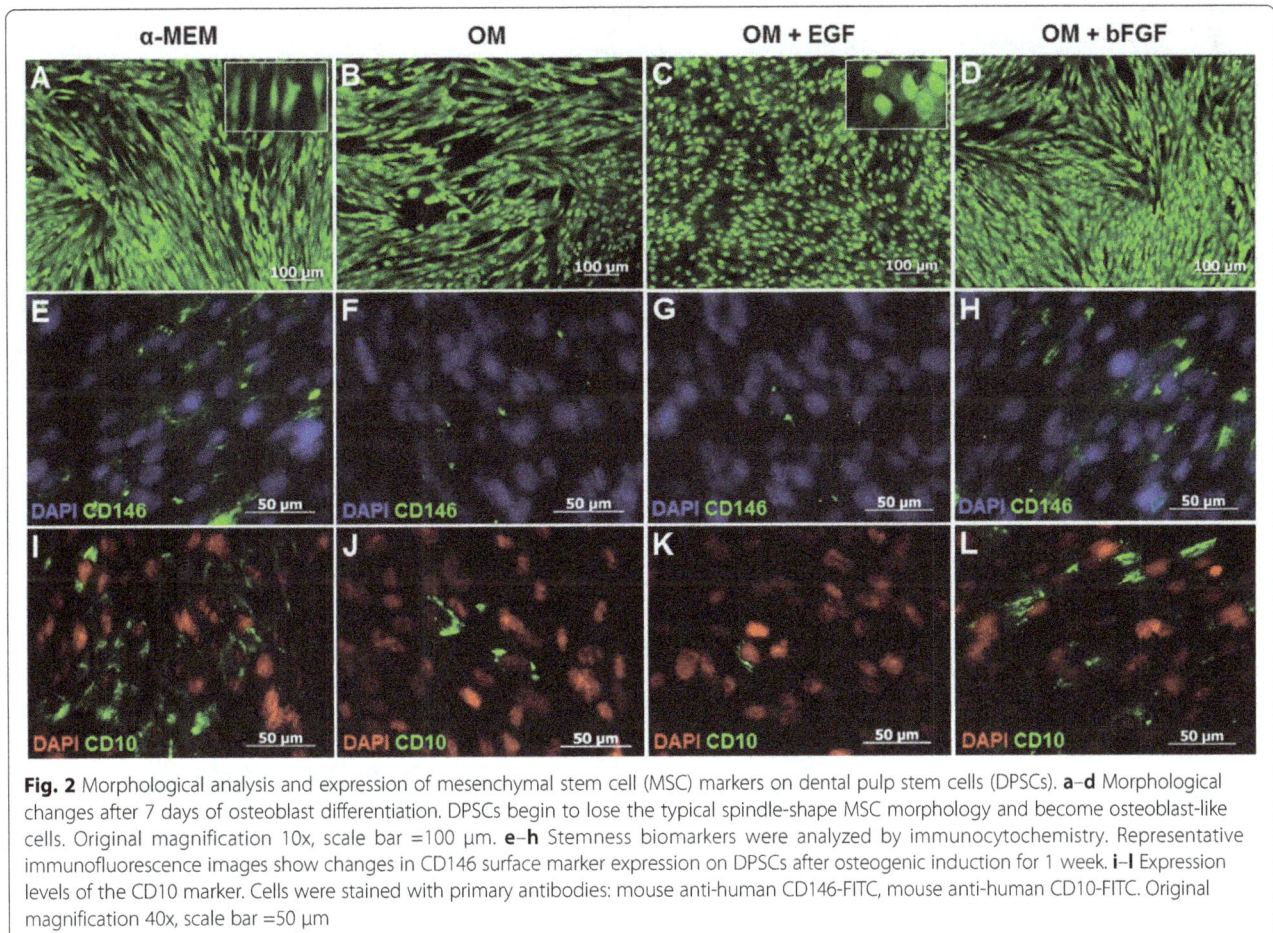

Fig. 2 Morphological analysis and expression of mesenchymal stem cell (MSC) markers on dental pulp stem cells (DPSCs). **a–d** Morphological changes after 7 days of osteoblast differentiation. DPSCs begin to lose the typical spindle-shape MSC morphology and become osteoblast-like cells. Original magnification 10x, scale bar =100 µm. **e–h** Stemness biomarkers were analyzed by immunocytochemistry. Representative immunofluorescence images show changes in CD146 surface marker expression on DPSCs after osteogenic induction for 1 week. **i–l** Expression levels of the CD10 marker. Cells were stained with primary antibodies: mouse anti-human CD146-FITC, mouse anti-human CD10-FITC. Original magnification 40x, scale bar =50 µm

difference with ARS (174.87 µg/ml) with respect to OM or OM + EGF, but the number of mineralized nodules were fewer than OM, suggesting an inhibitory effect (Fig. 3e).

Gene expression by RT-PCR
After 21 days of cell culture, gene expression of OCN was negative in the α-MEM group. In addition, the OM group was positive for this osteoblast-phenotypic marker; however, its expression level was superior due to the presence of EGF in the culture medium, suggesting its importance during osteogenesis. Contrary to these effects, the addition of bFGF resulted in a decrease in BSP, OCN and OPN expression with respect to OM treated-cells (Fig. 3g).

Discussion
Growth factors are recognized for their active participation in many biological processes such as cell migration, proliferation and differentiation [11, 28]. In the osteogenic context, it is also known that some of these factors play an essential role in bone regeneration since they are responsible for triggering cell specific signalling pathways that

allow expression of bone morphogenetic proteins (BMPs), which are molecules centrally involved in extracellular matrix mineralization and damage bone repair [29–31].

Our results provide evidence that supplementation with EGF enhances osteogenic mineralization on DPSCs during cell differentiation, suggesting its important role in favoring this cell fate. EGF and bFGF supplementation is commonly used to ensure survival and proliferation of MSCs cultured under serum-free conditions [32–34]; however, recent studies suggest that EGF added to traditional osteogenic medium not only promotes cell proliferation but also enhances mineralization of MSCs derived from bone marrow [24, 25, 35]. We have found that DPSCs are an excellent alternative to use instead of bone marrow for cell therapy; however, a challenge to overcome is the small amount of dental pulp tissue obtained; it is for this reason that in our study the cells were obtained from human premolars extracted for orthodontic purposes.

It is known that growth factors such as IGF-1, TGF-β and TNF-α enhance osteogenic differentiation of DPSCs [36–38]. Additionally, a recent study showed that 12 or 24 h of EGF treatment enhanced chemokine IL-8 and

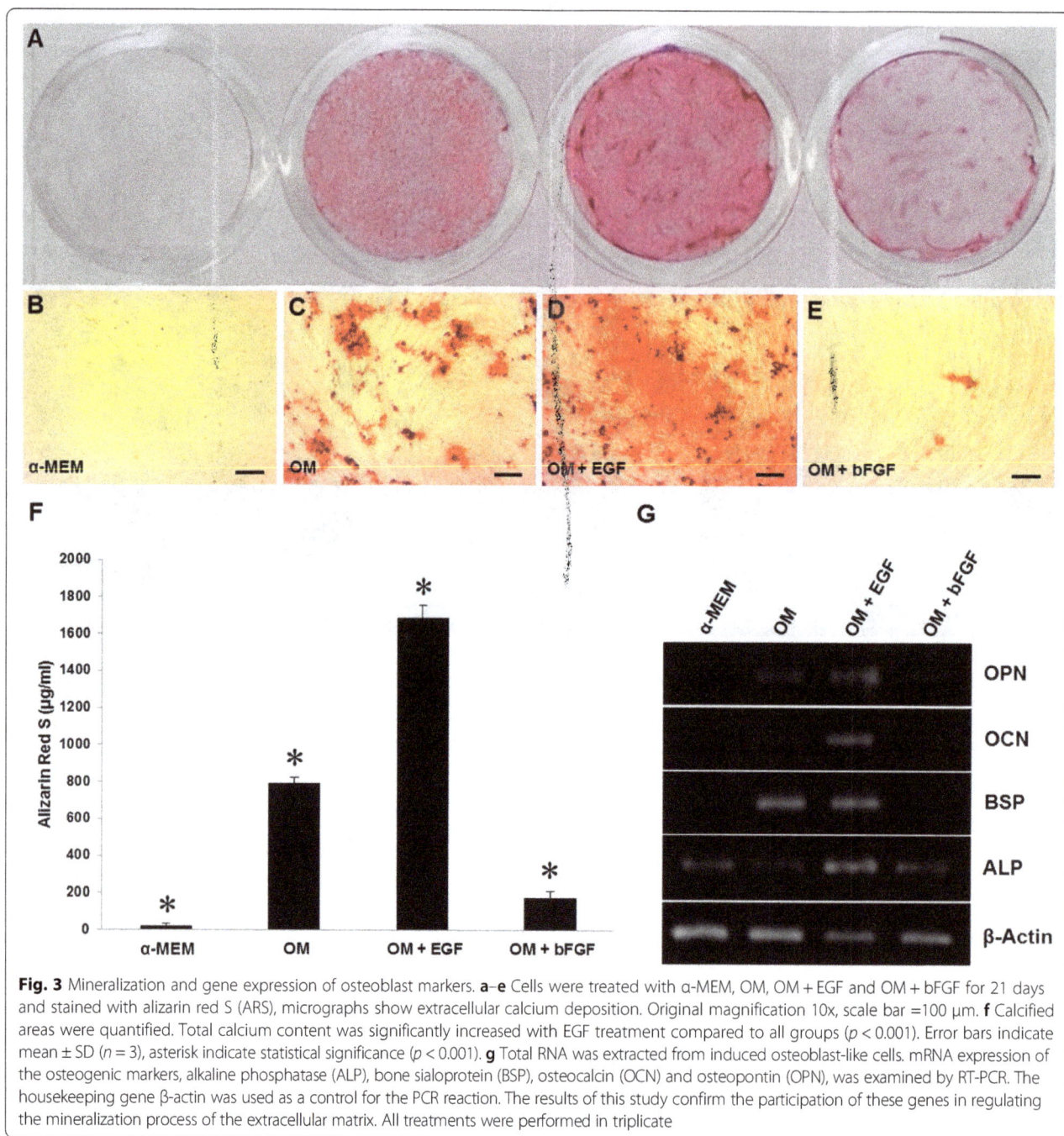

Fig. 3 Mineralization and gene expression of osteoblast markers. **a–e** Cells were treated with α-MEM, OM, OM + EGF and OM + bFGF for 21 days and stained with alizarin red S (ARS), micrographs show extracellular calcium deposition. Original magnification 10x, scale bar =100 μm. **f** Calcified areas were quantified. Total calcium content was significantly increased with EGF treatment compared to all groups ($p < 0.001$). Error bars indicate mean ± SD ($n = 3$), asterisk indicate statistical significance ($p < 0.001$). **g** Total RNA was extracted from induced osteoblast-like cells. mRNA expression of the osteogenic markers, alkaline phosphatase (ALP), bone sialoprotein (BSP), osteocalcin (OCN) and osteopontin (OPN), was examined by RT-PCR. The housekeeping gene β-actin was used as a control for the PCR reaction. The results of this study confirm the participation of these genes in regulating the mineralization process of the extracellular matrix. All treatments were performed in triplicate

BMP-2 expression in human periodontal ligament cells (HPDLCs) [39]. Since BMPs play a critical role in the mineralization process [40, 41], one can predict that the supernatant cell culture of EGF-treated cells could promote osteogenic differentiation more efficiently. Based on our findings, EGF can be used alone or in combination with any of these factors to achieve a synergistic effect. It is noteworthy that previous studies with EGF do not give similar results, but sometimes observations can be antagonistic. In this respect, some studies have

reported an inhibitory effect induced of EGF on osteogenic differentiation of MSCs not derived from dental pulp [42, 43]. A possible explanation for these heterogeneous results could be variation of cell origin of MSCs used in each study. This strengthens the importance of characterizing MSCs derived from dental pulp. Another possible reason for this discrepancy is the use of primary or immortalized cells as well as their heterogeneity. In order to reduce this heterogeneity, our experiments were performed using magnetically-labelled DPSCs CD105[+]

thus favoring the phenotype of primary cells, which could be closer to an *in vivo* situation than the experiments done with immortalized cells.

On the other hand, we also observed that bFGF was not able to exert effects similar to EGF and was a significant inhibitory factor for mineralization and differentiation towards osteoblast-like cells. This confirms that not all growth factors related to the proliferation and expan- sion of DPSCs are capable of enhancing osteogenic mineralization. Similarly, these effects were also observed by Li et al. [17–19] on SHED, although they evaluated a higher bFGF concentration (100 ng/ml), which is 10 times more concentrated than that of our experiments.

Cell morphology has been used as an important indicator to characterize and assess cell quality [44, 45]; we observed that morphological changes can also be used to follow mesenchymal-osteoblast cell transition from DPSCs at early stages (1 week). Here we found typical osteoblast morphology in advanced stages of cell differentiation (3 weeks) associated with high levels of calcium deposits. During the odontogenic differentiation, it is known that there is an up-regulation of odontoblast-specific genes, including dentin sialophosphoprotein (DSPP) and dentin matrix protein 1 (DMP1) [46, 47]. In our study due to dental origin of the cells is possible an odontogenic differentiation too; these results suggest that cell morphology in early stages of cell differentiation can be an important complementary data to assess cell lineage; however, in a confluent cell culture it is technically complicated to measure those morphological changes. It is noteworthy that after 1 week in osteogenic conditions, the DPSCs changed their colony-cell distribution; moreover, a greater cell adherence can be observed. As a general consensus, some surface markers are included within the minimum criteria for defining MSCs [48]; however, others markers have been associated with MSC lineage, such as CD146 and CD10, both expressed on DPSCs [49, 50] but their biological implication to the MSC lineage remains poorly known. Furthermore, *in vitro* EGF treatment was enough to reduce the expression of both cell markers, confirming an osteogenic role by EGF on DPSCs. The cell differentiation trigger changes in the immunophenotype of DPSCs, a test that can be used to monitor cell differentiation. We have found that there is a strong relationship between CD146 and CD10 expression levels and the osteogenic differentiation of DPSCs because these markers are related with the stemness of these cells. After 7 days, we observed stronger surface marker suppression with EGF but it is clear that this criterion is not enough to consider it as osteogenic differentiation; however, it can be useful to follow the

DPSC-osteoblast transition process. Nonetheless, it would be necessary to enlarge this kind of assays to characterize the behavior of other surface markers associated with the stemness of MSCs. Additionally, osteogenic *in vitro* differentiation of MSCs is commonly evidenced by early ALP activity, extracellular matrix mineralization and expression of typical osteoblast markers [51–53]. In agreement with our experiments, an increase of mRNA expression of ALP was observed in cells cultured with EGF. In addition, it is well known that OCN is an important osteogenic marker which regulates the formation of mineralization nodules and hence, leads to osteogenesis [54]. In this context, the upregulation of OCN expression as results from EGF treatment strengthen this study, suggesting its osteogenic effect. OPN, another important marker of late-stage osteoblast differentiation [55], was also overexpressed when cells were cultured with EGF, confirming its osteogenic role.

To our knowledge, this is the first report that evaluates the osteogenic effects of EGF on DPSCs; however, to elucidate the mechanism by which this occurs as well as its efficacy in animal models, further studies are required.

In conclusion, this study demonstrates that EGF plays an enhancer role on osteogenic differentiation of DPSCs because it is capable of increasing extracellular matrix mineralization. A low concentration of EGF (10 ng/ml) is sufficient to induce morphological and phenotypic changes; however, bFGF at an equal concentration exerts an inhibitory effect. These data suggests that DPSCs in combination with EGF could be an effective stem cell-based therapy to bone tissue engineering applications in periodontics and oral implantology.

Competing interests
The authors declare that they have no competing interests.

Authors' contributions
CDAM conceived the idea and designed the study; carried out cell culture experiments and drafted the manuscript; acquired and analyzed the data. YGP participated in the design and development of the experimental process; reviewed the data. APLL carried out immunocytochemistry experiments; acquired and analyzed the data. RERZ carried out PCR experiments; acquired and analyzed the data. AMJ carried out flow cytometry experiments; acquired and analyzed the data. CEMDLG participated in the design and development of experimental process; reviewed the data. MMM analysis and interpretation of data; drafted the manuscript. MADLGR analysis and interpretation of data; participated in the revision of the manuscript. All authors read and approved the final manuscript.

Acknowledgments
The first author, CDAM, thanks the Consejo Nacional de Ciencia y Tecnología (CONACYT), Mexico for funding through the PhD scholarship. All authors are grateful with Dr. José Luis Montiel Hernández and Dr. Sergio Lozano-Rodríguez for their assistance in editing the manuscript and Dr. Ismael Malagón Santiago for his help in the statistical analysis.

Funding

This work was supported by grant Proinnova No.141616 from Esteripharma de México, S.A.de C.V., Cancer Society in Stockholm, the King Gustav V Jubilee Fund, Stockholm and The Swedish Cancer Society.

Author details

[1]Unidad de Odontología Integral y Especialidades, Centro de Investigación y Desarrollo en Ciencias de la Salud, Universidad Autónoma de Nuevo León, Monterrey, Nuevo León, México. [2]Instituto de Biotecnología, Facultad de Ciencias Biológicas, Universidad Autónoma de Nuevo León, San Nicolás de los Garza, Nuevo León, México. [3]Departamento de Química, Facultad de Ciencias Biológicas, Universidad Autónoma de Nuevo León, San Nicolás de los Garza, Nuevo León, México. [4]Facultad de Odontología, Universidad Autónoma de Nuevo León, Monterrey, Nuevo León, México. [5]Facultad de Medicina, Universidad Autónoma de Nuevo León, Monterrey, Nuevo León, México. [6]Department of Oncology-Pathology, CCK, Karolinska Institutet, Stockholm, Sweden.

References

1. Bianco P, Robey PG. Stem cells in tissue engineering. Nature. 2001;414:118–21.
2. Pittenger MF, Mackay AM, Beck SC, Jaiswal RK, Douglas R, Mosca JD, et al. Multilineage potential of adult human mesenchymal stem cells. Science. 1999;284:143–7.
3. Gronthos S, Mankani M, Brahim J, Robey PG, Shi S. Postnatal human dental pulp stem cells (DPSCs) in vitro and in vivo. Proc Natl Acad Sci U S A. 2000;97:13625–30.
4. Gronthos S, Brahim J, Li W, Fisher LW, Cherman N, Boyde A, et al. Stem cell properties of human dental pulp stem cells. J Dent Res. 2002;81:531–5.
5. Miura M, Gronthos S, Zhao M, Lu B, Fisher LW, Robey PG, et al. SHED: stem cells from human exfoliated deciduous teeth. Proc Natl Acad Sci U S A. 2003;100:5807–12.
6. Riccio M, Resca E, Maraldi T, Pisciotta A, Ferrari A, Bruzzesi G, et al. Human dental pulp stem cells produce mineralized matrix in 2D and 3D cultures. Eur J Histochem. 2010;54:e46.
7. Langenbach F, Handschel J. Effects of dexamethasone, ascorbic acid and β-glycerophosphate on the osteogenic differentiation of stem cells in vitro. Stem Cell Res Ther. 2013;4:117.
8. Yu J, He H, Tang C, Zhang G, Li Y, Wang R, et al. Differentiation potential of STRO-1+ dental pulp stem cells changes during cell passaging. BMC Cell Biol. 2010;11:32.
9. Hoemann CD, El-Gabalawy H, McKee MD. In vitro osteogenesis assays: influence of the primary cell source on alkaline phosphatase activity and mineralization. Pathol Biol. 2009;57:318–23.
10. Huang Z, Nelson ER, Smith RL, Goodman SB. The sequential expression profiles of growth factors from osteoprogenitors [correction of osteroprogenitors] to osteoblasts in vitro. Tissue Eng. 2007;13:2311–20.
11. Rodrigues M, Griffith L, Wells A. Growth factor regulation of proliferation and survival of multipotential stromal cells. Stem Cell Res Ther. 2010;1:32.
12. Carpenter G, Cohen S. Epidermal growth factor. J Biol Chem. 1990;265:7709–12.
13. Mroczkowski B, Reich M, Chen K, Bell GI, Cohen S. Recombinant human epidermal growth factor precursor is a glycosylated membrane protein with biological activity. Mol Cell Biol. 1989;9:2771–8.
14. Tamama K, Fan VH, Griffith LG, Blair HC, Wells A. Epidermal growth factor as a candidate for ex vivo expansion of bone marrow-derived mesenchymal stem cells. Stem Cells. 2006;24:686–95.
15. Tsutsumi S, Shimazu A, Miyazaki K, Pan H, Koike C, Yoshida E, et al. Retention of multilineage differentiation potential of mesenchymal cells during proliferation in response to FGF. Biochem Biophys Res Commun. 2001;288:413–9.
16. Ito T, Sawada R, Fujiwara Y, Seyama Y, Tsuchiya T. FGF-2 suppresses cellular senescence of human mesenchymal stem cells by down-regulation of TGF-beta 2. Biochem Biophys Res Commun. 2007;359:108–14.
17. Qian J, Jiayuan W, Wenkai J, Peina W, Ansheng Z, Shukai S, et al. Basic fibroblastic growth factor affects the osteogenic differentiation of dental pulp stem cells in a treatment-dependent manner. Int Endod J. 2014;48(7):690–700.
18. Osathanon T, Nowwarote N, Pavasant P. Basic fibroblast growth factor inhibits mineralization but induces neuronal differentiation by human dental pulp stem cells through a FGFR and PLCγ signaling pathway. J Cell Biochem. 2011;112:1807–16.
19. Li B, Qu C, Chen C, Liu Y, Akiyama K, Yang R, et al. Basic fibroblast growth factor inhibits osteogenic differentiation of stem cells from human exfoliated deciduous teeth through ERK signaling. Oral Dis. 2012;18:285–92.
20. Osathanon T, Nowwarote N, Manokawinchoke J, Pavasant P. bFGF and JAGGED1 regulate alkaline phosphatase expression and mineralization in dental tissue-derived mesenchymal stem cells. J Cell Biochem. 2013;114:2551–61.
21. Fan VH, Tamama K, Au A, Littrell R, Richardson LB, Wright JW, et al. Tethered epidermal growth factor provides a survival advantage to mesenchymal stem cells. Stem Cells. 2007;25:1241–51.
22. Harris RC, Chung E, Coffey RJ. EGF receptor ligands. Exp Cell Res. 2003;284:2–13.
23. Schmidt MH, Furnari FB, Cavenee WK, Bogler O. Epidermal growth factor receptor signaling intensity determines intracellular protein interactions, ubiquitination, and internalization. Proc Natl Acad Sci U S A. 2003;100:6505–10.
24. Kratchmarova I, Blagoev B, Haack-Sorensen M, Kassem M, Mann M. Mechanism of divergent growth factor effects in mesenchymal stem cell differentiation. Science. 2005;308:1472–7.
25. Platt MO, Roman AJ, Wells A, Lauffenburger DA, Griffith LG. Sustained epidermal growth factor receptor levels and activation by tethered ligand binding enhances osteogenic differentiation of multi-potent marrow stromal cells. J Cell Physiol. 2009;221:306–17.
26. Stanford CM, Jacobson PA, Eanes ED, Lembke LA, Midura RJ. Rapidly forming apatitic mineral in an osteoblastic cell line (UMR 106–01 BSP). J Biol Chem. 1995;270:9420–8.
27. Sambrook J, Maccallum P, Russel D. Molecular Cloning: A Laboratory Manual. 3rd ed. Woodbury, NY: Cold Spring Harbor Press; 2001.
28. Discher DE, Mooney DJ, Zandstra PW. Growth factors, matrices, and forces combine and control stem cells. Science. 2009;324:1673–7.
29. Suzuki A, Ghayor C, Guicheux J, Magne D, Quillard S, Kakita A, et al. Enhanced expression of the inorganic phosphate transporter Pit-1 is involved in BMP-2-induced matrix mineralization in osteoblast-like cells. J Bone Miner Res. 2006;21:674–83.
30. Luppen CA, Smith E, Spevak L, Boskey AL, Frenkel B. Bone morphogenetic protein-2 restores mineralization in glucocorticoid-inhibited MC3T3-E1 osteoblast cultures. J Bone Miner Res. 2003;18:1186–97.
31. Rawadi G, Vayssière B, Dunn F, Baron R, Roman-Roman S. BMP-2 controls alkaline phosphatase expression and osteoblast mineralization by a Wnt autocrine loop. J Bone Miner Res. 2003;18:1842–53.
32. Bonnamain V, Thinard R, Sergent-Tanguy S, Huet P, Bienvenu G, Naveilhan P, et al. Human dental pulp stem cells cultured in serum-free supplemented medium. Front Physiol. 2013;4:357.
33. Tamama K, Kawasaki H, Wells A. Epidermal growth factor (EGF) treatment on multipotential stromal cells (MSCs). Possible enhancement of therapeutic potential of MSC. J Biomed Biotechnol. 2010;2010:795385.
34. Howard C, Murray PE, Namerow KN. Dental pulp stem cell migration. J Endod. 2010;36:1963–6.
35. Kim SM, Jung JU, Ryu JS, Jin JW, Yang HJ, Ko K, et al. Effects of gangliosides on the differentiation of human mesenchymal stem cells into osteoblasts by modulating epidermal growth factor receptors. Biochem Biophys Res Commun. 2008;371:866–71.
36. Huang CH, Tseng WY, Yao CC, Jeng JH, Young TH, Chen YJ. Glucosamine promotes osteogenic differentiation of dental pulp stem cells through modulating the level of the transforming growth factor-beta type I receptor. J Cell Physiol. 2010;225:140–51.
37. Feng X, Huang D, Lu X, Feng G, Xing J, Lu J, et al. Insulin-like growth factor 1 can promote proliferation and osteogenic differentiation of human dental pulp stem cells via mTOR pathway. Dev Growth Differ. 2014;56:615–24.
38. Feng X, Feng G, Xing J, Shen B, Li L, Tan W, et al. TNF-α triggers osteogenic differentiation of human dental pulp stem cells via the NF-κB signalling pathway. Cell Biol Int. 2013;37:1267–75.
39. Teramatsu Y, Maeda H, Sugii H, Tomokiyo A, Hamano S, Wada N, et al. Expression and effects of epidermal growth factor on human periodontal ligament cells. Cell Tissue Res. 2014;357:633–43.
40. Devescovi V, Leonardi E, Ciapetti G, Cenni E. Growth factors in bone repair. Chir Organi Mov. 2008;92:161–8.
41. Chen D, Zhao M, Mundy GR. Bone morphogenetic proteins. Growth Factors. 2004;22:233–41.

42. Krampera M, Pasini A, Rigo A, Scupoli MT, Tecchio C, Malpeli G, et al. HB-EGF/HER-1 signaling in bone marrow mesenchymal stem cells: inducing cell expansion and reversibly preventing multilineage differentiation. Blood. 2005;106:59–66.

43. Hu F, Wang X, Liang G, Lv L, Zhu Y, Sun B, et al. Effects of epidermal growth factor and basic fibroblast growth factor on the proliferation and osteogenic and neural differentiation of adipose-derived stem cells. Cell Rep. 2013;15:224–32.

44. Matsuoka F, Takeuchi I, Agata H, Kagami H, Shiono H, Kiyota Y, et al. Morphology-based prediction of osteogenic differentiation potential of human mesenchymal stem cells. PLoS One. 2013;8:e55082.

45. Leischner U, Schierloh A, Zieglgansberger W, Dodt HU. Formalin-induced fluorescence reveals cell shape and morphology in biological tissue samples. PLoS One. 2010;5:e10391.

46. Nam S, Won JE, Kim CH, Kim HW. Odontogenic differentiation of human dental pulp stem cells stimulated by the calcium phosphate porous granules. J Tissue Eng. 2011;2011:812547.

47. Sun HL, Wu YR, Huang C, Wang JW, Fu DJ, Liu YC. The effect of SIRT6 on the odontoblastic potential of human dental pulp cells. J Endod. 2014;40:393–8.

48. Dominici M, Le Blanc K, Mueller I, Slaper-Cortenbach I, Marini F, Krause D, et al. Minimal criteria for defining multipotent mesenchymal stromal cells. The International Society for Cellular Therapy position statement. Cytotherapy. 2006;8:315–7.

49. Gronthos S, Franklin DM, Leddy HA, Robey PG, Storms RW, Gimble JM. Surface protein characterization of human adipose tissue-derived stromal cells. J Cell Physiol. 2001;189:54–63.

50. Vishwanath VR, Nadig RR, Nadig R, Prasanna JS, Karthik J, Pai VS. Differentiation of isolated and characterized human dental pulp stem cells and stem cells from human exfoliated deciduous teeth: An in vitro study. J Conserv Dent. 2013;16:423–8.

51. Mori G, Brunetti G, Oranger A, Carbone C, Ballini A, Lo Muzio L, et al. Dental pulp stem cells: osteogenic differentiation and gene expression. Ann N Y Acad Sci. 2011;1237:47–52.

52. Stucki U, Schmid J, Hämmerle CF, Lang NP. Temporal and local appearance of alkaline phosphatase activity in early stages of guided bone regeneration. A descriptive histochemical study in humans. Clin Oral Implants Res. 2001;12:121–7.

53. Ling LE, Feng L, Liu HC, Wang DS, Shi ZP, Wang JC, et al. The effect of calcium phosphate composite scaffolds on the osteogenic differentiation of rabbit dental pulp stem cells. J Biomed Mater Res A. 2015;103:1732–45.

54. Shi X, Wang Y, Varshney RR, Ren L, Zhang F, Wang DA. In-vitro osteogenesis of synovium stem cells induced by controlled release of bisphosphate additives from microspherical mesoporous silica composite. Biomaterials. 2009;30:3996–4005.

55. McKee MD, Addison WN, Kaartinen MT. Hierarchies of extracellular matrix and mineral organization in bone of the craniofacial complex and skeleton. Cells Tissues Organs. 2005;181:176–88.

6

Frontalis suspension surgery to treat patients with essential blepharospasm and apraxia of eyelid opening-technique and results

Chrisanthi Karapantzou[1], Dirk Dressler[2], Saskia Rohrbach[3] and Rainer Laskawi[1,4*]

Abstract

Introduction: We describe the results of 15 patients suffering from essential blepharospasm with apraxia of eyelid opening who underwent frontalis suspension surgery.

Material and methods: Patients with apraxia of eyelid opening and unresponsive to botulinum toxin injections were studied. Bilateral frontalis suspension surgery was performed (sling operation) using polytetrafluoroethylene (Gore-Tex®) sutures. The patients reported the *degree of improvement* using a subjective rating scale to evaluate the benefit of the operation at two times after surgery (0-10 days and 180-360 days).

Results: The patients reported a high degree of subjective improvement. In the early postoperative period (0-10 days) the mean degree of subjective improvement was 74.6% (standard deviation (SD) 26.4%). At 180-360 days after surgery the mean improvement was 70.0% (SD 26.7%). Small hematomas of the upper lid occurred postoperatively in all patients. Other complications were suture extrusions (9.1%), suture granulomas (6.1%), lacrimation (5.0%) and local infections (7.5%). Postoperatively, all patients needed additional botulinum toxin injections for optimal outcome.

Conclusion: Frontalis suspension surgery is a minimally invasive and effective treatment option for apraxia of eyelid opening in patients with essential blepharospasm unresponsive to botulinum toxin injections alone.

Keywords: Blepharospasm, Apraxia of eye lid opening, Frontalis suspension surgery

Introduction

The treatment of essential blepharospasm with botulinum toxin (BoNT) is a well-established method [1,2]. However, some patients suffer from a special form of blepharospasm that renders them unable to open their eyes adequately despite local BoNT treatment. This phenomenon is due to the inability to raise the eyelid (see Figure 1). This is referred to in the literature as "apraxia of eyelid opening", "levator inhibition blepharospasm" or "dystonic eyelid opening disorder" [3-6]. It leads to a compensatory constrained posture such as retroflexion of the head to enable the patient to see through the narrow palpebral fissure. The patients frequently exhibit photophobia, and perform certain compensatory movements to keep the palpebral fissure as wide as possible. Many patients increase vertical

traction by contracting the frontalis muscle to widen the opening of the palpebral fissure. Since BoNT treatment alone will not provide any significant improvement of the eye opening, a number of more or less invasive surgical procedures have been introduced [3-5,7,8]. In our patients with this condition we perform frontalis suspension surgery ("sling operation") based on the technique of Roggenkämper and Nüssgens [3,4]. In this report we describe this surgical procedure and present our results of the operation as well as the assessments of the patients with regard to the success of the treatment and to their quality of life.

Patients and methods
General information

This retrospective analysis, which had the approval of our institutional ethics review board (University of Göttingen Medical Center), encompasses 15 patients, nine women and six men, who underwent bilateral frontalis suspension

---

* Correspondence: rlaskaw@gwdg.de
[1]ENT-Department, University of Göttingen Medical Center, Göttingen, Germany
[4]HNO-Klinik Universitätsmedizin Göttingen, Robert-Koch-Str. 40, 37075 Göttingen, Germany
Full list of author information is available at the end of the article

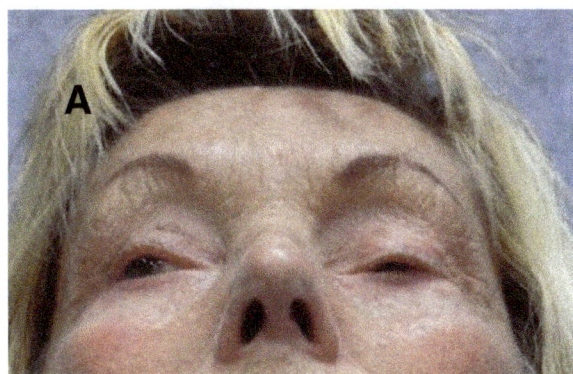

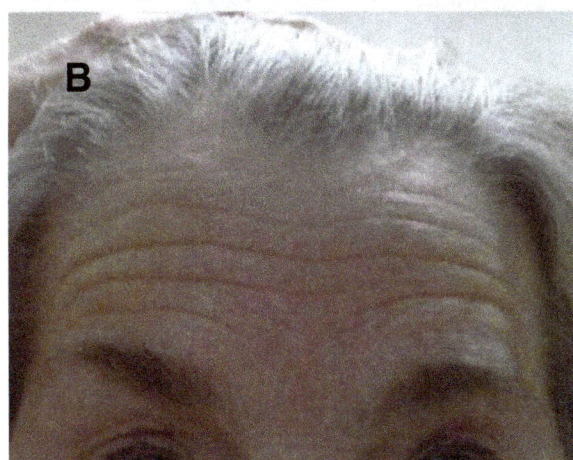

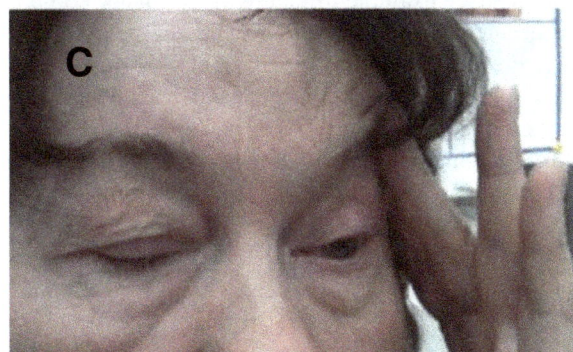

Figure 1 Clinical presentation and compensatory maneuvers in patients with blepharospasm and apraxia of eyelid opening.
A: Patient with apraxia of eyelid opening. Retroflexion of the head.
B: Innervation of the frontalis muscle as a compensatory maneuver to increase eye opening. **C**: Lifting the upper lid with a finger to open the eye.

surgery (surgical details given below) for insufficiency of the lid retractors. All patients had had preoperative BoNT therapy, which by itself had not enabled adequate eyelid opening. A total of 40 eyelid operations, including revisions (number see below) were performed. Seven patients were operated on in one session and eight in a two-stage procedure. A total of ten surgical revisions of five eyelids were necessary in three patients. Thirty-six operations (90%) were performed in general anesthesia with

intubation. The patients participated voluntarily in the postoperative interviews (see below). Photographs of patients are published with their written consent.

Surgical technique

All primary operations (based on [3,4], n = 30) were performed in general anesthesia. The eyebrows and the eyelids were infiltrated subcutaneously with a local anesthetic containing epinephrine (1% Ultracain®) to reduce local bleeding. After disinfecting the skin (Braunol®), and sketching the incision lines above the upper edge of the lid and slightly above the eyebrow (Figure 2) we made three skin incisions and locally undermined the skin so that the polytetrafluoroethylene (PTFE, Gore-Tex®) sutures and knots used for the suspension could be buried as deeply as possible (Figure 2). A lid plate was inserted under the eyelid during the incision to protect the eye. Depending on the thickness of the eyelid, a size 3-0 (87%) or 4-0 (13%) suture was passed through the medial caudal incision in the upper border of the eyelid cephalad to the medial incision just above the eyebrow. A needle was used to pass the suture subcutaneously (see Figure 2). On retraction, the needle was used to pull a second subcutaneous PTFE suture caudally through the medial incisions (Figure 2). Starting from the medial incision, two loops (squares) of rectangular shape were then formed with subcutaneous PTFE sutures (medial, lateral, Figure 2). In order to form an adequate angle, the sutures were led out of the other incisions (lateral, medial) and then reinserted subcutaneously in the desired direction. Finally, the ends of each suture were brought out through the medial upper incision for the first square and out of the lateral upper incision for the second square to be tied (Figure 2). The surgical site was disinfected after each step in placing the sutures. The skin incisions, except for the lateral and medial upper incisions above the eyebrow, were then closed (Figure 2). The position of the eyelid was assessed and adjusted to give a slight overcorrection with a discrete 2-3 mm wide palpebral fissure. The protruding sutures were knotted and buried subcutaneously. The lateral and medial upper incisions were then closed with skin sutures. We used thin, absorbable sutures (Vicryl® 7-0) for skin closure to avoid having to remove them later (Figure 2). Ointment (Polyspectran®) was applied to the eyes, and the forehead and upper eyelid were covered with a sterile dressing.

Subjective evaluation of treatment success

Postoperative "satisfaction" with the operation was assessed individually for each eye see [3,4]. The left and right side were evaluated separately because the patients might possibly register a difference, e.g. eye-opening not equally good or bad on both sides, or because the eyes were operated on separate occasions. The patients were requested

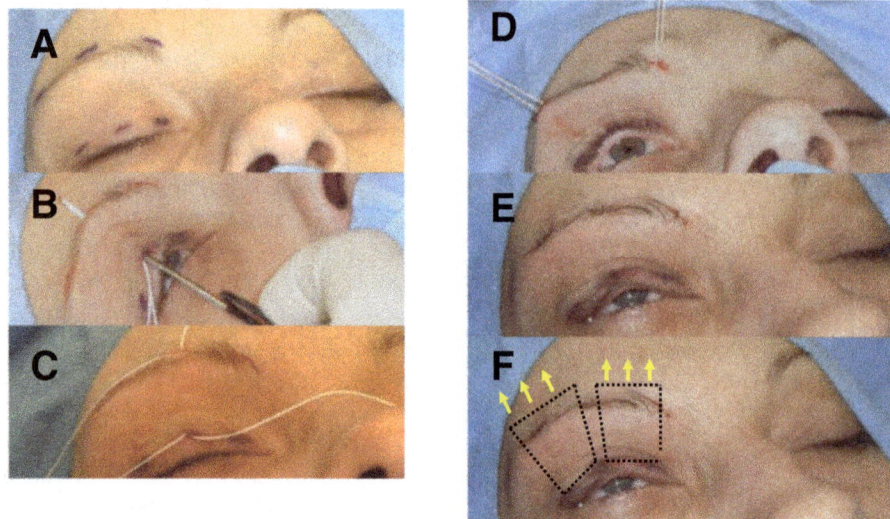

Figure 2 Steps in frontalis suspension operation. A: Typical incisions in the upper eyelid and above the eyebrow. **B**: Subcutaneous insertion of polytetrafluoroethylene (Gore-Tex®) sutures from the edge of the upper eyelid to the caudal portion of the frontalis muscle. **C**: The two sutures are positioned to form the lateral and medial two loops (squares) of rectangular shape. **D**: Sutures brought out laterally and medially before tying the knots. **E**: Final status with desired slight opening of the eyelid after tying and burying the knots and stitching the skin incisions. The final step is to apply eye ointment and a special dressing that allows both eyes to be opened immediately after surgery. **F**: The subcutaneous position of the polytetrafluoroethylene sutures is illustrated in an idealized manner. The arrows indicate the direction of force of the frontalis muscle. By suspending the upper eyelid from the caudal frontalis muscle, the upper eyelid can be actively raised by the patient.

to give a subjective evaluation of the success of treatment at two different time windows. Success was scored on a scale of zero to 100 percent. Zero percent was the "lack of any improvement after the operation", whereas 100% was "optimal treatment results and resolution of all complaints after the operation". The assessment periods were between day 1 to 10 (early postoperative period) and between day 180 to 365 (late postoperative period) after surgery. The percentage values for the left and the right eye were added for each patient, and the average and standard deviation (SD) were calculated. The average group value of each time period was obtained by calculating the average and standard deviation of the individual averages during that period.

Thirteen patients were able to assess the results in both time periods, while two patients were only able to assess the first period, since the required interval for the second period had not elapsed since the operation.

Results
General information

The average interval between the first manifestation of the disorder and the diagnosis was 2.9 years (SD 1.9 years; range 0 to 7.0 years). The average interval between initial diagnosis and begin of BoNT therapy was 0.73 years (SD 1.78; range 0 to 7.0 years).

The average interval between starting local BoNT treatment and the first frontalis suspension operation was 2.8 years (SD 1.7 years; range 1.0 to 6.0 years).

Surgical technique and complication rate

All patients initially reported an improvement of their symptoms (see example in Figure 3). No major complications occurred during surgery or in the immediate postoperative period. The typical and unavoidable postoperative local hematomas and discrete edema of the upper lid were seen in all patients. The relevant postoperative events are summarized in Table 1. During the study period, including revision operations, a total of 66 PTFE sutures or loops (squares) of rectangular shape were placed in the fifteen patients. Six sutures had to be removed during this period because of local tissue reaction giving an extrusion rate of 9.1% (see Table 1). The interval between surgery and reaction to the suture or to revision surgery was two weeks to five months (mean 2.6 months; SD 1.98 months).

BoNT treatment was continued in all patients, since the effect of the operation alone, although it greatly improved the situation, was not sufficient for an optimal result.

Individual observations

Several interesting details became apparent when the results of the individual patients who had undergone the frontalis suspension procedure were analyzed. These are presented in two short case reports.

Case 1

A 56-year old female patient underwent bilateral two-stage frontalis suspension surgery for typical blepharospasm with apraxia of eyelid opening (Figure 3). After

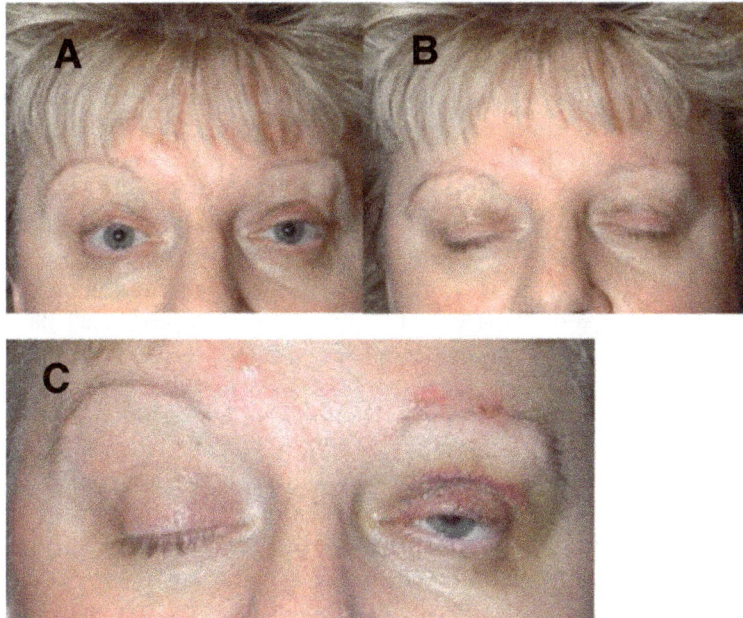

Figure 3 Patient after bilateral frontalis suspension surgery. The eyes can be opened **(A)** and closed **(B)** without difficulty. The patient's BoNT treatment was continued. Insert **C** shows the situation immediately after the unilateral operation of the left eye, identifiable by the small hematoma. One can clearly see that the apraxia persists in the non-operated right eye and that eye opening is not possible in spite of innervation of the frontalis muscle. The position of the eyebrow is higher and the upper eyelid is completely closed. After the suspension surgery, the left, operated eye is already partly opened with only a low-intensity innervation. This is consistent with a lateralized control of the apraxia.

the first operation we noticed that the levator inhibition effect appeared to differ between the two sides (Figure 3). When the patient attempted to raise her eyebrows we observed an increased innervation of the frontalis muscle on the non-operated side but without a resulting adequate lift of the eyelid. A markedly slighter innervation of the frontalis muscle of the treated side gave a much wider opening of the eyelid (Figure 3).

Case 2

A 73-year old male patient with multifocal dystonia presented with blepharospasm and apraxia of eyelid opening. Following successful frontalis suspension surgery the PTFE sutures were expulsed on both sides after two months (right side), respectively five months (left side). Despite repeated revision operations with the aim of burying the knots the sutures eventually had to be removed. Despite this the patient continued to be able to open his eyes.

Table 1 Type and incidence of postoperative complications

Postoperative complications	Frequency
Suture extrusion	6 of 66 sutures (9.1%)
Suture granuloma	4 of 66 sutures (6.1%)
Lacrimation	2 of 40 operated eyelids (5.0%)
Infection	3 of 40 operated eyelids (7.5%)

The effect persisted for seven months (right eye), respectively 11 months (left eye).

Subjective rating of success of treatment

All of the fifteen patients reported an initial postoperative improvement of eye opening.

The average early postoperative (0 to 10 days) subjective rating of therapeutic success was 74.6% (SD 26.4%; range 20 to 100%). The average rating at the later period (180 to 365 days) was 70.0% (SD 26.7%; range 0 to 100%).

Discussion

One main approach in the treatment of essential blepharospasm is to reduce muscle mass in the cranial portion of the orbicularis oculi muscle, often together with parts of the procerus and the corrugator supercilii muscles [7]. These procedures can be combined with suspension operations [8]. They are considerably more invasive than suspension operations alone, as performed in our own and other institutions [3-5].

The polytetrafluoroethylene (PTFE, Gore-Tex®) sutures gave satisfactory functional results. However, it is well known that PTFE sutures do not always integrate well into the tissue bed, and they can cause problems with tissue reactions and extrusion [9-11]. The extrusion rate of 9.1% and the 6.1% incidence of granulomas in our patients are similar to those described by other authors [5].

It should be mentioned that whenever a suture that was introduced using our method is extruded, a new one can be inserted without any problems after a waiting period of only a few weeks. In addition, if the traction effect of the suture decreases, it is possible to uncover the knot and "reposition" the upper eyelid.

Fascia lata gives very good functional results compared to other materials [12,13], but we prefer polytetrafluoroethylene because this is a minimally invasive option to elevate the upper lid in patients with blepharospam with apraxia of eye lid opening. The removal of fascia lata is more invasive, an additional skin incision is needed in another body region (thigh), and the results do not differ much from the use of polytetrafluoroethylene in this connection [12,13].

Our observations in individual patients were interesting. In our surgically treated patients, we did not observe the known effect that a unilateral BoNT injection can cause bilateral improvement of blepharospasm. The observed phenomenon of a lateralized change in the ability to raise the eyelid is an argument for a lateralized "organization" of the apraxia of eyelid opening. Another observation was that adequate eye opening could persist even after a suture had to be removed. This phenomenon has not been described previously in the literature. In the case described here, a new suture was implanted in a different position after an appropriate waiting period. The observed phenomenon could be due to the development of filiform scar tissue that, for a limited time, could still give traction on the upper eyelid when the frontalis muscle contracted. This could also be an effect of the remaining sutures if not all had been removed. In this case, the remaining sutures maintain a connection between the upper eyelid and the caudal part of the frontalis muscle.

All patients had preoperative BoNT therapy, but this alone was unable to allow sufficient elevation of the eyelids. The patients rated the treatment results as an improvement, which underscores the positive effect of the operation. It was not possible to discontinue BoNT treatment in any of the patients, since alleviation of the orbicularis oculi muscles spasms appears to be in varying degrees an essential component for optimal results. It is relevant in this context that the BoNT injections during postoperative treatment should not be placed in the caudal portion of the frontalis muscle. This is very important since the strength of the frontalis muscle and the ability to raise the upper eyelid would be reduced if this recommendation were to be ignored. The study by Grivet et al. [14] is of interest in this context. The authors reported that the immediate postoperative improvement of the "Functional Disability Scores" (FDS) was significantly greater in those patients with blepharospasm whose BoNT treatment had been discontinued postoperatively compared to those whose treatment had not been interrupted. But the FDS of the patients with postoperatively continued BoNT injections improved later to the level of the patients without postoperative BoNT treatment. In their analysis, however, the authors did not stratify their patients by subtypes or by surgical method. If such a total absence of spasms of the orbicularis oculi muscle is basically relevant in patients with apraxia of eyelid opening remains undecided. Our data, which show that continuing postoperative BoNT treatment was necessary in all patients, argue against that assumption.

The average subjective improvement ratings of our patients were between 75% and 70%, which is a relatively high level see [3-5]. Roggenkämper and Nüssgens [3,4] observed a stable effect for their patient population as a whole, a result that is similar to the analysis of the follow-up period of our study. But this retrospective study does have some limitations. The results would have been more robust had the improvement of eye opening described by the patients been confirmed by objective measurements. A validated questionnaire and score for the patients' self-assessment with focus on the degree of eye opening would also have been useful. A further study with a greater number of patients would be useful more detailed insights into this rare and complex disease and determine the therapy options.

In summary one can conclude that frontalis suspension surgery using polytetrafluoroethylene (Gore-Tex®) sutures is a minimally invasive and effective option for the treatment of apraxia of eyelid opening in patients with essential blepharospasm. The quality of daily life and general patient satisfaction is improved. The *combination* with *botulinum toxin* injections seems to be of advantage for an optimal treatment outcome.

Competing interests
The authors declare that they have no competing interests.

Authors' contributions
CK treatment of patients, conceived the study, acquisition of data, analysis and interpretation of data. DD treatment of patients, participated in the design of the study, revising manuscript for important intellectual input and content, statistical consultation. SR surgery of the patients, drafting manuscript, revising manuscript for important intellectual input and content. RL conceived the study, surgery of the patients, drafting manuscript, acquisition of data, analysis and interpretation of data. All authors read and approved the final manuscript.

Author details
[1]ENT-Department, University of Göttingen Medical Center, Göttingen, Germany. [2]Department of Neurology, University of Hannover Medical Center, Hannover, Germany. [3]Department of Audiology and Phoniatrics, University of Berlin Medical Center, Berlin, Germany. [4]HNO-Klinik Universitätsmedizin Göttingen, Robert-Koch-Str. 40, 37075 Göttingen, Germany.

Frontalis suspension surgery to treat patients with essential blepharospasm and apraxia of eyelid...

47

References

1. Nüssgens Z, Roggenkämper P: **Long-term treatment of blepharospasm with botulinum toxin type A.** *Ger J Ophthalmol* 1995, **4**:363–367.

2. Czyz CN, Burns JA, Petrie TP, Warkins JR, Cahill KV, Foster JA: **Long-term botulinum toxin treatment of benign essentaila blepharospasm, hemifacial spasm, and Meige syndrome.** *A J Ophthalmol* 2013, **156**:173–177.

3. Roggenkämper P, Nüssgens Z: **Frontalis suspension in the treatment of essential blepharospasm unresponsive to botulinum toxin therapy. First results.** *Ger J Ophthalmol* 1993, **2**:426–428.

4. Roggenkämper P, Nüssgens Z: **Frontalis suspension in the treatment of essential blepharospasm unresponsive to botulinum toxin therapy: long-term results.** *Graefe's Arch Clin Exp Ophthalmol* 1997, **235**:486–489.

5. Wabbels B, Roggenkämper P: **Long-term follow up of patients with frontalis sling operation in the treatment of essentail blepharospasm unresponsive to botulinum toxin therapy.** *Graefe's Arch Clin Exp Ophthalmol* 2007, **245**:45–50.

6. Reichel G, Stenner A, Herrman W: **Palpebrale Variante des Blepharospasmus - Abgrenzung zur Lidöffnungsapraxie und zur Inhibitionsstörung durch synchrone EMG-Ableitungen.** *Akt Neurol* 2009, **36**:60–64.

7. Georgescu D, Vagefi MR, McMullan TFW, McCann JD, Anderson RL: **Upper eyelid myectomy in blepharospasm with associated apraxia of lid opening.** *Am J Ophthalmol* 2008, **145**:541–547.

8. Patil B, Foss AJE: **Upper lid orbicularis muscle strip and sequential brow suspension with autologous fascia lata is benefiacial for selected patients with essential blepharospasm.** *Eye* 2009, **23**:1549–1553.

9. Lemagne JM, Liu C: **Complications of frontalis suspension using polytetrafluoroethylene (Gore-Tex).** *Orbit* 1991, **10**:29–31.

10. Takahashi Y, Leibovitch I, Kakzaki H: **Frontalis suspension surgery in upper eyelid blepharoptosis.** *Open Ophthamology J* 2010, **4**:91–97.

11. Hayashi K, Katori N, Kasai K, Kamisasanuki T, Kokubo K, Ohno-Matsui K: **Comparison of nylon monofilament suture and polytetrafluoroethylene sheet for frontalis suspension surgery in eyes with congenital ptosis.** *Am J ophthalmol* 2013, **155**:654–663.

12. Ben Simon GJ, Macedo AA, Schwarcz RM, Wang DY, McCann JD, Goldberg RA: **Frontalis suspension for upper eyelid ptosis: evaluation of different surgical designs and suture materials.** *Am J Ophthalmol* 2005, **140**:887–885.

13. Wasserman B, Springer DT, Helveston EM: **Comparison of materials used in frontalis suspension surgery.** *Arch Ophthalm* 2001, **118**:687–691.

14. Grivet D, Robert PY, Thuret G, De Feligonde OP, Gain P, Maugery J, Adenis JP: **Assessment of blepharospasm surgery using an improved disability scale: study of 138 patients.** *Ophthal Plast Reconstr Surg* 2005, **21**:230–234.

7

CANDLE SYNDROME: Orofacial manifestations and dental implications

T. Roberts[1][*], L. Stephen[1], C. Scott[2], T. di Pasquale[1], A. Naser-eldin[1], M. Chetty[1], S. Shaik[1], L. Lewandowski[3] and P. Beighton[2]

Abstract

A South African girl with CANDLE Syndrome is reported with emphasis on the orodental features and dental management. Clinical manifestations included short stature, wasting of the soft tissue of the arms and legs, erythematous skin eruptions and a prominent abdomen due to hepatosplenomegaly. Generalized microdontia, confirmed by tooth measurement and osteopenia of her jaws, confirmed by digitalized radiography, were previously undescribed syndromic components. Intellectual impairment posed problems during dental intervention. The carious dental lesions and poor oral hygiene were treated conservatively under local anaesthetic. Prophylactic antibiotics were administered an hour before all procedures.

Due to the nature of her general condition, invasive dental procedures were minimal. Regular follow-ups were scheduled at six monthly intervals. During this period, her overall oral health status had improved markedly.

The CANDLE syndrome is a rare condition with grave complications including immunosuppression and diabetes mellitus. As with many genetic disorders, the dental manifestations are often overshadowed by other more conspicuous and complex syndromic features. Recognition of both the clinical and oral changes that occur in the CANDLE syndrome facilitates accurate diagnosis and appropriate dental management of this potentially lethal condition.

Background

The CANDLE syndrome [MIM256040] is a rare autosomal recessive disorder in which autoinflammatory processes lead to multisystem complications. The acronym "CANDLE" pertains to Chronic Atypical Neutrophilic Dermatosis with Lipodystrophy and Elevated temperature. Other variable features include intellectual disability and short stature. Published reports are scanty and apart from macroglossia [1] no other oro-dental features have been mentioned in the literature.

The CANDLE syndrome, which is classified as a proteasome-associated autoinflammatory syndrome (PRAAS), and known as the Nakajo-Nishimura syndrome (NKJO) was delineated in 1939 by Nakajo, a medical staff member at Tohoku University in Japan. The initial syndromic features included erythematous skin lesions, clubbed fingers, periosteal thickening and cardiac insufficiency [2]. Thereafter, Nishimura et al. [3] expanded the phenotype to include hypertrophic pulmonary osteoarthropathy. Additional phenotypic features which have been reported included prominent eyes, enlarged nose and lips; elongated, broad fingers; gross wasting of the arms and legs, severe joint pains and fever that were alleviated by the use of steroids; muscle atrophy and weakness; mild mental retardation; hepatomegaly; macroglossia; short stature and calcifications of the basal ganglia are other documented syndromic manfestations [1, 4–6].

Garg et al., [7] described a syndrome with similar features to NKJO and coined the term "Joint contractures, Muscular Atrophy, Microcytic anemia, and Panniculitis-induced Lipodystrophy (JMP) syndrome". The main difference between the NKJO and JMP syndromes is the absence of fever in JMP syndrome and the absence of seizures in NKJO [6]. Toretello et al. [8] subsequently proposed the acronym "CANDLE" and drew attention to the fact that affected persons were homozygous for an autosomal recessive gene. In a further significant development, Wang et al. 2014 [9] suggested that the CANDLE syndrome, NakajoNishimura syndrome and JMP syndrome may be clinical variants of the same

* Correspondence: reseachcor@gmail.com
[1]Faculty of Dentistry, University of the Western Cape, Private Bag X08, Mitchell's Plain, 7785 Cape Town, South Africa
Full list of author information is available at the end of the article

genetic disorder reflecting intragenic heterogeneity in the determinant *PSMB8* gene mutations.

In this article, we have documented and reviewed the clinical manifestations in an affected girl with emphasis oro-facial features and dental implications. In this context previously undescribed abnormalities include microdontia, microstomia and diastemata have been documented. These observations will be of practical significance in dentistry.

Case report

A South African girl born in 2001 was seen in 2013 at the age of 12 years at the St Joseph's home for disabled children, Cape Town. She was referred to Tygerberg Dental Hospital for routine dental management.

In early childhood, the affected girl received medical attention for painful progressive panniculitis, myositis and arthritis. A presumptive diagnosis of the CANDLE syndrome had previously been established on a basis of the characteristic phenotypic features of CANDLE syndrome described in medical literature, including typical facial characteristics, marked hepatosplenomegaly, fevers, lymphadenopathy, calcification of her basal ganglia on CT, and episodes of intense inflammation without infectious cause. She also suffered from delayed growth together with pronounced lipodystrophic chondritis, which resulted in a flattened nasal bridge (Fig. 1). She

was severely immunocompromised as a result of immunosuppressant drugs. She also had type II diabetes mellitus, gastric reflux and had a history of tuberculosis during infancy.

Extra-oral examination

At the age of 12 years she had short stature, with broad, thick fingers, wasting of the soft tissue of her arms and legs and an enlarged abdomen due to hepatosplenomegaly. Her facial features were coarse. Diffuse erythematous skin plaques were evident on her arms and limbs. There was no previous history of dental problems but marked oedema was noted around the perioral and nasal area. The mandibular symphyses were prominent and microstomia was present. There was no evidence of jaundice, anemia, cyanosis or clubbing. Cervical lymph nodes were palpable on the right side of the neck.

Intra-oral examination

The oral soft tissues appeared unremarkable but bleeding occurred when probing the gingival margins corresponding to teeth 21, 37 and 47. Generalized spacing of her teeth and a Class III malocclusion (incisal classification) were evident. All teeth showed microdontia and mamelons were present on the incisal surfaces. (Fig. 2). Both first mandibular molars were absent possibly as a consequence of previous extractions.

Special investigations
Laboratory studies

Numerous investigations for autoimmune and infectious diseases had been undertaken. These included Anti-Nuclear antibodies *ANA* (3 consecutive tests), anti-DNA antibodies and other auto-antibodies. She had a normal white blood cell count, mild microcytic anemia, and mild elevation of platelet levels. These investigations all yielded negative results. Inflammatory markers and serum triglycerides were elevated. At times of flare, transient

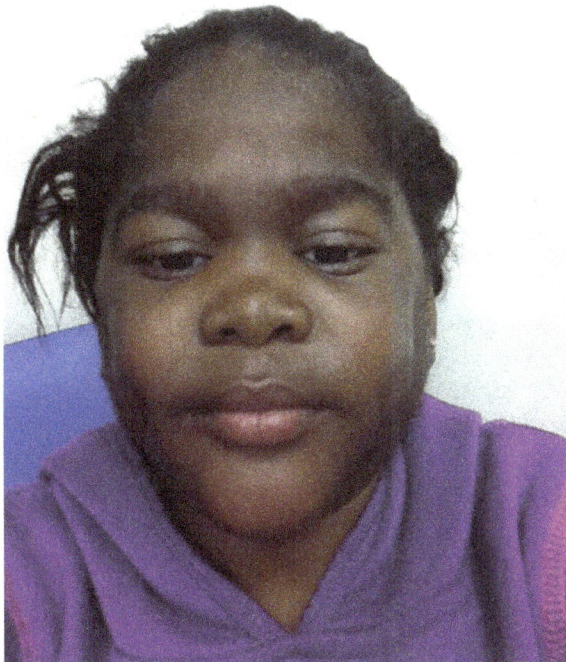

Fig. 1 The affected girl presenting with a flattened nasal bridge

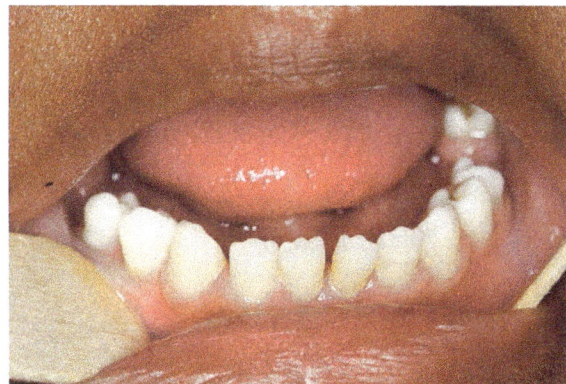

Fig. 2 Generalized microdontia, spacing of teeth and mammelons affecting the permanent dentition

elevation of muscle enzymes CK, AST and ALT had occurred. Her uric acid levels were normal. She had been investigated several times for HIV with negative results, given that these infections are highly prevalent in South Africa. Investigations for infectious disorders included tests for bacterial, viral, parasitic, and fungal infections; all were negative. The syphilis RPR test was non-reactive. Urine studies yielded normal results. Abdominal ultrasonic studies confirmed the presence of hepatosplenomegaly. A CT scan of her brain was undertaken shortly after a seizure, revealing calcifications of her basal ganglia, but no other signs of a mass lesion or inflammation. Histopathological investigations of multiple tissues showed diffuse neutrophilic infiltrates at multiple sites including muscle, liver and skin.

She had significantly increased levels of Interferon gamma (IFN-y).

Dental radiography

A panoramic view (64 kV, 112 mAs) confirmed missing teeth 36 and 46, and revealed caries on teeth 15, 25 and 21. There was generalized spacing of mandibular dentition and an overerupted first maxillary right molar (Fig. 3). The radiologist also noted generalized osteopenia of the mandible. Further investigations were undertaken to confirm the presence of osseous changes and to establish the magnitude of possible osteopenia\osteoporosis. According the WHO, osteopenia is defined as "bone density measurements (T score) between 1 and 2.5 standard deviations below the young adult mean" [10]. To avoid exposing the young patient to further radiation exposure and as the panorex radiograph was already available, the bone mineral density (BMD) was determined by digitalizing and analyzing the dental images. The BMD of the mandible correlates favourably with that found in the lumbar spine and neck of the femur which are the conventional sites of BMD measurements [11, 12]. Both linear and densitometric measurements were obtained using an analytical software package (J Image). The Panoramic Mandibular Index (PMI), Klemmeti Index and Mandibular Cortical Width (MCW) were measured as described by Mansour et al. [13]. The mean pixel intensity that is the amount of the radiolucency or radioopacity of a region on the radiograph on a gray scale from zero (complete radioopacity) to the highest value (complete radiolucency) was determined.

The Klemmeti Index measures the morphology of the mandibular cortex and is conventionally categorized as C1 (normal), C2 (osteopenic), or C3 (osteoporotic).

Since standard values for bone mineral density in children are available, the results were compared to two females of similar age and ethnicity using the same exposure values (Table 1). All results indicate that the BMD of the affected girl was much less than the two girls of same age, gender and ethnicity.

Cone beam tomography (CBCT; 110 kV, 3.46 mAs) was used to ascertain whether additional complications were present. The results of this investigation revealed that the frontal and sphenoidal sinuses were absent. Both maxillary sinuses were hypoplastic, the left side to a greater degree (Fig. 4). Bilateral opacification of the external auditory canals was noted. There was bilateral widening of the diploeic space in the lesser wing of the sphenoid bone and bilateral widening of the diploeic space of the maxilla, the left side being more prominent than the right.

Tooth size analysis

Alginate impressions of both the maxillary and mandibular arches were made and the impressions were immediately poured into a laboratory dental stone. All measurements were taken directly from the unsoaped plaster study models. The teeth measured included the maxillary and mandibular permanent central and lateral incisors, the maxillary and mandibular permanent canines, first and second premolars and the maxillary first molars.

A sliding manual caliper was used to measure the mesiodistal tooth width according to the guidelines defined by Hunter and Priest [14].

The results of the measurements were compared with unpublished data from a report of research conducted in South Africa (unpublished data di Pasquale 2012). All the affected girl's teeth were smaller than the mean of the sample (Table 2). There was a total reduction in the size of 7.47mm in each quadrant in the maxilla and 8.14 mm in each quadrant in the mandible. This is s a clinically important difference and could be considered to be diagnostic of microdontia.

Dental management

The carious lesions and poor oral hygiene were treated conservatively under local anaesthetic. Prophylactic

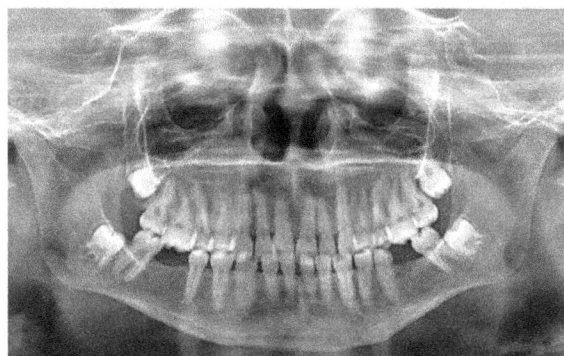

Fig. 3 A panorex image of the jaws showing generalized microdontia

Table 1 Bone mineral density measurements of the girl with Candle syndrome compared with two unaffected females of same age, ethnicity and gender

Densitometric analysis	Affected girl	Control 1	Control 2
Mean PI	78.65	94.2	96.3
Morphometric analysis			
Mandibular cortical width	0.66 mm (mean)	2.08 mm (mean)	2.81 mm (mean)
Klemmeti index	C 3	C 1	C2
Panoramic mandibular Index	Not applicable		

antibiotics were administered an hour before all interventions and due to the nature of her general condition, invasive procedures were .avoided where possible. Regular follow-ups were scheduled at six monthly intervals. During this period, her overall oral health status had improved markedly.

Consent

Written informed consent was obtained from the patient's legal guardian for publication of this case report and any accompanying special investigations and images. A copy of the written consent is available for review by the Editor-in-Chief of this journal.

Discussion

Our approach to the documentation and discussion of the orofacial and dental manifestations of the CANDLE syndrome was constrained by the rarity of the disorder as only approximately 30 cases have been reported in the literature. The strength of our approach is the combination of expertise of the authors, involving different scientific, dental and clinical disciplines.

Pathogenesis

The CANDLE syndrome is caused by homozygosity for mutations in the Proteasome (Prosome, Macropain) Subunit, Beta Type, 8 (PSMB8) gene that encodes for proteasomes that are responsible for the physiological degradation of proteins. Mutations of PSMB8 result in an accumulation of modified and oxidated proteins in cells and tissues, leading to an increase of cellular stress and increased apotosis occurring in muscle and fat [1, 15–17]. Recent developments indicate that not all

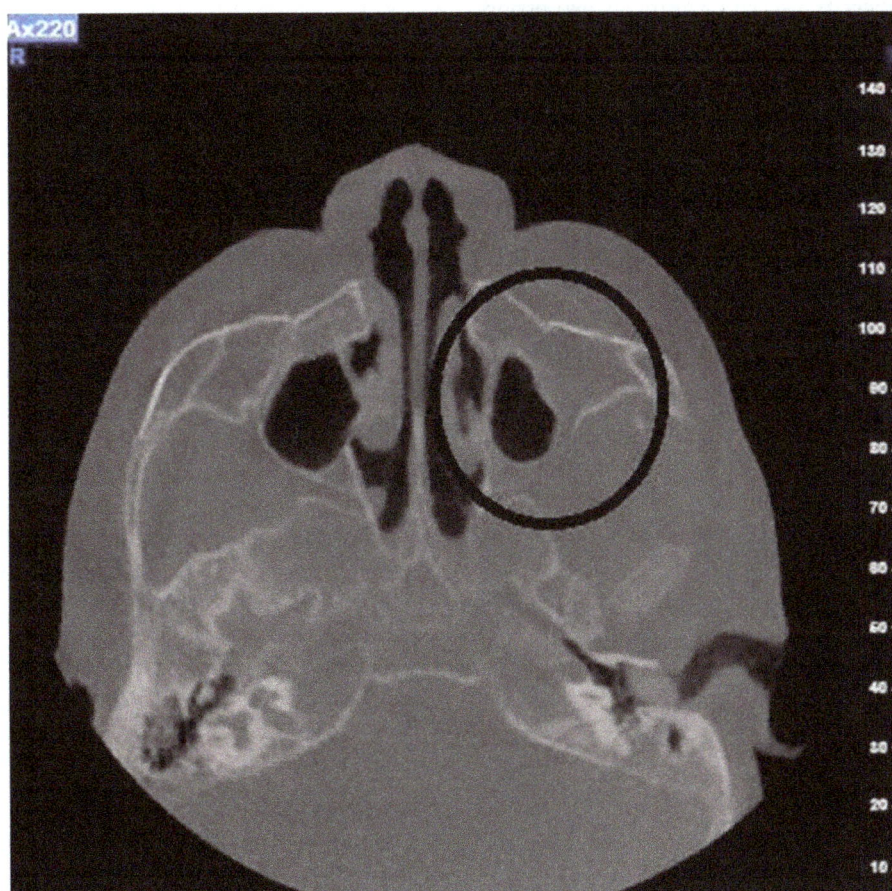

Fig. 4 Cone Beam Tomography showing hypoplasia of both maxillary sinuses

Table 2 Comparison of normal tooth size in black South African females with patient's tooth size

	Unpublished data			Patient's measurements				
Tooth	Mean	Std. deviation	Minimum	Maximum	Right	Left	Mean	Difference
Upper 6	10.50	0.41	9.65	11.15	9.50	10.20	9.85	0.65
Upper 5	6.97	0.38	6.21	7.67	5.50	5.10	5.30	1.67
Upper 4	7.55	0.43	6.70	8.54	6.00	6.50	6.25	1.30
Upper 3	7.88	0.41	6.83	8.74	7.00	7.00	7.00	0.88
Upper 2	7.28	0.53	5.85	8.01	6.20	6.10	6.15	1.13
Upper 1	9.04	0.49	7.80	10.20	6.80	7.60	7.20	1.84
Lower 6	11.47	0.56	10.36	12.77				
Lower 5	7.59	0.44	6.71	8.52	5.00	5.60	5.30	2.29
Lower 4	7.64	0.43	6.85	8.59	6.00	5.90	5.95	1.69
Lower 3	7.10	0.31	6.54	7.86	6.10	6.10	6.10	1.00
Lower 2	6.13	0.33	5.57	6.86	4.90	4.10	4.50	1.63
Lower 1	5.47	0.31	4.72	6.35	3.90	4.00	3.95	1.52

individuals affected by the CANDLE syndrome have *PSMB8* mutations [18]. Brehm et al. 2015 identified 8 mutations in 4 proteasome genes, *PSMA3*, *PSMB4*, *PSMB9*, and proteasome maturation protein (*POMP*), that have not previously been related to the disease. These mutations affect transcription, protein expression, protein folding, proteasome assembly, and, eventually, proteasome activity [19].

Microdontia

Microdontia has previously not been reported in CANDLE syndrome. This developmental abnormality can involve either the primary or permanent dentition and as a component of a few genetic syndromes (Table 3). Microdontia can also occur in non- genetic conditions notably as a complication of radiation or chemotherapeutic treatment [20].

Shafer et al. [21] classified microdontia into three categories viz:

a. True generalized microdontia in which all the teeth are smaller than normal is rare.

Table 3 Microdontia in genetic syndromes

Syndromic conditions	Reference
Gorlin-Chaudhry-Moss syndrome	[28]
William syndrome	[29]
Turner syndrome	[30]
Rothmund-Thomson syndrome	[31, 32]
Seckel syndrome	[33, 34]
Spondyloepiphyseal dysplasia	[35, 36]
Kenny-Caffey Syndrome.	[37]
Coffin-Lowry syndrome	[38]
Microcephalic osteodysplastic primordial dwarfism	[39, 40]

b. Relative generalized microdontia occurs when teeth are normal in size, but appear to be smaller than normal. For example, if the jaws are large and teeth are normal.
c. Microdontia involving a single tooth.

The genetic basis of microdontia

Over 300 genes are implicated in tooth development [22]. Many of these genes regulate ectodermal-mesenchymal interactions in a programmed sequence. In turn, these processes control the shape, number and sizes of teeth. Similar ectodermal-mesenchymal interactions occur throughout the developing fetus and in many instances, involve the same genes. For these reasons, the occurrence of dental anomalies in genetic syndromes could be an indicator of common developmental factors in both dental and other tissues [23].

The relationship between growth and tooth size indicates that repeated ectodermal– mesenchymal interactions occur during the initiation and morphogenesis phases of tooth development. Although epigenetic influences affect the position of tooth forming tissue within the jaw, scheduling of the communicating signals explains differences in tooth size. In this context, no particular gene has been implicated as the primary cause of microdontia.

Although a decrease in bone density is commonly associated with the long-term use of corticosteroids, there is no documented evidence to suggest that steroids influence odontogenesis.

Microstomia

Microstomia refers to a decrease in the size of the opening of the mouth. Although there are no standardized criteria to measure the extent of mouth opening, microstomia affects both function and aesthetics [24]. Microstomia can result in to difficulty in swallowing, speech impairment, deficient oral hygiene and dental caries. In the affected girl, small dimensions of the oral orifice compromised dental management scaling and polishing.

Diastemata

The term refers to increased spacing between teeth and is often caused by loss of interproximal contact between teeth. The most common site of diastemata is in the anterior maxilla between the cuspid teeth [25]. Generalized increase in interdental spacing occurs when there is a disproportionate relationship between the size of the teeth and that of the jaw [26]. Interproximal tooth wear may be a contributing factor. The generalized spacing of the affected girl's teeth was probably the result of the microdontia.

Hypoplastic air sinuses

Hypoplasia of the cranial sinuses was evident on CBCT investigation of the affected girl. Sinuses serve several functions: they decrease the weight of the anterior aspect of the skull, increase the resonance of the voice, have a protective role by dampening pressure (e.g. due to trauma to the face), increase the rigidity of the facial bones and serve to protect structures such as the eyes. They also filter and humidify the air during respiration [27].

Osteopenia

The results of the both densometric and linear measurements suggest that osteopenia was present in the affected girl. It is uncertain however, whether the osteopenia resulted from the long-term use of systemic corticosteroid or whether it is a previously unreported syndromic component. Periodontal disease, decreased alveolar bone density and edentulism are frequent in persons affected by osteoporosis. Fractures of the jaw can result in impaired function, affecting the individual's quality of life.

Dental management considerations in the CANDLE syndrome

The presence of severe immunosuppression that was compounded by diabetes mellitus in the affected girl was a matter of concern. In these circumstances, a multidisciplinary approach was necessary for the provision of dental management. Factors that warranted consideration when planning her dental treatment included diet, blood glucose levels, reduced leukocyte function Decreased integrity of the blood vessels, which is a common complication of diabetes mellitus was also relevant. In addition, immunosuppressive drugs could result in bone marrow suppression and decrease the production of platelets and leukocytes as well as induce osteopenic changes that could predispose to jaw fractures. Together, these factors increase the risk of developing infection,

delayed wound healing and prolonged bleeding times. In these circumstances, the dental management of the affected girl was by conventional procedures with an increased awareness of the risks of possible complications.

Conclusion

The CANDLE syndrome is a rare condition with grave complications including immunosuppression and diabetes mellitus. As with many genetic disorders, the dental manifestations are often overshadowed by other more conspicuous and complex syndromic features. Recognition of both the clinical and oral changes that occur in the CANDLE syndrome facilitates accurate diagnosis and appropriate management of this potentially lethal condition.

All investigations were undertaken with full ethical approval in accordance with the Declaration of Helsinki as updated in the version promulgated in June 2013 and the Singapore Statement on Research Integrity. Ethics approval was received from the University of Cape Town Faculty of Health Sciences Institutional Ethics Committee (no. 203/2013).

Competing interests

The authors declare that they have no competing interests.

Authors' contributions

TR made substantial contributions to examining the patient, acquisition of dental records, conception, drafting and revising the manuscript. LS participated in the design and drafting of the report and assisted in revising it for critical content. CS managed the medical condition of the patient and contributed to the content. Tdi P provided the data on tooth size prediction and also undertook comparative analysis of the tooth sizes. NA assisted in the interpretation of the radiographs, was responsible for the dental management of the patient, took the impressions for orthodontic models and measured the teeth. MC participated in the examination of the patient and revising intellectual content. SS was responsible for the interpretation and writing the reports of the CBCTs and Panorex radiograph. LL undertook the molecular investigations and provided expert guidance during the project and in the compilation of the manuscript. PB contributed significantly to the conception, drafting and revision of the manuscript. He also made considerable contributions to the intellectual content and gave final approval of the version to be published. All authors read and approved the final manuscript.

Acknowledgements

The authors wish to acknowledge the following:
Dr M Kumar, University of the Western Cape, for the analysis of the digital radiographs Financial support was available from the National Research Foundation and the Medical Research Council of South Africa via grants received by Prof Beighton (MRC: 415882 and NRF: 443503).
The content of this article is the sole work of the authors. No benefits of any form have been or are to be received from a commercial party related directly or indirectly to the subject of this article.

Author details

[1]Faculty of Dentistry, University of the Western Cape, Private Bag X08, Mitchell's Plain, 7785 Cape Town, South Africa. [2]Faculty of Health Sciences, University of Cape Town, Observatory, 7925 Cape Town, South Africa. [3]Duke Global Health Institute, Pediatric Rheumatology, Global Health, Duke University Medical Center, Durham, USA.

References

1. Yamada S, Toyoshima I, Mori S, Tsubaki T. Sibling cases with lipodystrophic skin change, muscular atrophy, recurrent skin eruptions, and deformities and contractures of the joints: a possible new clinical entity. Rinsho Shinkeigaku. 1984;24:703–10.

2. Nakajo A. Secondary hypertrophic osteoperiostosis with pernio. J Derm Urol. 1939;45:77–86.

3. Nishimura N, Deki T, Kato S. Hypertrophic pulmonary osteo-arthropathy with pernio-like eruption in the two families: report of the three cases. Jpn J Derm Venereol. 1950;60:136–41.

4. Kitano Y, Matsunaga E, Morimoto T, Okada N, Sano S. A syndrome with nodular erythema, elongated and thickened fingers, and emaciation. Arch Derm. 1985;121:1053–6.

5. Tanaka M, Miyatani N, Yamada S, Miyashita K, Toyoshima I, Sakuma K, et al. Hereditary lipo-muscular atrophy with joint contracture, skin eruptions and hyper-gamma-globulinemia: a new syndrome. Intern Med. 1993;32:42–5.

6. Arima K, Kinoshita A, Mishima H, Kanazawa N, Kaneko T, Mizushima T, et al. Proteasome assembly defect due to a proteasome subunit beta type 8 (PSMB8) mutation causes the autoinflammatory disorder, Nakajo-Nishimura syndrome. Proc Nat Acad Sci. 2011;108:14914–9. doi:10.1073/pnas.1106015108.

7. Garg A, Hernandez MD, Sousa AB, Subramanyam L, Martinez de Villarreal L, dos Santos HG, et al. An autosomal recessive syndrome of joint contractures, muscular atrophy, microcytic anemia, and panniculitis-associated lipodystrophy. J Clin Endocr Metab. 2010;95:E58–63. doi:10.1210/jc.2010-0488.

8. Torrelo A, Patel S, Colmenero I, Gurbindo D, Lendinez F, Hernandez A, et al. Chronic atypical neutrophilic dermatosis with lipodystrophy and elevated temperature (CANDLE) syndrome. J Am Acad Derm. 2010;62:489–95. doi:10.1016/j.jaad.2009.04.046.

9. Wang H, Das L, Tan Hung Tiong J, Vasanwala RF, Arkachaisri T. CANDLE syndrome: an extended clinical spectrum. Rheumatology 2014;53:2120-2122 doi:10.1093/rheumatology/keu297.

10. WHO. WHO scientific group on the assessment of osteoporosis at primary health care level. Geneva: WHO Press; 2004.

11. Klemetti E, Kolmakov S, Heiskanen P, Vainio P, Lassila V. Panoramic mandibular index and bone mineral densities in postmenopausal women. Oral Surg Oral Med Oral. 1993;75:774–9.

12. Devlin H. Identification of the risk for osteoporosis in dental patients. Dent Clin N Am. 2012;56:847–61. doi:10.1016/j.cden.2012.07.010.

13. Mansour S, AlGhamdi AS, Javed F, Marzouk H, Khan EA. Panoramic radiomorphometric indices as reliable parameters in predicting osteoporosis. Am J Med Sci. 2013;346(6):473–8. doi:10.1097/MAJ.0b013e3182972148.

14. Hunter WS, Priest WR. Errors and discrepancies in measurement of tooth size. J Dent Res. 1960;39:405–14.

15. Agarwal AK, Xing C, DeMartino GN, Mizrachi D, Hernandez MD, Sousa AB, et al. PSMB8 encoding the beta-5i proteasome subunit is mutated in joint contractures, muscle atrophy, microcytic anemia, and panniculitis-induced lipodystrophy syndrome. Am J Hum Genet. 2010;87:866–72. doi:10.1016/j.ajhg.2010.10.031.

16. Kitamura A, Maekawa Y, Uehara H, Izumi K, Kawachi I, Nishizawa M, et al. A mutation in the immunoproteasome subunit PSMB8 causes autoinflammation and lipodystrophy in humans. J Clin Invest. 2011;121:4150–60. doi:10.1172/JCI58414.

17. Cavalcante MP, Brunelli JB, Miranda CC, Novak GV, Malle L, Aikawa NE, et al. CANDLE syndrome: chronic atypical neutrophilic dermatosis with lipodystrophy and elevated temperature-a rare case with a novel mutation. Eur J Pediatr. 2015. [Epub ahead of print].

18. Liu Y, Ramot Y, Torrelo A, Paller AS, et al. Mutations in proteasome subunit β type 8 cause chronic atypical neutrophilic dermatosis with lipodystrophy and elevated temperature with evidence of genetic and phenotypic heterogeneity. Arthritis Rheum. 2012;64(3):895–907. doi:10.1002/art.33368.

19. Brehm A, Liu Y, Sheikh A. et. Additive loss-of-function proteasome subunit mutations in CANDLE/PRAAS patients promote type I IFN production. J Clin Invest. 2015;125(11):4196–211. doi:10.1172/JCI81260. Epub 2015 Oct 20.

20. Van der Waal I, Van der Kwast WAM. Developmental anomalies and eruption disturbances and some acquired disorders of the teeth. In: Oral pathology. Chicago: Quintessence Publishing Co Inc; 1988. p. 114.

21. Shafer WG, Hine MK, Levy BM. Develpmental Disturbances of oral and paraoral structures, A Textbook of Oral Pathology. Philadelphia: W. B. Saunders Co; 1983. p. 37.

22. Galluccio G, Castellano M, La Monaca C. Genetic basis of non-syndromic anomalies of human tooth number. Arch Oral Biol. 2012;57(7):918–30. doi:10.1016/j.archoralbio.2012.01.005.

23. Brook AH. Multilevel complex interactions between genetic, epigenetic and environmental factors in the aetiology of anomalies of dental development. Arch Oral Biol. 2009;54 Suppl 1:3–17. doi:10.1016/j.archoralbio.2009.09.005.

24. Garnett MJ, Nohl FS, Barclay SC. Management of patients with reduced oral aperture and mandibular hypomobility (trismus) and implications for operative dentistry. BMJ. 2008;204:125–31. doi:10.1038/bdj.2008.47.

25. Steigman S, Weissberg Y. Spaced dentition. An epidemiologic study. Angle Orthod. 1985;55(2):167–76.

26. Boushell LW. Diastema. J Esthet Restor Dent. 2009;21(3):209–10. doi:10.1111/j.1708-8240.2009.00261.x.

27. Gallup AC, Hack GD. Human paranasal sinuses and selective brain cooling: a ventilation system activated by yawning? Med Hypotheses. 2011;77(6):970–1003. doi:10.1016/j.mehy.2011.08.022.

28. Ippel PF, Gorlin RJ, Lenz W, van Doorne JM, Bijlsma JB. Craniofacial dysostosis, hypertrichosis, genital hypoplasia, ocular, dental, and digital defects: confirmation of the Gorlin-Chaudhry-Moss syndrome. Am J Med Genet. 1992;44(4):518.

29. Poornima P, Patil P, Subbareddy V, Arora G. Dentofacial characteristics in William's syndrome. Contemp Clin Dent. 2012;3 Suppl 1:41–S44. doi:10.4103/0976-237X.95103.

30. Gunther DF, Sybert VP. Lymphatic, tooth and skin manifestations in Turners syndrome. Int Congr Series. 2006;1298:58–62.

31. Haytaç MC, Oztunç H, Mete UO, Kaya M. Rothmund-Thomson syndrome: a case report. Oral Surg Oral Med Oral Pathol Oral Radiol Endod. 2002;94(4):479–84.

32. Canger EM, Celenk P, Devrim I, Avşar A. Oral findings of Rothmund-Thomson syndrome. Case Rep Dent . 2013;2013:935716. doi: 10.1155/2013/935716.

33. Seymen F, Tuna B, Kayserili H. Seckel syndrome: report of a case. J Clin Pediatr Dent. 2002;26(3):305–9.

34. De Coster PJ, Verbeeck RM, Holthaus V, Martens LC, Vral A. Seckel syndrome associated with oligodontia, microdontia, enamel hypoplasia, delayed eruption, and dentin demineralization: a new variant? J Oral Pathol Med. 2006;35(10):639–41.

35. Rajab A, Kunze J, Mundlos S. Spondyloepiphyseal dysplasia Omani type: a new recessive type of SED with progressive spinal involvement. Am J Med Genet A. 2004;126A(4):413–9.

36. Singhal A, Singhal P, Gupta R, Jarial KD. True generalized microdontia and hypodontia with spondyloepiphyseal dysplasia. Case Rep Dent. 2013;2013:685781. doi:10.1155/2013/685781.

37. Moussaid Y, Griffiths D, Richard B, Dieux A, Lemerrer M, Léger J, et al. Oral manifestations of patients with Kenny-Caffey Syndrome. Eur J Med Genet. 2012;55(8–9):441–5. doi:10.1016/j.ejmg.2012.03.005.

38. Norderyd J, Aronsson J. Hypoplastic root cementum and premature loss of primary teeth in Coffin-Lowry syndrome: a case report. Int J Paediatr Dent. 2012;22(2):154–6. doi:10.1111/j.1365-263X.2011.01160.x.

39. Lin HJ, Sue GY, Berkowitz CD, Brasel JA, Lachman RS. Microdontia with severe microcephaly and short stature in two brothers: osteodysplastic primordial dwarfism with dental findings. Am J Med Genet. 1995;58(2):136–42.

40. Kantaputra PN, Tanpaiboon P, Unachak K, Praphanphoj V. Microcephalic osteodysplastic primordial dwarfism with severe microdontia and skin anomalies: confirmation of a new syndrome. Am J Med Genet A. 2004;130A(2):181–90.

8

Accuracy evaluation of CAD/CAM generated splints in orthognathic surgery: a cadaveric study

Thomas Schouman[2], Philippe Rouch[3], Benoît Imholz[1], Jean Fasel[4], Delphine Courvoisier[5] and Paolo Scolozzi[1*]

Abstract

Introduction: To evaluate the accuracy of CAD/CAM generated splints in orthognathic surgery by comparing planned versus actual post-operative 3D images.

Methods: Specific planning software (SimPlant® OMS Standalone 14.0) was used to perform a 3D virtual Le Fort I osteotomy in 10 fresh human cadaver heads. Stereolithographic splints were then generated and used during the surgical procedure to reposition the maxilla according to the planned position. Pre-operative planned and postoperative 3D CT scan images were fused and imported to dedicated software (MATLAB® 7.11.) for calculating the translational and rotational (pitch, roll and yaw) differences between the two 3D images. Geometrical accuracy was estimated using the Root Mean Square Deviations (RMSD) and lower and upper limits of accuracy were computed using the Bland & Altman method, with 95 % confidence intervals around the limits. The accuracy cutoff was set at +/− 2 mm for translational and ≤ 4° for rotational measurements.

Results: Overall accuracy between the two 3D images was within the accuracy cutoff for all values except for the antero-posterior positioning of the maxilla (2.17 mm). The translational and rotational differences due to the splint were all within the accuracy cutoff. However, the width of the limits of agreement (range between lower and upper limits) showed that rotational differences could be particularly large.

Conclusion: This study demonstrated that maxillary repositioning can be accurately approximated and thus predicted by specific computational planning and CAD/CAM generated splints in orthognathic surgery. Further study should focus on the risk factors for inaccurate prediction.

Keywords: Orthognathic surgery, Computer-assisted surgery, CAD/CAM splints

Introduction

Treatment planning in orthognathic surgery is based on a combination of clinical, radiological and plaster casts analyses. These analyses allow for a simulation of the ideal repositioning of the skeletal pieces of the facial skeleton that should be reproduced during the surgery as closely as possible to the simulation. Usually, surgical intermediate and final occlusal acrylic splints made on plaster models mounted on a semi-adjustable articulator, after facebow transfer, are used to reproduce the planning during surgery. This method has numerous and inherent sources of

* Correspondence: paolo.scolozzi@hcuge.ch
[1]Department of Surgery, Service of Maxillofacial and Oral Surgery, University Hospital and Faculty of Medicine, Geneva, Switzerland
Full list of author information is available at the end of the article

non-controllable errors. The succession of manipulations and the multiple stakeholders implied make this handmade planning reliability questionable [1–5]. The accuracy of this method cannot be estimated by making preoperative and postoperative clinico-radiological comparisons. Such comparisons only provide a global approximation of the whole process and do not allow differentiating the errors due to patient registration, model surgery, surgical technique, and method of comparison itself [1–5].

New methods of 3D virtual planning integrating fully digitized clinical and radiological data are now fully efficient and surgical wafers can also be generated from these data, without the need for additional human interference [6–16]. These methods presumably offer the highest accuracy of treatment planning, but the overall accuracy of the planning and of its surgical reproducibility has not yet been quantified. The aim of the present cadaveric study was to evaluate the accuracy of CAD/CAM generated splints in orthognathic surgery.

Materials and methods

To address the research purpose, the authors designed and implemented an experimental study using 10 fresh human cadaver heads for evaluating the accuracy of CAD/CAM stereolithographic surgical splints. The specimens were obtained from the Division of Anatomy of our University after the required authorization was given by the legally responsible person and the study was approved by our hospital ethical board (Study 10–274).

Technical procedure

3D coordinate system and reference points

Nine 1.5 mm diameter titanium monocortical screws (*Synthes®-CH 4436 Oberdorf, Switzerland*) were inserted in each human cadaver head as follows: a) three screws within the skull (one within the nasion and one within the left and right infraorbital rim). These screws were used as points of reference (fiducial markers) to define a three-dimensional coordinate system; b) three screws within the maxilla (one within the maxillary midline underneath the anterior nasal spine and one above the roots of the left and right upper first molars); c) three screws in the mandible (one within the mental midline underneath the lower

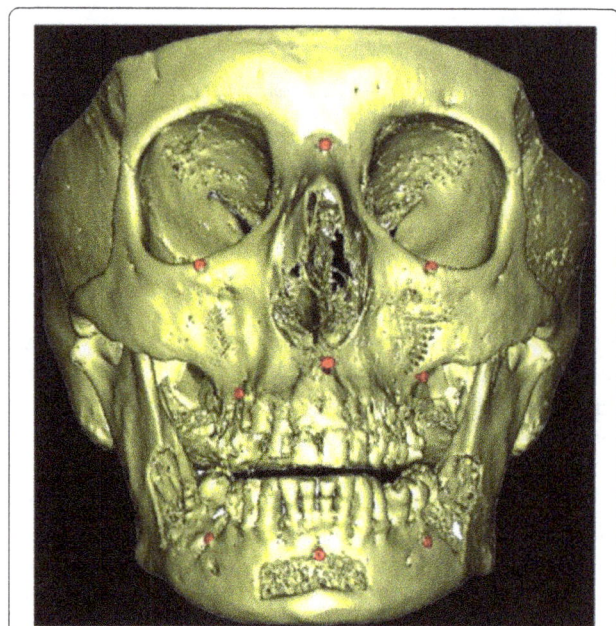

Fig. 1 Frontal 3D CT scan image view showing the nine cortical bone screws (*in red*) placed as references to define a three-dimensional coordinate system (3 in the skull, 3 in the maxilla and 3 in the mandible)

central incisors and one underneath the roots of the lower left and right first molars) (Fig. 1).

Image acquisition

Preoperative imaging was performed with a 64-slice CT scanner (Siemens Sensation 64; Germany: 120 kV; 240 mAS; 2 9 32 detectors; increment, 0.7 mm; collimation, 64 9 0.6; slice thickness, 1 mm; matrix, 512 9 512 pixels; gantry tilt, 0°).

Pre-operative computational image analysis

CT scan images in DICOM (Digital Imaging and Communications in Medicine) format were processed using SimPlant OMS Standalone 14.0 software (SIMPLANT Business Unit, Technologielaan 15, 3001 Leuven, Belgium www.materialisedental.com). The dental casts obtained from alginate dental impressions were scanned using a high-resolution 3D optical scanner (Dental 3D Scanner D-200™, http://www.3shape.com). The dental scan images were then imported to the software and superimposed on the CT scan images by means of a semi-automated 3D surface registration (*Iterative Closest Point registration*). In two partially edentulous cases, the missing teeth were replaced by a prosthesis fixed with bone screws to obtain a stable occlusal platform.

3D virtual surgical planning

The 3D-coordinate system was integrated into the 3D-model with X, Y, and Z axes corresponding respectively to the medio-lateral axis, antero-posterior axis and infero-superior axis. The plane for the virtual Le Fort I osteotomy was first generated (Fig. 2a) and then the 3D maxillary bone was segmented (Fig. 2b). The maxillary digitally osteotomized segment was repositioned to simulate the planned and arbitrarily chosen movements as follows (Fig. 2c):

a) *Maxillary advancement:* 5 mm
b) *Superior maxillary repositioning on the left side:* 4 mm at the pterygo-maxillary and 3 mm at the naso-maxillary buttresses
c) *Inferior maxillary repositioning on the right first side:* 3 mm at the pterygo-maxillary buttress.

The intermediate splint was thus designed according to the new maxillary position as well as specific maxillary cutting guides to reproduce the planned virtual Le Fort I-type osteotomy (Fig. 2d).

CAD/CAM surgical splint

Stereolithographic splints were generated based upon the treatment planning as follows:

The .STL file (*Standard Tesselation Language or Stereolithography format*) of the new maxillo-mandibular relationship was converted into a layer-by-layer contour model.

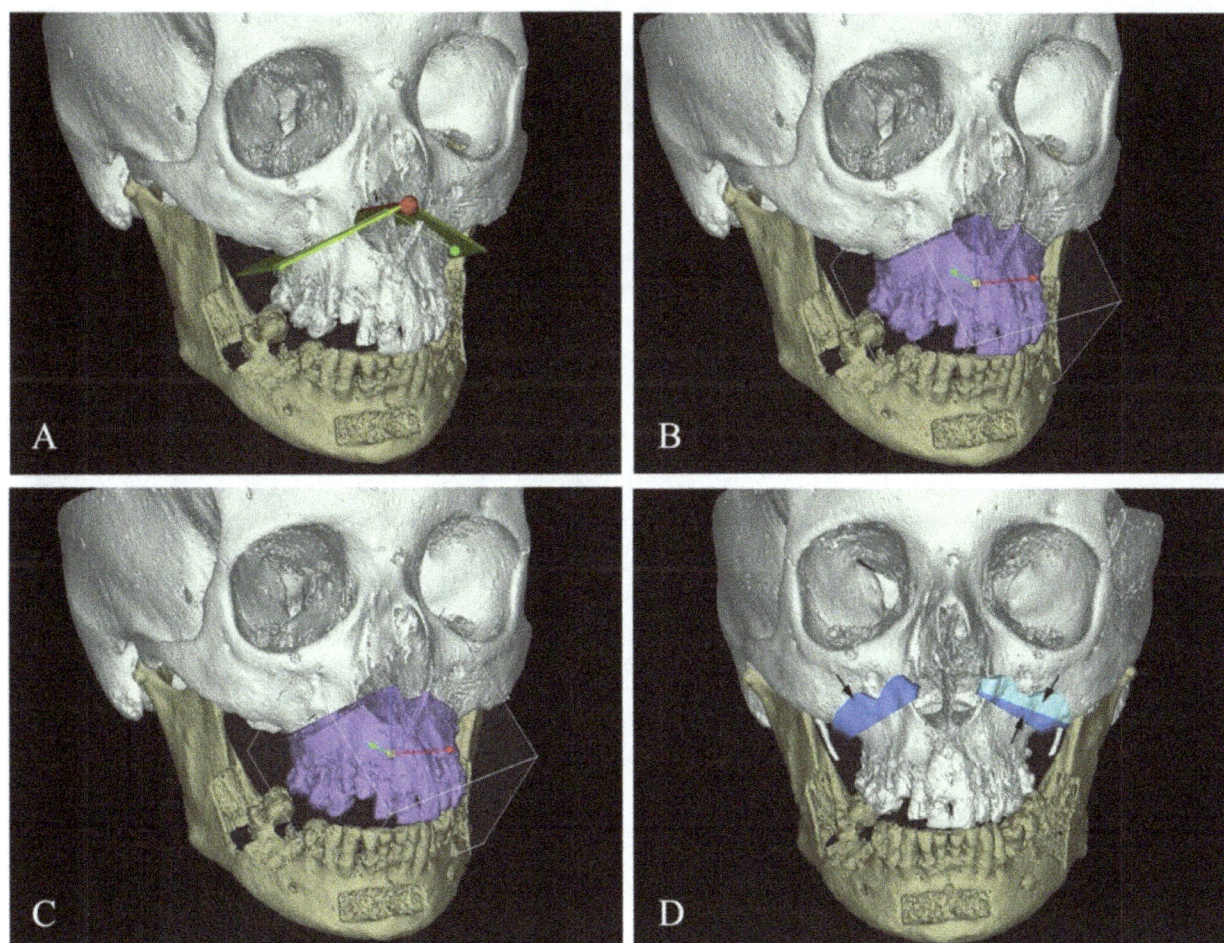

Fig. 2 a Generation of the plane for the virtual maxillary's osteotomy (**b**) Segmentation of 3-D bone segments corresponding to the Le Fort I osteotomy (**c**) Repositioning of the maxillary osteotomized segment according to the planned movements (**d**) Generation of specific maxillary cutting guides to reproduce the planned virtual Le Fort I-type osteotomy (*arrows*)

A new part-specific file was generated to be run on the stereolithographic machine. The splints were then fabricated (3D printing) by using Triad®TranSheet™ material from DentSply (http://www.dentsply.com/en).

Data were used then to create the specific surgical cutting guides (Fig. 3).

Surgical procedure

The surgical procedure has been performed by the same surgeon (T.S). A complete Le Fort I-type osteotomy was performed with a reciprocating saw by using specific maxillary cutting guides. The maxilla was then down fractured. The bone resection on the left side of the maxilla needed for asymmetrical intrusion was carried out according to the measurements made at the internal reference points following the virtual surgical planning. To secure the maxilla in its new position, a maxillo-mandibular fixation (MMF) with the intermediate stereolithographic occlusal splint was performed using peri-zygomatic non-metallic

ligatures posteriorly and a ligature between a screw within the nasion and a screw within the symphysis anteriorly (Fig. 4a–c).

Post-operative computational image analysis

Post-operative CT-scans with the intermediate splint in place were taken using the pre-operative protocol. Planned pre- and post-operative 3D CT scan images were fused by means of an automated surface matching method by using the skull, which was not repositioned by the surgery, as reference for registration (Fig. 5). The differences between the two images were calculated by using MATLAB® 7.11 (R2010b) software (MathWorks 92190 Meudon France http://fr.mathworks.com/products/matlab/) as follows:

1) The three following 3D anatomical regions were defined for the final evaluation: a) skull, b) maxilla, and c) mandible.

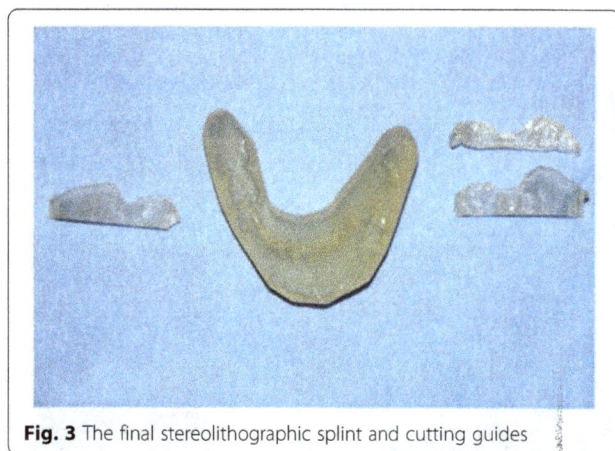

Fig. 3 The final stereolithographic splint and cutting guides

2) The position of three fixed points (screws) within the 3D-coordinate system of the CT scan was determined on the planned pre- (Pt_{plan1} Pt_{plan2} Pt_{plan3})[*1] and post-operative (Pt_{ppop1} Pt_{ppop2} Pt_{ppop3})[*2] 3D CT scan images. [*1] $_{plan:}$ = *planned*; [*2] $_{ppop:}$*post-operative*

3) A landmark (*barycenter*) "rigidly" related to the three fixed points (screws) was then calculated for each anatomical region (skull, maxilla and mandible) in the planned and post-operative images as follows: (XPt_1 XPt_2 XPt_3) (Y_{Pt1} YPt_2 YPt_3) (Z_{Pt1} ZPt_2 ZPt_3) represented the spatial coordinates of the three points (screws) within each anatomical region.

4) The pre- and post-operative barycenters ($Bary_{plan}$ and $Bary_{ppop}$) corresponding to the three anatomical regions (skull, maxilla and mandible), whose axis were collinear to those of the CT scan, were thus taken as references for determining the translational and rotational (pitch, roll and yaw) measurements (Fig. 6).

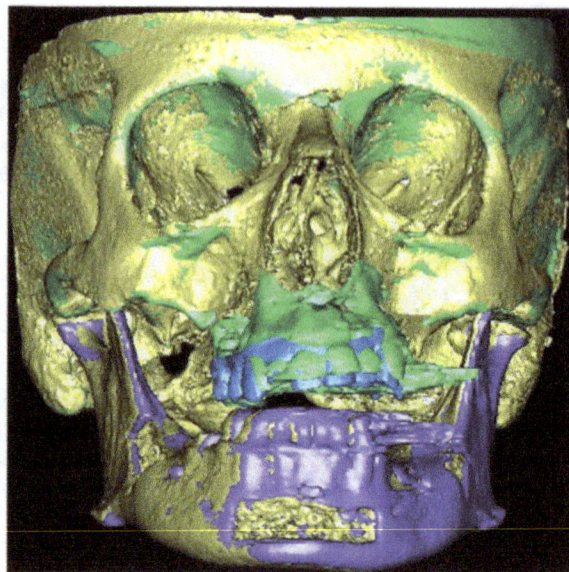

Fig. 5 Planned pre- and post-operative 3D CT scan images fused by means of an automated surface matching method by using the skull, which was not repositioned by the surgery, as reference for registration

5) Three vectors on the planned pre- ($\underline{V}_{plan1};\underline{V}_{plan2};\underline{V}_{plan3}$) and post-operative ($\underline{V}_{ppop1};\underline{V}_{ppop2};\underline{V}_{ppop3}$) were then determined to describe the space of the three anatomical regions (Fig. 7):

6) Finally, the measurements of the translational movements were calculated from the length of the corresponding vector connecting the pre- and post-operative barycenters ($\underline{Mov}$ = $\underline{Bary}_{plan}$ $\underline{Bary}_{ppop}$) whereas the measurements of rotational (pitch, roll and yaw) movements were calculated from the following transfer matrices:

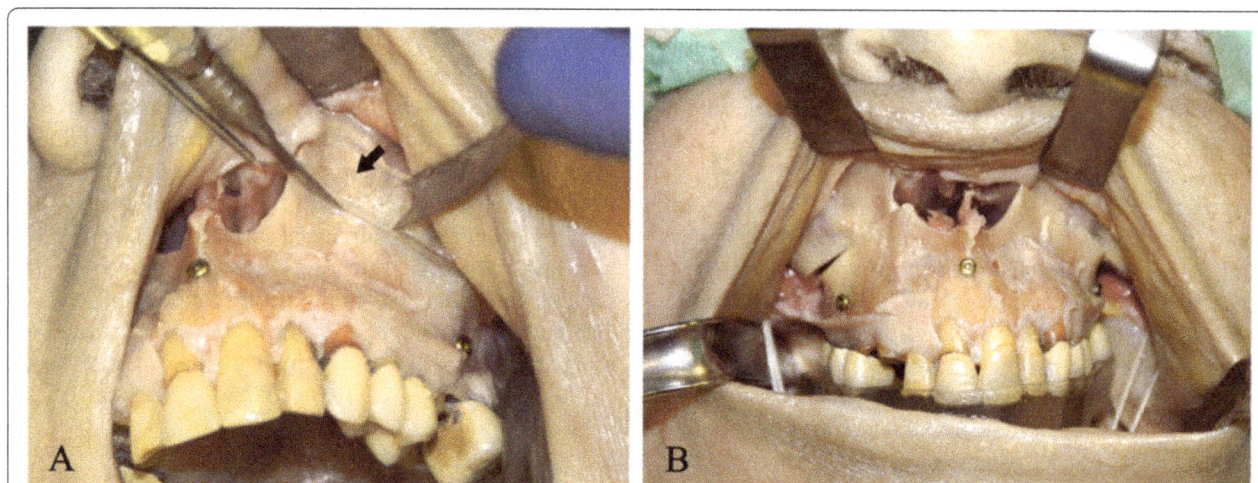

Fig. 4 a Complete Le Fort I-type osteotomy performed with a reciprocating saw by using specific maxillary cutting guides (*black arrow*) (**b**) Maxillo-mandibular repositioning according to the planned movements with the intermediate stereolithographic occlusal splint

$X_{bary} =$	$\dfrac{XPt_{plan1} + XPt_{plan2} + XPt_{plan3}}{3}$	$X_{bary} =$	$\dfrac{XPt_{ppop1} + XPt_{ppop2} + XPt_{ppop3}}{3}$
$Y_{bary} =$	$\dfrac{YPt_{plan1} + YPt_{plan2} + YPt_{plan3}}{3}$	$Y_{bary} =$	$\dfrac{YPt_{ppop1} + YPt_{ppop2} + YPt_{ppop3}}{3}$
$Z_{bary} =$	$\dfrac{ZPt_{plan1} + ZPt_{plan2} + ZPt_{plan3}}{3}$	$Z_{bary} =$	$\dfrac{ZPt_{ppop1} + ZPt_{ppop2} + ZPt_{ppop3}}{3}$

$$\text{pitch} = \arctan\left[\frac{Yppop\ z}{Yppop\ y}\right]$$

$$\text{roll} = \arctan\left[\frac{Yppop\ x}{Yppop\ y}\right]$$

$$\text{yaw} = \arctan\left[\frac{Yppop\ y}{Yppop\ x}\right]$$

7) The difference between the positions of the screws on the pre- versus post-operative images due to the screw's deformation related to the MMF as well as to the skull's manipulations was also calculated for the three anatomical regions and was labeled as the *inter-points distance (IPD)*.

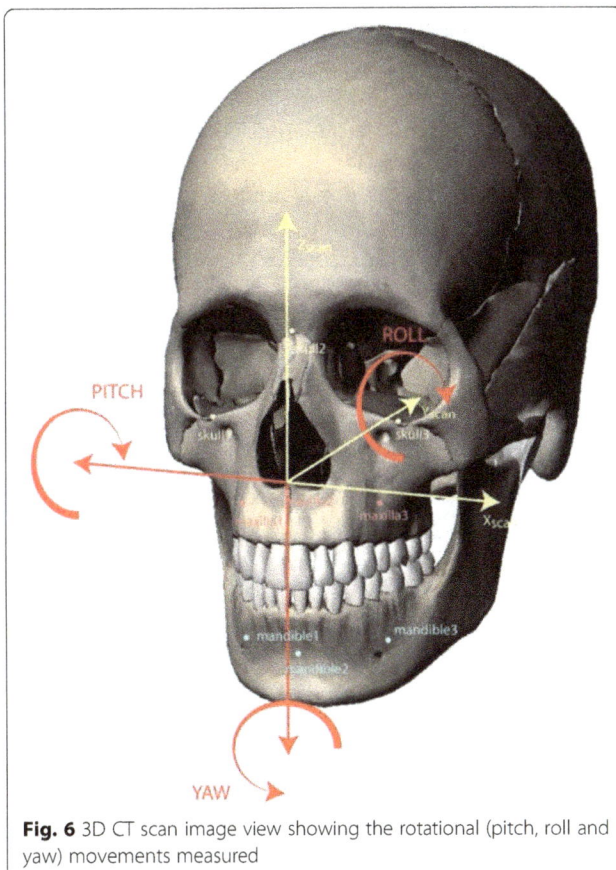

Fig. 6 3D CT scan image view showing the rotational (pitch, roll and yaw) movements measured

Statistical analysis

Data were analyzed using R 3.1.1 statistical software (R Development Core Team, Vienna, Austria). Geometrical accuracy was estimated using Root Mean Square Deviations (RMSD = square root (1/n sum (d²)), which were computed for each axis on the orientation and angle differences for the mandible and the maxilla. In addition, lower and upper limits of accuracy were computed using the Bland & Altman method, with 95 % confidence intervals around the limits. The upper and lower limits l are given by $d \pm 1.96\times$ SD, and the confidence interval around the limits are given by:

$$l\text{-}t\sqrt{\frac{3SD^2}{n}}$$

where $\sqrt{\frac{3SD^2}{n}}$ is the standard error of the limit and t is the critical value for the t distribution (2-tailed at 0.05).

Overall accuracy as a function of each head was estimated by calculating the translational and rotational differences in the three-dimensional coordinate system (x: medio-lateral; y: antero-posterior and z: supero-inferior) between pre- and post-operative skull, maxilla and mandible and represented the imprecision related to the whole procedure (computational, manufacturing and surgical). The differences determined for each cranial region accounted for the accuracy of the computational process used for determining splint accuracy. The differences determined for the mandible resulted from the accuracy of the computational process and the condylar mandibular repositioning error. Finally, the differences determined for the maxilla resulted from the accuracy of the computational process, the condylar mandibular repositioning error plus the intrinsic error related to the splint and could be calculated as follows: MxRE = Md RE + SE*. Thus, the intrinsic error due to the splint could be estimated by calculating the difference in 3D deviations between maxilla and mandible as follows:

SE = MxRE - Md RE * .

According to the literature, a translational difference of less than 2 mm and an orientation difference of less than 4° were considered to be good accuracy [16–18].

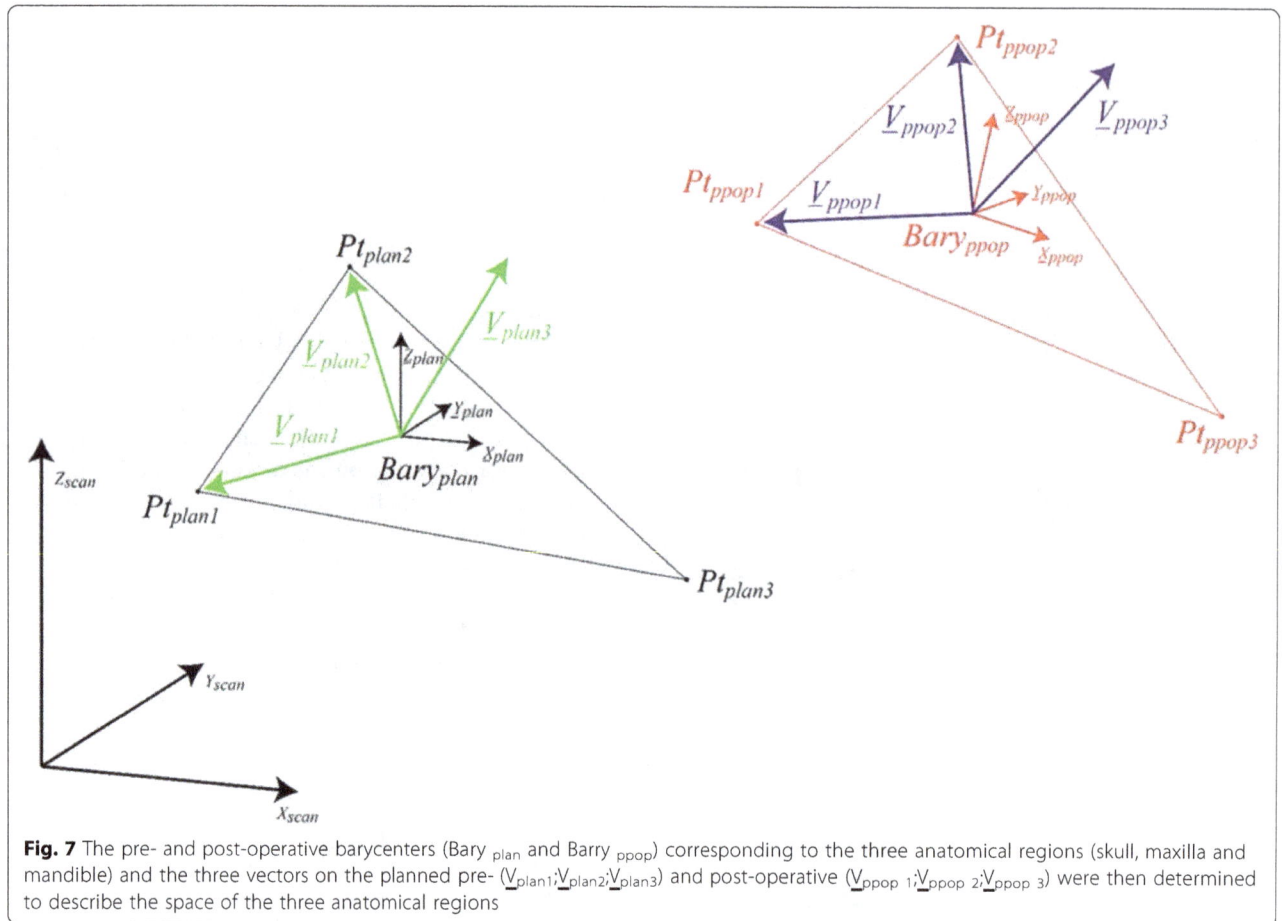

Fig. 7 The pre- and post-operative barycenters (Bary $_{plan}$ and Barry $_{ppop}$) corresponding to the three anatomical regions (skull, maxilla and mandible) and the three vectors on the planned pre- (V$_{plan1}$;V$_{plan2}$;V$_{plan3}$) and post-operative (V$_{ppop\ 1}$;V$_{ppop\ 2}$;V$_{ppop\ 3}$) were then determined to describe the space of the three anatomical regions

Finally, the RMSD of the *inter-points (IPD)* was calculated and compared to the overall RMSD.

MxRE: Maxillary repositioning error, MdRE: Mandibular repositioning error, SRE: Splint error

Results

The 3D translational and rotational differences measured between planned and post-operative cranial region demonstrated good accuracy of the whole imaging computational process ranging from 0.00 to 0.20 mm for translational and 0.10° to 0.67° for rotational movements. The 3D translational and rotational differences measured between planned and post-operative mandible and maxilla were found to be within the permitted accuracy cutoff except for the antero-posterior positioning of the maxilla, which was slightly beyond this limit (2.17 mm) (Table 1). However, the Bland & Altman method showed a greater variability of the extreme values with the lower limits of the translational differences exceeding 2 mm in the medio-lateral axis for both the mandible and the maxilla. Conversely, the upper limits were all beyond the admitted values except in the supero-inferior axis for the maxilla (Table 2). With respect to rotational differences, the lower limits were all within 4° for the mandible and for roll and yaw for the maxilla. The upper limits were

$\underline{V}_{plan1} = \underline{Bary}_{plan}\underline{Pt}_{plan1}$ $\underline{V}_{ppop1} = \underline{Bary}_{ppop1}\underline{Pt}_{ppop1}$

$\underline{V}_{plan2} = \underline{Bary}_{plan}\underline{Pt}_{plan2}$ $\underline{V}_{ppop\ 2} = \underline{Bary}_{ppop2}\underline{Pt}_{ppop2}$

$\underline{V}_{plan3} = \underline{Bary}_{plan}\underline{Pt}_{plan3}$ $\underline{V}_{ppop\ 3} = \underline{Bary}_{ppop3}\underline{Pt}_{ppop3}$

Table 1 Overall accuracy (*Root Mean Square Deviation*) of 3D translational and rotational differences between the planned and post-operative images

	Translational difference		Rotational difference	
Skull	Mediolateral	0.05	Pitch	0.67
	Anteroposterior	0.17	Roll	0.31
	Superoinferior	0.20	Yaw	0.10
Mandible	Mediolateral	2.00	Pitch	1.03
	Anteroposterior	1.69	Roll	0.63
	Superoinferior	1.23	Yaw	1.09
Maxilla	Mediolateral	1.55	Pitch	3.70
	Anteroposterior	2.17	Roll	2.06
	Superoinferior	0.81	Yaw	0.93

Table 2 Overall accuracy (*Bland-Altman upper and lower limits*) of 3D translational and rotational differences between the planned and post-operative images

		Translational difference (95 % CI)			Rotational difference (95 % CI)		
		Lower limit	Upper limit		Lower limit	Upper limit
Skull	Mediolateral	−0.08 (−0.14 to −0.02)	0.11 (0.05 to 0.17)	Pitch	−1.52 (−2.25 to −0.79)	0.83 (0.10 to 1.56)
	Anteroposterior	−0.39 (−0.61 to −0.18)	0.29 (0.08 to 0.51)	Roll	−0.65 (−1.05 to −0.25)	0.64 (0.24 to 1.04)
	Superoinferior	−0.33 (−0.58 to −0.08)	0.46 (0.21 to 0.71)	Yaw	−0.22 (−0.34 to −0.10)	0.17 (0.05 to 0.29)
Mandible	Mediolateral	−3.21 (−5.63 to −0.79)	4.56 (2.14 to 6.98)	Pitch	−2.17 (−3.50 to −0.84)	2.09 (0.77 to 3.42)
	Anteroposterior	−1.82 (−3.57 to −0.07)	3.81 (2.06 to 5.56)	Roll	−1.16 (−1.95 to −0.37)	1.38 (0.59 to 2.18)
	Superoinferior	−1.42 (−2.73 to −0.10)	2.80 (1.49 to 4.11)	Yaw	−1.35 (−2.54 to −0.15)	2.49 (1.30 to 3.69)
Maxilla	Mediolateral	−2.67 (−4.59 to −0.75)	3.50 (1.58 to 5.42)	Pitch	−5.46 (−9.81 to −1.12)	8.49 (4.15 to 12.84)
	Anteroposterior	−1.84 (−3.90 to 0.22)	4.77 (2.71 to 6.83)	Roll	−2.76 (−5.09 to −0.44)	4.72 (2.39 to 7.04)
	Superoinferior	−1.55 (−2.58 to −0.51)	1.78 (0.74 to 2.81)	Yaw	−1.92 (−3.11 to −0.72)	1.92 (0.73 to 3.12)

all within 4° for the mandible and only for yaw for the maxilla.

Compared to this overall accuracy, the translational and rotational differences due only to the splint were lower and were all within the accuracy cutoff (Table 3). Nevertheless, the width of the limits of agreement (range between lower and upper limits) showed that rotational differences could be particularly large (Table 4).

The translational difference due to screw deformation was higher for the mandible than for the skull or the maxilla and represented a relatively large source of error since it varied from 25.5 % (medio-lateral axis of the mandible: 0.51/2.00) to 66.9 % (antero-posterior axis of the mandible, 1.13/1.69) (Table 5).

Discussion

The aim of this cadaveric study was to evaluate the accuracy of computer-assisted design and manufacturing (CAD/CAM) generated splints used for maxillary repositioning during a Le Fort I osteotomy. Our results provide the following considerations. First, the accuracy related to the imaging process evaluated by the differences between pre- and post-operative translational and rotational movements as measured on the only structure that was not repositioned during the surgery such as the skull was found to be excellent. The calculation of the accuracy was directly influenced by: a) the imaging acquisition error related to the multi-slice CT scan used (CT-Sensation 64 = within 0.3 mm); b) the intrinsic

Table 3 Splint accuracy (*Root Mean Square Deviation*) of 3D translational and rotational differences between the planned and post-operative images

Translational difference		Rotational difference	
Mediolateral	1.18	Pitch	1.03
Anteroposterior	1.63	Roll	0.63
Superoinferior	1.03	Yaw	1.09

software error related to the procedure of 3D segmentation and fusion between planned pre-operative and post-operative CT scan images. This step was made by powerful algorithms that allowed for a very rapid automated calculation. The precision rate of the surgical planning software used in the present study as given by the manufacturers was within 1 mm; c) the technical error in determining the position of the screws within the CT images for measurement calculation; d) the human errors that may potentially occur at every step of either the computer planning or the surgical procedure cannot be ignored although it is very difficult to quantify them; e) the whole procedure of the accuracy assessment itself. Second, maxillary repositioning was found to be accurate according to the standard permitted by several researchers who have set the accuracy cutoff for translational movements at 2 mm considering that differences that are not larger than 2 mm may not likely be noticeable to the naked eye or even be perceived by patients and 4° for the rotational movements of the occlusal plane [16–18]. Conversely, other investigated have reported the accuracy between the actual and planned facial landmark measurements permitted for clinical use to be within 0.5 mm [19]. To the best of our knowledge, there is no consensus on the tolerable margin of error for a specific technique to be considered accurate. Moreover, it should also be pointed out that using mean difference resulted in an overly optimistic accuracy assessment since positive and negative differences cancel each other. In fact, when using the Bland & Altman method to establish the lower and upper limits of accuracy with 95 % confidence intervals around these limits, the results showed greater variability and thus showcased a lower overall accuracy. Thus, the differences measured for the maxilla quantify the error related to the surgical procedure as well as the error related to the splints. No doubt this was the most important information, since this is finally what is

Table 4 Splint accuracy (*Bland-Altman upper and lower limits*) of 3D translational and rotational differences between the planned and post-operative images

Translational difference (95 % CI)			Rotational difference (95 % CI)		
	Lower limit	Upper limit		Lower limit	Upper limit
Mediolateral	−2.71 (−4.12 to −1.30)	1.83 (0.41 to 3.24)	Pitch	−9.33 (−14.16 to −4.49)	6.22 (1.38 to 11.06)
Anteroposterior	−2.23 (−4.09 to −0.37)	3.74 (1.88 to 5.60)	Roll	−4.60 (−6.92 to −2.27)	2.87 (0.54 to 5.19)
Superoinferior	−1.63 (−2.87 to −0.39)	2.35 (1.11 to 3.59)	Yaw	−1.51 (−2.81 to −0.22)	2.65 (1.35 to 3.94)

obtained when applying such a surgical procedure onto the patient. The calculation of this accuracy was determined by: a) the difference of the condylar repositioning in the centric relation between the planned and the actual post-operative images; b) the error of the 3D optical scans used for registering the dental models; c) the error of the registration process of the digital models after 3D optical scanning within the CT images; and d) the error of the manufacturing process of the splint.

Third, the main part of the differences between the post-operative and planned position of the maxilla was due to a difference in mandibular position and not due to inaccuracies of the splint itself (e.g., splint design, fit of splint onto teeth, positioning of the splint onto teeth). In fact, by calculating the difference between the maxillary and mandibular deviations, we obtained the true error related to the splint, which was less than 2 mm, thus confirming an acceptable accuracy of the digital splints. These results were confirmed by a re-analysis matching post-operative onto pre-operative planning scan images of the mandible and not onto the pre-operative planning scan images of the skull. By doing so, the deviations between planned and post-operative images of the maxilla were only related to the splint itself and thus to the above-mentioned sources of errors related to the manufacturing process. In fact, with this analysis, the surgical errors due to the difference in condylar positioning between planning and

Table 5 RMSD to estimate inaccuracy due to screw deformation

	Distance	
Skull	Mediolateral	0.14
	Anteroposterior	0.22
	Superoinferior	0.18
Mandible	Mediolateral	0.51
	Anteroposterior	1.13
	Superoinferior	0.40
Maxilla	Mediolateral	0.24
	Anteroposterior	0.17
	Superoinferior	0.20

surgery could be excluded and were thus not taken into account in the final calculation.

The CAD/CAM splints have been described in the literature as the most accurate and reliable method for orthognathic treatment, especially for asymmetrical cases [6–16]. Previous clinical studies on the CAD/CAM splints have highlighted several factors that could potentially have a non negligible impact on the overall accuracy measurement. These include the osteosynthesis procedure that may influence the final position of the maxilla, the image's metal artifacts related to the plates, which can cause aberrant values that are difficult to take into account during the registration and fusion process, the errors related to the virtual mandibular autorotation necessary to obtain a centric relation in cases where the postoperative CT-scan has been taken with the patient's mouth open, the timing of post-operative imaging that could also influence the results as the bone segments may suffer some slight displacements and remodeling under muscular loading [16]. In our study, the mobilized maxillo-mandibular complex was locked into the splint and secured to the skull base with non-metallic bone wiring and the post-operative CT scan was taken a few days after the surgery.

Hsu et al. concluded that a combination of the computer-aided surgical simulation and the CAD/CAM splint resulted in excellent positional and orientation accuracy for the maxilla and mandible and excellent accuracy for the maxillary dental-midline position [16]. In this multicenter clinical study, the authors measured linear and angular deviations between the centroids of mobilized bone segments using dental landmarks. Similar to our study, the authors reported large differences (>4 mm) between planned and actual outcomes in some cases. The authors stated that this was due to failure to capture centric relation of the mandibular condyle. Our results were similar and showed that CAD/CAM splints were reliable for replicating the 3D virtually planned maxillo-mandibular relation and that the error related to the surgical mandibular repositioning was predominant [16]. As long as the maxillary repositioning remains rigidly tied to the mandible via a splint, the maxillary repositioning's accuracy will always be dependent on the mandibular repositioning during surgery. For this reason, the unsolved difficulty of reproducing the planned centric relation of the condyles has always played a major role in limiting the potential benefit of 3D-virtual planning and CAD-CAM splints.

The present study has demonstrated that digital CAD/CAM splints resulted in acceptable accuracy with respect to the capacity of reproducing the planned maxillo-mandibular repositioning. However the inaccuracy in the maxilla-mandibular repositioning was mainly related to the difference in the condylar post-operative repositioning compared to the pre-operative position and negligibly to the splint itself.

Competing interests
The authors declare that they have no competing interests.

Authors' contributions
TS carried out the technical procedure and drafted the manuscript. PR carried out the computer analysis. BI has participated in acquisition of data and carried out the technical procedure. JF provided the cadaveric specimens and the technical infrastructure. DC participated in the design of the study and performed the statistical analysis. PS conceived of the study, and participated in its design and coordination. All authors read and approved the final manuscript.

Acknowledgements
The authors wish to thank Veerle Pattijn, MSc Eng, PhD (Application Engineering Manager Materialise Dental Leuven, Belgium - Veerle.Pattijn@materialise.be for the computational assistance.

Author details
[1]Department of Surgery, Service of Maxillofacial and Oral Surgery, University Hospital and Faculty of Medicine, Geneva, Switzerland. [2]Hôpital Pitié-Salpêtrière, Service de Chirurgie Maxillofaciale et Stomatologie, UPMC Université Paris, Paris, France. [3]Arts et Métiers ParisTech, LBM, 151, Boulevard de l'hôpital, Paris, France. [4]Department of Anatomy, Faculty of Medicine - University of Geneva, Geneva, Switzerland. [5]CRC & Division of Clinical Epidemiology, Department of Health and Community Medicine, University of Geneva & University Hospitals of Geneva, Geneva, Switzerland.

References
1. Olszewski R, Reychler H. Limitations of orthognathic model surgery: theoretical and practical implications. Rev Stomatol Chir Maxillofac. 2004;105:165–9.
2. Gil JN, Claus JD, Manfro R, Lima Jr SM. Predictability of maxillary repositioning during bimaxillary surgery: accuracy of a new technique. Int J Oral Maxillofac Surg. 2007;36:296–300.
3. Schneider M, Tzscharnke O, Pilling E, Lauer G, Eckelt U. Comparison of the predicted surgical results following virtual planning with those actually achieved following bimaxillary operation of dysgnathia. J Craniomaxillofac Surg. 2005;33:8–12.
4. Xia JJ, Shevchenko L, Gateno J, Teichgraeber JF, Taylor TD, Lasky RE, et al. Outcome study of computer-aided surgical simulation in the treatment of patients with craniomaxillofacial deformities. J Oral Maxillofac Surg. 2011;69:2014–24.
5. Bouchard C, Landry PE. Precision of maxillary repositioning during orthognathic surgery: a prospective study. Int J Oral Maxillofac Surg. 2013;42:592–6.
6. Gateno J, Xia J, Teichgraeber JF, Rosen A, Hultgren B, Vadnais T. The precision of computer-generated surgical splints. J Oral Maxillofac Surg. 2003;61:814–7.
7. Mischkowski RA, Zinser MJ, Kübler AC, Krug B, Seifert U, Zöller JE. Application of an augmented reality tool for maxillary positioning in orthognathic surgery - a feasibility study. J Craniomaxillofac Surg. 2006;34:478–83.
8. Metzger MC, Hohlweg-Majert B, Schwarz U, Teschner M, Hammer B, Schmelzeisen R. Manufacturing splints for orthognathic surgery using a three-dimensional printer. Oral Surg Oral Med Oral Pathol Oral Radiol Endod. 2008;105:e1–7.
9. Swennen GRJ, Mollemans W, Schutyser F. Three-dimensional treatment planning of orthognathic surgery in the era of virtual imaging. J Oral Maxillofac Surg. 2009;67:2080–92.
10. Xia JJ, Gateno J, Teichgraeber JF. New clinical protocol to evaluate craniomaxillofacial deformity and plan surgical correction. J Oral Maxillofac Surg. 2009;67:2093–106.
11. Bai S, Bo B, Bi Y, Wang B, Zhao J, Liu YF, et al. CAD/CAM surface templates as an alternative to the intermediate wafer in orthognathic surgery. Oral Surg Oral Med Oral Pathol Oral Radiol Endod. 2010;110:e1–7.
12. Aboul-Hosn Centenero S, Hernandez-Alfaro F. 3D planning in orthognathic surgery: CAD/CAM surgical splints and prediction of the soft and hard tissues results - our experience in 16 cases. J Craniomaxillofac Surg. 2012;40:162–8.
13. Bai S, Shang H, Liu Y, Zhao J, Zhao Y. Computer-aided design and computer-aided manufacturing locating guides accompanied with prebent titanium plates in orthognathic surgery. J Oral Maxillofac Surg. 2012;70:2419–26.
14. Zinser MJ, Mischkowski RA, Sailer HF, Zoller JE. Computer-assisted orthognathic surgery: feasibility study using multiple CAD/CAM surgical splints. Oral Surg Oral Med Oral Pathol Oral Radiol. 2012;113:673–87.
15. Polley JW, Figueroa AA. Orthognathic positioning system: intraoperative system to transfer virtual surgical plan to operating field during orthognathic surgery. J Oral Maxillofac Surg. 2013;71:911–20.
16. Hsu SS, Gateno J, Bell RB, Hirsch DL, Markiewicz MR, Teichgraeber JF, et al. Accuracy of a computer-aided surgical simulation protocol for orthognathic surgery: a prospective multicenter study. J Oral Maxillofac Surg. 2013;71:128–42.
17. Padwa BL, Kaiser MO, Kaban LB. Occlusal cant in the frontal plane as a reflection of facial asymmetry. J Oral Maxillofac Surg. 1997;55:811–6.
18. Kaipatur N, Al-Thomali Y, Flores-Mir C. Accuracy of computer programs in predicting orthognathic surgery hard tissue response. J Oral Maxillofac Surg. 2009;67:1628–39.
19. Schendel SA, Jacobson R, Khalessi S. 3-dimensional facial simulation in orthognathic surgery: is it accurate? J Oral Maxillofac Surg. 2013;71:1406–14.

9

Correlation between preoperative predictions and surgical findings in the parotid surgery for tumors

Michael Vaiman[1*], Judith Luckman[2], Tal Sigal[3] and Inessa Bekerman[3]

Abstract

Background: To compare preoperative CT/MRI based predictions with real surgical findings for deep lobe parotid gland surgery.

Methods: The study analyzed 122 parotidectomies (2004–2014) for benign tumor removal. The facial nerve, the Utrecht line, the Conn's arc, and the retromandibular vein were used as landmarks for CT/MRI presurgical evaluation of patients. We assessed 106 CT images and 86 MRI images. The study compared preoperative evaluation of tumor location with its actual location that was revealed during the operation and assessed the importance of the landmarks.

Results: In general, the agreement between preoperative CT prediction and actual location of the parotid tumors was achieved in 88.7 % ($n = 94/106$) when facial nerve line was used as a landmark. However, out of 14 tumors in the deep lobe only 5 were located correctly (35.7 %). Of the other existing CT landmarks, none showed more precision over others. The agreement between MRI based prediction and surgical results on actual location of the tumor was achieved in 94.2 %. Out of 12 MRI-investigated tumors in the deep lobe nine were located correctly that gives 75 % agreement with surgical results.

Conclusion: Our data suggests that no existing CT landmark can be accepted as completely reliable in cases when selective deep lobe parotidectomy is planned. If tumor location is suspected in the deep lobe of the gland, MRI imaging is necessary to confirm the diagnosis. An operating surgeon should be prepared that in some cases the true location of the tumor would be revealed only during surgery.

Keywords: Parotidectomy, Parotid tumors, CT, MRI, Deep lobe parotidectomy

Background

The precise identification of location of benign tumors of the parotid gland in the superficial or deep lobes can help to avoid total parotidectomy. In addition to gland preservation, in cases when only the deep lobe is affected selective parotidectomy can help to preserve the facial nerve, avoid Frey's syndrome (gustatory sweating), and provide better aesthetic/cosmetic results.

Various landmarks were used in computed tomography (CT) and magnetic resonance imaging (MRI) investigations for precise localization of the tumor and of the facial nerve. Among these landmarks, the facial nerve line (FNL) is the line between the lateral surface of the posterior belly of *m. digastricus* and the lateral surface of the cortex of the ramus part of the mandible [1, 2]. The Utrecht line (UL) runs from the most dorsal point of the ipsilateral half of the first vertebra to the most dorsal point of the retromandibular vein [3, 4]. The Conn's arc (CA) is a 8.5 mm radius semicircle with the center on the most distant point of the posterior edge of the ramus [1, 5]. In addition to these lines, the retromandibular vein (RV), the styloid process, the lateral border of the masseter, the lateral border of the mandible, and the Stensen's duct were used as landmarks also [3, 6, 7]. Definitely some disagreement exists on the question which landmark or line is the most reliable for preoperative diagnostics. While some authors

* Correspondence: vaimed@yahoo.com
[1]Department of Otolaryngology – Head and Neck Surgery, Assaf Harofe Medical Center, Affiliated to Sackler Faculty of Medicine, Tel Aviv University, Zerifin, Israel
Full list of author information is available at the end of the article

name FNL as the most reliable landmark [2, 3], the other suggest UL [1] or the Stensen's duct [6]. These landmarks are presented at the Fig. 1a-d.

To answer this question, we compared preoperative CT/MRI based predictions with real surgical findings for parotid gland surgery.

Methods
Study design and setting
The retrospective study analyzed 122 surgical operations (2004–2014) for different types of partial parotidectomy.

The study compared preoperative evaluation of tumor location with its actual location that was revealed during the operation and assessed the importance of the landmarks. The study protocol conformed to the ethical guidelines of the 1975 Declaration of Helsinki (amended 2000) as reflected a priori after approval by the institution's Helsinki committee.

The *inclusion criteria* were as follows. All selected patients had primary benign parotid tumors. From 2004 to 2014, 142 parotidectomies were performed to remove benign tumors. Of them, CT or CT + MRI were performed

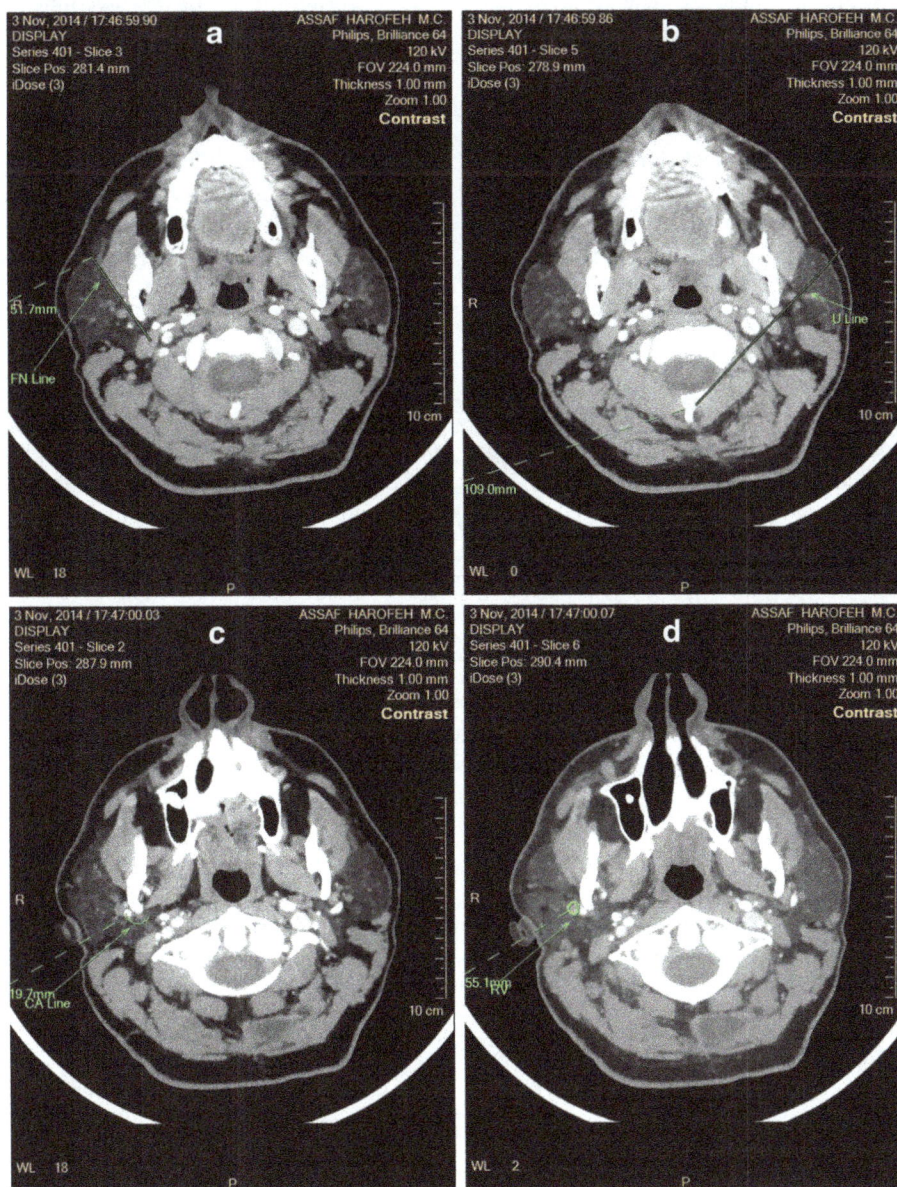

Fig. 1 a The facial nerve line (FNL) is the line between the lateral surface of the posterior belly of *m. digastricus* and the lateral surface of the cortex of the ramus part of the mandible as seen at CT scan image. **b** The Utrecht line (UL) runs from the most dorsal point of the ipsilateral half of the first vertebra to the most dorsal point of the retromandibular vein as seen at CT scan image. **c** The Conn's arc (CA) is a 8.5 mm radius semicircle with the center on the most distant point of the posterior edge of the ramus as seen at CT scan image. **d** The retromandibular vein line (RV) as seen at CT scan image

for 122 patients and in 20 cases clinical picture, ultrasonography and FNAB was enough to confirm the diagnosis. These 122 cases were selected for analysis. We analysed data that was obtained by the operating surgeons before the surgery and compared preoperative CT/MRI based predictions with real surgical findings for parotid gland surgery. The cases with malignant tumors were excluded from the analysis because total parotidectomies were performed disregarding the location of the tumor.

Data sources and measurements

All the CT scans were obtained by the 256-slice CT scanner (Brilliance iCT, Philips Healthcare, The Netherlands) with NanoPanel 3D spherical detectors in axial (transverse) plane that were used further for reconstruction of coronal (frontal) and sagittal planes (spine window, middle third; window parameters: WW 60, WL 360, accuracy 1 pixel). The standard Philips protocols for head and neck imaging were implemented in all cases with slices performed at 25° to the skull base. When the CT scans were obtained, the parotid glands were analyzed using FNL, UL, CA, and RV landmarks. All measurements were made using the same window, contrast and brightness.

The MRI parameters were as follows: Precontrast: a coronal TIRM sequence: TR, 5580 ms; TE, 61 ms; section thickness, 3 mm; FOV, 287 mm; resolution, 624; an axial T2 fs-dixon sequence: TR, 4010 ms; TE, 79 ms; section thickness, 3 mm; FOV, 280 mm; resolution, 739; an axial T1-weighted fs-dixon TSE sequence: TR, 590 ms; TE, 11 ms; section thickness, 3 mm; FOV, 586 mm; resolution, 1215; a coronal T1-weighted fs-dixon TSE sequence: TR, 670 ms; TE, 10 ms; section thickness, 3 mm; FOV, 548 mm; resolution, 1132. Post contrast: an axial gadolinium-enhanced T1 VIBE fat-saturated sequence 1 + 4; TR, 3.78 ms; TE, 1.25 ms; section thickness, 4 mm; FOV, 192 mm; resolution, 439; an axial T1 fs-dixon TSE fat-saturated sequence; a coronal gadolinium-enhanced T1 TSE fat-saturated sequence: TR, 613 ms; TE, 12 ms; section thickness, 3 mm; FOV 410 mm; resolution, 871 and a sagittal gadolinium-enhanced T1 TSE fat-saturated sequence: TR, 628 ms; TE, 8.7 ms; section thickness, 3 mm; FOV, 400 mm; resolution, 868.

While CT scans were performed in 106 cases, the MRI was performed in 86 cases for further confirmation of the diagnosis. Of them, both CT and MRI were performed in 70 cases and in 16 cases only MRI was performed.

Analysis

The error margin was expressed by means of the technical error of measurement (TEM) to calculate the inter-evaluator variability between two initial evaluators (authors 3 and 4 of the submission). The same equipment and methodological procedures for measurements were adopted by both evaluators. When the initial results were obtained, an independent evaluator was invited from another institution to re-evaluate the results (author 2 of the submission).

The questions put to be answered by the CT/MRI investigation were as follows: 1) the location of the tumor (deep lobe/superficial lobe), 2) encapsulation of the tumor (yes/no), 3) tumor's progression into the parapharyngeal space (yes/no). The data were statistically evaluated by three-dimensional analysis of variance, SPSS, Standard version 17.0 (SPSS, Chicago, IL, 2007), and χ^2 criterion using 95 % confidence interval. The level of significance for all analyses was set at $p < 0.05$.

Results

From 2004 to 2014, 450 patients underwent CT/MRI of the parotid region. Of them, 106 patients were diagnosed with benign neoplasms of the parotid gland and 11 were diagnosed with malignant neoplasms. In addition to CT, MRI, or CT/MRI investigations performed for 122 cases selected for analysis, the diagnosis was confirmed by ultrasonography and FNAB for all these patients. Among these selected cases, there were 58 (47.55 %) females and 64 (52.45 %) males with a mean age of 43 years (18–80 years) in the analyzed cohort of benign tumors. Three different surgeons experienced in salivary gland surgery operated on these patients. The patients selected for surgery were diagnosed with pleomorphic adenoma ($n = 60$; 49.2 %), Warthin's tumor ($n = 32$; 26.2 %), lipoma ($n = 26$; 21.3 %), and hemangioma ($n = 4$; 3.3 %). Successful parotidectomy was achieved in 97.5 % ($n = 119$) of the operated cases. In three cases reoperation with gland excision was needed.

Based on ultrasonography, CT, or MRI data, the type of the surgery was chosen. All surgeries were performed under general anaesthesia. In all cases, after-surgery follow-up was scheduled at 1, 3, 6, 12, and 24 months after the procedure, however only 64 patients were under follow-up for 12 month and only 33 appeared after 24 month after the surgery. The six-month follow-up revealed an absence of symptoms in all cases. Recovery of three patients with gland excision was successful.

Comparison between CT/MRI findings and the surgery results

For inter-evaluator TEM, difference between evaluators varied from 3.38 to 3.75 for different questions (acceptable). For TEM between the initial conclusions and the independent evaluator re-evaluation difference varied from 3.5 to 4.2 (acceptable).

By preoperative CT prediction with the help of FNL landmark, eight of the patients had the tumor located in the deep lobe of the gland and in 98 cases the lesion was diagnosed in the superficial lobe. As it was found during surgery, out of 106 cases 92 tumors were located in the superficial lobe of the gland and 14 tumors appeared to be in the deep lobe. In addition to this, out of eight cases initially diagnosed in the deep lobe only five were found there and another three were found in the superficial lobe. Therefore, general agreement between preoperative prediction and actual location of the superficial or deep lobe tumors was achieved in 88.7 % (12 mistakes out of 106 cases). However, out of 14 tumors in the deep lobe only five were located correctly (35.7 %).

The other existing landmarks were less precise:

Utrecht line (UL) vs. surgery 83 % (18 mistakes/106 cases);

The Conn's arc (CA) vs. surgery 71.7 % (30 mistakes/ 106 cases);

Retromandibular vein (RV) vs. surgery 73.6 % (28 mistakes/106 cases);

The main body of mistakes concerned cases with tumors in the deep lobe. Data on specificity and sensitivity of the above mentioned CT landmarks are presented in Table 1.

Analysis of MRI imaging presented excellent results in detecting encapsulation of the tumor and tumor's progression into the parapharyngeal space (100 % agreement with surgical results). Agreement between preoperative prediction and actual location of the tumor was achieved in 94.2 % (5 mistakes/86 cases). The four mistakes however were made in deep lobe cases. Out of 12 MRI-investigated tumors in the deep lobe nine were located correctly that gives 75 % agreement with surgical results. Data on

specificity and sensitivity of MRI imaging analysis are presented in Table 2.

Discussion

The location of the tumor proportional to the retromandibular vein, the styloid process, the lateral border of the masseter, the lateral border of the mandible, and the Stensen's duct was detected and the relation to the facial nerve was analyzed by the surgeons before the operation and further clarified during the operation. Analyzing the obtained data we can see that while both CT and MRI are very sensitive and specific in questions of tumor encapsulation and progression to the spaces out from the parotid gland itself, the abilities of these investigative methods to localize a lesion within the glandular tissue are less impressive, especially for CT.

One may say that FNL landmark for CT images was satisfactory precise by achieving 88.7 % agreement with surgical data. However, its precision for deep lobe location was only 35.7 % that is not satisfactory at all. Other landmarks showed worse agreement. It means that if a surgeon suspects a tumor in the deep lobe and plans selective deep lobe parotidectomy with superficial lobe preservation, he/she cannot completely rely on obtained CT imaging and is forced to add MRI data.

Some previous publications indicate high sensitivity and specificity (up to 100 %!) of CT based preoperative location of the parotid tumor [1, 2, 8]. We understand it as a wrong interpretation of statistical reports. Finding general sensitivity/specificity for cases of the tumor has sense if tumor distribution is equal in all parts of a gland or any other organ. In case of the parotid gland, most of the cases of tumor, up to 81-90 %, are found in the superficial lobe [9–13]. Suppose, a researcher had 100 cases of a tumor, of them 90 cases were located in the superficial lobe and 10 were located in the deep lobe. Suppose, a radiologist indicated all 100 cases to be located in the superficial lobe and is satisfied with 90 % agreement, but for a surgeon who could perform selective deep lobe parotidectomy instead of total or superficial parotidectomy this would be a total failure. This particular surgeon will not welcome such "90 % agreement" with any visible outburst of joy.

Table 1 Specificity and sensitivity of CT investigation for tumors of the parotid gland (n = 106). The variables investigated: (1) *tumor location in the superficial lobe (yes/no)*, (2) *tumor location in the deep lobe (yes/no)*, (3) *encapsulation of the tumor (yes/no)*, and (4) *progression into the parapharyngeal space (yes/no)*

Variable	TP	FP	TN	FN	specificity	sensitivity
Location: superficial lobe						
Facial nerve line	87	3	5	11	0.88	0.94
Utrecht line	56	7	7	36	0.5	0.6
The Conn's arc	55	8	6	37	0.57	0.59
Retromandibular vein	64	7	7	28	0.5	0.69
Location: deep lobe						
Facial nerve line	5	3	89	9	0.84	0.36
Utrecht line	6	8	84	8	0.79	0.43
The Conn's arc	7	5	87	7	0.82	0.5
Retromandibular vein	9	10	82	5	0.77	0.64
Encapsulation	101	0	4	1	0.95	0.99
parapharyngeal space	4	2	97	3	0.8	0.95

Abbreviations: TP true positive, *FP* false positive, *TN* true negative, *FN* false negative

Table 2 Specificity and sensitivity of MRI investigation for tumors of the parotid gland. Tumor location was assessed using the facial nerve line as the most sensitive

Variable	specificity	sensitivity
Tumor location in the superficial lobe (yes/no)	0.95	0.95
Tumor location in the deep lobe (yes/no)	1	0.8
Encapsulation of the tumor (yes/no)	1	1
progression into the parapharyngeal space (yes/no)	1	1

Precise localization of the tumor is very important. Rarely today but still parotidectomy may cause permanent damage to nerve such as facial paralysis and Frey's syndrome after surgery due to the anatomical interralations between the parotid gland and the facial nerve (FN). Currently, superficial parotidectomy causes minimal risk to the FN in most of the cases, whereas surgery for tumors in the deep lobe of the gland has a higher rate of FN injury. If total parotidectomy is necessary, however, the FN would be injured because of exposing FNs even when they are not sacrificed. Therefore, accurate preoperative evaluation of the location of the parotid gland tumor is important for the surgical outcomes and prognosis of patients because its location significantly affects the time and difficulty of operation.

As it was said above, various researchers commented on many predicting methods, such as CA, FN line, U line, and RV, to identify the location of the parotid gland tumor before operation using CT imaging and predicted the relationship between the location of the tumor and these landmarks. Satisfactory results were reported but in practice the idea did not work out quite so well. That is why we agree with those authors who stated that MRI is dominant for determining tumor location and facial nerve involvement [14]. When identifying tumor location using CT or MRI imaging, the FN branches in the CT image cannot be detected even with contrast media. It is common sense that MRI is more sensitive than CT but we inclined to agree with those authors who indicated that even MRI cannot achieve 100 % correct diagnosis [3, 15].

Recently, another approach to the problem was introduced suggesting the suprahyoid neck to be divided into characteristic anatomic spaces, which allow for the accurate localization of both normal and abnormal elements in the neck [16]. While dealing mostly with sublingual and submandibular glands, this method might be extrapolated to the parotid region and perhaps practitioners and radiologists will obtain more precise method for localization of deep lobe lesions.

Limitations of the research
All the CT scans and MRI images were obtained as described above. It might be possible that scanners of different trademarks could provide slightly different results of measurements as well as sonography evaluation. We evaluated benign tumors of the gland and different approach might be applied to malignant tumors.

Generalisability
External validity of the study results is based on recent efforts in standardization of CT and MRI nomenclature and protocols for various scanner manufacturers (GE, Philips, Toshiba, Hitachi, Siemens). All these manufacturers provide features to automatically initiate a prescribed axial, helical or dynamic scan when a threshold level of contrast enhancement is reached at a specified region of interest (in our case, the parotid gland) [17].

Conclusion
Our data suggests that no existing CT landmark can be accepted as completely reliable in cases when selective deep lobe parotidectomy is planned. If tumor location is suspected in the deep lobe of the gland, MRI imaging is necessary to confirm the diagnosis. An operating surgeon should be prepared that in some cases the true location of the tumor would be revealed only during surgery.

Competing interests
None of the authors has conflict of interest with the submission
No financial support was received for this submission

Authors' contributions
MV study concept, study design, analysis of the data, manuscript draft, approved manuscript final version; TS and IB collection of the data, data analysis, approved manuscript final version; JL acted as independent judge, approved manuscript final version.

Author details
[1]Department of Otolaryngology – Head and Neck Surgery, Assaf Harofe Medical Center, Affiliated to Sackler Faculty of Medicine, Tel Aviv University, Zerifin, Israel. [2]Department of Radiology, Neuroradiology section, Beilinson campus, Rabin medical center, Holon, Israel. [3]Department of Radiology, Assaf Harofe Medical Center, Affiliated to Sackler Faculty of Medicine, Tel Aviv University, Zerifin, Israel.

References
1. Lim CY, Chang HS, Nam KH, Chung WY, Park CS. Preoperative prediction of the location of parotid gland tumors using anatomical landmarks. World J Surg. 2008;32(10):2200–3. doi:10.1007/s00268-008-9663-0.
2. Lee CO, Ahn CH, Kwon TG, Kim CS, Kim JW. Preoperative prediction of the location of parotid gland tumors using radiographic anatomical landmarks. J Korean Assoc Oral Maxillofac Surg. 2012;38:38–43.
3. Ariyoshi Y, Shimahara M. Determining whether a parotid tumor is in the superficial or deep lobe using magnetic resonance imaging. J Oral Maxillofac Surg. 1998;56(1):23–6.
4. de Ru JA, van Benthem PP, Hordijk GJ. The location of parotid gland tumors in relation to the facial nerve on magnetic resonance images and computed tomography scans. J Oral Maxillofac Surg. 2002;60(9):992–4.
5. Conn IG, Wiesenfeld D, Ferguson MM. The anatomy of the facial nerve in relation to CT/sialography of the parotid gland. Br J Radiol. 1983;56(672):901–5.
6. Kurabayashi T, Ida M, Ohbayashi N, Ishii J, Sasaki T. Criteria for differentiating superficial from deep lobe tumours of the parotid gland by computed tomography. Dentomaxillofac Radiol. 1993;22(2):81–5.
7. Bryan RN, Miller RH, Ferreyro RI, Sessions RB. Computed tomography of the major salivary glands. AJR Am J Roentgenol. 1982;139(3):547–54.
8. Ulku CH, Uyar Y, Unaldi D. Management of lipomas arising from deep lobe of the parotid gland. Auris Nasus Larynx. 2005;32(1):49–53.
9. Bron LP, O'Brien CJ. Facial nerve function after parotidectomy. Arch Otolaryngol Head Neck Surg. 1997;123(10):1091–6.
10. Leverstein H, Van der Wal JE, Tiwari RM, Van der Waal I, Snow GB. Results of the surgical management and histopathological evaluation of 88 parotid gland Warthin's tumours. Clin Otolaryngol Allied Sci. 1997;22(6):500–3.
11. O'Brien CJ. Current management of benign parotid tumors–the role of limited superficial parotidectomy. Head Neck. 2003;25(11):946–52.

12. Hussain A, Murray DP. Preservation of the superficial lobe for deep-lobe parotid tumors: a better aesthetic outcome. Ear Nose Throat J. 2005;84(8): 518–520-2, 524.

13. Zhang NS, Wei W, Sun JY. Parotidectomy of deep-lobe tumors. Zhonghua Er Bi Yan Hou Tou Jing Wai Ke Za Zhi. 2007;42(10):757–9.

14. Popovski V. Massive deep lobe parotid neoplasms and parapharyngeal space-occupying lesions: contemporary diagnostics and surgical approaches. Prilozi. 2007;28(1):113–27.

15. Zaghi S, Hendizadeh L, Hung T, Farahvar S, Abemayor E, Sepahdari AR. MRI criteria for the diagnosis of pleomorphic adenoma: a validation study. Am J Otolaryngol. 2014;35(6):713–8. doi:10.1016/j.amjoto.2014.07.013.

16. Gamss C, Gupta A, Chazen JL, Phillips CD. Imaging evaluation of the suprahyoid neck. Radiol Clin North Am. 2015;53(1):133–44. doi:10.1016/j.rcl.2014.09.009.

17. Kalra MK, Saini S. Standardized nomenclature and description of CT scanning techniques. Radiology. 2006;241:657–60.

10

The validity of three neo-classical facial canons in young adults originating from the Arabian Peninsula

Maisa O Al-Sebaei

Abstract

Introduction: Understanding facial harmony and proportions is essential for facial reconstructive procedures and orthognathic surgery planning. In the literature, the neoclassical facial canons have been revisited in populations including North American whites and African Americans. The purpose of this study was to establish a baseline for selected facial anthropometric measurements and test the validity of 3 neoclassical facial canons in a cohort of young Saudi adults originating from the Arabian Peninsula.

Methods: The study group consisted of 168 healthy, esthetically pleasing Saudi Arabian dental students originating from the Arabian Peninsula (93 males and 75 females, age 20–24 years). Using a caliper, three neoclassical facial canons were measured; the vertical thirds of the face, the orbital canon (intercanthal distance = eye fissure length), and the orbito-nasal canon (intercanthal distance = nasal width) and analyzed using Student's t-test, general linear modeling, and pairwise comparison of means.

Results: The upper, middle, and lower thirds were not equal in measurement to each other ($p < 0.0001$). Sex dimorphism was observed in the lower facial third and nasal width measurements, with both larger in men (both $p < 0.0001$). The majority of subjects had longer upper and lower thirds than middle thirds, with 91.4% of males and 88% of females demonstrating a larger lower third than middle third. The most frequent variation in the orbital canon was a wider intercanthal distance than eye fissure length (55.9% of males and 74.7% of females). The most frequent variation in the orbito-nasal canon was a wider nasal width than intercanthal distance (92% of males and 56% of females).

Conclusions: Although these individuals are esthetically pleasing, they do not exhibit equal facial thirds or conform to orbital or orbito-nasal canons. The three neoclassical canons studied could not be validated in young adults originating from the Arabian Peninsula. Thus, the esthetic goals in reconstructive and orthognathic surgery should respect this ethnic variation.

Keywords: Neo-classical canons, Facial anthropometry, Direct anthropometry, Facial proportions

Introduction

The human sculptures created in ancient Greece were derived from proportions that followed established rules or so called "canons" [1]. These canons are based on the hypothesis that in a harmonious face, certain fixed ratios exist between different parameters. Leonardo da Vinci described the body and facial canons in the late 1400s. This work was followed by Albrecht Dürer in the 1500s, who defined the three equal lengths of the face (the forehead, the nose, and the mouth and chin), as well as the intercanthal distance being equal to the eye fissure length [2]. These neoclassical facial canons can be regarded as precursors to the current anthropometric facial indices, which were used by anatomists, medical artists, maxillofacial and esthetic surgeons, orthodontists, and esthetic dentists [3-11].

In the twentieth century, orthodontists continued to define facial proportions through the popularization of cephalometrics (an indirect method of anthropometry) [12]. It was not until the 1980s that Leslie Farkas, the father of modern facial anthropometry, revisited the classic canons for facial proportions as he measured and compared

Correspondence: Moalsebaei@kau.edu.sa
Department of Oral and Maxillofacial Surgery, King AbdulAziz University,
Faculty of Dentistry, PO Box 80209, Jeddah 21589, Kingdom of Saudi Arabia

the neoclassical canons in different ethnicities and craniofacial deformities such as clefts [10,13-15]. The validity of these canons was rejected in the races studied, with only a minor percentage of the studied population actually exhibiting the neoclassical canons [16].

Evaluation of facial esthetics is essential during treatment planning of prosthodontic, orthodontic, plastic facial reconstructive surgery, and orthognathic surgery. Several textbooks and journal articles use derivatives of neoclassical canons such as the facial thirds, where the face is divided vertically into three regions of equivalent height, which is used instead of the facial three-section canon. Additionally, the rule of fifths, which divides the face in the transverse dimension into five equal parts by assuming that the intercanthal distance is equal to the nasal width and widths of the eyes, incorporates orbital and orbito-nasal canons [17,18].

Thus far, no data have been published on the validity of neoclassical facial canons in a Saudi Arabian population. Therefore, this study aimed to determine the validity of the neoclassical canons for young adults in Saudi Arabia originating from the Arabian Peninsula, as well as to establish a baseline for the norms and explore sexual dimorphism in this population.

Methods

This study was approved by the Research Ethics Committee of the Faculty of Dentistry (REC-FD, King AbdulAziz Faculty of Dentistry, Jeddah, Saudi Arabia). Participation in the study was voluntary and each subject signed a consent form explaining the procedure.

Subjects

The study group consisted of 168 healthy, esthetically pleasing Saudi Arabians: 93 males and 75 females ranging in age from 20 to 24 years old. All subjects were dental students at King AbdulAziz University, Jeddah.

The following criteria were used to determine if the subject was "esthetically pleasing": (1) Angle class I molar and canine relationship, (2) mild convex to straight profile on clinical examination (3) normal growth and development, and (4) no obvious craniofacial or dentofacial deformities. The inclusion criteria were as follows: (1) esthetically pleasing as defined above; (2) all teeth present and erupted into occlusion excluding the third molars; and (3) the subject's parents and maternal and paternal grandparents all originating from the Arabian Peninsula. The exclusion criteria consisted of (1) previous history of orthodontic treatment and (2) previous history of any cosmetic, reconstructive, or corrective facial surgery.

Facial measurements

A sliding caliber (Seritex, Inc. Tinton Falls, NJ) was used to measure selected anthropometric facial components

directly on each study subject. Measurements were performed in accordance with the well-established methods published by Farkas [19]. All measurements were collected by the author (MOS) with the subject's head in the neutral position and recorded in millimeters. To evaluate reproducibility of the reading, an intra-reliability test was performed. Ten subjects were selected at random and their measurements were recorded at two different times, two weeks apart. A kappa test indicated significant agreement between both recorded measurements, with kappa = 0.783, p < 0.001.

The following measurements were assessed:

Vertical canon

The face is divided into equal thirds by a horizontal line passing through the trichion, nasion, subnasale, and gnathion (tr-n = n-sn = sn-gn) (Figure 1).

- Upper facial third: trichion to nasion (tr-n).
- Middle facial third: nasion to subnasale (n-sn).
- Lower facial third: subnasale to gnathion (sn-gn).

Horizontal canon 1 (orbital canon)

The intercanthal distance (ICD) equals the width of the eye or eye fissure length (EFL) (ex-en = en-en) (Figure 2).

- EFL: exocanthion to endocanthion (ex-en).
- ICD: endocanthion to endocanthion (en-en).

Horizontal canon 2 (Orbito-nasal canon)

The ICD equals the nasal width (NW) (en-en = al-al) (Figure 2).

- ICD: endocanthion to endocanthion (en-en).
- NW: alare to alare (al-al).

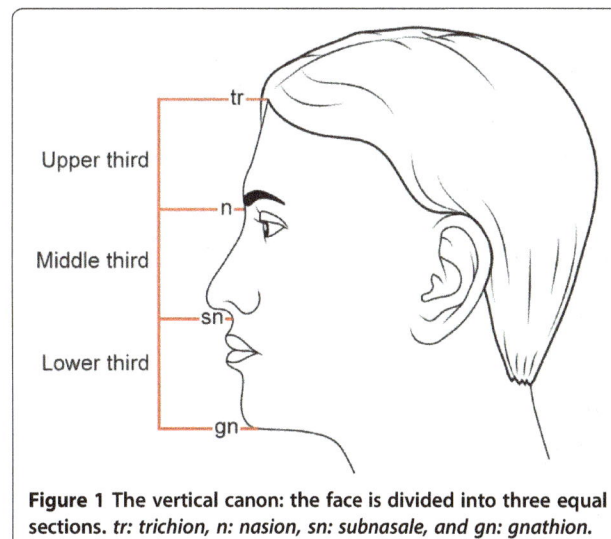

Figure 1 The vertical canon: the face is divided into three equal sections. *tr: trichion, n: nasion, sn: subnasale, and gn: gnathion.*

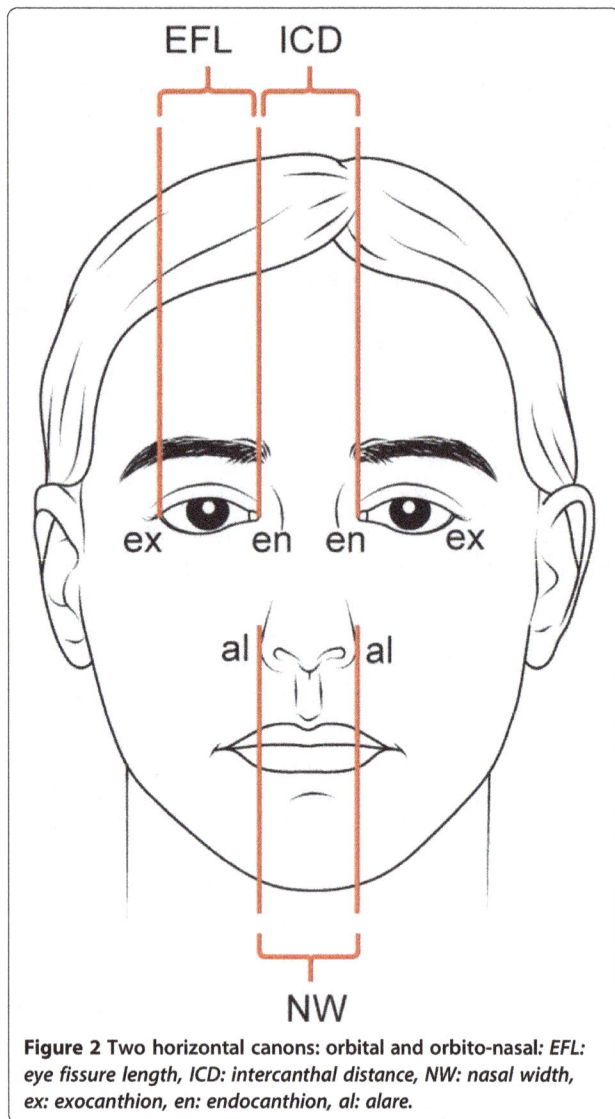

Figure 2 Two horizontal canons: orbital and orbito-nasal: *EFL: eye fissure length, ICD: intercanthal distance, NW: nasal width, ex: exocanthion, en: endocanthion, al: alare.*

Data analysis

The data were entered into a datasheet and analyzed using the SAS package (version 9.2, Cary, N.C). Values were expressed as means ± standard deviation (SD). The level of significance was set at $p < 0.05$.

A Student's t-test was used to compare the male and female mean measurements. A general linear model test (GLM) was used to compare the measurements of the vertical canons overall and according to sex. A pairwise comparison of mean measurements was performed using the least significant difference test separately for each sex.

A facial canon was accepted as *equal* if the difference between the measurements was 0–1 mm [10,20]. The chi-square test was used to compare sexes with regard to the vertical canon (*tr-n = n-sn, n-sn = sn-gn and tr-n = sn-gn*), orbital canon (*ex-en = en-en*), and orbito-nasal canon (*en-en = al-al*). The level of significance was set at $p < 0.05$.

Results

The mean measurements for the vertical and horizontal canons are shown in Table 1. When comparing the three measurements of the vertical canon of the face in all subjects (both sexes combined), the upper, middle, and lower thirds were not equal to each other; instead they significantly differed ($p < 0.0001$). Similarly, both the orbital and orbito-nasal canon measurements were significantly different from each other (both $p < 0.001$).

When the sexes were analyzed separately, a similar result was observed. In both men and women, the thirds of the face were also found to significantly differ from each other (both $p < 0.0001$). The orbital (EFL and ICD) and orbito-nasal canons (ICD and NW) also significantly differed from each other (both $p < 0.0001$).

The only sex differences in the measurements in our study were in the lower third of the face (*sn-gn*) and nasal base (*al-al*), with males exhibiting a larger lower third and nasal width than females.

Pairwise comparison indicated that the mean difference was significantly different from 0 for all paired measurements, except the upper and lower thirds of the face, which did not significantly differ among men ($p = 0.7261$). In Saudi men, the lower third was larger than the middle third by a mean difference of 10.9 mm (Table 2).

Variation from the neo-facial canons is shown in Table 3. The vertical canons and the orbital canon demonstrated no sexual dimorphism. However, a sex difference was observed in the orbito-nasal canon. None of the tested neoclassical facial canons were valid for the majority of the sample population. In men, the most frequently occurring neoclassical canon was the orbital canon, observed in 29% of the participants, and the least frequently observed was the equal length of the middle and lower thirds, seen in only 5.4% of the participants. In women, the most frequently met neoclassical canon was the orbito-nasal canon, in 33.3% of participants, whereas the least frequent was the equal length of the upper and middle thirds, seen in only 9.3% of the subjects.

Overall, the majority of males and females demonstrated a larger upper than middle third, a larger lower

Table 1 Mean measurements for males and females and comparison between sexes

Measurement	Males N = 75	Females N = 93	p value
Upper third	64.71 (7.51)	65.46 (6.90)	0.51
Middle third	54.12 (4.34)	53.19 (4.13)	0.16
Lower third	65.02 (5.16)	60.27 (4.62)	<0.0001*
Eye fissure length	32.85 (2.73)	32.41 (3.44)	0.37
Inter-canthal distance	30.30 (3.10)	30.32 (2.40)	0.97
Nasal width	36.85 (3.16)	32.87 (3.29)	<0.0001*

Significant at p < 0.05.

Table 2 The mean difference in measurements between the vertical, orbital, and orbito-nasal canons as a pairwise comparison

Canon	Males	p value	Females	p value
Vertical Canons				
Upper third – middle third tr-n = n-sn	10.6	<0.0001*	12.3	<0.0001 *
Middle third – lower third n-sn = sn-gn	−10.9	<0.0001*	−7.1	<0.0001*
Upper third – lower third tr-n = sn-gn	−0.3	<0.0001*	5.2	0.7261
Orbital canon				
Eye fissure length –intercanthal distance ex-en = en-en	−2.8	<0.0001*	−2.0	<0.0001*
Orbito-nasal canon				
Intercanthal distance –Nasal width en-en = al-al	−7.1	< 0.0001*	−2.3	< 0.0001*

Statistically significant difference between the measurements.

than middle third, a larger upper than lower third, a wider EFL length than ICD, and a predominately wider NW than ICD.

Discussion

The objective of esthetic and reconstructive surgery is to restore ideal and acceptable facial proportions with

Table 3 Comparison of neo-canons and their variation according to sex by a difference of more than or less than 1 mm

Canon	Males N = 75	Females N = 93	p value
Vertical Canon			
tr-n = n-sn	9.7	9.3	0.9398
tr-n > n-sn	**81.7**	**88**	
tr-n < n-sn	8.6	2.7	
n-sn = sn-gn	5.4	10.7	0.2020
n-sn > sn-gn	3.2	1.3	
n-sn < sn-gn	**91.4**	**88**	
tr-n = sn-gn	21.5	14.7	0.2560
tr-n > sn-gn	**39.8**	**72**	
tr-n < sn-gn	38.7	13.3	
Orbital Canon			
ex-en = en-en	29.0	25.0	0.5930
ex-en > en-en	**55.9**	**74.7**	
ex-en < en-en	15.1	17.3	
Orbito-Nasal Canon			
en-en = al-al	6.5	33.3	<.0001*
en-en > al-al	1.1	10.7	
en-en < al-al	**92.4**	**56.0**	

Bold font *denotes the most predominant variation of the canons in both sexes.*
* Statistically significant at p < 0.05.

respect to the ethnic background of the individual. In orthognathic surgery, where osteotomies of the maxilla and mandible are performed to establish dental and facial balance and harmony, facial proportions serve as a guide to the movement of the maxilla-mandibular complex. Maxillofacial surgeons are always on a quest to find more objective guides to facial harmony and balance.

Farkas and his co-workers are credited for extensive work in recording anthropometric facial measurements of healthy individuals from different ethnic backgrounds. These studies have revealed the variability of facial proportional relationships [10,11,20-22].

Based on the work of Farkas and others, facial anthropometric findings in healthy North American white, Chinese, and African American populations have indicated that the neoclassical facial canons were not valid [11]. Farkas found the equal facial thirds originally described by Albrecht Dürer in the 1500s [2,10] to be present only in a small percentage of African and white Americans [10,11,20].

In one multi-center study published in 2005, Farkas et al. assessed 14 anthropometric measurements in 1470 healthy individuals drawn from five regions of the world, 53.1% of whom were of Caucasian origin and the remainder from 13 countries in Europe and three countries in the Middle East (Egypt, Iran, and Turkey) [16]. To our knowledge, that report is the only large-scale study of these anthropometric measurements in subjects from the Middle East. However, these "Middle Eastern" ethnicities are different from that of the Arabian Peninsula, which has distinct and unique facial features. A summary of the results of the current study, compared to those in other Saudi samples, Arab samples, and other ethnicities is shown in Table 4.

With regard to the Saudi population, very few studies have addressed anthropometric facial measurement. In 2011, Bukhari [23] assessed four anthropometric eye measurements in Saudi men and women. In comparison to our results, the previously reported EFL was lower and ICD was higher (both statistically significant at p <0.05). The difference between our study and Bukhari's results might be due to the different sample populations. Our study cohort consisted of young adults, while their subjects ranged from 15 to over 70 years old.

Another study that assessed anthropometric measurements of the Saudi Arabian nose was conducted by Al-Qattan et al. [24], who reported a higher ICD and lower NW in both sexes and a shorter middle third of the face in women in comparison to our study. However, due to differences in measurement technique, with the previous study using the indirect anthropometry method of photogrammetry, the results of the two studies cannot be directly compared.

Table 4 Comparison between the mean anthropometric facial measurements in the current study and other studies of Arab populations and other ethnicities

Ethnic group		N	Upper Third tr-n		Middle third n-sn		Lower third sn-gn		EFL en-ex		ICD ex-ex		NB al-al	
			M	F	M	F	M	F	M	F	M	F	M	F
Current Study	Saudi	M = 75 F = 93	64.7 (7.5)	65.5 (6.9)	54.1 (4.3)	53.2 (4.1)	65.0 (5.2)	60.3 (4.6)	32.9 (2.7)	32.4 (3.4)	30.3 (3.1)	30.3 (2.4)	36.6 (3.2)	32.9 (3.3)
Dharap et al. 2013	Gulf Arabs	M = 51 F = 117	N/A	N/A	N/A	N/A	N/A	N/A	N/A	N/A	N/A	N/A	37.1 (3.4)	33.2 (2.4)
Algaidi et al. 2012	Egyptian	M = 108 F = 88	N/A	N/A	54.7 (0.5)	45.8 (0.2)*	63.8 (0.6)*	56.4 (0.6)*	N/A	N/A	N/A	N/A	39.8 (0.4)*	32.8 (0.5)
Bokhari 2011	Saudi	M = 276 F = 392	N/A	N/A	N/A	N/A	N/A	N/A	30.8 (2.9)*	29.5 (2.8)*	32.7 (2.8)*	31.3 (3.5)*	N/A	N/A
Husein et al. 2010	Indian American	F = 102	N/A	63.9 (7.4)	N/A	58.1 (5.5)*	N/A	57.8 (7.5)*	N/A	30.6 (2.4)*	N/A	31.2 (3.7)*	N/A	35.6 (3.3)*
Farkas et al. 2005	Egyptian	M = 30 F = 30	63.6 (9.5)	61.2 (6.0)*	54.6 (5.6)	47.4 (5.2)*	64.1 (6.4)	57.8 (4.5)*	31.5 (1.8)*	30.8 (1.8)*	31.8 (2.1)*	30.9 (2.3)	32.4 (4.0)*	29.3 (3.7)*
Farkas et al. 2005	Iranian	M = 30 F = 30	53.4 (8.2)*	56.9 (8.3)*	62.6 (3.2)*	66.2 (4.4)*	73.3 (4.3)*	66.2 (4.4)*	37.2 (3.5)*	24.4 (3.3)*	27.3 (2.7)*	24.6 (3.5)*	35.3 (3.0)	32.1 (2.5)
Farkas et al. 2005	Turkish	M = 30 F = 30	61.9 (6.1)	60.7 (7.0)*	58.1 (3.5)*	55.2 (4.0)*	65.9 (4.2)	59.1 (3.8)	30.6 (1.2)*	29.8 (1.6)*	32.8 (2.6)*	31.7 (2.2)*	36.8 (2.3)	32.9 (2.1)
Farkas 2005	North American white	M = 109 F = 200	67.1 (7.5)*	63.0 (6.0)*	54.8 (3.3)	50.6 (3.1)*	72.6 (4.5)*	64.3 (4.0)*	31.3 (1.2)*	30.7 (1.2)*	33.3 (2.7)*	31.8 (2.3)*	34.9 (2.1)*	31.4 (2.0)*
Farkas et al. 2005	Chinese	M = 30 F = 30	67.1 (6.9)	64.1 (7.5)	53.5 (2.8)	51.7 (3.3)	72.7 (5.2)*	66.4 (5.6)*	29.4 (1.2)*	28.5 (1.8)*	37.9 (3.3)*	36.5 (3.2)*	39.2 (2.9)	37.2 (2.1)*
Farkas et al. 2007	African American	M = 50 F = 50	72.0 (7.8)*	67.1 (5.9)	51.8 (3.1)*	48.8 (3.7)*	78.7 (7.3)*	71.5 (5.2)*	32.9 (1.7)	32.4 (2.4)	35.8 (2.9)*	34.4 (3.4)*	44.1 (3.4)*	40.1 (3.2)*

Values are expressed as mean measurements and standard deviation in parenthesis. EFL: eye fissure length, ICD: intercanthal distance, NB: nasal base. *Statistically significant at $p < 0.05$.

The mean nasal width of an Arab cohort from the Gulf region measured in a study by Dharap et al. [25] is consistent with that of our study, although the term "Arabian Gulf" was used loosely by the authors, since the subjects were from five countries of the Gulf Cooperation Council. The origin of people from the Gulf is not uniform; it can be Persian, Turkish, East Asian, or other.

Anthropometric studies in regions such as the Gulf are very difficult because of the possible influence of inter-racial marriage and immigration on anthropometric facial measurements. The term "Saudi" is a nationality and not an ethnicity. Saudi Arabia is located in the Arabian Peninsula, and although most Saudis are ethnically Arab, originating from tribes in the Arabian Peninsula, people of the Kingdom of Saudi Arabia are mixed and can be descended from Iran, Turkey, East Asia, Russia, and Africa. We were unable to find a previous study involving a cohort of young Saudi Arabian adults originating purely from the Arabian Peninsula. Additionally, none of the studies involving Saudi populations observed or tested the validity of the neoclassical facial canons. Therefore, the present study tested the validity of the neo-classical canons on young adults from the Arabian Peninsula, with the aim to define a cohort of individuals with the same ethnic origins.

The only sex differences observed among the measurements in this study were the longer lower facial third and NW demonstrated by men. The majority of the population, both men and women, had longer upper and lower thirds than middle third, which is consistent with the findings of Farkas et al. that North American white and African American faces exhibited a larger chin than the canonical face [10,11].

The validity of the vertical canon of equal facial thirds was not confirmed in our sample. The middle third was the smallest of the three, and the majority of participants (91.4% of men and 88% of women) demonstrated a larger lower third than middle third. This observation is also consistent with the findings of Farkas et al. (2000), where the middle third was the smallest third in both North American whites and African Americans. In that study, the lower third of the face was larger than the middle third in 100% of both populations, and the upper third was larger than the middle third in 100% of African American and 95% of North American white participants [11].

Farkas et al. [11] also found the orbital canon (palpebral fissure length equal to ICD) to be valid in only 33% of North American white and 13% of African American participants. The ICD was predominately wider than EFL in African Americans (73%). The opposite was true in our study population, in whom the majority (55.9% of men and 74.7% of women) had wider EFL than ICD. Thus, those individuals in our study with valid orbital canons (25% of women and 29% of men) fall between

African Americans and North American whites. By contrast, in a Chinese Han population, Dawaei et al. found that the most predominant variation of the orbital canon was a wider intercanthal distance than eye fissure length. The measurements were equal in about 35.5 percent of the Chinese Han population [20].

The most frequently validated canon among those tested was the nasoorbital canon (NW equal to ICD) in females (33.3%), but this canon was valid in only 6.5% of men. This finding is in contrast to the results of Farkas et al. (1985), where 40.8% of North American whites and 3% of African Americans demonstrated a valid orbito-nasal canon [10]. In Chinese subjects, an equal nasoorbital canon was found in approximately one-third of the population studied (35.4%) [20].

The most predominant variation in our sample was a wider NW than ICD (56% in females and 92% in males). Similarly, this was the most predominant variation of the nasoorbital canon in African Americans (94%), whereas in North American whites, the wider nose was seen in 27.9% of participants [10,11].

Conclusions

To date, no studies testing the validity of the neo-classical facial cannons originally described by artists of the Renaissance and adopted by plastic, maxillofacial, and reconstructive surgeons in an ethnically homogenous Saudi population. Our study sample was carefully selected to consist of young adults originating only from the Arabian Peninsula. In general, we observed a trend for a longer lower third in comparison to middle third of the face, a wider eye fissure length than intercanthal distance, and a wider nasal base in comparison to intercanthal distance. Men had a significantly larger lower third and nasal width measurement than women.

The neoclassical facial canons could not be validated in this cohort of young adults originating from the Arabian Peninsula. Like any ethnicity, facial norms and measurements of other Caucasian populations cannot be applied to the Arab population. This distinction has a great impact on treatment planning for corrective, reconstructive, and orthognathic procedures. Further studies in our region should aim at establishing baseline values for all the facial anthropometric measurements recommended by Farkas and his colleagues among people from the Arabian Peninsula.

Abbreviations

ICD: Intercanthal distance (en-en); EFL: Eye fissure length (ex-en); NW: Nasal width (al-al).

Competing interests

The author declares no competing interests.

Author's contributions
MOA designed the study, acquired the measurement data, performed data interpretation, drafted the manuscript, and wrote the final manuscript.

Acknowledgment
This project was funded by the Deanship of Scientific Research (DSR), King AbdulAziz University, Jeddah, Saudi Arabia, under grant no. (442/254/1431). The author, therefore, acknowledges with thanks the DSR technical and financial support.
The author would like to acknowledge Prof. Saad Al-Sowayan, a Saudi Arabian anthropologist, for his valuable advice during the preparation of the study design and manuscript. I would also like to acknowledge Dr. Khalid Zawawi for his valuable assistance and advice during the preparation of the manuscript.

References
1. Edler RJ. Background considerations to facial aesthetics. J Orthod. 2001;28:159–68.
2. Vegter F, Hage JJ. Clinical anthropometry and canons of the face in historical perspective. Plast Reconstr Surg. 2000;106:1090–6.
3. Prokopakis EP, Vlastos IM, Picavet VA, Nolst Trenite G, Thomas R, Cingi C, et al. The golden ratio in facial symmetry. Rhinology. 2013;51:18–21.
4. Seghers M, Longacre J, Destefano G. The golden proportion and beauty. Plast Reconstr Surg. 1964;34:382–6.
5. Mizumoto Y, Deguchi Sr T, Fong KW. Assessment of facial golden proportions among young Japanese women. Am J Orthod Dentofacial Orthop. 2009;136:168–74.
6. Pini NP, de-Marchi LM, Gribel BF, Ubaldini AL, Pascotto RC. Analysis of the golden proportion and width/height ratios of maxillary anterior dentition in patients with lateral incisor agenesis. J Esthet Restor Dent. 2012;24:402–14.
7. Sunilkumar LN, Jadhav KS, Nazirkar G, Singh S, Nagmode PS, Ali FM. Assessment of Facial Golden Proportions among North Maharashtri-an Population. J Int Oral Health. 2013;5:48–54.
8. Levin EI. Dental esthetics and the golden proportion. J Prosthet Dent. 1978;40:244–52.
9. Zlataric DK, Kristek E, Celebic A. Analysis of width/length ratios of normal clinical crowns of the maxillary anterior dentition: correlation between dental proportions and facial measurements. Int J Prosthodont. 2007;20:313–5.
10. Farkas LG, Hreczko TA, Kolar JC, Munro IR. Vertical and horizontal proportions of the face in young adult North American Caucasians: revision of neoclassical canons. Plast Reconstr Surg. 1985;75:328–38.
11. Farkas LG, Forrest CR, Litsas L. Revision of neoclassical facial canons in young adult Afro-Americans. Aesthet Plast Surg. 2000;24:179–84.
12. Ricketts RM. Divine proportion in facial esthetics. Clin Plast Surg. 1982;9:401–22.
13. Farkas LG, Hajnis K, Posnick JC. Anthropometric and anthroposcopic findings of the nasal and facial region in cleft patients before and after primary lip and palate repair. Cleft Palate Craniofac J. 1993;30:1–12.
14. Farkas LG, James JS. Anthropometry of the face in lateral facial dysplasia: the unilateral form. Cleft Palate J. 1977;14:193–9.
15. Farkas LG, Katic MJ, Forrest CR. Comparison of craniofacial measurements of young adult African-American and North American white males and females. Ann Plast Surg. 2007;59:692–8.
16. Farkas LG, Katic MJ, Forrest CR, Alt KW, Bagic I, Baltadjiev G, et al. International anthropometric study of facial morphology in various ethnic groups/races. J Craniofac Surg. 2005;16:615–46.
17. Proffit WR, Fields HW, Sarver DM. Contemporary Orthodontics. 4th ed. St. Louis, MO: Mosby Elsevier; 2007.
18. Naini FB, Gill DS. Facial aesthetics: 1. Concepts Canons Dent Update. 2008;35:102–4.
19. Farkas LG. Anthropometry of the Head and Face. 2nd ed. New York: Raven; 1994.
20. Wang D, Qian G, Zhang M, Farkas LG. Differences in horizontal, neoclassical facial canons in Chinese (Han) and North American Caucasian populations. Aesthet Plast Surg. 1997;21:265–9.
21. Borman H, Ozgur F, Gursu G. Evaluation of soft-tissue morphology of the face in 1,050 young adults. Ann Plas Surg. 1999;42:280–8.
22. Jayaratne YS, Deutsch CK, McGrath CP, Zwahlen RA. Are neoclassical canons valid for southern Chinese faces? PLoS One. 2012;7:e52593.
23. Bukhari AA. The distinguishing anthropometric features of the Saudi Arabian eyes. Saudi J Ophthalmol. 2011;25:417–20.
24. Al-Qattan MM, Alsaeed AA, Al-Madani OK, Al-Amri NA, Al-Dahian NA. Anthropometry of the Saudi Arabian nose. J Craniofac Surg. 2012;23:821–4.
25. Dharap AS A, Fadel R, Osman M, Chakravarty M, Abdul Latif N, Abu-Hijlrh M. Facial anthropometry in Arab population. Bahrain Medical Bulletin. 2013;35:69–77.

11

Lip closing force of Class III patients with mandibular prognathism: a case control study

Sihui Chen[†], Ying Cai[†] and Fengshan Chen[*]

Abstract

Introduction: To compare the lip closing force of patients with mandibular prognathism to that of patients without dentofacial anomalies.

Methods: The subject group included 62 female patients of Class III relationship with mandibular prognathism. The control group been comprised of 71 patients of Class I relationships without skeletal deformities. Maximum lip closing force and average lip closing force were measured using a Y-meter. Student's t-test was carried out to analyse the differences between the groups. Correlation and stepwise multiple linear regression analyses were performed to analyse the relationship between lip closing force and craniofacial morphology.

Results: The lower lip closing force of subjects with mandibular prognathism was significantly greater than that of patients in the control group ($P < 0.001$), while the upper lip closing force showed no difference ($P > 0.05$). The lower lip closing force of patients with mandibular prognathism was strongly correlated with IMPA (Lower Incisor - Mandibular Plane angle, $P < 0.001$) and FMA (Frankfort Plane-Mandibular Plane angle, $P < 0.001$). Multiple regression equations: (MaxLL) = 12.192 - 0.125 * (IMPA) + 0.082 (FMA); (AveLL) = 9.112 - 0.091 * (IMPA) + 0.054 (FMA).

Conclusions: The lower lip closing force was markedly increased in Class III patients with mandibular prognathism and was strongly correlated with lower incisor position and mandibular plane angle.

Keywords: Lip closing force, Mandibular prognathism, Class III, Perioral force

Introduction

High prevalence of Class III malocclusions has been found in Asian populations. Kitai [1] reported that 5-20% of the Japanese population possessed the characteristics of Class III malocclusion. Similarly, Johnson [2] discovered a prevalence of 23% in Chinese children.

Studies have indicated that 63–73% of Class III malocclusions are of the skeletal type [3], while in the research of Mackay [4], those patients who required surgical correction of Class III conditions all had some degree of mandibular prognathism, which has long been viewed as one of the most severe maxillofacial deformities [5]. Indeed, mandibular prognathism, which is commonly related to Class III malocclusion, is a facial disharmony for which patients frequently seek treatments [6].

However, the etiological mechanisms of this condition still remain unrevealed. Class III malocclusion is not a distinct clinical entity, and it can exist in with any number of combinations of skeletal and dental components. Among the possibilities, muscular factors could constitute a vital component, based on commonly held perspectives.

Complex interdependence exists among teeth, perioral force and jaws. Ideal dentition arises from an equilibrate system composed of intraoral forces, represented by the tongue, and extraoral forces, represented by the lip force. If the force balance collapses, for example the lip force is less powerful than a normal condition, teeth inclination would change towards the weaker side. More complicated mechanism may be involved, but similar force system is very important to the growth and development of the dentoalveolar morphology. These soft tissue matrices, and particularly labial pressure from the circumoral musculature, may influence the outcome of craniofacial growth [7]. For example, hypofunction of mentalis muscle, resulting in less restriction on mandibular

* Correspondence: orthodboy@126.com
[†]Equal contributors
Department of Orthodontics, Laboratory of Oral Biomedical Science and Translational Medicine, School of Stomatology, Tongji University, Middle Yanchang Road 399, Shanghai, P. R. China

growth, appears to be related to mandibular protrusion [8]. A sound understanding of the surrounding soft tissues and their biological behaviour, especially labial pressure, which is represented by lip closing force [4], could help to reveal the etiology of dentoalveolar dysplasia.

Concerning the relationship between lip-closing force and craniofacial morphology, the closing force of the upper lip has a great influence on maxillary incisor angulation, vertical skeletal pattern and lip protrusion [9,10]. As to the skeletal pattern, most of the previous researches have focused on both Class I and Class II malocclusions [9,11-15]. Hardly any research has concentrated on Class III malocclusions, except Ueki [16], who demonstrated that the LCF of postoperative Class III patients were higher than the preoperative status. After all, the related data remain incomplete.

Our research group restricted our subjects to those with simplex mandibular prognathism to eliminate confounding factors, such as maxillary retrognathism and asymmetry, so that we could define a possible mechanism regarding how LCF influences the ultimate outcomes of craniofacial growth in Class III conditions.

The purposes of this study were to define both the upper and lower LCFs acting in Class III malocclusion patients with mandibular prognathism and to indicate the possible relationships between LCF and craniofacial morphology.

Materials and methods

All the patients who took part in this study were newly diagnosed patients who requested orthodontic treatment over a three-year period in the Orthodontic Department of Tongji Stomatological Hospital. The subject group (Group 1) consisted of 62 female patients (average age 17.92 ± 1.65 y) with Class III malocclusion. All the cases were diagnosed as skeletal Class III, characterized by mandibular prognathism but with relatively normal positioning of the maxilla on the basis of lateral cephalographic analysis. The control group (Group 2) consisted of 71 female patients (average age 18.20 ± 1.46 y) in our department with Class I skeletal patterns and Class I occlusal relationships without skeletal deformity. The inclusion criteria were: no loss of permanent teeth; no missing or supernumerary teeth; no history of orthognathic surgery or previous orthodontic treatment; no congenital craniofacial anomalies; and no occlusal canting or other asymmetric skeletal patterns.

To evaluate the occlusal and skeletal patterns of each subject, cephalograms were obtained. The measurement landmarks were SNA (Sella–Nasion-A Angle, represent maxilla position toward cranium), SNB (Sella-Nasion-B Angle, represent mandible position toward cranium), ANB (A-Nasion-B Angle, represent mandible position toward maxilla), PP-FH (Palatal Plane - Frankfort Plane

Angle), OP-FH (Occlusal Plane - Frankfort Plane Angle), overbite, overjet, UI-FH (Upper Incisor - Frankfort Plane Angle), FMA (Frankfort Plane - Mandibular Plane Angle), IMPA (Lower Incisor - Mandibular Plane Angle), ANS-Ptm (length of maxilla) and Co-Pog (length of mandible). All the landmarks (Figure 1 and Figure 2) were identified and digitized by the same investigator, utilizing Dolphin Imaging software (version 10.5, Dolphin, Imaging and Management Solutions, Chatsworth, CA, USA).

The Y-meter, the instrument for LCF measurement, has previously been used in other studies [9,10] (Figure 3). The biteplate was coated with baseplate wax before each measurement to help the subjects to hold with their incisors in position. The Slimline Sensor (9131A49, Kistler Co. Winterthur, Switzerland) was located on the upper surface of the horizontal plate of the Y-meter, with which the lip under measurement status maintained contact. The quartz sensor was intended to measure dynamic and quasi-static forces. Its characteristics, high resolution, high rigidity and extremely small dimensions render it ideal for measuring the vertical vector of the lip closing force. A base charge amplifier (5034A10, Kistler Co.) and DASY-LAB (DASYTEC, Amherst, NH, USA) software, version 5.50, were also applied for data acquisition. The Y-meter was stored at 37°C to minimize temperature-induced errors.

After a brief explanation was provided and several practice measurements were taken, each subject was requested to close his or her lips as tightly as possible. The LCF was monitored for 5 seconds. The maximum value and the average value for 5 seconds were measured with the DASYLAB software. Measurements were generated three times at 3-minute intervals. After measuring the upper LCF, the identical procedure was used to evaluate the closing force of the lower lip with the Y-meter upside down. We recorded the LCF values with the patients in the natural head position.

Student's t-test was carried out to analyse the differences between the groups. Pearson's product moment correlation test was used to analyse the relationship between lip force and craniofacial morphology. Stepwise multiple linear regression analysis, with the average and maximum values of both LCFs, was further performed. All the statistical analyses were performed with SPSS software (SPSS Inc., Chicago, IL, USA), version 20 for Windows.

To evaluate the magnitude of measurement error involved in this study, lateral cephalograms of 12 randomly selected subjects were retraced, redigitized and reanalyzed after a 2-week interval, and the error was calculated by Dahlberg's formula [17]. The error ranged between 0.04 mm and 0.20 mm for the linear measurements and between 0.15° and 0.90° for the angular measurements. All the measurement procedures and

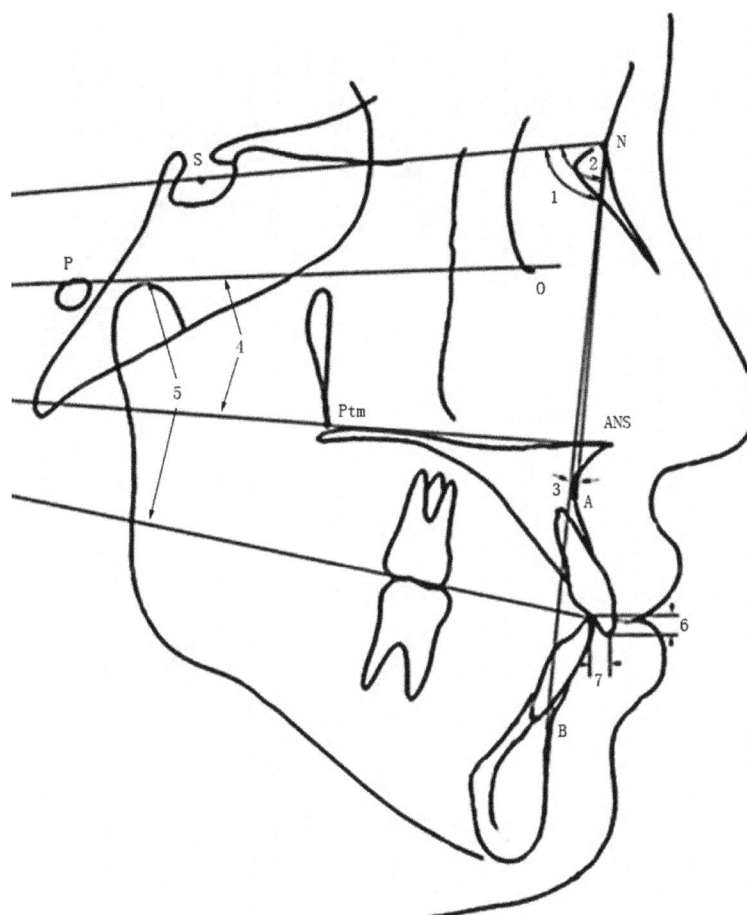

Figure 1 Measurements used in this study. 1, SNA (Sella–Nasion-A Angle); 2, SNB (Sella-Nasion-B Angle); 3, ANB (A-Nasion-B Angle); 4, PP-FH (Palatal Plane - Frankfort Plane Angle); 5, OP-FH (Occlusal Plane - Frankfort Plane Angle); 6, overbite; 7, overjet.

cephalometric analyses were performed by the same researcher.

This study took the Declaration of Helsinki on medical protocol and ethics and the regional Ethical Review Board of Tongji University approved the study. The researcher previously obtained the informed consent of all the subjects. The rights of our subjects were protected, and the data were only for research use.

Results

The means and standard deviations for each variable are shown in Table 1. All the cases in the subject group were diagnosed as skeletal Class III, characterized by mandibular prognathism (average ANB -3.67 ± 0.86, SNB 84.63 ± 1.16) and normal positioning of the maxilla (average SNA 80.96 ± 1.37). No skeletal deformities existed among the patients in the control group (average SNA 81.98 ± 1.23, SNB 80.87 ± 1.29 and ANB 1.11 ± 0.79).

The results of Levene's test and Student's t-test of LCF are provided in Table 2, from which we can discover unequal variance in variable MaxLL and AveLL, but not in

variable MaxUL and Ave UL. We adopted the adjusted data according to the Levene's test. Both the maximum and average lower LCFs in the subject group (Group 1) was significantly different from those of the patients in the control group (Group 2, $P < 0.001$). The upper LCF showed no discernible differences between the two groups ($P > 0.05$).

In the correlation analyses (Table 3), the IMPA angle showed a high level of negative correlation with both the maximum and average lower LCFs of the patients in the subject group ($P < 0.001$). The IMPA produced r values of -0.789 (vs. MaxLL) and -0.697 (vs. AveLL), respectively. The FMA angle showed a significant positive relationship with the lower LCFs of patients with mandibular prognathism ($P < 0.001$) and produced r values of 0.672 (vs. MaxLL) and 0.582 (vs. AveLL), respectively.

The result of stepwise multiple linear regression analysis is presented in Table 4. 3-D scatter plots are showed in Figure 4 and Figure 5. With regard to the results of stepwise regression analysis, the maximum lower LCF was determined by an equation using the

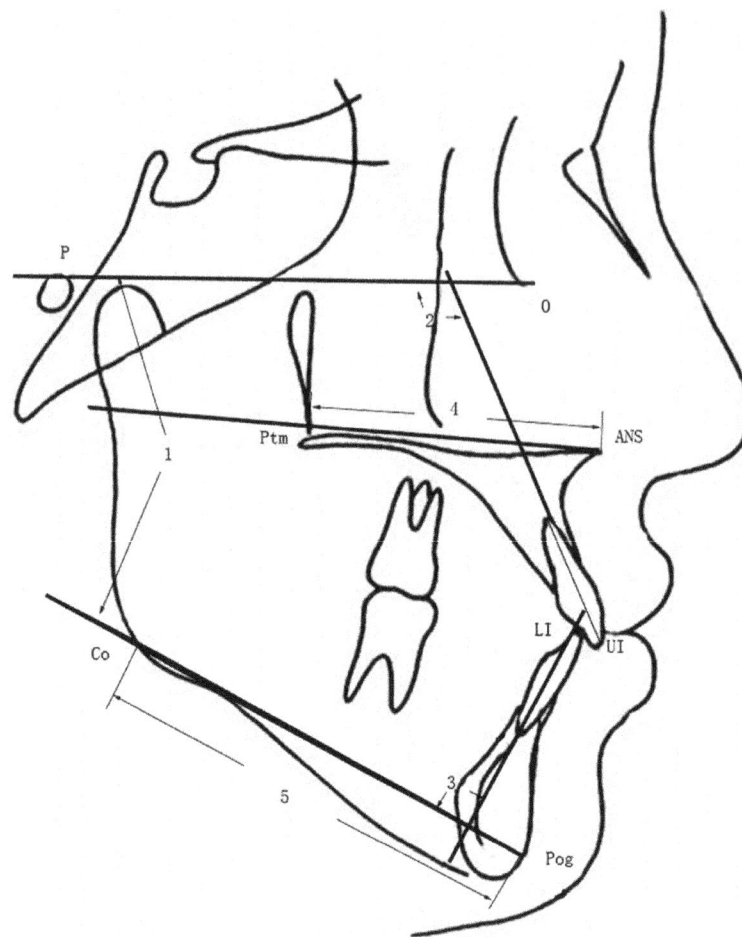

Figure 2 Measurements used in this study (continued). 1, FMA (Frankfort Plane - Mandibular Plane Angle); 2, U1-FH (Upper Incisor - Frankfort Plane Angle); 3, IPMA (Lower Incisor - Mandibular Plane Angle); 4. ANS-Ptm (length of maxilla); 5, Co-Pog (length of mandible).

IMPA and FMA as follows: (MaxLL) = 12.192 - 0.125 * (IMPA) + 0.082 (FMA). The average lower LCF was determined by an equation using the IMPA and FMA as follows: (AveLL) = 9.112 - 0.091 * (IMPA) + 0.054 (FMA).

Discussion

Phenotypic heterogeneity and variation in clinical severity typify the diversity found within the complex class of occlusal morphologies grouped under the umbrella term of "Class III malocclusion" [18]. Definitions of the condition have varied throughout the orthodontic, dental, anatomical, and anthropological literature. Mackay [4] identified five Class III subgroups, all of which exhibited mandibular prognathism. Because of the high prevalence of mandibular prognathism in Class III patients, we chose this group of patients as our target subjects. A greater degree of lip pressure was noted in men than in women in previous studies [16,19], so all the subjects in our study were women to eliminate this type of variation.

Etiologic constituents of Class III malocclusion have turned out to be quite complex. It might appear that the variations in dental arch morphology, tooth position and skeletal components could account for Class III relationships; also, the contribution of the soft tissue matrices cannot be overlooked. It is conceivable that Class III malocclusions might result from the activity of the circumoral musculature, to some degree. For example, hypofunction of mentalis muscle appears to be related to mandibular protrusion [8]. Bardach [20] et al. tested the hypothesis that cleft lip repair contributed to maxillofacial growth aberrations. They found that undermining the soft tissue of the upper lip on the surface of the maxilla was detrimental to maxillofacial growth in beagles.

Teeth encounter even bigger force during oral functions, such as chewing, speaking and swallowing. The impact of perioral force under functional circumstance is rather significant, but it is technically difficult to measure it. Large interindividual variation is a common finding in studies of muscle pressure [21,22]. It would be very difficult to control the interindividual variation

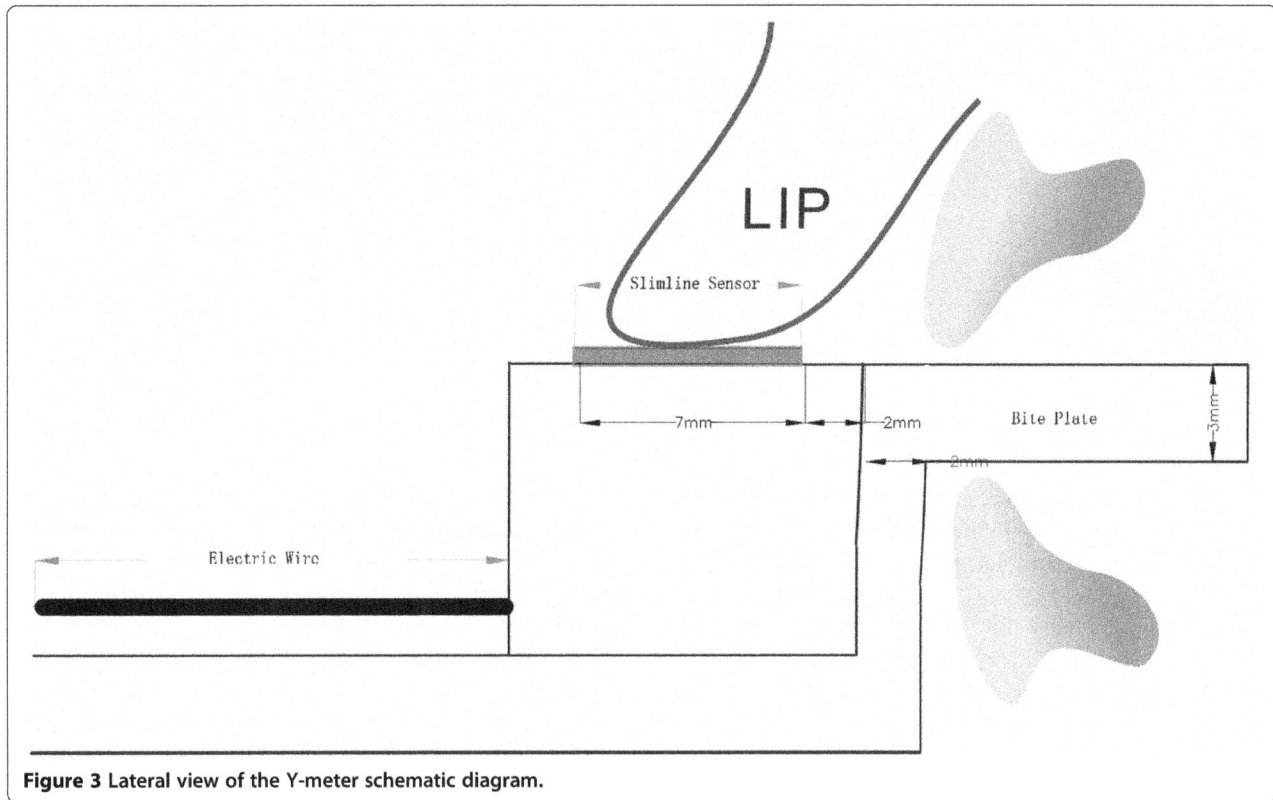

Figure 3 Lateral view of the Y-meter schematic diagram.

because of the varied functional response among individuals. Bundgaard [23] stated that similarities in occlusion and facial morphology do not account for similarities in the functional pattern. Due to the variation of functional position status, we chose peak passive lip pressure to represent it. It is also undeniable that most of the time lips are at rest, so that the static pressure for the lips also generates remarkable influence on the teeth and jaws.

Preceding studies [9-16] have shown higher upper LCF in Class I malocclusion. Among our subjects, both the average and maximum upper LCF of Class I patients showed no differences with those of the patients in the subject group (Table 2, $P > 0.05$). The different result possibly arose from distinct eligibilities of experimental design. According to Ruan's [24] theory, decreased upper lip pressure was due to maxillary retrognathia, which is one of etiologies of Class III malocclusion. However, many factors may lead to Angle Class III condition, including maxillary hypodevelopment, mandibular overdevelopment or a combination of these two. To remove the confounding factors, the subjects in our study were of normal maxillary development (average SNA 80.96 ± 1.37, within the normal range), so it may be explicable that the upper LCF showed no difference with that of control group in our study.

Lip force pattern has been demonstrated to be related to skeletal dysplasia in the maxillofacial region [9,11-15]. Thüer and Ingervall [15] measured the lip pressure of children with varying types of malocclusions and indicated that the lip pressure exerted on the upper incisors was higher in Class II division 1 than in Class I malocclusions and was lowest in children with Class II division 2 malocclusions. In our study, both average and maximum lower LCFs of the patients with mandibular prognathism

Table 1 Mean and SD of each variable

	Group 1	Group 2
SNA	80.96 ± 1.37	81.98 ± 1.23
SNB	84.63 ± 1.16	80.87 ± 1.29
ANB	−3.67 ± 0.86	1.11 ± 0.79
PP-FH	2.35 ± 0.72	1.95 ± 0.47
OP-FH	11.93 ± 1.19	12.18 ± 1.23
overbite	1.86 ± 1.05	2.65 ± 0.77
overjet	−3.24 ± 0.84	2.52 ± 0.79
UI-FH	74.07 ± 2.25	71.71 ± 2.17
FMA	34.43 ± 3.03	30.55 ± 2.56
IMPA	78.54 ± 3.88	87.77 ± 4.58
Ans-Ptm	46.77 ± 1.90	47.05 ± 1.87
MaxUL	7.59 ± 1.00	7.63 ± 0.67
AVeUL	5.94 ± 1.25	6.22 ± 0.60
MaxLL	5.19 ± 0.80	4.65 ± 0.97
AveLL	3.80 ± 0.65	3.12 ± 0.85

Table 2 Levene's test and student's *t*-test of LCF

| | Levene's test | | *t*-test for equality of means | | | | | | |
| | F | Sig. | t | df | Sig. (2-tailed) | Mean difference | Std. error difference | 95% confidence interval of the difference | |
								Lower	Upper
MaxUL	17.233	.000	-.282	131	.778	-.041	.146	-.331	.248
AveLL	35.573	.000	−1.677	131	.096	-.281	.167	-.612	.050
MaxLL	1.196	.276	3.513	130.674	.001	.541	.154	.236	.845
AveLL	2.853	.094	5.204	128.774	.000	.681	.131	.422	.940

Max UL indicates maximum upper lip closing force; Ave UL, average upper lip closing force; Max LL, maximum lower lip closing force; Ave LL, average lower lip closing force;
The *t*-test result of MaxLL and AveLL were adjusted according to the Levene's Test.

was considerably higher than those of the control group (Table 2, P < 0.001). In terms of biomechanics, the lower lip closing force was generated by the contraction of orbicularis oris muscle and mentalis muscle. The orbicularis oris muscle, annular and flat, is located in the lips around the rima oris. The mentalis muscle makes its insertion from the mandible and they interlace the orbicularis oris to an extensive degree. Overdevelopment of the mandible in vertical direction resulted in downwards and backwards rotation, which may initiate the growth remodelling of

Table 3 Results of pearson correlations

		MaxUL	AVeUL	MaxLL	AveLL
SNA	r	-.121	.039	-.223	-.174
	Sig.	.349	.764	.082	.175
SNB	r	.002	.126	-.177	-.095
	Sig.	.987	.328	.168	.463
ANB	r	-.195	-.108	-.116	-.150
	Sig.	.128	.405	.371	.245
pp-FH	r	.003	.040	-.043	-.049
	Sig.	.980	.757	.740	.705
op-FH	r	-.217	-.064	-.078	.013
	Sig.	.091	.622	.544	.922
overbite	r	.033	.028	-.425**	-.255*
	Sig.	.797	.831	.001	.045
overjet	r	-.144	-.072	-.337**	-.131
	Sig.	.265	.577	.007	.312
U1-FH	r	-.134	-.090	.032	.043
	Sig.	.299	.486	.808	.740
FMA	r	.001	-.003	.672**	.582**
	Sig.	.995	.981	.000	.000
IMPA	r	.110	.083	-.789**	-.697**
	Sig.	.396	.523	.000	.000
Ans_Ptm	r	-.003	-.094	.220	.065
	Sig.	.980	.466	.086	.615

**. Correlation is significant at the 0.01 level.
*. Correlation is significant at the 0.05 level.

these two muscles by their contraction direction and pressure tension.

Most authors have accepted the equilibrium theory of tooth position [13,25]. The tongue, cheeks, and lips are the most critical environmental determinants of tooth position. LCF plays a significant role in guiding tooth eruption and in maintaining dental arch formation and stability. In our research, the IMPA angle was significantly negatively correlated with the lower LCF (Table 3, P < 0.001). IMPA, standing for the lower incisor-mandibular plane angle, reflects the relative inclination of the lower incisor towards the mandible. Different from the normal condition, the overdevelopment of the mandible positioned the lower incisors in front of the upper incisors. This kind of situation will make the incisors lose their normal function of biting and cutting. The compensatory mechanism thus arose to make the lower incisors leaning in the lingual direction to match the upper teeth, so that the patients can eat normally.

The ANB angle usually serves as an eminent representative of the skeletal pattern, while the SNB angle has commonly been used to describe the mandibular antero-posterior relationship to the cranial base. In our research, LCF showed no discernible relationship with these skeletal indicators (Table 3, P > 0.05), indicating that LCF might have little relationship with the formation of the skeletal pattern. More likely, compared to lip force, heredity plays a more substantial role in contributing to the skeletal pattern development of MP [26] through gene function [27,28] or other neuromuscular factors.

Class III patients with long faces are widespread in Asia [2,29]. In our research, the FMA angle was substantially correlated with lower LCF (Table 3, P < 0.001). FMA, standing for the Frankfort Horizontal-Mandibular Plane Angle, reflects vertical relation of facial hard tissue and development direction of mandible. With the FMA getting larger, followed by an increase in the anterior face height, the mandible rotated downwards and backwards. That change may influence the direction and tension of perioral muscles. However, some studies have

Table 4 Stepwise multiple linear regression analysis

Dependent variable		Unstandardized coefficients		Standardized coefficients	t	Sig.
		B	Std. error	Beta		
MaxLL	(Constant)	12.192	2.119		5.753	.000
	IMPA	-.125	.019	-.602	−6.538	.000
	FMA	.082	.024	.308	3.348	.001
AveLL	(Constant)	9.112	2.096		4.347	.000
	IMPA	-.091	.019	-.544	−4.840	.000
	FMA	.054	.024	.253	2.253	.028

indicated that patients with low mandibular plane angles have greater development of their perioral and masticatory musculature than those with high angles [30,31]. Their results contained the development of masticatory musculature, including masseter, medial, lateral pterygoid muscle, etc. However, in our research, the object was restricted to the lip closing force, which is mainly generated by the orbicular muscle and the mentalis. In addition to this, the data varies significantly among different races and ethnicities, and also different test instrument could make a contribution to the discrepancy.

It was reasonable that causal relationships were more critical than correlations in explaining disease mechanism. In our research, we found that lower lip closing force of mandibular prognathism patient was related to their craniofacial structure. Base on the existing data, we cannot conclude whether it was the skeletal deformity gave rise to the abnormal lip closing force or the opposite. The deep mechanism needs our further research design and practice. A longitudinal study may be engaged.

Variations in tissue growth and the development and function of force within the oral environment often result in different types of malocclusion [16]. A better understanding of the forces in tooth-adjacent areas could contribute to diagnosing, treating, and maintaining outcomes in orthodontic patients. Further research should be focused on the causal relationships and the means to intervene in dysfunctional lip forces in the early stages of different types of malocclusion, to reduce the difficulty of subsequent treatments. Further studies in molecular biology are also needed to identify gene-environment interactions so that we can undertake research to uncover the etiology of MP.

Conclusions

The lower LCF of patients with mandibular prognathism was significantly higher than that of patients with Class I.

LCF had little impact on the formation of the jaws, but it had an influence on the position of incisors to a certain extent. The lower LCF was significantly negatively correlated with the IMPA.

The lower LCF was significantly positively correlated with the FMA.

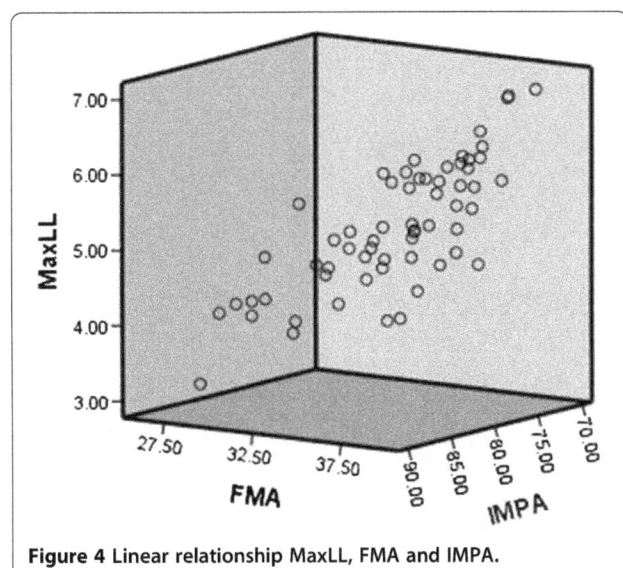

Figure 4 Linear relationship MaxLL, FMA and IMPA.

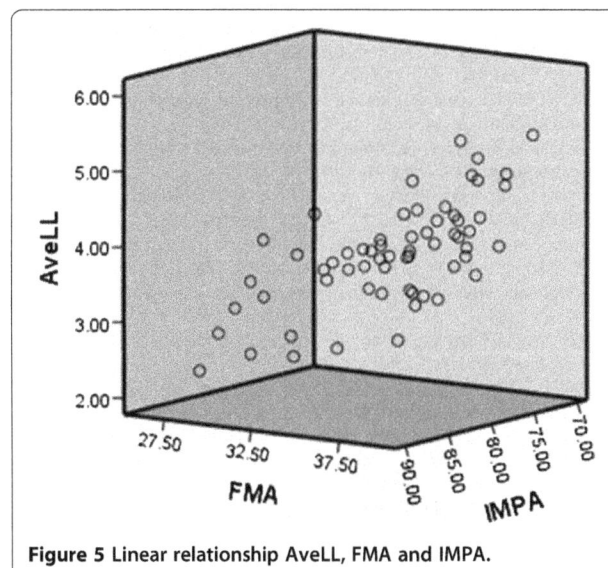

Figure 5 Linear relationship AveLL, FMA and IMPA.

Abbreviation
MP: Mandibular prognathism; LCF: Lip closing force; FMA: Frankfort
Mandibular Plane Angle; IMPA: L1 to mandibular plane angle.

Competing interests
The authors declare that they have no competing interests.

Authors' contributions
SC participated in the design of the study and acquisition of data, and
carried out the manuscript drafting. YC performed the statistical analysis and
coordination and contributed to draft the manuscript. FC conceived of the
study, and participated in its design. All authors read and approved the final
manuscript.

Acknowledgements
This work was supported by the National Natural Science Foundation of
China (No. 81170942,81371129) and the Natural Science Foundation of
Shanghai (No. 10JC1415500).

References
1. Kitai N, Takada K, Yasuda Y: School health database and its application [in Japanese]. *J Kin-To Orthod Soc* 1989, 24:33–38.
2. Johnson JS, Soetamat A, Winoto NS: A comparison of some features of the Indonesian occlusion with those of two other ethnic groups. *Br J Orthod* 1978, 5:183–188.
3. Susami R: A cephalometric study of dentofacial growth in Class III subjects with anterior crossbite [In Japanese]. *J Jpn Orthod Soc* 1967, 26:1–34.
4. Mackay F, Jones JA, Thompson R, Simpson W: Craniofacial form in Class III cases. *Br J Orthod* 1992, 19:15–20.
5. Graber LW: Chin cup therapy for mandibular prognathism. *Am J Orthod* 1977, 72:23–41.
6. Capelozza Filho L, Martins A, Mazzotini R, da Silva Filho OG: Effects of dental decompensation on the surgical treatment of mandibular prognathism. *Int J Adult Orthod* 1996, 11:165–180.
7. Singh GD: Morphologic determinants in the Etiology of class III Malocclusions: a review. *Clin Anat* 1999, 12:382–405.
8. Seren E: EMG investigation on mentalis, masseter and OOS muscles of adults with Class III malocclusion. *Turk Ortodonti Derg* 1990, 3:85–93.
9. Jung MH, Yang WS, Nahm DS: Maximum closing force of mentolabial muscles and type of malocclusion. *Angle Orthod* 2010, 80:72–79.
10. Jung MH, Yang WS, Nahm DS: Effects of upper lip closing force on craniofacial structures. *Am J Orthod Dentofacial Orthop* 2003, 123:58–63.
11. Proffit WR: Equilibrium theory revisited: factors influencing position of the teeth. *Angle Orthod* 1978, 48:175–186.
12. Lear CS, Deco RE, Ng DH: Threshold levels for displacement of human maxillary central incisors in response to lingual directed forces. *J Dent Res* 1974, 53:942.
13. Proffit WR: Muscle pressures and tooth position: North American Whites and Australian aborigines. *Angle Orthod* 1975, 45:1–11.
14. Posen AL: The influence of maximum perioral and tongue force on the incisor teeth. *Angle Orthod* 1972, 42:285–309.
15. Thüer U, Ingervall B: Pressure from the lips on the teeth and malocclusion. *Am J Orthod Dentofacial Orthop* 1986, 90:234–242.
16. Ueki K, Mukozawa A, Okabe K, Miyazaki M, Moroi A, Marukawa K, Nakagawa K: Changes in the lip closing force of patients with Class III malocclusion before and after orthognathic surgery. *Int J Oral Maxillofac Surg* 2012, 41:835–838.
17. Dahlberg G: *Statistical Methods for Medical and Biological Students*. New York: Interscience Publications; 1940.
18. Ellis E 3rd, McNamara JA Jr: Components of adult class III malocclusion. *J Oral Maxillofac Surg* 1984, 42:295–305.
19. Ruan WH, Chen MD, Gu ZY, Lu Y, Su JM, Guo Q: Muscular forces exerted on the normal deciduous dentition. *Angle Orthod* 2005, 75:785–790.
20. Bardach J, Kelly JM, Salyer KE: The effects of lip repair with and without soft-tissue undermining and delayed palate repair on maxillary growth: an experimental study in beagles. *Plast Reconstr Surg* 1994, 94:343–351.
21. Thüer U, Jason T, Ingervall B: Application in children of a new method for the measurement of forces from the lips on the teeth. *Eur J Orthod* 1985, 7:63–78.
22. Kato Y, Kuroda T, Togawa T: Perioral force measurement by a radiotelemetry device. *Am J Orthod Dentofacial Orthop* 1989, 95:410–414.
23. Bundgaard M, Bjerregard J, Melsen B, Terp S: An electro-myographic study of the effect of the mandibular lip bumper. *Eur J Orthod* 1983, 5:149–156.
24. Ruan WH, Ye XW, Su JM: Pressure from the lips and the tongue in children with Class III malocclusion. *J Zhejiang Univ Sci B* 2007, 8:296–301.
25. Weinstein S, Haack DC, Morris LY: On an equilibrium theory of tooth position. *Angle Orthod* 1963, 35:1–25.
26. Chang HP, Tseng YC, Chang HF: Treatment of Mandibular Prognathism. *J Formos Med Assoc* 2006, 105:781–790.
27. Jeong J, Li X, McEvilly RJ, Rosenfeld MG, Lufkin T, John LR: Rubenstein: Dlx genes pattern mammalian jaw primordium by regulating both lower jaw-specific and upper jaw-specific genetic programs. *Development* 2008, 135:2905–2916.
28. Balic A, Adams D, Mina M: Prx1 and Prx2 cooperatively regulate the morphogenesis of the medial region of the mandibular process. *Dev Dyn* 2009, 238(10):2599–2613.
29. Tomes CS: The bearing of the development of the jaws on irregularities. *Dental Cosmos* 1873, 15:292–296.
30. Ingervall B, Janson T: The value of clinical lip strength measurements. *Am J Orthod* 1981, 80:496–507.
31. Proffit WR, Fields HW: Occlusal forces in normal and long-face children. *J Dent Res* 1983, 62:571–574.

12

Management and prevention of acute bleedings in the head and neck area with interventional radiology

Katharina Storck[1*], Kornelia Kreiser[2], Johannes Hauber[1], Anna-Maria Buchberger[1], Rainer Staudenmaier[1], Kilian Kreutzer[3] and Murat Bas[1]

Abstract

Background: The Interventional Neuroradiology is becoming more important in the interdisciplinary treatment of acute haemorrhages due to vascular erosion and vascular tumors in the head and neck area. The authors report on acute extracranial haemorrhage in emergency situations but also on preventive embolization of good vascularized tumors preoperatively and their outcome.

Methods: Retrospective analysis of 52 patients, who underwent an interdisciplinary approach of the ORL Department and the Interventional Neuroradiology over 5 ½ years at the Department of Otorhinolaryngology, Klinikum Rechts der Isar, Technical University of Munich, Germany. Their outcome was analysed in terms of success of the embolization, blood loss, survival rate and treatment failures.

Results: 39/52 patients were treated for acute haemorrhage. Twenty-five of them attributable to vascular erosion in case of malignant tumors. Affected vessels were the common carotid artery as well as its internal and external parts with branches like the ascending pharyngeal, the facial and the superior thyroid artery.
Altogether 27/52 patients were treated for malignant tumors, 25/52 were attributable to acute haemorrhage due to epistaxis, after tonsillectomy, benign tumors and bleeding attributable to inflammations. Treatment of all patients consisted either of an unsuccessful approach via exposure, package of the bleeding, electrocoagulation or surgical ligature followed by embolization or the primary treatment via interventional embolization/stenting.

Conclusions: The common monitoring of patients at the ORL and interventional neuroradiology is an important alternative especially in the treatment of severe acute haemorrhage, following vascular erosion in malignant tumors or benign diseases. But also the preoperative embolization of good vascularized tumors must be taken into account to prevent severe blood loss or acute intraoperative bleeding.

Keywords: Interventional neuroradiology, Haemorrhage, Embolization, Head and neck, Vascular erosion

Background

The incidence of the therapeutical use of interventional neuroradiology in the head and neck is increasing especially in acute bleeding situations. The first description of therapeutic percutaneous embolization in intractable epistaxis appeared as early as 1974 [1]. Because of the intimate anatomy of the extracranial and intracranial vascular system, the treatment of acute haemorrhage and also the preoperative treatment of hypervascular tumors by an endovascular or transcutaneous technique is still reserved for specific indications and, in most cases, is still not the first choice of treatment. Classic indications may include acute arterial haemorrhage attributable to vascular erosions in carcinomas, refractory epistaxis or bleeding after tonsillectomy. But also the preoperative "downstaging" of benign and malign tumors represents a considerable amount of cases, in order to prevent severe blood loss or intraoperative haemorrhage. We present a retrospective study of 52 patients who attended the Department of Otolaryngology (ORL) of the Technical University of Munich

* Correspondence: katharina.storck@mri.tum.de
[1]Department of Otorhinolaryngology, Klinikum Rechts der Isar, Technische Universität München, Ismaningerstrasse 22, 81675 Muenchen, Germany
Full list of author information is available at the end of the article

(TUM) and who underwent intra-arterial embolization treatment at the Department of Interventional Neuroradiology, TUM, during a time span of January 2007 to May 2012 (5 ½ years).

Methods
Patients
Data were collected during a 5.5-year period. Charts were reviewed for demographics, range of indications for embolization, tumor localization and size, initial oncological treatment, localization of bleeding, tumor recurrence, survival outcome (Munich cancer register) and failure rates of the embolization. All research has been approved by the authors' ethic committee of the Technical University of Munich (Permit Number: 251/15). Fifty-two patients underwent interventional procedures including selective angiographic or transcutaneous embolization/stenting. The mean age of the entire cohort was 54.9 ± 19.7 years (Range 11–94 years). Of these patients, 35 were male and 17 were female; 38 patients presented with tumors ($n = 27$ malignant tumors, $n = 11$ benign tumors), nine patients with refractory epistaxis, three patients with refractory bleeding after tonsillectomy and two patients with bleeding because of inflammation.

The mean age of 64.8 ± 11.8 years was the highest in patients with malignant tumors and the lowest with 27.3 ± 4.8 years in patients with bleeding after tonsillectomy. Patients of the ORL, who underwent other intracranial interventions, e.g. attributable to apoplexy, were excluded.

Embolization
Generally, percutaneous embolization was performed under general anaesthesia after imaging diagnostics such as magnetic resonance imaging (MRI) or computerized tomography (CT)-scan. In every case a guiding catheter (e.g. 6 F Envoy® [Codman]) was positioned supra-aortic in the internal carotid artery (ICA), external carotid artery (ECA), vertebral artery (VA) or branches of the thyrocervical trunk by a transfemoral, transarterial access over a hydrophilic guide wire (e.g. 0.35 Glidewire® [Terumo]). The bleeding or the pathological vessels could be localized by injection of a contrast agent (Imeron 300® [Bracco]) into the vessels. In cases of solid tumorous masses with a subcutaneous or intranasal superficial localization, direct transcutaneous or transnasal respectively puncture was considered; therefor a 20 G, 88 mm coaxial needle (Spinocan® [B.Braun]) was placed under biplane fluoroscopy by means of a transarterial "roadmap". The correct position was checked by an injection of contrast agent directly through the needle. If the ICA ran nearby the target lesion a balloon was temporarily inflated in the ICA to prevent embolization of the liquid into intracranial vessels (Copernic®, BALT).

In cases of a more diffuse bleeding or multiple rather separated affected vessels the intra-arterial access was the approach of choice, in doing so a microcatheter (Prowler select® [Codman], Nautica™, Rebar™, Echelon™, Marathon™, Apollo™ [ev3]) was delivered to the target vessel over a microwire (syncro²standard® [Boston scientific], Traxcess® [Microvention]).

Embolization liquids were synthetic glue (Glubran2, [GEM S.r.l.], Histoacryl® [B. Braun]) diluted with an oily contrast agent (Lipiodol®UltraFluid [Guerbet]) at a ratio of 1:3 or an ethylene vinyl alcohol copolymer dissolved in dimethyl sulfoxide (Onyx®LES [Covidien]). Solid embolization devices were polyvinyl alcohol (PVA) particles of different sizes (150–355, 250–350, 500–700 µm; BeadBlock™ [Terumo]; Contour™ [Boston Scientific]) or bare metal coils (Axium™, Helix™ Coils, [ev3]; Deltaplush™ [Codman]), fibered coils (Helix™Fibered Coils, [ev3]) respectively. In three cases stent grafts (Fluency® [BARD]) were implanted in the common carotid artery, in one of these patients five days later the same vessel was occluded with vascular plugs (Amplatzer® [St.Jude Medical]) proximal and distal of the lesion.

Results
Acute versus elective embolization
39/52 patients (75 %) developed acute arterial haemorrhage. In 25 cases due to vascular erosion in malignant tumors, followed by refractory epistaxis ($n = 9$) and haemorrhage after tonsillectomy ($n = 3$). Only one benign tumor and one haemorrhage due to inflammation led to an acute intervention. Figure 1 shows the distribution of emergency and elective embolization depending on the diagnosis. Especially with respect to the emergency embolization of acute haemorrhage, 34/39 were successful and five unsuccessful in terms of stopping the haemorrhage.

13/52 patients underwent elective intra-arterial embolization mostly to prevent intraoperative severe blood loss due to good vascularized tumors. The elective embolization was successful in 9/13 cases in terms of "downstaging" the vascularization and successful resection of the tumor within 48 h after the embolization and failed in four cases all due to the lack of feeding vessels.

Figure 2 shows the success rate based on the diagnosis. One benign tumor resulted in a papilloma without feeding vessels. Seven failures occurred in malignant tumors, of which no feeding vessels could be detected in five cases, a palliative and only uncompleted embolization via direct puncture could be accomplished in one case and no stable embolization position could be found in one case. The last case was an unclear pharyngeal bleeding without feeding vessels with

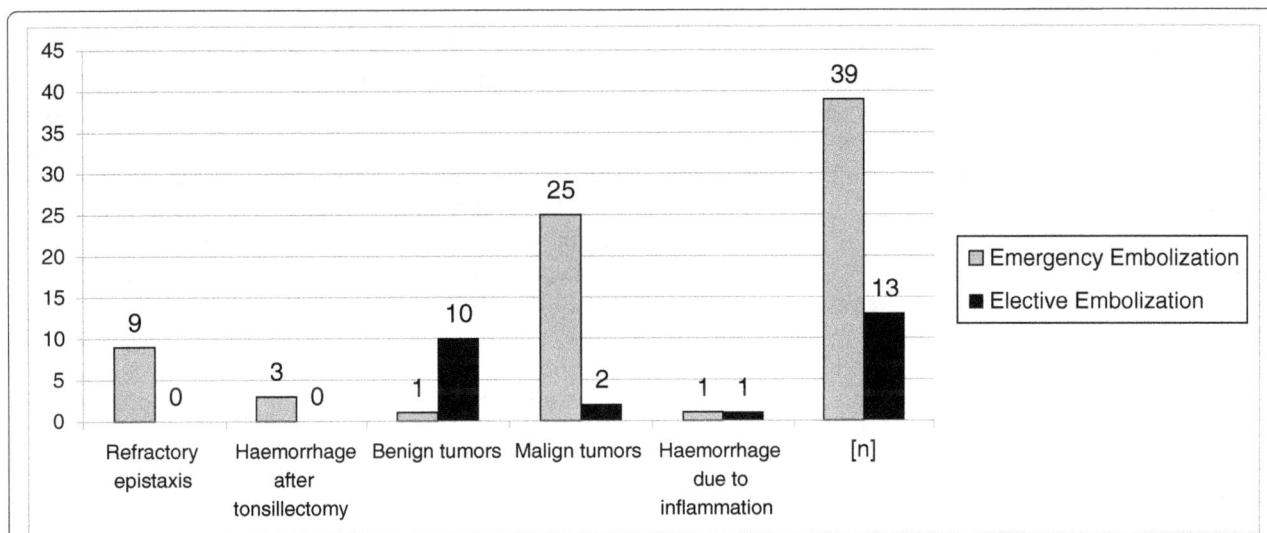

Fig. 1 Distribution of diagnosis-related emergency versus elective embolization

spontaneous suspension.Table 1 shows the reasons for the failure of the embolization.

Malignant tumors

27/52 patients were treated for malignant tumors, 25/27 of them for acute haemorrhage. Only two patients were treated for the preoperative downstaging of malignant tumors; 21/27 patients presented with head and neck squamous cell carcinoma (HNSCC) classified T1 through T4, three with thyroid carcinoma and three with other malignant tumors. Of the 21 HNSCC, 12 presented oropharyngeally, three hypopharyngeally, three laryngeally, one oro-, hypopharyngeally (2-stage carcinoma) and one oro-, hypopharyngeally and laryngeally (3-stage carcinoma). In four patients, bleeding came from the primary tumor (initial diagnosis). In 18 cases, the bleeding was attributable to a recurrence of the primary tumor

(three thyroid carcinomas, 15 HNSCC). Only three patients presented with haemorrhage without histological evidence of a recurrence of the tumor. In two patients the preoperative attempt to downstage the tumor by embolization was used without success, due to missing pathological afferent vessels. Of the 21 HNSCC patients, 13 developed acute arterial haemorrhage after primary radiotherapy, seven after surgery with adjuvant radiotherapy and only one patient after primary surgery. We also analysed the embolized vessels. A total of 36 vessels were embolized/stented: in 31 cases, branches of the external carotid artery (12 times superior and inferior thyroid artery) and in five cases, branches of the subclavian artery.

Due to a tumorous erosion of the common carotid artery a covered fluency stent graft was used for the reconstruction in two cases. Another covered fluency stent

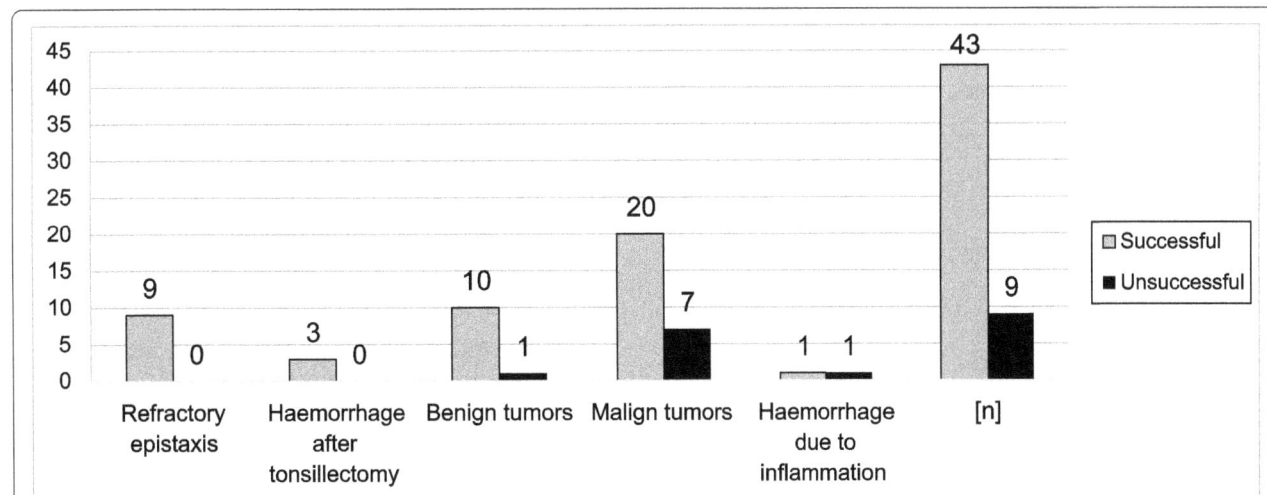

Fig. 2 Diagnosis-related success rate of the embolization

graft was used for an erosion of the common carotid artery due to a chronical inflammation.

With the assistance of the Munich Cancer Register we also obtained data concerning the survival rate of all tumor patients. The long-term follow-up of a maximum of 60 months post-interventional showed an overall survival rate of 38 % (Fig. 3).

Benign tumors

Eleven patients were treated for benign tumors preoperatively by embolization in order to minimize the vascularization and the intra-surgery bleeding. 10/11 underwent preoperative embolization, one an acute intervention due to acute intraoperative bleeding. Four patients had tumors of the glomus caroticum. All patients described an increasing not painful swelling of the neck.

Three young male patients with juvenile nasopharyngeal angiofibromas describing the typical symptoms as nose blockade, swelling of the face, headache or epistaxis. In all three patients the preoperative embolization of the tumors resulted in a satisfying resectability of the nasopharyngeal angiofibroma via midfacial degloving without remarkable side effects. Within the follow-up time span of this research none of these young patients presented with the recurrence of the tumor. Two patients presented with haemangioma with a progredient swelling of the temporal or submandibular region and one each of papilloma and chondroma. In Fig. 4, the preoperative MRI scans of a 17-year-old boy with a juvenile nasopharyngeal angiofibroma are shown. Figure 5 shows the embolization via direct puncture of the tumor.

Epistaxis

All patients ($n = 9$) who underwent emergency intra-arterial embolization for epistaxis were first treated conservatively via nasal packing and/or cautery under local anaesthesia and local vasoconstrictors or under general anaesthesia via endoscopic surgery or by septumplasty, all without success. In eight cases, posterior epistaxis could

be seen. In one case, an anterior/ posterior epistaxis in a patient with Osler's disease could be detected. In seven cases, the sphenopalatine artery was embolized, in one case the maxillary artery, in one case the ascending palatine artery and in one case the descending palatine artery. Three of the patients suffered from hypertension, two of them being additionally treated with anticoagulants. One patient suffered from Osler's disease and is well known in our department, since he presents with epistaxis at frequent intervals.

Haemorrhage after tonsillectomy

Three patients presented with severe haemorrhage after tonsillectomy. None of them were operated upon in our department. All three cases were refractory to the primary attempt of operative haemostasis through the oral cavity under general anaesthesia via ligation, cautery and oral packing. As in all three cases the colleagues of the interventional neuroradiology were already prepared for a possible intervention, embolization of the arteries was performed immediately after the operation, instead of ligating the external carotid artery via a cervical approach. The facial artery was embolized with success and neck surgery to prepare and ligate the carotid artery or it's branches was not necessary.

Blood loss

Malignant tumors

We additionally analysed the blood loss as it is one of the main reasons for the intervention to be considered. Concerning the malignant tumors, the blood loss due to acute haemorrhage was high. Of 27 patients, 15 were unsuccessfully treated by surgical haemostasis primarily. In three patients, no blood transfusion was needed. In these cases the preoperative haemoglobin level was 11.0 (± 1.5) [g/dL] and 10.1 (± 2.0) [g/dL] after the unsuccessful surgery. The preoperative haemoglobin level of the other twelve patients was 9.0 (± 2.5) [g/dL] and postoperatively 9.2 (± 2.3) [g/dL]. These twelve patients all together received 16 fresh frozen plasma and 74 red cell concentrates. 12 patients were treated by primary embolization without a primary surgical intent due to the dramatic bleeding. 10/14 did not receive blood transfusion since the haemoglobin level before the embolization was 12.2 (± 1.9) [g/dL] and after the procedure 10.9 (± 2.0) [g/dL]. In two patients, a blood transfusion was needed. The haemoglobin level was 9.8 (± 1.0) [g/dL] before and 11.1 (± 2.3) [g/dL] after the embolization. These two patients received twelve red cell concentrates all together.

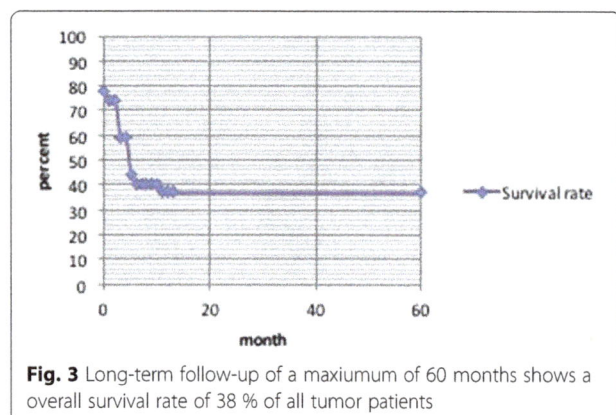

Fig. 3 Long-term follow-up of a maxiumum of 60 months shows a overall survival rate of 38 % of all tumor patients

Benign tumors

Especially in the preventive preoperative embolization of good vascularized benign tumors, the minimization of

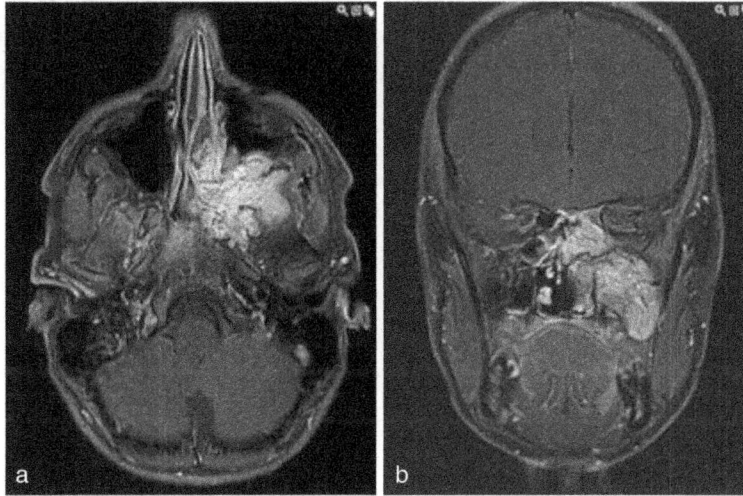

Fig. 4 Preoperative MRI Scan of a 17-year-old boy with a juvenile nasopharyngeal angiofibroma: **a** shows the axial view and **b** shows the coronary scan

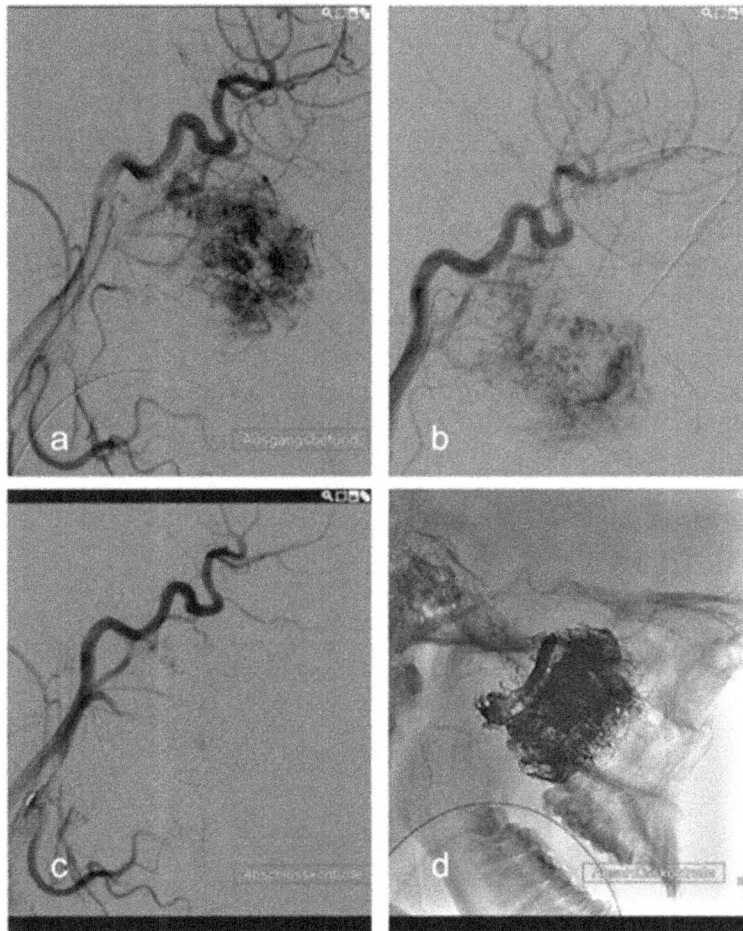

Fig. 5 Embolization of the juvenile nasopharyngeal angiofibroma via direct puncture, all in lateral view: **a** pre-interventional digital subtraction angiography. **b** example of the needle position in lateral view. **c** post-interventional control via digital subtraction angiography. **d** post-interventional digital subtraction angiography without image subtraction

Table 1 Reasons for the failure of embolization

Dignity	Diagnosis	Reason for failure
Benign tumor	Papilloma of the soft palate	No feeding vessel
Malign tumor	Hypopharyngeal HNSCC	Palliative and incomplete embolization via direct puncture
	CUP-Syndrom	No feeding vessel
	Oropharyngeal HNSCC	No feeding vessel
	Oropharyngeal HNSCC	No feeding vessel
	Plasmozytoma of the sphenoid sinus	No feeding vessel
	Oropharyngeal HNSCC	No feeding vessel
	Oropharyngeal HNSCC	No stable embolization position
Hemorrhage due to inflammation		No feeding vessel with spontaneous suspension of the bleeding

the intraoperative blood loss and the occurrence of an acute intra- or postoperative bleeding was a major issue of the embolization. One was primarily treated surgically and afterwards by embolization due to acute intraoperative bleeding. In this case, the preoperative haemoglobin level was 15 [g/dL] and after the operation 12.2 [g/dL]. Before embolization, we measured a value of 12.2 [g/dL] and afterwards a value of 9.4 [g/dL]. Hence, blood loss in total was 5.6 [g/dL]. 10/11 benign tumors received a preoperative embolization of the tumor. In eight cases, no blood transfusion was needed. The haemoglobin level before the embolization was 13.4 (±1.1) [g/dL] and after the embolization 12.3 (±1.9) [g/dL]. Surgical procedures were then performed within 48 h. The haemoglobin level was then preoperatively 14.3 (±0.8) [g/dL] and after the surgery 13.4 (±1.1) [g/dL]. In two cases, blood transfusion intraoperatively was necessary (one tumor of the glomus caroticum and one juvenile nasopharyngeal angiofibroma). Here, the haemoglobin level was 13.0 [g/dL] and after the embolization 12.1 [g/dL]. Before surgery, the haemoglobin level was 11.4 [g/dL] and after surgery and three erythrocyte concentrates 8.1 [g/dL].

One special case that needs to be mentioned was a young girl following the ingestion of an alkali liquid in an attempt of suicide and a subsequent infection of the neck due to recurrent fistulas. A severe haemorrhage of the common carotid artery attributable to inflammation occurred with dramatic blood loss. The preoperative

haemoglobin level was 9.1 [g/dL] and postoperative 6.5 [g/dL] after 20 RCCs (red cell concentrates) and 20 packed blood plasma.

The Table 2 shows the total need of RBCs and blood plasma.

Selective angiography and embolization versus direct puncture

In 52 patients, 44 received selective angiography and embolization or stenting due to active haemorrhage. Only 8 % were treated by direct puncture of the tumor. All of them were elective preoperative procedures (6 benign tumors, 2 malign tumors) for the minimization of the vasculature. Table 3 shows the distribution between the two strategies relating to the diagnosis.

Since various materials for the embolization or stenting of vessels are available, we also determined the frequencies of these possibilities. In total, materials were used in 45 cases. In seven cases, bare metal coils were used, in nine cases a mixture of acrylic glue (Glubran2®:-Lipidol (1:3)), in one case ethylene vinyl alcohol (Onyx®) and in three cases fibre coils. To ensure the patency of the carotids and to seal the outgoing vessels, covered stentgrafts (Fluency®) were used in two patients. In all other cases ($n = 23$), combinations of the above-mentioned materials were employed. No statistical significance was seen between the different materials, the outcome concerning the haemorrhage and the complications and side effects.

Table 2 Diagnosis-related need of RBCs and blood plasma

	Total number of patients [n] = 52	Number of patients with transfusions [n] = 21	Amount of RCC's [n] = 120	Amount of fresh frozen plasma [n] = 32
Epistaxis	9	3	8	2
Haemorrhage after tonsillectomy	3	2	3	0
Benign tumors	11	2	3	0
Malign tumors	27	14	86	16
Haemorrhage attributable to inflammation	2	1	20	14

Table 3 Direct puncture versus selective angiography and embolization

	Direct puncture	Selective angiography and embolization
Epistaxis	0	9
Haemorrhage after tonsillectomy	0	3
Benign tumors	6	5
Malign tumors	2	25
Haemorrhage attributable to inflammation	0	2

Discussion

In situations of acute haemorrhage and the preoperative management of vascular tumors in the extracranial head and neck area, an interdisciplinary approach of head and neck surgeons and interventional neuroradiologists sometimes offers the best therapy options. However, the selection of those patients who are suitable for this approach requires deep considerations of the pros and cons concerning their risk profile. The insertion of a microcatheter into the tumor or haemorrhage feeding vessels and the following embolization via various materials under general anaesthesia requires wide experience and a profound knowledge of the anatomy. In particular, anastomoses between the extracranial and intracranial circulations are potentially dangerous and, hence, a thorough knowledge of anatomy is essential to minimize the risk of cranial nerve palsies, blindness or stroke to name just a few. Liquid agents and small particles of < 150 μm should be used with caution because of the previously mentioned risks [2]. Our aim was to provide a broad analysis of all the data from 52 patients who underwent interventional procedures as an interdisciplinary approach between the ORL and Department of Interventional Neuroradiology of the "Klinikum Rechts der Isar", Technical University of Munich, during a 5.5-year period. The data obtained in this analysis comprises a rather heterogeneous patient population. The same applies to the choice of embolization material and interventional radiological techniques used. Taking into account that situations of acute haemorrhages are predominant with 75 % a continuous and recurring workflow could not be abstracted from the medical records. Unfortunately, this study is addressing a question which is for clinical an ethical reasons not transferable in a blinded and controlled trail and so has to deal with the limitations of retrospective gained data. To our knowledge there is no comparable data published so far.

The indications for interventional radiology can be divided into three categories [3]. The first category includes acute haemorrhage such as acute carotideal bleeding and also epistaxis. The carotid blowout can be defined as "bleeding from the carotid artery or its branches" and is one of the most feared complications, especially in advanced head and neck malignancy, whether treated surgically or with radiotherapy [4]. In our cohort, three patients suffered from tumors or inflammatory diseases which spreaded straight to the carotid arteries. The second category includes vascular lesions (e.g. tumors such as haemangioma, paraganglioma or juvenile nasopharyngeal angiofibroma or arteriovenous malformations and fistulas). The third category includes venous sampling for parathyroid hormones in the diagnostics of primary hyperparathyroidism, which is not considered in this paper [3]. Another field is the intra-arterial chemo-embolization of oral and oropharyngeal cancer, which is also not considered in this study because of the lack of patients treated by this option [5].

In our cohort nine patients (17 %) were treated for refractory epistaxis by embolization. Compared with an average of 669 (±24.8) patients a year presenting to our service with moderate to severe epistaxis and 31 of them who needed treatment under general anesthesia, the total number of nine patients in 5.5 years is small. We think it is a good alternative especially in posterior epistaxis but as shown by the results it is reserved to special refractory bleeding which can not be stopped even by an endonasal surgical approach circumventing an extracranial approach. We have not seen any of the complications described in the literature such as apoplexy, facial nerve paresis, blindness or haematomas [6]. However, a total amount of nine is too small for a reliable statement to be made. Based on long-term follow-up, we had to exclude one patient with Osler's disease who repeatedly presents to us with epistaxis. Nevertheless, the interventional embolization in the case of refractory epistaxis can be a secure and effective alternative [7–9].

Consistent with the literature, the occurrence of refractory bleeding after tonsillectomy needing to be treated by embolization is extremely low [10]. From an average of 79 (±19.53) patients per year presenting with haemorrhage after tonsillectomy and 32 of them treated under general anaesthesia, the total of three patients in 5.5 years is gladly very low. It is a good minimal invasive alternative to the conventional ligation of the afferent carotideal branches by open neck surgery if available.

In benign vascular tumors in particular, the preoperative embolization of the feeding vessels might be a good option to minimize the risk of intraoperative bleeding and to increase the possibility of resecting the whole tumor. The embolization of nasopharyngeal angiofibromas and other benign tumors has previously been described in the literature [11, 12]. In the case of juvenile angiofibromas, preoperative embolization might minimize intraoperative bleeding. In such cases, the operation site for endoscopic resection is clearer and the possibility for resecting the whole tumor and minimizing the risk of recurrence is higher. A comparison of patients with angiofibromas with or without preoperative embolization in 1975 showed that, in cases of preoperative embolization, the blood loss was halved [13].

The study of Tang et al. showed a medium range of 1 ½ litres of blood loss intraoperatively after embolization in 13 patients and only 500 ml in cases of transnasal resection. The average range of blood reserve usage was 4 l [14]. Similar results have been shown for paragangliomas and vascular malformations [15, 16]. Since, in our department, all patients with the mentioned tumors are embolized before the operation, we cannot compare the blood loss with or without the preoperative embolization, but as seen in our results only two patient needed in total three red blood cell concentrates during surgery.

The largest number of interventions involved haemorrhage attributable to malignant tumors. Of 27 patients, eight women and 19 men underwent intra-arterial or transcutaneous embolization for oncological reasons. Consistent with the known distribution of malignomas in the head and neck area, 21 patients had HNSCCs [17]. Concerning the 25 patients with haemorrhage, 21 only developed acute arterial bleeding after specific time intervals following primary therapy. Of these patients 18 patients revealed evidence of recurrent tumor disease as established by biopsy and imaging techniques (14 after previous primary R(C)T and only four after previous surgery and adjuvant R(C)T). Only three patients did not present a recurrent tumor. In comparison with these data, Greve et al. found no recurrence of tumor in all presented 10 cases [18].

In our patients, haemorrhage in malignant tumors had two different reasons. On the one hand, the recurrence of the tumor in many cases might cause an infiltration of the vessels with leakage and haemorrhage. On the other hand, bleeding is caused by long-term effects of irradiation on the vessels such as arteriosclerosis and necrotizing vasculitis [19]. These late irradiation effects might be attributable to chronic oxidative stress [20]. Especially after primary R(C)T due to inoperable tumors the doses of the radiotherapy is higher.

In four cases, haemorrhage occurred as early as the primary diagnosis of cancer. In these cases, the tumor had already infiltrated the surrounding vessels causing the bleeding.

In the long-term follow-up at 60 months, the survival rate was still 38 %, despite the high rate of recurrent tumors and the inoperability of most of the tumors. So we can assume that the embolization/stenting of the acute haemorrhage in malignant tumors can prolong the survival rate in some cases where the conventional surgery has its limits. Regarding blood loss, patients with malignant tumors and primary unsuccessful surgery had the highest need of red blood cell concentrates, with 74 RBC and 16 packs fresh frozen plasma in only twelve patients.

Conclusion

Interventional radiology has an increasingly important position in the treatment especially of acute haemorrhages but also vascular tumors in the head and neck area. In the treatment of acute bleeding due to benign diseases it minimizes the necessity of large incisions and in malignant tumors it sometimes reveals a good treatment alternative in chronical altered soft tissue due to radiotherapy or surgery. The common monitoring of these patients at the ORL, the anaesthesiologists and the Department of Interventional Radiology is necessary, especially in the treatment of severe haemorrhage following not only vascular erosion in malignant tumors, but also benign diseases such as epistaxis. However, the indication for embolization or stenting of the tumor or feeding vessels must be considered carefully because of specific complications.

Competing interest

The authors declare that they have no competing interests.

Authors' contributions

Conceived and designed the study: KS, KK(1), JH, MB(2), RS. Performed the study and analysed the data: KS, KK(1), KK(2), JH, MB(1). Wrote the paper: KS, KK(2), KK(1), MB(2). All authors read and approved the final manuscript.

Acknowledgements

The corresponding author states no financial or other relationships with other people or organizations, which may lead to a conflict of interest.

Author details

[1]Department of Otorhinolaryngology, Klinikum Rechts der Isar, Technische Universität München, Ismaningerstrasse 22, 81675 Muenchen, Germany. [2]Department of Diagnostic and Interventional Neuroradiology, Klinikum Rechts der Isar, Technische Universität München, Ismaningerstrasse 22, 81675 Muenchen, Germany. [3]Department of Maxillofacial Surgery, Universitaetsklinikum Eppendorf, Martinistraße 52, 20246 Hamburg, Germany.

References

1. Sokoloff J, Wickbom I, McDonald D, Brahme F, Goergen TC, Goldberger LE. Therapeutic percutaneous embolization in intractable epistaxis. Radiology. 1974;111:285–7.
2. Cooke D, Ghodke B, Natarajan SK, Hallam D. Embolization in the head and neck. Semin Interv Radiol. 2008;25:293–309.
3. Broomfield S, Bruce I, Birzgalis A, Herwadkar A. The expanding role of interventional radiology in head and neck surgery. J R Soc Med. 2009;102:228–34.
4. Cohen J, Rad I. Contemporary management of carotid blowout. Curr Opin Otolaryngol Head Neck Surg. 2004;12:110–5.
5. Kovacs AF, Turowski B. Chemoembolization of oral and oropharyngeal cancer using a high-dose cisplatin crystal suspension and degradable starch microspheres. Oral Oncol. 2002;38:87–95.
6. Cullen MM, Tami TA. Comparison of internal maxillary artery ligation versus embolization for refractory posterior epistaxis. Otolaryngol Head Neck Surg. 1998;118:636–42.
7. Elden L, Montanera W, Terbrugge K, Willinsky R, Lasjaunias P, Charles D. Angiographic embolization for the treatment of epistaxis: a review of 108 cases. Otolaryngol Head Neck Surg. 1994;111(1):44–50.
8. Moreau S, De Rugy MG, Babin E, Courtheoux P, Valdazo A. Supraselective embolization in intractable epistaxis: review of 45 cases. Laryngoscope. 1998;108(6):887–8.
9. Siniluoto TM, Leinonen AS, Karttunen A, Karjalainen HK, Jokinen KE. Embolization for the treatment of posterior epistaxis. An analysis of 31 cases. Arch Otolaryngol Head Neck Surg. 1993;119:837–41.

10. Levy EI, Horowitz MB, Cahill AM. Lingual artery embolization for severe and uncontrollable postoperative tonsillar bleeding. Ear Nose Throat J. 2001;80:208–11.
11. Siniluoto TM, Luotonen JP, Tikkakoski TA, Leinonen AS, Jokinen KE. Value of pre-operative embolization in surgery for nasopharyngeal angiofibroma. J Laryngol Otol. 1993;107:514–21.
12. Tikkakoski T, Luotonen J, Leinonen S, Siniluoto T, Heikkilä O, Päivänsälo M, et al. Preoperative embolization in the management of neck paragangliomas. Laryngoscope. 1997;107:821–6.
13. Pletcher JD, Newton TH, Dedo HH, Norman D. Preoperative embolization of juvenile angiofibromas of the nasopharynx. Ann Otol Rhinol Laryngol. 1975; 84:740–6.
14. Tang IP, Shashinder S, Gopala Krishnan G, Narayanan P. Juvenile nasopharyngeal angiofibroma in a tertiary centre: ten-year experience. Singapore Med J. 2009;50:261–4.
15. Persky MS, Berenstein A, Cohen NL. Combined treatment of head and neck vascular masses with preoperative embolization. Laryngoscope. 1984;94:20–7.
16. Valavanis A. Preoperative embolization of the head and neck: indications, patient selection, goals, and precautions. AJNR Am J Neuroradiol. 1986;7:943–52.
17. Wittekind C. Prognostic factors in patients with squamous epithelium carcinoma of the head and neck area and their evaluation. Laryngorhinootologie. 1999;78:588–9.
18. Greve J, Bas M, Schuler P, Turowski B, Scheckenbach K, Budach W, et al. Acute arterial hemorrhage following radiotherapy of oropharyngeal squamous cell carcinoma. Strahlenther Onkol. 2010;186:269–73.
19. Okamura HO, Kamiyama R, Takiguchi Y, et al. Histopathological examination of ruptured carotid artery after irradiation. ORL J Otorhinolaryngol Relat Spec. 2002;64:226–8.
20. Zhao W, Diz DI, Robbins ME. Oxidative damage pathways in relation to normal tissue injury. Br J Radiol. 2007;80(Spec No 1):23–31.

13

Eggshells as natural calcium carbonate source in combination with hyaluronan as beneficial additives for bone graft materials, an *in vitro* study

Jörg Neunzehn[1], Thomas Szuwart[2*] and Hans-Peter Wiesmann[1]

Abstract

Introduction: In bone metabolism and the formation especially in bone substitution, calcium as basic module is of high importance. Different studies have shown that the use of eggshells as a bone substitute material is a promising and inexpensive alternative. In this *in vitro* study, the effects of eggshell granulate and calcium carbonate towards primary bovine osteoblasts were investigated. Hyaluronan (HA) was used as artificial extracellular matrix (ECM) for the used cells to facilitate proliferation and differentiation and to mimic the physiological requirements given by the egg *in vivo*.

Methods: Hyaluronan, eggshells, a combination of hyaluronan and eggshells and $CaCO_3$ were applied to the cells as additive to the used standard medium (modified High Growth Enhancement Medium) in a concentration of 0,1 g/l. The effect of the additives in the culture medium was examined by proliferation tests, immunohistochemical staining (anti-collagen type I, anti-osteopontin, anti-osteonectin and anti-osteocalcin) and kinetic oxygen measurements.

Results: Our investigations revealed that all investigated additives show beneficial effect on osteoblast activity. Cell proliferation, differentiation and the metabolic activity of the differentiated cells could be influenced positively. Especially in the case cell cultures treated with eggshells the strongest effects were detected, while for the hyaluronan compared with eggshells, a weaker increase in cell activity was observed.

Conclusion: In summary, it can be stated that the investigated components come into consideration as beneficial supplements for bone graft materials especially for maxillo facial surgery application.

Keywords: Calcium carbonate, Eggshell, Hyaluronan, Osteoblast, Bone, Bone graft material

Introduction

In the last years, a lot of different methods and materials were used to find a proper alternative to autologous bone to treat osseous defects. The use of autologous bone is the preferred augmentation method and is therefore furthermore the gold standard.

A range of bone graft substitutes are used as alternatives to autologous grafts. The ideal bone graft material should be biocompatible, osteoinductive, osteoconductive and should have satisfactory mechanical properties. A very good solution could be the production of a composite of biomaterials which could build up all the properties needed for complete bone regeneration.

In this study, three different substances, hyaluronan, calcium carbonate and eggshell-powder were tested concerning their impact towards osteoblasts.

The mean weight of hen's eggshells is about 5.5 g and its mean thickness is between 280 – 400 µm. The essential part of eggshell is represented by mineral with 95.1%, proteins (3.3%) and water (1.6%) of the constituents. With 37.3% of the total weight, calcium is the main mineral component (the mostly in crystalline form existing calcium is calcium carbonate ($CaCO_3$) with 93.6% followed by calcium triphosphate (0.8%) and magnesium carbonate).

According to the different structures of the egg, the protein content in the eggshell could vary. The organic

* Correspondence: szuwart@uni-muenster.de
[2]Department of Cranio-Maxillofacial Surgery, University Hospital of Muenster, Research Group Vascular Biology of Oral Structures (VABOS), Waldeyerstr 30, Muenster 48149, Germany
Full list of author information is available at the end of the article

matrix of the eggshell consists mainly of a protein-polysaccharide complex containing 11% polysaccharides and at least 70% proteins [1]. Hydroxyproline isn't a component of the matrix protein [2], but in amino acid composition it is close to cartilage-protein-polysaccharides [3]. Chondroitin sulphates A and B are present in the matrix and account for approximately 35% of the total polysaccharides [1].

The calcified eggshell contains an organic matrix constituting of about 3% of the eggshells weight. Furthermore, this organic part contains proteoglycans and proteins like ovocleidin 116, ovotransferrin, ovalbumin, ovocalyxin-32, ovocleidin-17, osteopontin (OPN), and lysozyme, in which some of them are able to modify eggshell calcite crystal morphology and the rate of precipitation [4,5]. Of high interest in the context of bone metabolism is OPN. This specific protein plays a significant role in calcification by increasing osteoblast adhesion onto the matrix and binds to hydroxyapatite [4,6]. Anymore two functional roles of the eggshell proteins are the regulation of eggshell mineralization, and also the antimicrobial protection of the egg and its contents [7].

As alternative for bone substitute materials eggshells have been recently used in different in vivo studies [8,9]. Preliminary studies have focused on the biological behavior of this natural material and, more particularly, its biocompatibility and its ability to bond to the recipient bone [10]. No toxicity or inflammatory effects of this natural material are proven. In addition to its biocompatibility, avian eggshells are more than only a kind of calcium carbonate reserve. The organic components, with a special view to the proteins represented in the eggshell could be of special interest concerning osteointegration, cell migration, cellproliferation and other important steps of bone regeneration.

With approximately 95% of calcium carbonate hen eggshell has a similar mineral composition to coral. This coralline calcium carbonate is used for years to treat bone defects in dentistry and orthopedics in a converted form as hydroxyapatite and in its natural aragonite form. Because of its application as bone graft material in form of eggshells or coralline component, calcium carbonate is another investigated substance in this study [11,6,9,12-14].

Furthermore, in this study osteoblasts are also treated with hyaluronan. Hyaluronan (HA) is a natural occurring linear polysaccharide of the extracellular matrix of nearly all vertebrate animals and also as a kind of special "biofilm" around bacteria [15]. Because of its specific biochemical and physical properties hyaluronan is a quite interesting biomaterial. Its viscoelasticity is the reason why this material is one of the most important substances of different tissues and organ systems [16]. The special feature to build up hydrogen bonding

between adjacent carboxyl and N-acetyl groups when it is incorporated into aqueous solution, allows HA to maintain conformational stiffness and to retain water. In this way it is possible, that up to six liters of water could be bound up by about one gram of HA. Its physiological functions in body are shock absorption, lubrication, space filling and protein exclusion. Either more, biochemical properties of HA contain the interaction with different proteoglycans of the extracellular matrix, modulation of inflammatory cells, and scavenge of free radicals [16,17].

The in vivo application of HA and in combination with other biomaterials, bone graft materials and autologous bone has also shown good results concerning the wound healing process and bone remodeling [18,19].

Based up on these data the aim of this in vitro study is to investigate the effect of eggshells, calcium carbonate and hyaluronan as a bone substitute material by the use of proliferation tests, histological staining and cell activity/viability monitoring. The investigated substances were applied to the cells as additive to the used standard medium in a concentration of 0,1 g/l.

Methods and materials
Cell culture
The needed osteoblasts were derived from periosteum of calf metacarpus. It was cut into 3–6 mm^2 pieces and transferred into culture dishes. The osteogenic layer of the periosteum specimen were placed face downwards. Osteoprogenitor cells migrate from these tissue explants [20]. For 3 weeks the explants were cultured in High Growth Enhancement Medium (ICN Biomedicals GmbH, Eschwege, Germany) supplemented with 10% fetal calf serum, 250 µg/ml amphotericin B, 10,000 IU/ml penicillin, 10,000 µg/ml streptomycin, 200 mM L-glutamine (Biochrom KG seromed(R), Berlin, Germany) and 10 mM β-glycerophosphate, at 37°C and 5% CO_2 in humidified air. The cell culture medium was replaced once a week. Cells of the first passage were used for this study. The osteoblastic character of the cells used in this study was positively proven by immune histological staining (ALP, osteopontin, osteocalcin) during cultivation.

The cells were harvested by incubation with collagenase (Biochrom KG seromed(R)) and tyrode solution, collected and pelleted by centrifugation. The resuspended cells were seeded on the bottom of culture dishes with densities used for the different investigations. For the tests, the cell culture conditions were equal to those used for the periosteum outgrowth culture.

The substances investigated in this study were hyaluronan (HA), eggshells, a combination of hyaluronan and eggshells and $CaCO_3$. The substances were applied to the cells as additive to the used standard medium in a concentration of 0,1 g/l. The hyaluronan specimens in this study were diluted out of Ostenil® (TRB Chemedica, Germany).

Proliferation

For the proliferation tests the cells were seeded into cell culture dishes at a concentration of approximately 10 000 cells/cm². Cultures were examined regularly by light microscopy and counted at defined positions in each cell culture dish after 1d, 2d, 3d, 6d and 7d.

Histology and Immunohistochemistry

The differentiation of the osteoblasts was characterized by determination of the synthesis of bone matrix proteins. Cells were seeded at a concentration of 60 000 cells per cm² and cultivated for 4 weeks. For immunohistochemistry, the cell culture medium was decanted. The specimens were washed three times with phosphate-buffered saline (PBS). Specific antibodies were used to detect extracellular matrix proteins by immunohistochemical staining.

Anti-collagen type I, polyclonal was obtained from Bio-Trend Chemikalien GmbH, Germany, the antibodies anti-osteocalcin and anti-osteonectin were obtained from Takara, Shiga, Japan and anti-osteopontin from CHEMI-CON International Inc., Temecula, USA. For immunohistochemical staining, the DAKO EnVisionTM + –system was applied. The stained cell cultures were controlled and analysed by light microscopy. Richardson staining was accomplished with a blue dye (Methylen blue Azur II).

Cell activity/Kinetic oxygen measurement

To monitor and analyze the cell activity the CVC-96 Cell culture monitoring system (O2-Scan GmbH, Germany) in combination with the fluorescence reader FLx800 TBI (Bio-Tek, Germany) was used. The CVC96 system allows observing and evaluating the cells metabolic rate of oxygen. CVC96 is a special lid, provided with pins for each well of a 96-well plate dipping in the culture medium without penetrating the cells. The tops of these pins are covered with gas permeable membrane including a fluorescent dye, which shows its fluorescence depending of the O_2 content.

Low level of the O_2 content in the medium detects higher cell activity because the oxygen in the medium is consumed by the cells in culture [21].

The cells were seeded at a concentration of 60 000 cells per cm², cultivated up to the state of confluence and supplied with the different treated media and a standard medium. The cell activity of the cultures was measured after 30, 60 and 90 hours.

Statistics

One way analysis of variance (ANOVA) was applied for statistical analysis by the use of SigmaPlot®12 (Systat Software, Inc.). P values < 0.05 were considered significant and indicated by one*. Furthermore **indicate P < 0.01, and ***P < 0.001.

The validity and applicability of the different case groups and the appropriate values for the statistical analytic was proved by the used software Sigma Plot ®12 automatically.

Results

General findings show, that all additives investigated in this study have a beneficial effect towards osteoblast like cells activity. The cell proliferation, cell differentiation and the metabolic activity of the differentiated cells could be influenced positively.

In particular, for the cultures treated with eggshell particles the strongest effect was detected, while for the hyaluronan compared with eggshells, a weaker increase in cell activity was observed.

Proliferation

In the studies on cell proliferation, the cells in the reference culture with standard medium developed in the typical way for osteoblast like cells.

The influence of different medium supplements on the proliferation of bovine osteoblasts is observed and evaluated over a period of seven days.

Figure 1 shows the proliferation profiles of the different case groups over the whole test period of seven days. The left graph represents the results of the cell counts with the corresponding standard deviations. Also in this cell proliferation study the cell numbers of the first measuring point were normalized to 100 to revise differences in the total cell amount during cell cultivation (Figure 1 right diagram).

All cell cultures treated with the active ingredients show higher cell numbers than those of the control cultures at nearly all time points (2nd, 3rd, 5th, 7th day).

While the counts of the cells treated only by the addition of hyaluronic acid (HA) increases in a negligent way, the values of the cultures treated with eggshell (ES), calcium carbonate (CC) and the combination of eggshell with hyaluronan (HAES) significantly increases for the most time points, especially after seven days. Particularly mentionable is the cell number doubling in the samples with eggshells as medium additive from fifth to seventh day.

In addition to the proliferation curves of the different treated cell cultures shown in Figure 1, the proliferation factors related to the cell populations on day 1, clarify the high cell number increases in the groups CC, HAES and PO in relation to the control cultures and the case group HA (Figure 2). This has apparently no significant proliferation-enhancing effect on the primary osteoblasts.

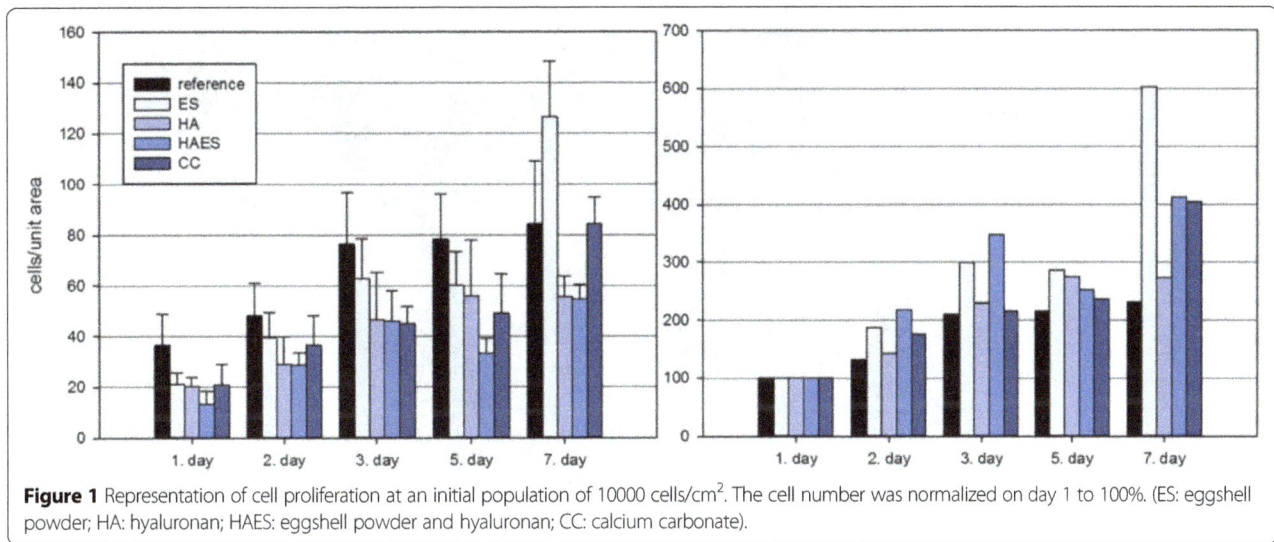

Figure 1 Representation of cell proliferation at an initial population of 10000 cells/cm². The cell number was normalized on day 1 to 100%. (ES: eggshell powder; HA: hyaluronan; HAES: eggshell powder and hyaluronan; CC: calcium carbonate).

Cell morphology and cell differentiation

All cultures are vital over the experimental period of 4 weeks. The cell cultures treated with eggshells and the combination eggshell/hyaluronan showed clear signs of aging. After that period the cultures were not as rich in cells and show first indication of imminent mineralization. After two weeks, all cultures are still rich in cells, but they differ occasionally significantly concerning their level of development and differentiation. Therefore, this point in time was chosen for the comparative representation. The synthesis and characterization of the degree of differentiation of the cells is shown in a Richardson overview staining and analysis of the expression pattern of the bone-specific markers collagen I, osteonectin and osteocalcin.

In all cultures, from the first week osteonectin and collagen type I are expressed clearly. From the second week, all cultures provided with a supplemented medium show distinct but partially still weak and not area-covering osteocalcin signals. Osteocalcin as an indicator for possible mineralization is particularly represented at this points.

Richardson staining

Figure 3 shows the results of the overview staining of a control culture and investigated case groups treated with eggshell powder, calcium carbonate, hyaluronan and hyaluronan combined with the eggshell powder as medium supplement.

In contrast to the cultures treated with the medium additives, the control group shows a very homogeneous stained cell layer with relatively even distributed nuclei, which appear very uniform in size and round-oval shape (Figure 3a). The clearest difference from the control is shown in Figure 3e, representing the HAES starved cells with a high nuclear density. The cell nuclei appear much smaller and have lost their round shape. They seem to be edgier than the nuclei of the other case groups. Intercellular open spaces have been built, streaked with a fibrillar network (Figure 3e). The cultures treated with hyaluronan (Figure 3d) and CC (Figure 3c) are very similar. Their nuclei have variations in relation of their form, but are not as small and edgy as the nuclei of the HAES cultures. In contrast to the control cultures, both treated cultures show extra- and intercellular free spaces that are filled with a fine, blue stained network structure (Figures 3c and d). The cell cultures supplied with ES represent the highest cell density with relatively closely spaced and intensively stained cell nuclei. These are surrounded by a very pronounced intercellular network structure (Figure 3b).

Expression of type I collagen

Figure 4 illustrates the comparable collagen expression of the control cultures (Figure 4a) and the cell cultures treated with ES (Figure 4b) concerning the collagen structure formation. Intercellular unstained areas are

medium additive	ES	ESHA	CC	HA	reference
proliferation factor	6,03	4,13	4,05	2,73	2,31

Figure 2 Proliferation factors of the different cell cultures (ES/eggshell, ESHA/eggshell + hyaluronan, CC/calcium carbonate, HA/hyaluronan) after seven days of cultivation.

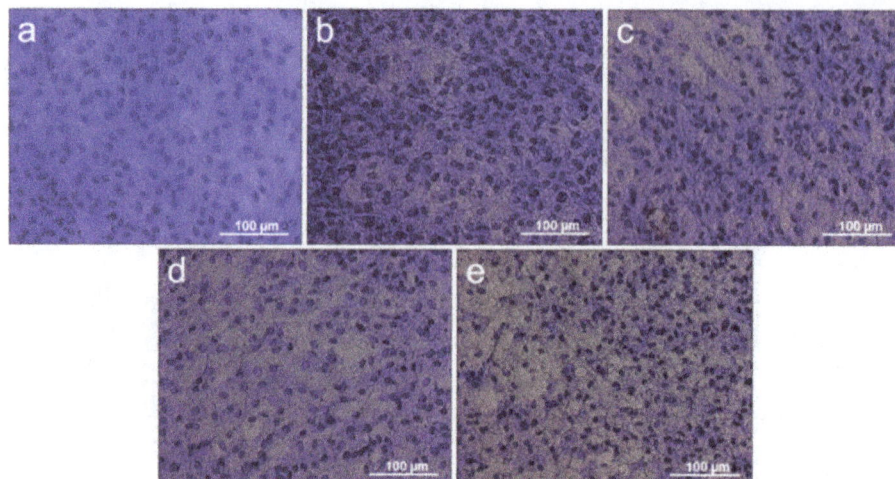

Figure 3 Richardson overview staining. **a)** control culture, cell cultures treated with **b)** eggshell powder (ES), **c)** calcium carbonate (CC), **d)** hyaluronan (HA), **e)** hyaluronan + eggshell powder (HAES) as cell culture medium supplement.

recognizable. The collagen appears more stained in the control group (Figure 4a).

Apart from the intensity of the color, the other three case groups appear very similar. The collagen network seems to be more pronounced than the collagen structures of the control and ES cultures. The infrequent intercellular, not collagenous open spaces of the case groups HA (Figure 4d) and HAES (Figure 4e) are slightly stained in contrast to all other investigated specimens. With HAES treated cells appear to be stained more intensely than those whose medium was enriched with HA.

Expression of osteonectin

The expression pattern of osteonectin of control, HA, CC and ES cultures are similar concerning their basic

structure as shown in Figure 5. They differ, however, considerably in the intensity of staining.

The staining intensity of reference culture (Figure 5a) is less pronounced than that of HA- (Figure 5d) and CC-cultures (Figure 5c). The expression patterns of the ES sample show a much more intense staining (Figure 5b). The staining of the HAES-cultures (Figure 5e) is comparable in intensity with the HA and CC samples. However, the weaker and stronger regions of stained HAES-culture are not as clearly distinguished from each other, as in the other cultures. The different intensities merge into each other (Figure 5e).

Expression of osteocalcin

After the culture period of two weeks, all especially treated cultures partially represent still weak and not

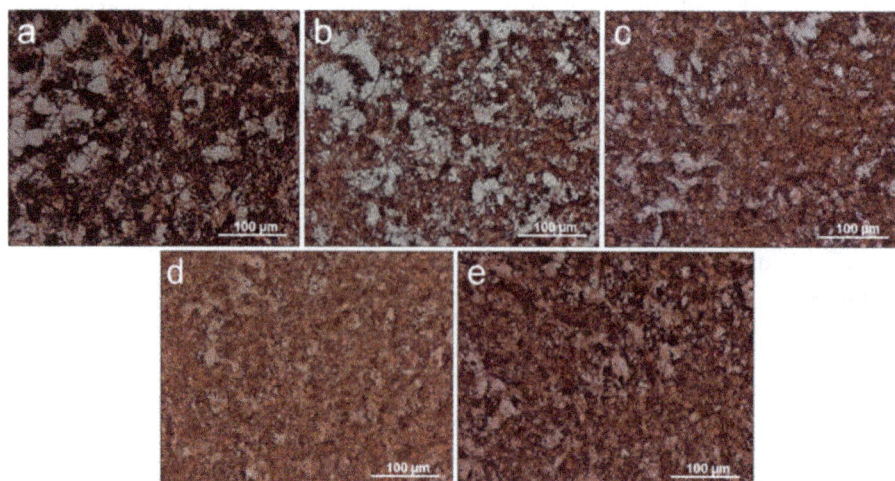

Figure 4 Immunohistochemistry staining with type I collagen on polystyrene. **a)** control culture, cell cultures treated with **b)** eggshell powder (ES), **c)** calcium carbonate (CC), **d)** hyaluronan (HA), **e)** hyaluronan + eggshell powder (HAES) as cell culture medium supplement.

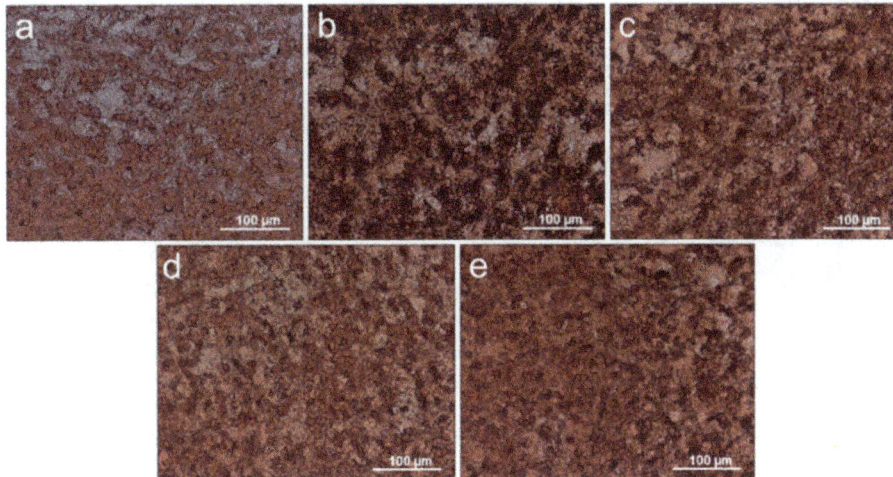

Figure 5 Immunohistochemistry staining with osteonectin on polystyrene. **a)** control culture, cell cultures treated with **b)** eggshell powder (ES), **c)** calcium carbonate (CC), **d)** hyaluronan (HA), **e)** hyaluronan + eggshell powder (HAES) as cell culture medium supplement.

comprehensive osteocalcin detections. The control and the HA-cultures show the least detectable osteocalcin expression (Figure 6a and d). The osteocalcin expression of the cells treated with CC seems to be a little bit higher (Figure 6c).

The highest attested osteocalcin expression is represented in the staining of the ES (Figure 6d) and HAES (Figure 6e) starved cells. These dark stained regions can be discerned over the entire surface of the cell culture dishes. Cells treated with HAES (Figure 6e) have significantly larger stained areas, indicating an imminent mineral formation.

Cell activity

The diagram in Figure 7 represents the results of the oxygen concentration in the different culture media of the investigated case groups. The oxygen uptake rates of the cell cultures demonstrate the cell activity. In particular, the cell cultures treated with eggshell powder, hyaluronan and calcium carbonate show at all three time points (30, 60 and 90 hours) higher cell activities compared to the reference cell culture.

The most significant effect on the oxygen consumption, and thus the cell viability of the osteoblasts, is given by hyaluronan (HA) as medium additive followed by the medium additives ES and CC. The oxygen consumption of the cells in the cultures with the drug combination HAES is similar to these of the reference. During the whole time of 90 h a slight decrease of cell activity can be observed in all case groups.

On the last measurement time point after 90 hours the fluorescence values of the three case groups ES, HA

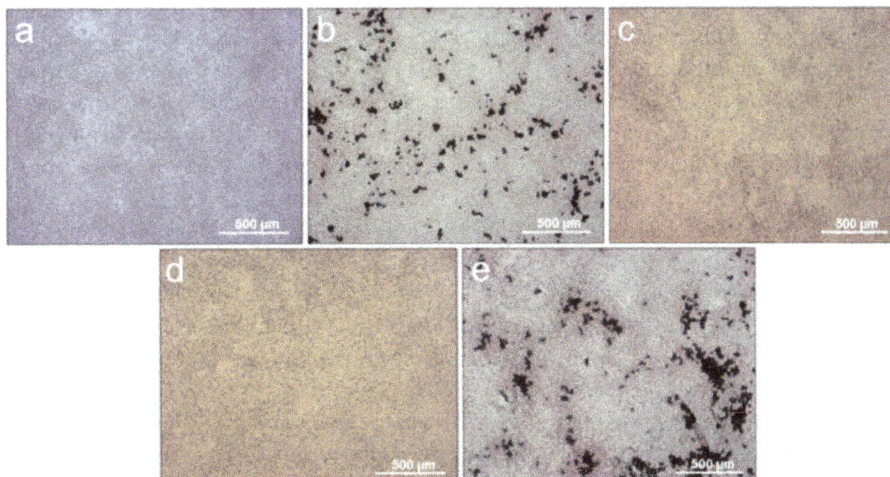

Figure 6 Immunohistochemistry staining with osteocalcin on polystyrene. **a)** control culture, cell cultures treated with **b)** eggshell powder (ES), **c)** calcium carbonate (CC), **d)** hyaluronan (HA), **e)** hyaluronan + eggshell powder (HAES) as cell culture medium supplement.

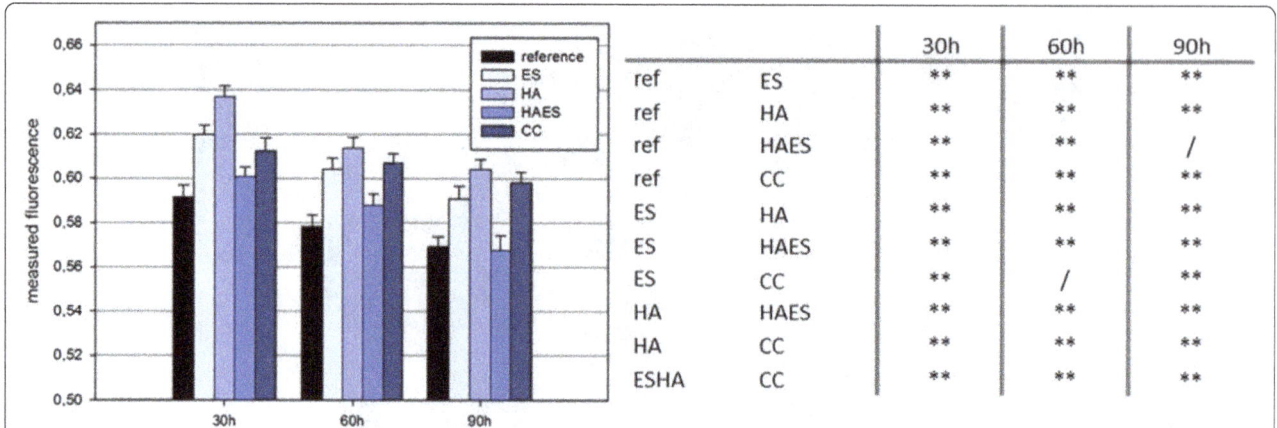

Figure 7 Representation of the fluorescence after 30 h, 60 h and 90 h, at an initial population of 60000 cells/cm^2. Note: the oxygen extinguishes the fluorescence; a high fluorescence signal indicates a low oxygen level and thus a high cell activity. Results of the pairwise one-way analysis of variance (Anova) for the different case groups at the measured time points after 30, 60 und 90 hours P values < 0.05 were considered significant and indicated by one asterisk. Furthermore **indicate P < 0.01, and ***P < 0.001 (table on the right side) (ES: eggshell powder; HA: hyaluronan; HAES: eggshell powder and hyaluronan; CC: calcium carbonate, ref: reference).

and CC is still above the measuring values of the control cultures after 30 hours.

The tabular presentation of the statistical analysis in Figure 7, in which the results of the cell activity measurements of the individual case groups are compared pairwise with each other, represents the high significance of the results, which highlights the accuracy of the results of all case groups.

Discussion

The basic approach of using eggshell particles for bone regeneration is not new, and some positive effects of the material were shown in different *in vivo* studies [22,6,23,11,9,10,1,24,25].

However, the procedure carried out in the past studies is usually limited to the filling of bone defects with different sized eggshell units. The proven effectiveness of the eggshell used usually depends on the particle size and type of particle treatment in these studies.

Dupoirieux et al. were able to demonstrate that smaller particles (with a diameter of approximately 50 μm) led to a more rapid bone healing *in vivo* than bigger ones (about 150 and 300 μm in diameter). The larger ostrich eggshell particles didn't resorb completely in the same time period [10].

The bio-inspired approach to develop a bone regeneration material in which the eggshell, as natural calcium carbonate supplier is embedded in a hyaluronan hydrogel like in this study is a new promising approach.

In this approach the hyaluronan is intended to support the active transport the released ingredients of the eggshell particles to the corresponding cells and defect edges to promote the vascularization of tissue defects as well as the wound healing *in vivo*.

Huang et al. demonstrated that hyaluronan, depending on its molecular weight, promotes a significant increase in matrix mineralization of osteoblasts [26]. One further study found that the specific application of hyaluronan normalizes the osteocalcin production in osteoarthritic osteoblasts [27]. Other authors show a promoting effect of HA on bone formation and suggest that the molecular weight and concentration of HA the differentiation behavior of the cells have a decisive influence [28,29].

Due to the large number of positive, *in vitro* confirmed properties of hyaluronan, it has also been used in combination with bone replacement materials and bone matrix for bone regeneration *in vivo*. On the field of *in vivo* studies there are no results or data found in literature were hyaluronan is combined with eggshell powder to investigate its potential concerning bone regeneration, only with eggshell in combination with carrageena gel or xanthan gum gel as support system [25]. An increase of osteoid formation was shown by the use of the different carrier materials compared towards the negative control in bone defects of rats *in vivo*. Hyaluronan was as additive in this combination was not investigated in any studies before.

The basic evaluation criteria or procedures regarding the biocompatibility and efficacy of tissue replacement and regenerative materials include cell culture experiments in which the cell activity and the response of tissue cells on the materials or substances are investigated with different methods.

Each cell activity, regardless of whether migration, proliferation or differentiation consumes oxygen. Therefore, the oxygen consumption of cells in the medium, an indicator for proliferation and differentiation is also, especially in the case of primary osteoblasts, which do not divide after formation of a confluent monolayer and start to differentiate an indicator of the cell metabolic activity. The oxygen consumption of the osteoblasts was measured by CVC96-System (O2-Scan GmbH, Germany). The analysis method and the applicability of this system was shown by Plate et al. [21].

The measurement of the cell activity that has been determined from the measured amount of oxygen in the cell culture medium clearly shows that in particular the hyaluronan treated cells show an increased cellular activity. However, the "metabolic" stimulation of the primary cells under the effect of the hyaluronan, documented in Figure 7 appears to have no significant effect on cell proliferation of the treated cells shown in Figure 1.

The cell activity measurement with a starting population of 60 000 cells per cm^2 clearly shows for all additives used in this experiment, a significantly proven increase cell activity compared to the reference cell cultures (table in Figure 2). Due to the high number of cells, it could be assumed that the cells at the differentiation level, they stopped proliferation before this measurements. Cell cultures treated with the active medium ingredients, are metabolically active in a different way, they metabolize "more" than the cells without any special treatment.

The results of the histological- and immunohistochemical detection reactions shown in Figures 3 to 6, particularly at the end of the differentiation immediately before mineral formation (shown by the high expression of osteocalcin in Figure 6) underline these findings.

In comparison to the control cultures and with hyaluronan treated cell, the investigated samples with the eggshell-powder as medium additive show a proliferation-enhancing impact towards the osteoblasts.

The higher cellular activity of the hyaluronan treated cells compared with the eggshell and calcium carbonate cell cultures are reflected both in cell proliferation and differentiation. With a proliferation factor of 6.03 after seven days cells represent the highest increase in cell number in this experimental approach.

Cell proliferation is a very important criterion for assessing the biological response to a drug in the phase prior to the actual cell differentiation. A slightly increased proliferation rate induced by eggshell powder is known both from preliminary *in vitro* studies and literature [30]. Studies concerning the mode of action of hyaluronan in combination with eggshell particles don't exist in literature.

The results of this study provide evidence that in the late phase of proliferation a beneficial effect of the additives towards the cells is provable. The first few days and the subsequent phase of the cell behavior in *in vitro* studies mainly differ in two aspects. In the first phase of the experiment, the cells adhere to the substrate, in this case the cell culture dish, and adapt to their environment. Conditioned by the relatively small number of resettlement the cells are mainly represented as single cells. Cell-cell contacts are barely detectable in this state. At this early stage, directly after cell passage, the cells exist in a limited way as osteoblasts. Their cell type specific differentiation takes place in the following days, after reaching a confluent cell monolayer with distinct cell-cell contacts.

Despite the shown unusual cell activity and proliferation factor of 4.13 (egg shell: 6.03; control: 2.31), the cells of the case group treated with hyaluronan and eggshell-powder appear, with respect to their phenotype after two weeks compared to the other groups, significantly changed. In the overview staining in Figure 3, the cell density of these cultures appears distinctly reduced and the original round-oval shape of the nuclei is irregular, partially edged and reduced in their size. These are indicators for a far advanced osteogene differentiation. This assumption is confirmed by the analysis of the immunohistochemical investigations concerning the staining of osteocalcin in Figure 6. Osteocalcin is expressed in a much higher way and a positive response towards this antibody is proven in a higher way than in the other case groups.

The cultures treated with HAES as culture medium additive additionally represent signs of imminent mineralization and compared to the other cultures a clearly increased osteocalcin expression. The osteocalcin enriched areas are strong and significantly bordered toward their surroundings. Slightly lower but also more dominant than in the other cultures the number of comparable areas of positive osteocalcin staining is recognizable in the cells supplied with the eggshell powder without hyaluronan.

The impact of the combination of eggshell powder with hyaluronan (HAES) concerning the cell phenotype and the immunohistochemical detection of osteocalcin underline the pronounced osteogene differentiation of the cells treated with HAES, compared with the eggshell treated cells, and confirms the differentiation-enhancing effect of hyaluronan-eggshell combination on tested osteoblasts.

The present cell culture study also shows a much higher efficiency of egg shell compared with the tested calcium carbonate particles with respect to cell proliferation and differentiation. An effect which could be caused by the eggshell specific proteins embedded in the calcit mineral layers of the shell. These eggshell specific proteins like ovocleidin-17, ovocleidin-116, ococalyxin-21, −25, −32 and −36, which are responsible for the biomineralization during the eggshell development in the hen's uterus are still represented in the eggshell and are also released in the eggshell degradation process during the embryo genetic development of the chick [10,31-36]. The allergenic potential and the influence of the eggshell's organic components towards immune response have to be investigated *in vivo*.

Conclusion

The results of the current *in vitro* study demonstrate the high potential of the combination of eggshell particles and hyaluronan as basic components for bone regeneration and tissue engineering.

In this study the addition of hyaluronan to eggshell particles enhances the osteogene differentiation of the cells, shown by the immunhistochemical staining, especially the osteocalcin measurements. These results correspond with the finding of other studies, where beneficial effects concerning matrix mineralization, cell differentiation and osteocalcin regulation were shown.

Competing interests
The authors declare that they have no competing interests.

Authors' contributions
All experiments were arranged and accomplished by JN supported by TS and HPW. The final manuscript was read and approved by all authors. The whole project was supervised by HPW.

Acknowledgements
The authors would like to thank the laboratory staff members of the involved groups and the members of the Department of Tissue Engineering and Biomineralization of the University of Muenster, for excellent technical assistance.
We acknowledge support by Deutsche Forschungsgemeinschaft and Open Access Publication Fund of University of Muenster.

Author details
[1]Technische Universität Dresden, Institute of Material Science, Chair for Biomaterials, Budapester Strasse 27, D-01069 Dresden, Germany.
[2]Department of Cranio-Maxillofacial Surgery, University Hospital of Muenster, Research Group Vascular Biology of Oral Structures (VABOS), Waldeyerstr 30, Muenster 48149, Germany.

References
1. Dupoirieux L, Pourquier D, Souyris F. Powdered eggshell: a pilot study on a new bone substitute for use in maxillofacial surgery. J Craniomaxillofac Surg. 1995;23(3):187–94.
2. Leach RM. Biochemistry of the organic matrix of the eggshell. Poult Sci. 1982;61(10):2040–7.
3. Baker JR, Balch DA. A study of the organic material of hen's-egg shell. Biochem J. 1962;82:352–61.
4. Pines M, Knopov V, Bar A. Involvement of osteopontin in egg shell formation in the laying chicken. Matrix Biol. 1995;14(9):765–71.
5. Panheleux M, Bain M, Fernandez MS, Morales I, Gautron J, Arias JL, et al. Organic matrix composition and ultrastructure of eggshell: a comparative study. Br Poultry Sci. 1999;40(2):240–52. doi: 10.1080/00071669987665.
6. Durmus E, Celik I, Aydin MF, Yildirim G, Sur E. Evaluation of the biocompatibility and osteoproductive activity of ostrich eggshell powder in experimentally induced calvarial defects in rabbits. J Biomed Mater Res B Appl Biomater. 2008;86(1):82–9. doi:10.1002/jbm.b.30990.
7. Rose ML, Hincke MT. Protein constituents of the eggshell: eggshell-specific matrix proteins. Cell Mol Life Sci. 2009;66(16):2707–19. doi:10.1007/s00018-009-0046-y.
8. Park JW, Jang JH, Bae SR, An CH, Suh JY. Bone formation with various bone graft substitutes in critical-sized rat calvarial defect. Clin Oral Implants Res. 2009;20(4):372–8.
9. Dupoirieux L. Ostrich eggshell as a bone substitute: a preliminary report of its biological behaviour in animals–a possibility in facial reconstructive surgery. Br J Oral Maxillofac Surg. 1999;37(6):467–71. doi:10.1054/bjom.1999.0041.
10. Dupoirieux L, Pourquier D, Neves M, Teot L. Resorption kinetics of eggshell: an in vivo study. J Craniofac Surg. 2001;12(1):53–8.
11. Baliga M, Davies P, Dupoirieux L. Powdered eggshell in the repair of cystic cavities of the jaw. Preliminary study. Rev Stomatol Chir Maxillofac. 1998;99 Suppl 1:86–8.
12. Dupoirieux L, Costes V, Jammet P, Souyris F. Experimental study on demineralized bone matrix (DBM) and coral as bone graft substitutes in maxillofacial surgery. Int J Oral Maxillofac Surg. 1994;23(6 Pt 2):395–8.
13. Schopper C, Moser D, Sabbas A, Lagogiannis G, Spassova E, Konig F, et al. The fluorohydroxyapatite (FHA) FRIOS Algipore is a suitable biomaterial for the reconstruction of severely atrophic human maxillae. Clin Oral Implants Res. 2003;14(6):743–9.
14. Schopper C, Moser D, Wanschitz F, Lagogiannis G, Spassova E, Ewers R. Histomorphologic findings on human bone samples six months after bone augmentation of the maxillary sinus with Algipore. J Long Term Eff Med Implants. 1999;9(3):203–13.
15. Pirnazar P, Wolinsky L, Nachnani S, Haake S, Pilloni A, Bernard GW. Bacteriostatic effects of hyaluronic acid. J Periodontol. 1999;70(4):370–4. doi:10.1902/jop.1999.70.4.370.
16. Laurent TC, Fraser JRE. Hyaluronan. Faseb J. 1992;6(7):2397–404.
17. Laurent UBG, Fraser JRE, Engstromlaurent A, Reed RK, Dahl LB, Laurent TC. Catabolism of hyaluronan in the knee-joint of the rabbit. Matrix. 1992;12(2):130–6.
18. Rehbein M. Hyaluronsäure als Trägersubstanz für bioaktive Proteine zur Optimierung der Knochendefektheilung. Aachen: Publikationsserver der RWTH Aachen University; http://publications.rwth-aachen.de/record/49976/files/Rehbein_Marcus.pdf; 2008.
19. Hulbert S, Morrison S, Klawitter J. Tissue reaction to three ceramics of porous and non-porous structures. J Biomed Mater Res. 1972;6(5):347–74.
20. Jones SJ, Boyde A. The migration of osteoblasts. Cell Tissue Res. 1977;184(2):179–93.
21. Plate U, Polifke T, Sommer D, Wunnenberg J, Wiesmann HP. Kinetic oxygen measurements by CVC96 in L-929 cell cultures. Head Face Med. 2006;2:6. doi:10.1186/1746-160X-2-6.
22. Schaafsma A, van Doormaal JJ, Muskiet FA, Hofstede GJ, Pakan I, van der Veer E. Positive effects of a chicken eggshell powder-enriched vitamin-mineral supplement on femoral neck bone mineral density in healthy late post-menopausal Dutch women. Br J Nutr. 2002;87(3):267–75. doi:10.1079/BJNBJN2001515.
23. Durmus E, Celik I, Ozturk A, Ozkan Y, Aydin MF. Evaluation of the potential beneficial effects of ostrich eggshell combined with eggshell membranes in healing of cranial defects in rabbits. J Int Med Res. 2003;31(3):223–30.
24. Dupoirieux L, Neves M, Pourquier D. Comparison of pericranium and eggshell as space fillers used in combination with guided bone regeneration: an experimental study. J Oral Maxillofac Surg. 2000;58(1):40–6. discussion 7–8.
25. Uraz A, Gultekin SE, Senguven B, Karaduman B, Sofuoglu IP, Pehlivan S, et al. Histologic and histomorphometric assessment of eggshell-derived bone graft substitutes on bone healing in rats. J Clin Exp Dent. 2013;5(1):e23–9. doi:10.4317/jced.50968.
26. Huang L, Cheng YY, Koo PL, Lee KM, Qin L, Cheng JC, et al. The effect of hyaluronan on osteoblast proliferation and differentiation in rat calvarial-derived cell cultures. J Biomed Mater Res A. 2003;66(4):880–4. doi:10.1002/jbm.a.10535.
27. Lajeunesse D, Delalandre A, Martel-Pelletier J, Pelletier JP. Hyaluronic acid reverses the abnormal synthetic activity of human osteoarthritic subchondral bone osteoblasts. Bone. 2003;33(4):703–10.
28. Pilloni A, Bernard GW. The effect of hyaluronan on mouse intramembranous osteogenesis in vitro. Cell Tissue Res. 1998;294(2):323–33.
29. Sasaki T, Watanabe C. Stimulation of osteoinduction in bone wound healing by high-molecular hyaluronic acid. Bone. 1995;16(1):9–15.
30. Neunzehn J, Wiesmann H. Putamen Ovi enhances biomineral formation of osteoblasts in vitro. Int J Curr Microbiol App Sci. 2014;3(3):924–36.
31. Gautron J, Hincke MT, Mann K, Panheleux M, Bain M, McKee MD, et al. Ovocalyxin-32, a novel chicken eggshell matrix protein. isolation, amino acid sequencing, cloning, and immunocytochemical localization. J Biol Chem. 2001;276(42):39243–52. doi:10.1074/jbc.M104543200.

Eggshells as natural calcium carbonate source in combination with hyaluronan as beneficial...

103

32. Gautron J, Hincke MT, Panheleux M, Garcia-Ruiz JM, Boldicke T, Nys Y. Ovotransferrin is a matrix protein of the hen eggshell membranes and basal calcified layer. Connect Tissue Res. 2001;42(4):255–67.

33. Gautron J, Murayama E, Vignal A, Morisson M, McKee MD, Rehault S, et al. Cloning of ovocalyxin-36, a novel chicken eggshell protein related to lipopolysaccharide-binding proteins, bactericidal permeability-increasing proteins, and plunc family proteins. J Biol Chem. 2007;282(8):5273–86. doi:10.1074/jbc.M610294200.

34. Hincke MT. Ovalbumin is a component of the chicken eggshell matrix. Connect Tissue Res. 1995;31(3):227–33.

35. Hincke MT, Gautron J, Panheleux M, Garcia-Ruiz J, McKee MD, Nys Y. Identification and localization of lysozyme as a component of eggshell membranes and eggshell matrix. Matrix Biol. 2000;19(5):443–53.

36. Nys Y, Gautron J, Garcia-Ruiz JM, Hincke MT. Avian eggshell mineralization: biochemical and functional characterization of matrix proteins. Comptes Rendus Palevol. 2004;3(6–7):549–62. doi: 10.1016/j.crpv.2004.08.002.

14

Headache prevalence and its characterization amongst hospital workers

Ikenna Onwuekwe[1], Tonia Onyeka[2*], Emmanuel Aguwa[3], Birinus Ezeala-Adikaibe[1], Oluchi Ekenze[1] and Elias Onuora[4]

Abstract

Background: Headaches are probably the commonest neurological complaint worldwide. Amongst workers it contributes significantly to loss of productive time and work efficiency. It is an important cause of disability and reduced quality of life. The prevalence and pattern amongst health workers in Africa has not been extensively studied.

Objective: This epidemiological sampling-based preliminary study examined the frequency and pattern of headache in a population of health workers of a tertiary hospital in Enugu, South East Nigeria.

Methods: Study participants, recruited by balloting, completed a self-administered questionnaire to screen for headache and its associations (defined as headache unrelated to fever and experienced within 6 months prior to the date the questionnaire was administered). Data analysis was by SPSS version 16. Ethical approval was obtained from the Hospital Ethical Review Committee.

Results: One hundred and thirty-three workers aged 18 – 70 years, were evaluated (males 53.4%, n = 71 and females 46.6%, n = 62). Headache was experienced by 88% of workers with primary headaches constituting more than 70% of cases. Females were more affected in both instances. Primary and secondary headaches occurred more in younger and older workers respectively and the association was significant (P <0.05). Headaches were not a significant cause of disability and loss of productivity.

Conclusion: Headaches are very prevalent in hospital workers in Enugu, Nigeria. In older workers screening for underlying causes is indicated. Disability, work absenteeism and loss of productive time are minimal despite the high headache prevalence.

Keywords: Headache, Pattern, Health workers, Nigeria

Introduction

Headache is the commonest neurological disorder in the community with variable intensity, ranging from a trivial nuisance to a severe, disabling, acute or chronic disorder, and may impose a substantial burden on sufferers and on society [1,2]. It is one of the commonest reasons for visiting the neurology clinics worldwide [3-5], exerting significant burden on its sufferers and impairing daily function especially when accompanied by other symptoms, hence

adversely affecting quality of life [6]. According to the World Health Organisation (WHO), 1.7 – 4% of the adult population of the world have headaches on 15 or more days every month [7] and a lifetime prevalence of more than 90% has been attributed to headache disorders in most populations of the world [8].

It is known that Africans have a higher threshold for pain and may not present to the clinic just for an 'ordinary headache' [9]. Local experiences show that patients suffering from other chronic neurological disorders present very late to doctors and sometimes never do so [9]. Chronic headaches produce individual and societal burdens, the former referring to its effect on family, social and

* Correspondence: doctortoniaonyeka@gmail.com
[2]Department of Anaesthesia/Pain & Palliative Care Unit, University of Nigeria Teaching Hospital, Ituku-Ozalla, PMB 01129 Enugu, Nigeria
Full list of author information is available at the end of the article

recreational activities and the latter referring to effects on healthcare cost (direct costs) and work and function (indirect costs), including absenteeism and reduced effectiveness [10].

There is limited data for headache prevalence in Africa. In 2004, the 1-year prevalence of headache from a door-to-door survey of rural south Tanzania was 23.1% (18.8% males and 26.4% females) [11]. Getahu and colleagues in Ethiopia found a 1-year prevalence rate of 73.2% [12]. A 1992 study from Ibadan, South West Nigeria, found the crude life-time prevalence for at least one episode of headache to be 51% [13].

In Nigeria, there is a paucity of data on the national prevalence and burden of chronic headaches [14] despite the fact that it is the commonest presenting neurological disorder in the authors' environment [1,3], and therefore the possibility that a big headache problem exists in Nigeria. There are also no known studies of the prevalence and characterization of headache among Nigerian healthcare workers or healthcare workers in South East Nigeria hence the relevance of this study.

Aim of the study

The aim of this preliminary study was to determine the frequency and pattern of headaches among a population of healthcare workers in a tertiary health institution located in South East Nigeria.

Methods

This was an epidemiological sampling-based study (Figure 1) using a semi-structured questionnaire. The questionnaire was pre-tested in another health facility at Nsukka (a local government area similar to the study area) for content validity. English language was used to reduce cross- cultural misinterpretations and wrong understanding of terms.

The questionnaire was self- administered to all various cadres of health workers in medical unit of University of Nigeria Teaching Hospital, a tertiary health institution located in Enugu, South- East Nigeria, over a 3- month period from September – November 2013, selected by simple random method out of the various units in the hospital e.g. surgical, medical, laboratory, physiotherapy, nutrition, administrative, laundry, transport, security, and medical record. Within these are various cadres of hospital staff: physicians, nurses, pharmacists and cleaners. Out of a total of 141 only 133 gave consent and hence were studied, giving a response rate of 94.3%. To ascertain the overall prevalence of headache, subjects were asked if they have ever had a headache within the previous six months and to note any association. They were to rate the severity of headache based on a scale of mild, moderate and severe. The impact of these severe headaches on the daily activity and the number of days they occur in a month were recorded. The character of the pain, location,

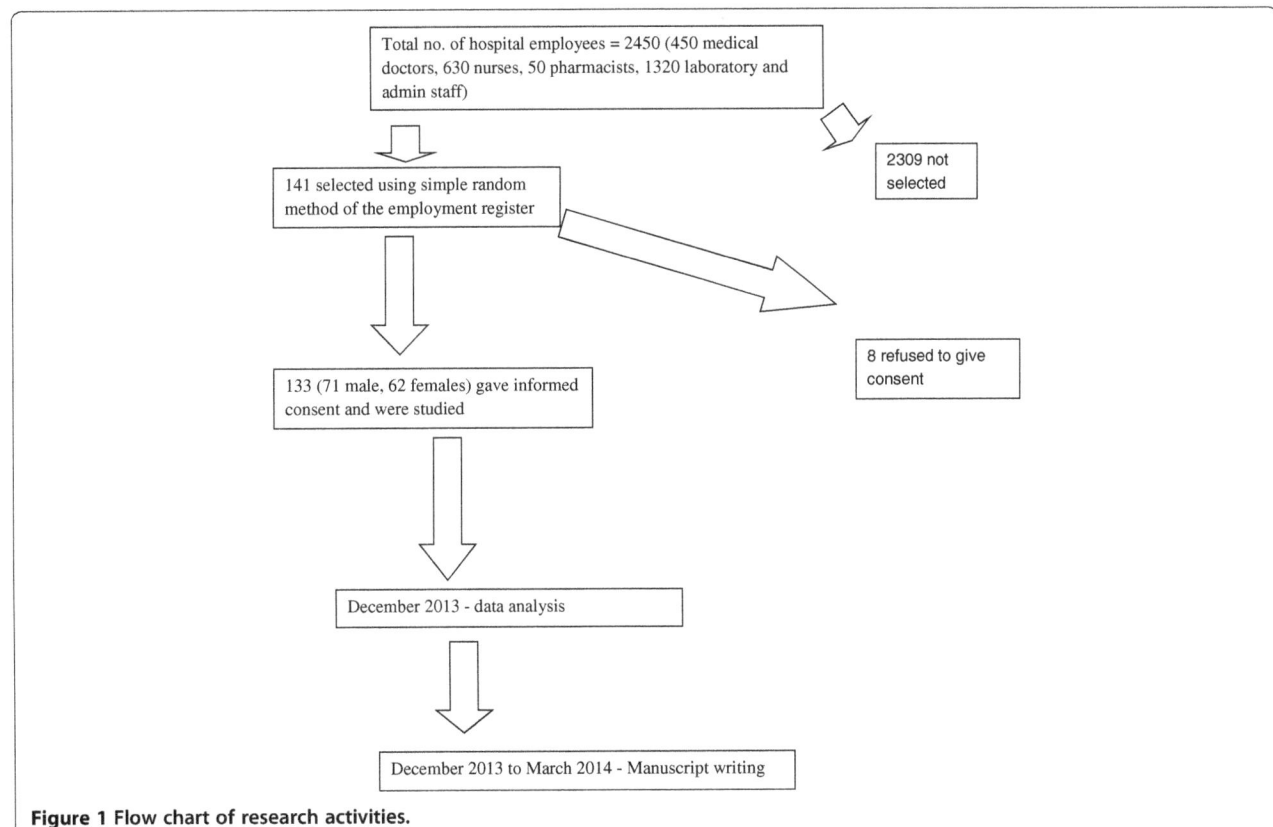

Figure 1 Flow chart of research activities.

duration, and the total numbers of times in the 6 months preceding the date of administering the questionnaire were also noted.

Statistical Package for Social Sciences version 16 was used in statistical analysis. Comparison of multiplex groups was carried out with One Way ANOVA test. On the other hand comparison of two distinct groups was carried out with student t test. Chi-square test (and/or Fisher's exact test) was used in analysis of categorical variables. The results were revealed as mean ± SD. P value <0.05 was interpreted as statistically meaningful. Ethical approval was obtained from the hospital ethics committee.

Results

Of the 2,450 hospital employees (450 medical doctors, 630 nurses, 50 pharmacists, and 1320 laboratory and administrative staff), 141 were selected using simple random method from the employment register and eventually only 133 health workers (71 males and 62 females) gave informed consent and were studied (response rate 94.3%). More of the respondents were males (53.4%) and most were within the 25 - 34 years age group (46.6%). Most of the workers had worked for only ≤5 years (72.9%). Table 1 illustrates.

The prevalence of headache in the past 6 months was 88.0% (among males the prevalence was 87.3% while in

Table 1 Demographic distribution and work experience of health workers

Variable	Frequency	Percent
Sex		
Male	71	53.4
Female	62	46.6
Total	133	100.0
Age Group		
15 – 24	13	9.8
25 – 34	62	46.6
35 – 44	36	27.1
45 – 54	15	11.3
55 – 64	6	4.5
65 and above	1	0.7
Total	133	100.0
Number of years worked		
1 – 5	97	72.9
6 – 10	18	13.5
11 – 15	7	5.3
16 – 20	4	3.0
21 – 25	5	3.8
26 – 30	2	1.5
Total	133	100.0

females it was 88.7%). There was no significant difference observed between the sexes (p = 0.806). In both sexes, primary headaches were more prevalent (71.0% in males and 76.4% in females). There was also no significant difference in the prevalence of the primary headaches among the sexes (p = 0.509). See Table 2.

Most respondents reported ≤5 episodes of headache in the last 6 months (74.4%) and these were typically of short-lasting durations, <60 minutes (44.4%). There was no observed periodicity to the headaches in 57.3% of cases (see Table 3). Most of the headaches were not located in any particular part of the head or side-locked (71.7%); were described as mildly severe in 59.8% of cases while 88.0% of respondents did not suffer any sleep disruption. The headaches were often not significantly disabling (73.4%) and in 93.2% of respondents did not lead to absenteeism or affect productivity at work (Table 4).

Stress (35.0%) and head trauma/illness/infection (18.8%) were the commonest predisposing conditions to the headache (Table 5). Refractive errors were present in 16.2% of respondents with headaches. In 25.6% there were headache prodromes and these included irritability (10.3%) and fatigue (5.1%). During the headaches, associated symptoms occurred in 30.8% of respondents and these included nasal congestion, redness of eyes, sinusitis or allergies (26.5%) as depicted in Table 6. In most cases, there was no known family history of migraines or other chronic headaches (Figure 2).

Management of headache was varied among respondents. In most cases (47.9%) no intervention was required. However in other instances, investigations (11.1%) and eye

Table 2 Prevalence of headache among the health workers

General prevalence of headache in the past 6 months		
Variables	Frequency	Percent
Headache present	117	88.0
Headache absent	16	12.0
Sex prevalence of headache		
	Male (%)	Female (%)
Headache present	62 (87.3)	55 (88.7)
Headache absent	9 (12.7)	7 (11.3)
Total	71 (100.0)	62 (100.0)
$\chi^2 = 0.060$; P value = 0.806		
Type of headache		
Primary	44 (71.0)	42 (76.4)
*Secondary	18 (29.0)	13 (23.6)
Total	62 (100.0)	55 (100.0)
$\chi^2 = 0.436$; P value = 0.509		

*Secondary headache is headache with a definitive and identifiable cause found for it i.e. those with pre-existing conditions that may cause the headache e.g. hypertension, cervical spondylosis, refractive error, sleep apnoea, malaria and other febrile conditions [15].

Table 3 Characterization of the headaches

Variable/Characteristics	Frequency (N =117)	Percent
Number of episodes in past 6 months		
1 – 5	87	74.4
6 – 10	25	21.4
11 – 15	3	2.6
16 – 20	2	1.6
Usual duration of headaches		
Seconds	19	16.2
Minutes	52	44.4
Hours	36	30.9
Days	10	8.5
Usual time of day of the headache		
Morning	18	15.4
Afternoon	15	12.8
Night	13	11.1
Continuous	4	3.4
No particular time	67	57.3
Is the headache becoming stronger, last longer or occur more frequent?		
Yes	22	18.8
No	95	81.2
What is the commonest nature of the headache?		
Throbbing/exploding	43	36.8
Sharp	4	3.4
Tightness	5	4.3
Dull	6	5.1
Aching	24	20.5
Pressure in head	32	27.3
Grinding	3	2.6

Table 4 Usual location and severity of the headache

Usual Location of headache	Frequency	Percent
Left side	3	2.6
Forehead	9	7.7
Around the head/ill-defined	11	9.4
Right side	2	1.7
Both Temples	2	1.7
Top of the head	1	0.9
Neck	2	1.7
Back of head	3	2.6
No particular side	84	71.7
Severity of headache		
Mild	70	59.8
Moderate	45	38.5
severe	2	1.7
Is the headache strong enough to wake you from sleep?		
Yes	14	12.0
No	103	88.0
Effect of headache on daily activities		
No significant disability	16	13.7
Mild disability	86	73.4
Moderate	3	2.6
Severe disability	12	10.3
Headache –related work absenteeism or reduced productivity?		
Yes	8	6.8
No	109	93.2

checks (7.7%) were done. The over-the counter- available analgesic, paracetamol, (83.8%) was the commonest treatment received (Table 7).

The health workers' ages did not significantly affect both the presence and treatment of headache (p = 0.483 and 0.293 respectively) but significantly affected the type of headache (p = 0.005) i.e. whether it was primary or secondary headache (Table 8). Years of working in the hospital did not significantly affect the prevalence of headache (P = 0.123), type of headache (P = 0.423) or treatment of the headaches (P = 0.535) as shown in Table 9. There was no correlation between the number of headache episodes and the number of years worked in the hospital [Pearson Correlation (r) = - 0.066] or age of the health worker [r = 0.001].

Discussion

Headache is the commonest presenting neurological disorder in most communities and clinical settings worldwide [2,12]. Studies from Nigeria, including Enugu, also support this [1,3,13]. The prevalence of headache in health care workers has been variously reported from Western countries [16,17] but there is a paucity of similar data from Nigeria and Africa. There was an inability to assess headaches as distinctly experienced in the various cadres of hospital workers and it was also not possible in this study to ascertain distinct headache entities and their roles. Other limitations of this study were its small sample size, the possibility of recall bias arising from patients' answers to occurrences of headaches in the past 6 months, and use of a 3-point pain scale instead of the 10-point Visual Analogue Scale (VAS) which has greater scale refinement and discrimination power. VAS has been noted to be a valid instrument for measurement of pain intensity in patients with headaches [18].

A prevalence of 88.0% was obtained for headaches amongst the hospital workers, with slightly higher rates

Table 5 Predisposing conditions to the headache

Factors preceding the headache	Frequency (N =117)	Percent
Accident, illness or infection	22	18.8
Odours	5	4.3
Fatigue	34	29.1
School	2	1.7
Hunger	17	14.5
Noise	4	3.4
Stress	41	35.0
Exercise	1	0.9
Family problem	2	1.7
Menstrual flow	2	1.7
Lack of sleep	8	6.8
Hot weather	2	1.7
None	49	41.9
Existing chronic medical conditions that may cause headache		
Hypertension	10	8.5
Cervical spondylosis	3	2.6
Refractive errors	19	16.2
Diabetes mellitus	2	1.7
Sleep apnoea	1	0.9
None	97	82.9

Note that some respondents filled more than one option.

Table 6 Headache prodromes and other features associated with the headaches

	Frequency (N =117)	Percent
Presence of warning signs before headache		
Yes	30	25.6
No	87	74.4
Warning signs		
Pallor	1	0.9
Mood swing	6	5.1
Irritability	12	10.3
Dizziness	3	2.6
Tired/sleepy	6	5.1
Rings around the eyes	1	0.9
Hyperactivity	1	0.9
Eye problems	2	1.7
None	104	88.9
Other symptoms associated with the headaches		
Presence of other symptoms during the headaches		
Yes	36	30.8
No	81	69.2
Nasal congestion, redness of eyes, sinusitis or allergies associated with the headache	31	26.5
Nausea.	2	1.7
Stomach pain	9	7.7
Vomiting	1	0.9
Confusion	3	2.6
Numbness in arms and legs	6	5.1
Diarrhoea	1	0.9
Dropping of the eyes	1	0.9
Fever	12	10.3

Note that some respondents filled more than one option.

in females than males. Though the study periods vary, the figure compares favourably with the rate of 84.4% obtained amongst from health workers in the United States [16] but is significantly higher than the 54.7% and 27.1% prevalence rates obtained from Italian and Turkish health workers respectively [16,19]. A survey of headache in Ethiopian textile workers found a prevalence of 73% [12]. The headache prevalence of 88% for hospital workers in this study compares favourably with the 88.3% prevalence found in a study of medical students in the same locality [20]. The prevalence is also higher than the community prevalence rates of 51% and 23.1% seen in Ibadan, South West Nigeria and rural south Tanzania respectively [11,13]. It is possible that the different figures may reflect a combination of environmental challenges, durations of study and varied survey instruments used.

It is well noted that females tend to have higher rates for headache prevalence across cultures and continents [1,3,12,16,17,19] and while this seemed to be the case in our study, the difference was not statistically significant. Reasons adduced for the higher female prevalence include the influence of oestrogens and progesterone on headaches after menarche and the greater propensity for females to seek medical attention for headaches [21].

Most of our subjects had probable primary headaches although no further attempts were made in this study to distinguish between the various different types (which include the trigeminal associated cephalalgias (TACs), migraine and tension- type headaches). Headaches were of short duration (<60 minutes) and were not side –locked in most instances unlike the longer duration (>6 hours) migraine headaches noted in the Turkish study [19]. Migraine headache prevalence rate is uniformly low across much of Africa but was found to be significantly high in a cohort of textile mill workers in Ethiopia [12,22].

Stress, probably related to challenges in the work environment, played the greatest role (35.0%) in this study and this reflected in the calming role attributed to relaxation techniques utilized by the health workers (40.2%) to manage their headaches. Besides life and work stress, personality traits such as aggression, anger and type A behaviour are factors that may aggravate stress and are

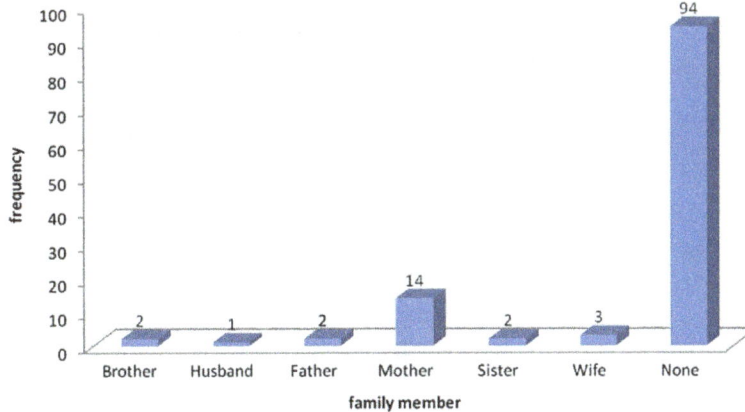

Figure 2 Family member with history of headaches, migraines, sick headaches, motion sickness or had trouble taking birth control pills because of headaches.

Table 7 Management received for the last headache episode

Management actions	Frequency (N =117)	Percent
Headache was managed by –		
Health worker	19	16.2
Self	42	35.9
No treatment received	56	47.9
A. Investigations done		
Laboratory	13	11.1
Eye check	9	7.7
B. Treatment received		
Anti-malaria	7	6.0
Ergotamine	1	0.9
Food	1	0.9
Ibuprofen	5	4.3
Other NSAIDs*	2	1.7
Paracetamol	98	83.8
Tramadol (narcotic analgesic)	1	0.9
Eye glasses were prescribed	16	13.7
Relaxation	1	0.9
Other actions that relieve the headaches		
Cold compress	13	11.1
Eating	20	17.1
Massage	3	2.6
Moving around	3	2.6
Relaxation	47	40.2
Sleep	31	26.5
Vomiting	1	0.9
Others	1	0.9

*NSAIDs = non-steroidal anti-inflammatory agents.
Note that some respondents filled more than one option.

frequently found in headache patients but were not sought for in this study [22-24].

There was no significant association or correlation found between the prevalence of headaches and years of working experience in this study. Non-pharmacological treatment was suitable for almost half of respondents (47.9%) while the over-the –counter medicine, paracetamol, was the most utilised drug treatment. This finding is essentially similar to that of health workers with headaches in the Unites States but contrasts with the use of NSAIDs in a Turkey study [17,19]. Despite working in a health facility, self-medication was commonly practised (35.9%) but this was even more significant among Turkish health workers (54.6%) [19].

The low rate of medical consultation for headache in hospital workers is of interest. In this study centre, headache ranks low among the disorders seen at both the Pain Clinic and Neurology Clinic accounting for only 2.7% of all neurological cases seen in the latter and 9th of the top 10 disorders encountered [3]. Some reasons adduced for the low rate of presentations to clinics for headaches as well as low rates of success in headache treatment amongst Africans include underdiagnoses or misdiagnoses due to lack of adequate knowledge by healthcare professionals, headache sufferers being ignorant of effective prophylaxis and treatment, perception of headaches as a trivial problem, and great tolerance to pain [25-29]. Other reasons include poor healthcare facilities [30], low economic power [25], gender/child discrimination [28], and unavailability of effective medication [28,29]. The authors are of the opinion that African patients' preference for/reliance on non-drug options (complementary and alternative medicine, CAM) [25,28,30] for pain relief may also be contributory.

Of important economic interest is the rarity of absenteeism from work or loss of productive time as reported in this study. These factors are important because many

Table 8 Age group and management of headache

Variables	Age group in years					
	15 -24	25 - 34	35 - 44	45 - 54	55 - 64	≤ 65
Presence of headache						
Yes	12(92.3)	53(85.5)	34(94.4)	13(86.7)	4(66.7)	1(100.0)
No	1(7.7)	9(14.5)	2(5.6)	2(23.3)	2(33.3)	0(0.0)
Total	13 (100.0)	62(100.0)	36(100.0)	15(100.0)	6(100.0)	1(100.0)
	Likelihood-ratio χ^2 = 4.480; P value = 0.483					
Type of headache						
Primary	7(58.3)	45(84.9)	27(79.4)	6(46.2)	1(33.3)	0(0.0)
Secondary	5(41.7)	8(15.1)	7(20.6)	7(53.8)	3(66.7)	1(100.0)
Total	12(100.0)	53(100.0)	34(100.0)	13(100.0)	4(100.0)	1(100.0)
	Likelihood-ratio χ^2 = 16.995; P value = 0.005 (significant)					
Treatment of headache						
Other health worker	10(83.3)	33(62.3)	18(52.9)	10(76.9)	3(66.7)	1(100.0)
Self	2(16.7)	20(37.7)	16(47.1)	3(23.1)	1(33.3)	0(0.0)
Total	12(100.0)	53(100.0)	34(100.0)	13(100.0)	4(100.0)	1(100.0)
	Likelihood-ratio χ^2 = 6.135; P value = 0.293					

headache sufferers are at the peak of their work-productive life [26]. Employers may lose an average of 12 days per year because of an employee headache syndrome [27]. The authors relate reason for the rarity of work absenteeism and loss of productive time to the majority of headaches being of a mild nature with low disabling rates. A similar negligible rate of absenteeism was the outcome among Italian health workers with headache [16].

Table 9 Number of years worked in the hospital and management of headache

Variables	Number of years worked in the hospital		
	1 - 10	11 - 20	21 - 30
Presence of headache			
Yes	101(87.8)	11(100.0)	5(71.4)
No	14(12.2)	0(0.0)	2(28.6)
Total	115(100.0)	11(100.0)	7(100.0)
	Likelihood-ratio χ^2 = 4.199; P value =0.123		
Type of headache			
Primary	75(65.2)	8(72.7)	3(42.9)
Secondary	40(34.8)	3(27.3)	4(57.1)
Total	115(100.0)	11(100.0)	7(100.0)
	Likelihood-ratio χ^2 = 1.719; P value = 0.423		
Treatment of headache			
Other health worker	78(67.8)	7(63.6)	6(85.7)
Self	37(32.2)	4(36.4)	1(14.3)
Total	115(100.0)	11(100.0)	7(100.0)
	Likelihood-ratio χ^2 = 1.250; P value = 0.535		

Conclusion

This preliminary study has revealed headaches to be common in this community of healthcare workers. However, the seemingly low effect of headache on health workers productivity in this study, despite its high prevalence rate and contrary to views [28] from other African studies, is of notable relief in a developing economy like Nigeria where health indicators are unimpressive and medical services still face huge challenges. In addition, presentation to Pain or Neurology clinic for headache disorders by respondents in this study has been shown to be low, demonstrating the need for increased and continuous health awareness on headache disorders as well as enhanced occupational health services in Nigerian hospitals. By the findings of this work, the authors encourage more robust studies on headache disorders among healthcare workers in African countries with a view to informing better practice decisions and reducing the global headache burden.

Competing interest
The authors declare that they have no competing interests.

Authors' contributions
TO and IO conceptualised the study; TO, IO, EA, BE, OE and EO designed the questionnaire and collected data; TO, EA and IO analysed the data; all authors participated in drafting the manuscript; all authors read and approved the final manuscript.

Acknowledgement
The authors are grateful to Dr. Ada Shirley for her co-operation with data collection.

Declaration
This study was not supported by a grant.

Author details

[1]Neurology Unit, Department of Medicine, University of Nigeria Teaching Hospital, Ituku-Ozalla, Enugu, Nigeria. [2]Department of Anaesthesia/Pain & Palliative Care Unit, University of Nigeria Teaching Hospital, Ituku-Ozalla, PMB 01129 Enugu, Nigeria. [3]Department of Community Medicine, University of Nigeria Teaching Hospital, Ituku-Ozalla, Enugu, Nigeria. [4]Department of Anaesthesia, University of Nigeria Teaching Hospital, Ituku-Ozalla, Enugu, Nigeria.

References

1. Onwuekwe IO, Ezeala-Adikaibe B, Ekenze OS: **Neurological disease burden in two semi-urban communities in South East Nigeria.** *Nig J Med* 2012, **1**(3):317–319.
2. Scher AL, Stewart WF, Lipton RB: **Migraine and headache: a meta-analytic approach.** In *Epidemiology of Pain.* Edited by Crombie IK, Croft PR, Linton SJ. Seattle: IASP Press; 1999:159–170.
3. Onwuekwe IO, Ezeala-Adikaibe B: **Prevalence and distribution of neurological disease in a Neurology Clinic in Enugu, Nigeria.** *Annals Med Health Science Res* 2011, **1**(1):63–68.
4. Vas J, Rebollo A, Perea-Milla E, Mendez C, Font C, Gomez-Rio M, Martin-Avila M, Cabrera-Iboleon J, Caballero MD, Olmos MA, Aguilar I, Faus V, Martos F: **Study protocol for a pragmatic randomised controlled trial in general practice investigating the effectiveness of acupuncture against migraine.** *BMC Compl Alternative Med* 2008, **8**:12.
5. Fowler TJ, Scadding JW: **Introduction.** In *Clinical Neurology.* 3rd edition. Edited by Fowler TJ, Scadding JE. London: Arnold; 2003:1–20.
6. Manack AN, Buse DC, Lipton RB: **Chronic migraine: epidemiology and disease burden.** *Curr Pain Headache Rep* 2011, **15**(1):70–78.
7. World Health Organisation (WHO): *Headache Disorders*; 2014. Available at: http://www.who.int/mediacentre/factsheets/fs277/en/ [Accessed 31 May 2014]
8. Pinder RM: **Migraine – a suitable case for treatment?** *Neuropsychiatr Dis Treat* 2006, **2**(3):245–246.
9. Patel V, Simbine AP, Soares IC, Weiss HA, Wheeler E: **Prevalence of severe mental and neurological disorders in Mozambique: a population-based survey.** *Lancet* 2007, **370**(9592):1055–1060.
10. Hu H, Markson LE, Lipton RB, Stewart WF, Berger ML: **Burden of migraine in the United States: disability and economic costs.** *Arch Intern Med* 1999, **159**:813–818.
11. Dent W, Spiss HK, Helbok R, Matuja WBP, Sheunemann S, Schmutzard E: **Prevalence of migraine in a rural area in South Tanzania: a door-to-door survey.** *Cephalalgia* 2004, **24**:960–966.
12. Takele GM, Haimanot RT, Martelleti P: **Prevalence and burden of headache in Akaki Textile Mill Workers, Ethiopia.** *J Headache Pain* 2008, **9**(2):119–128.
13. Osuntokun BO, Adeuja AO, Nottidge VA, Bademosi O, Olumide AO, Ige O, Yaria F, Schoenberg BS, Bolis CL: **Prevalence of headache and migrainous headache in Nigerian Africans: a community-based study.** *East Afr Med J* 1992, **69**(4):196–199.
14. Owolabi LF, Gwaram B: **Clinical Profile of Primary Headache disorders in Kano, Northwestern Nigeria.** *J Med Tropics* 2012, **14**(2):109–115.
15. ICHD: **International classification of headache disorders (ICHD) 3rd edition (beta version).** *Cephalalgia* 2013, **33**:629–808.
16. Hughes MD, Wu J, Williams TC, Loberger JM, Hudson MF, Burdine JR, Wagner PJ: **The experience of headaches in health care workers: opportunity for care improvement.** *Headache* 2013, **53**(6):962–969.
17. Sokolovic E, Riederer F, Szucs T, Agosti R, Sandor PS: **Self-reported headache among the employees of a Swiss University Hospital: prevalence, disability, current treatment and economic impact.** *J Headache Pain* 2013, **14**:29.
18. Lundqvist C, Benth JS, Grande RB, Aaseth K, Russel MB: **A vertical VAS is a valid instrument for monitoring headache pain intensity.** *Cephalalgia* 2009, **29**(10):1034–1041.
19. Dikici S, Baltaci D, Arslan G, Atar G, Ercan N, Yilmaz A, Kara IH: **Headache frequency among the health care workers and the relationship working conditions.** *Abant Med J* 2013, **2**(2):106–113.
20. Ezeala-Adikaibe B, Ekenze OS, Onwuekwe IO, Ulasi II: **Frequency and pattern of headache among medical students at Enugu, South East Nigeria.** *Nig J Med* 2012, **21**(2):205–208.
21. Martin BC, Dorfman JH, McMillan CA: **Prevalence of migraine headache and association with sex, age, race, and rural/urban residence: a population-based study of Georgia Medicaid recipients.** *Clin Ther* 1994, **16**:854–872.
22. Sjösten N, Nabi H, Westerlund H, Singh-Manoux A, Dartigues J, Goldberg M, Zins M, Oksanen T, Salo P, Pentti J, Kivimäki M, Vahtera J: **Influence of retirement and work stress on headache prevalence: a longitudinal modelling study from the GAZEL cohort.** *Cephalalgia* 2011, **31**(6):696–705.
23. Fichera LV, Andreassi JL: **Stress and personality as factors in women's cardiovascular reactivity.** *Int J Psychophysiol* 1998, **28**:143–155.
24. Abbate-Daga G, Fassino S, Lo Giudice R, Rainero I, Gramaglia C, Marech L, Amianto F, Gentile S, Pinessi L: **Anger, depression and personality dimensions in patients with migraine without aura.** *Psychother Psychosom* 2007, **76**:122–128.
25. Haimanot RT: **Burden of headache in Africa.** *J Headache Pain* 2003, **4**:S47–S54.
26. Vinding G, Zeeberg P, Lyngberg A, Nielsen R, Jensen R: **The burden of headache in a patient population from a specialized headache centre.** *Cephalalgia* 2007, **27**(3):263–270.
27. Von Korff M, Stewart WF, Simon D, Lipton RB: **Migraine and reduced work performance: A population-based diary study.** *Neurology* 1998, **50**(6):1741–1745.
28. Mengistu G, Alemayehu S: **Prevalence and burden of primary headache disorders among a local community in Addis Ababa, Ethiopia.** *J Headache Pain* 2013, **14**(1):30.
29. Takele GM, Tekle Haimanot R, Martelletti P: **Prevalence and burden of primary headache in Akaki textile mill workers, Ethiopia.** *J Headache Pain* 2008, **14**:119–128.
30. Haimanot RT: **Headache in the Tropics: Sub-Saharan Africa.** In *Handbook of Headache: Practical Management.* Edited by Martelletti P, Steiner T. Milan: Springer; 2011:533–540.

15

Reconstruction of facial defects with local flaps – a training model for medical students?

Florian Bauer*, Steffen Koerdt, Niklas Rommel, Klaus-Dietrich Wolff, Marco R. Kesting and Jochen Weitz

Abstract

Introduction: The lack of surgeons will be a future major problem in patient care for multifaceted reasons. Niche specialties such as OMFS face an additional drawback because of the need for dual qualification. Special surgical training that gives students the opportunity to gain experience in the techniques of plastic-reconstructive surgery (PRS) has therefore been established to promote interest in OMFS.

Methods: Two hands-on courses with 8 modules of 2 h for 10 students were established. Course modules included surgical techniques of PRS, such as local flaps in a complex facial defect on pig heads, and were supervised by two OMFS surgeons. The identical initial and final tests examined theoretical knowledge and practical skills. Questionnaires concerning basic demographic data, future career goals, and perception of surgical disciplines before and after the completion of the course were handed out.

Results: The 19 participating students (12 female, 7 male; median age 24 ± 2.24) were in their 8.31 ± 1.20 semester. Results of the tests showed improvement in knowledge following the courses (before 52.68 ± 12.64 vs. after 77.89 ± 11.37; $p < 0.05$). Based on the Likert scale, an increase in interest in a career in OFMS was observed (3.90 ± 1.18 vs. 2.72 ± 1.33; $p < 0.05$), but this was not so marked with regard to a career in a surgical discipline in general (1.93 ± 1.30 vs. 1.62 ± 1.19; $p > 0.05$). Perception of OMFS as a surgical discipline changed (3.68 ± 1.09 vs. 1.80 ± 0.64; $p < 0.05$). The following values also changed: students' perception of PRS in OMFS (14 (74.68 %) vs. 5 (25.32 %); 19 (100 %) vs. 0 (0 %)), evaluation of PRS as a study subject for medical students (7 (36.84 %) vs. 12 (63.16 %); 19 (100 %) vs. 0 (0 %)), and the interest in an OMFS elective subject (6 (31.58 %) vs. 13 (68.42 %); 18 (94.74 %) vs. 1 (5.26 %)) and as a final clinical year subject (4 (21.05 %) vs. 15 (78.95 %); 14 (73.68 %) vs. 5 (26.32 %)).

Conclusions: Hands-on courses with complex facial defects can be used to gain new professionals, even in niche specialties such as OMFS. Moreover, a hands-on course design, including innovative teaching methods and structured objective tests combined with a close student-teacher relationship and motivated instructors, is able to promote complex surgical skills in PRS.

Keywords: Teaching, Plastic-reconstructive surgery, facial defects, OMFS

Introduction

In the past, much effort has been made to interest young medical students in a career in academic surgery [1]. This seems to be especially important, as general interest in a surgical career is declining over time in medical schools [2]. Commonly, interest in surgery as a medical discipline is at a low level amongst medical students and young professionals [3]. Previous studies have shown that teaching itself has a major impact on the awareness of a medical discipline and, consequently, the attitude towards that specialty [4–6]. In course evaluations, in particular, concepts that involve practical tutorials and participation in operative procedures are rated as extremely valuable and account for a positive appreciation of the speciality [5, 7]. Even short workshops that are of only one hour in length and that convey a positive representation of the discipline are significantly able to change attitudes towards and perceptions of surgery [8, 4]. This seems especially true for plastic surgery as a report from the literature by Davis et al. proved [9]. The imminent shortage of surgeons in the near future illustrates the need

* Correspondence: florian.jm.bauer@tum.de
Department of Oral and Maxillofacial Surgery at the Klinikum rechts der Isar, Technische Universität München, Ismaningerstrasse 22, 81675 Munich, Germany

to motivate young professionals with regard to a career in surgery or a surgically orientated specialty [10]. This is especially true for the surgical field of Oral and Maxillofacial Surgery (OMFS). In many countries, dual degrees from medical and dental school are a prerequisite for the successful completion of residency. The long educational period, which comprises two complete university degree courses, might argue against choosing this subject as a future residency. Indeed, OMFS is a highly diversified specialty, which includes traumatology, cleft-lip-palate surgery, surgical oncology, orthognathic surgery, and especially plastic reconstructive surgery (PRS). However, many students associate only dental implantology with OMFS [11]. The various subspecialties within OMFS are usually affiliated with neighboring disciplines such as Otolaryngology, Pediatrics, and Plastic Surgery. The surgical reconstruction of facial defects following procedures such as ablative cancer surgery involve complex and advanced techniques that can fascinate young medical professionals and medical students alike. Therefore, an innovative curriculum has been developed that is aimed at teaching basic principles of reconstructive facial surgery to medial students in a hands-on course at university. Previous studies by Davis et al. were able to show the impact of a one day training course for a career in plastic surgery in general. 121 participants improved significantly in different key themes [9]. However, especially the reconstruction of facial defects using local flaps in OMFS is challenging for medical students. Therefore, the main goal of the current study has been to investigate the extent to which such complex surgical techniques are suitable for university medial courses and to determine the impact that a hands-on practical course can have on the perception of a surgical subspecialty such as OMFS.

Methods

Ethical approval and participants

All courses took place at the Department of Oral and Maxillofacial Surgery at the University of Technology, Munich, Germany. This study followed the Declaration of Helsinki on medical protocol and ethics, and the Institutional Review Board (IRB) of the University of Technology, Munich, Germany approved the study (No. 153/15). All participants were informed extensively and gave consent.

Course design

Two hands-on courses with 10 students each were undertaken. Each course consisted of an initial written test, eight modules of 2 h, and a final test. Course modules included basic surgical techniques, namely the radial forearm flap (RFF) as an example of microvascular free flaps, neck dissection (ND), full-thickness and split-thickness skin grafts, and local flaps such as the U-flap, kite-flap, rotation-flap, biloped-flap, and z-plasty. Each module was supervised by two OMFS surgeons. This enabled a close 1:5 student:teacher ratio. The identical first and final tests examined theoretical knowledge, which was available for self-instruction on a university-owned online platform. Practical skills were tested by using the Direct Observation of Procedural Skills (DOPS) method. Theoretical modules on RFF and ND were taught by using specially designed anatomical models [12]. Practical course modules consisted of a short theoretical introduction followed by practical tutorials with animal cadaver models, as shown in Fig. 1. Cadaver models were purchased from a local slaughterhouse. Ethical approval for use in medical education was obtained from the local IRB (No. 153/15).

Additionally, access to an online video tutorial was offered for further self-instruction. In the context of the tests, the participants were asked to answer questionnaires on various aspects concerning basic demographic data, future career goals, and perception of surgical disciplines before and after completion of the course (Table 1).

Statistical analysis

All data were analyzed by using IMB®SPSS® for Mac (version 22.0; IMB Corp., USA). Means and standard deviation (SD) were calculated, and tests of significance were performed. For normally distributed values, the t-test was performed. For values not normally distributed, the Mann–Whitney test was used. Statistical significance was defined as $\alpha = 0.05$. All p-values are local and given as two-tailed.

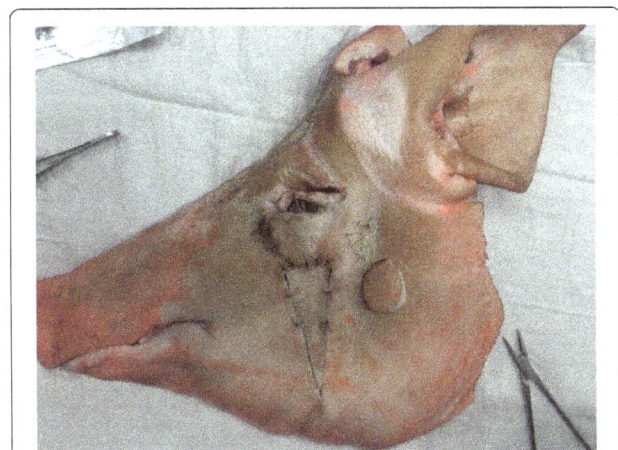

Fig. 1 Animal model used in the hands-on course for practicing local skin flaps

Table 1 Questionaire used for course evaluation

Item	Scale
Basic demographic data	
Age	
Semester	
Gender	
Possible career in surgery	Likert (1 = strongly agree to 5 = strongly disagree)
Possible career in OMFS	Likert (1 = strongly agree to 5 = strongly disagree)
Because of dual degree[1]	Yes/No
Because of speciality itself[1]	Yes/No
Perception of OMFS	Likert (1 = very good to 5 = very bad)
Is PRS part of OMFS	Yes/No
Are PRS techniques lernable for student	Yes/No
Interest in further OMFS courses	Yes/No
Interest in an externship in OMFS	Yes/No
Interest in OMFS as part of final year	Yes/No

OMFS: Oral and Maxillofacial Surgery; PRS: Plastic-Reconstructive Surgery
[1]Only had to be answered, if answer to previous question was 4 or 5 on the Likert scale

Results

A total of 19 students participated in the course and complete the evaluations. Students (12 female, 7 male; median age 24 ± 2.24 years) were in their 8.31 ± 1.20 semester in medical school at the University of Technology, Munich, Germany.

Based on the Likert scale, a statistically significant increase in students who were interested in a career in OFMS could be observed after completion of the course (3.90 ± 1.18 vs. 2.72 ± 1.33; $p < 0.05$; Fig. 2). A smaller increase could be observed concerning a career in a surgical discipline in general (1.93 ± 1.30 vs. 1.62 ± 1.19; $p > 0.05$; Fig. 2). The perception of OMFS as a surgical discipline also changed before and after completion of the course (before: 3.68 ± 1.09 vs. After: 1.80 ± 0.64; $p < 0.05$). Figure 3 visualizes the students´ perception of PRS in OMFS (before: 14 (74.68 %) vs. 5 (25.32 %); after: 19 (100 %) vs. 0 (0 %)), the evaluation of PRS as a subject in teaching for medical students (before: 7 (36.84 %) vs. 12 (63.16 %); after: 19 (100 %) vs. 0 (0 %)), and the interest in an OMFS elective subject (before: 6 (31.58 %) vs. 13 (68.42 %); after: 18 (94.74 %) vs. 1 (5.26 %)) and rotation during the final year at medical school (before: 4 (21.05 %) vs. 15 (78.95 %); after: 14 (73.68 %) vs. 5 (26.32 %)). Results of the tests also showed statistically significant improvement in the knowledge of the students (52.68 ± 12.64 vs. 77.89 ± 11.37; $p < 0.05$).

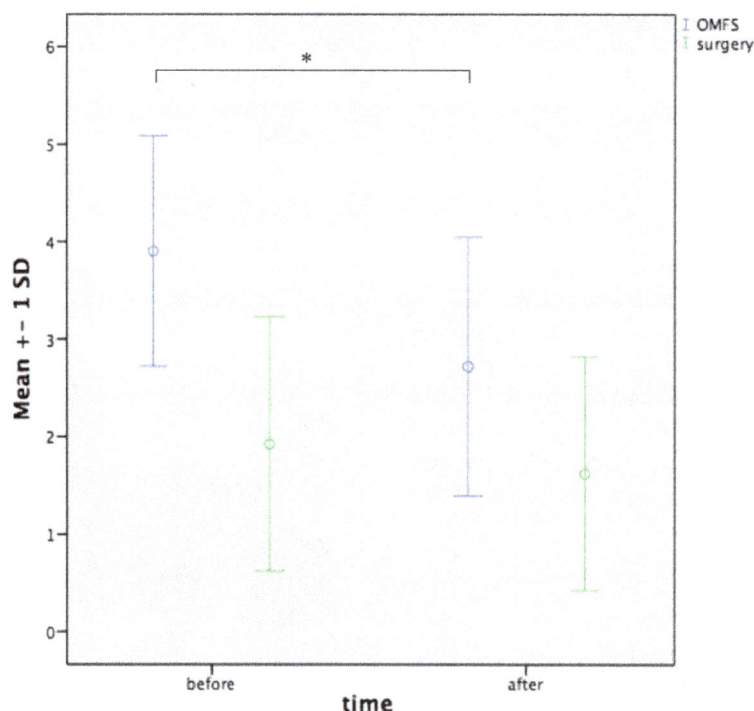

Fig. 2 Graphical illustration of students´ perception of OMFS and surgery in general, before and after completion of the course. OMFS: Oral and Maxillofacial Surgery; SD: Standard Deviation; * = $p < 0.05$

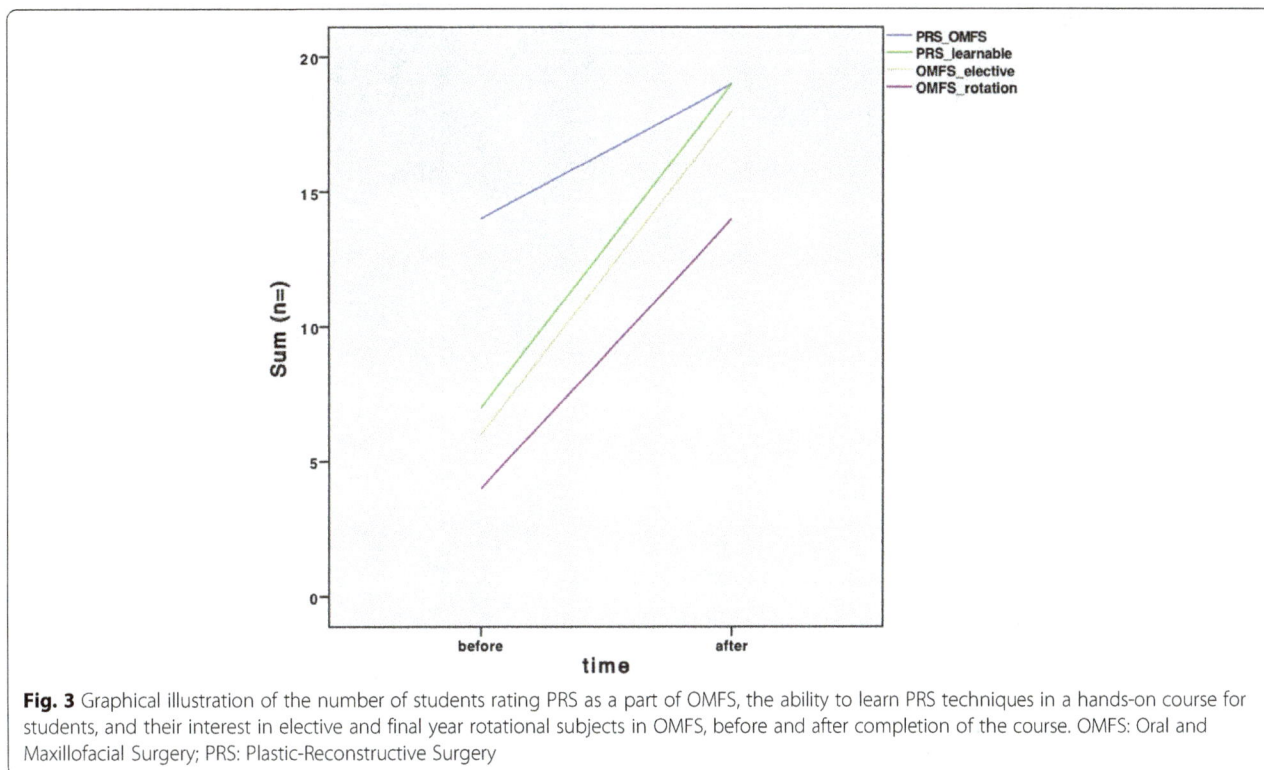

Fig. 3 Graphical illustration of the number of students rating PRS as a part of OMFS, the ability to learn PRS techniques in a hands-on course for students, and their interest in elective and final year rotational subjects in OMFS, before and after completion of the course. OMFS: Oral and Maxillofacial Surgery; PRS: Plastic-Reconstructive Surgery

Results of the final DOPS exam are displayed in Fig. 4 (all $p < 0.05$).

Discussion

In addition to patient care and research, the teaching and education of students are two of the core responsibilities in an academic medical setting. However, especially in surgery, the duties and tasks necessary in everyday patient care often collide with aims in research and teaching. Therefore, the evaluation and analysis of current concepts in teaching are of great importance [13]. The attractiveness of surgery has to be improved as a potential discipline for medical students, as a shortage of surgeons is imminent in the near future. Reasons for this are manifold. Surgical departments face new laws on working hours, an increased demand for a balanced work-life ratio, but also rising expectations for the individual academic surgeon [14]. Only about 9 % of all medical school graduates pursue a career in surgery. During medical school, potential interest in surgery can even decrease over time. Overall, more males than females are interested in the surgical field [10], despite the percentage of female medical students having continuously increased within the last few years [15]. Of all medical students, 60 % are female, whereas only 33 % of young female professionals start a career in surgery [16]. What are the reasons for this development Other studies have been able to show that an early connection with a specialty plays a major role in decision-making by young

professionals. Therefore, the satisfaction that results from working in this specialty has to be communicated to students early in their studies. Such emotional aspects can convince young professionals to chose a career in this discipline, despite all other cofactors [17]. Positive experiences and inspiring teachers are able to persuade students to become surgeons [18]. The course presented in this current study with 63 % female participation supports these ideas.

What is essential for a successful educative concept in surgery other workers have emphasized that the establishment of hand-on courses in combination with training courses has a positive effect on education [13]. In particular, the teaching of small groups in surgical courses is evaluated as significantly better than that in large groups. Furthermore, continuity and didactical training of the teaching assistants is important in a successful course design [1]. Our study group has been able to show that a structured hands-on course significantly improves the surgical skills of medical students and their self-assessment of these skills [5].

All participants in the current course were in the 7th to 10th semester in medical school. We assumed inhomogeneous previous knowledge and skills. An initial test checked the students' level according to the Kirkpatrik Level II "Learning". The results showed a certain basic theoretical knowledge, but students only possessed rudimentary practical surgical skills, including basic surgical skills. Is the teaching of complex surgical skills

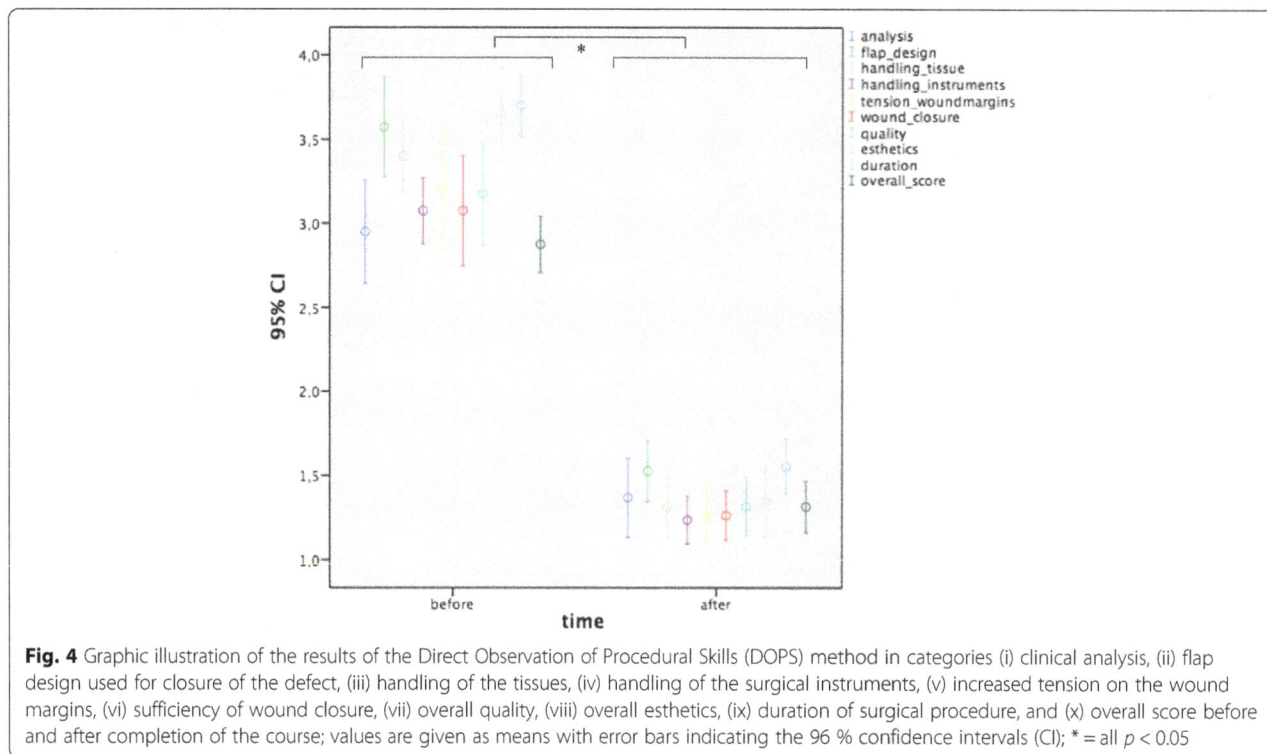

Fig. 4 Graphic illustration of the results of the Direct Observation of Procedural Skills (DOPS) method in categories (i) clinical analysis, (ii) flap design used for closure of the defect, (iii) handling of the tissues, (iv) handling of the surgical instruments, (v) increased tension on the wound margins, (vi) sufficiency of wound closure, (vii) overall quality, (viii) overall esthetics, (ix) duration of surgical procedure, and (x) overall score before and after completion of the course; values are given as means with error bars indicating the 96 % confidence intervals (CI); * = all $p < 0.05$

such as those required in PRS suitable for student courses, when a lack in basic surgical skills exists Challenges with surgical problems have been shown to represent positive factors in career decision-making of medical graduates [3]. Even the complex surgical techniques needed in PRS, such as the RFF, are suitable for student education purposes [12].

Initially, basic surgical techniques were taught in a two-hour module. Further modules consisted of advanced surgical skills in PRS. Wanzel et al. have shown that a one-on-one hands-on training of just 5 min significantly improves surgical skills of residents in local skin flaps in an animal model [19]. Other studies on local flap techniques in plastic reconstructive surgery described teaching options using foam models for example [20–22].

The results of the final test and the evaluation verify that PRS techniques are suitable for medical student education and can be conveyed in a hands-on course design as described in the current study. This course has been developed and carried out in a department specializing in OMFS. OMFS is a highly diverse surgical subspecialty that involves traumatology, cleft-lip-palate surgery, surgical oncology, orthognathic surgery, and especially PRS. In many countries, dual degrees from a medical and dental school are a prerequisite for the successful completion of residency; this results in a long training period. The combination of a professional and family life is particularly challenging in surgery. This is certainly an aspect

that has a major influence on young female and increasingly also on young male professionals when making a decision regarding their career [23]. A variety of important factors influences graduates to chose a career in surgery. These include role models and career chances. Other factors such as lifestyle, long working hours, and the long period of study are rated detrimentally [24]. Results from the current study confirm these findings. However, students had a significantly improved perception of OMFS after completion of the course and could even imagine choosing OMFS as an elective or rotational subject within their final year at medical school. Nevertheless, a certain selection bias certainly has to be kept in mind, as participation in this course was by choice. A fundamental interest in surgery presumably previously existed in this group. The finding that significantly more students were interested in the elective or rotational study of OMFS after completion of this course suggests that an interest in a surgical career can be fostered throughout medical studies. In particular, elective and rotational subjects can improve an interest in surgery significantly [25]. Participation in the operating theater, positive interactions with staff, and integration into a team are experiences that, during an elective study period, can convince students to chose a certain discipline. The high work load and long working hours remain as negative experiences during such an elective subject [26]. Final year rotational subjects, on the other hand, have a dramatic influence on future career development [27]. Therefore, well-structured final year rotational and elective subjects are essential [28].

Conclusions

Hands-on courses dealing with complex facial defects as presented in this study can gain the interest of young professionals, even for niche specialties such as OMFS. Moreover, a hands-on course design, including innovative teaching methods and structured and objective tests combined with a close student-teacher relationship and motivated instructors, is able to demonstrate even complex surgical skills in PRS. Further studies are necessary to investigate the long-term results as to whether these students did indeed choose OMFS as their future career, whether this kind of training had a positive influence, and the nature of its effects.

Competing interests
The authors declare, that they have no competing interests.

Authors' contributions
FB, NR, and JW conceived of the study and participated in its design and coordination. FB, NR, and SK made substantial contributions to conception and design of the manuscript as well as statistical analysis. FB, NR and SK have been involved in drafting the manuscript. KDW, MRK and JW were involved in revising the manuscript. All authors read and approved the final manuscript.

Acknowledgements
This publication was funded by the University of Technology, Munich, Germany in the funding program Open Access Publishing.

References

1. Schurer S, Schellberg D, Schmidt J, Kallinowski F, Mehrabi A, Herfarth C, et al. Evaluation of traditional German undergraduate surgical training. An analysis at Heidelberg University. Chirurg. 2006;77(4):352–9. doi:10.1007/s00104-005-1123-x.
2. Kaderli R, Buser C, Stefenelli U, Businger A. Students' interest in becoming a general surgeon before and after a surgical clerkship in German-speaking Switzerland. Swiss Med Wkly. 2011;141:w13246. doi:10.4414/smw.2011.13246.
3. Pikoulis E, Avgerinos ED, Pedeli X, Karavokyros I, Bassios N, Anagnostopoulou S. Medical students' perceptions on factors influencing a surgical career: the fate of general surgery in Greece. Surgery. 2010;148(3):510–5. doi:10.1016/j.surg.2010.01.013.
4. Kozar RA, Lucci A, Miller CC, Azizzadeh A, Cocanour CS, Potts JR, et al. Brief intervention by surgeons can influence students toward a career in surgery. J Surg Res. 2003;111(1):166–9.
5. Bauer F, Rommel N, Kreutzer K, Weitz J, Wagenpfeil S, Gulati A, et al. A novel approach to teaching surgical skills to medical students using an ex vivo animal training model. J Surg Educ. 2014;71(4):459–65. doi:10.1016/j.jsurg.2014.01.017.
6. Lund B, Fors U, Sejersen R, Sallnas EL, Rosen A. Student perception of two different simulation techniques in oral and maxillofacial surgery undergraduate training. BMC Med Educ. 2011;11:82. doi:10.1186/1472-6920-11-82.
7. Kadmon G, Schmidt J, De Cono N, Kadmon M. A Model for Persistent Improvement of Medical Education as Illustrated by the Surgical Reform Curriculum HeiCuMed. GMS Z Med Ausbild. 2011;28(2):Doc29. doi:10.3205/zma000741.
8. Smith AA, Duncan SF, Esparra BC. Can brief interventions by hand surgeons influence medical students toward a career in hand surgery? J Hand Surg Am. 2007;32(8):1267–70. doi:10.1016/j.jhsa.2007.06.004.
9. Davis CR, O'Donoghue JM, McPhail J, Green AR. How to improve plastic surgery knowledge, skills and career interest in undergraduates in one day.

10. Journal of plastic, reconstructive & aesthetic surgery : JPRAS. 2010;63(10):1677–81. doi:10.1016/j.bjps.2009.10.023.
10. Ganschow P. Attitude of medical students towards a surgical career - a global phenomenon? Zentralbl Chir. 2012;137(2):113–7. doi:10.1055/s-0031-1283983.
11. Jarosz KF, Ziccardi VB, Aziz SR, Sue-Jiang S. Dental student perceptions of oral and maxillofacial surgery as a specialty. J Oral Maxillofac Surg. 2013;71(5):965–73. doi:10.1016/j.joms.2011.05.014.
12. Nobis CP, Bauer F, Rohleder NH, Wolff KD, Kesting MR. Development of a haptic model for teaching in reconstructive surgery–the radial forearm flap. Simul Healthc. 2014;9(3):203–8. doi:10.1097/SIH.0000000000000000.
13. Ruesseler M, Schill A, Stibane T, Damanakis A, Schleicher I, Menzler S, et al. "Practical clinical competence" - a joint programme to improve training in surgery. Zentralbl Chir. 2013;138(6):663–8. doi:10.1055/s-0032-1328180.
14. Bell Jr RH, Banker MB, Rhodes RS, Biester TW, Lewis FR. Graduate medical education in surgery in the United States. Surg Clin North Am. 2007;87(4):811–23. doi:10.1016/j.suc.2007.06.005. v-vi.
15. Borman KR, Vick LR, Biester TW, Mitchell ME. Changing demographics of residents choosing fellowships: longterm data from the American Board of Surgery. J Am Coll Surg. 2008;206(5):782–8. doi:10.1016/j.jamcollsurg.2007.12.012. discussion 8–9.
16. Hill E, Vaughan S. The only girl in the room: how paradigmatic trajectories deter female students from surgical careers. Med Educ. 2013;47(6):547–56. doi:10.1111/medu.12134.
17. Hill EJ, Giles JA. Career decisions and gender: the illusion of choice? Perspect Med Educ. 2014;3(3):151–4. doi:10.1007/s40037-014-0128-x.
18. Riska E. Gender and medical careers. Maturitas. 2011;68(3):264–7. doi:10.1016/j.maturitas.2010.09.010.
19. Wanzel KR, Matsumoto ED, Hamstra SJ, Anastakis DJ. Teaching technical skills: training on a simple, inexpensive, and portable model. Plast Reconstr Surg. 2002;109(1):258–63.
20. Nicolaou M, Yang GZ, Darzi A, Butler PE. An inexpensive 3-D model for teaching local flap design on the face and head. Annals of the Royal College of Surgeons of England. 2006;88(3):320.
21. Davis CR, Fell M, Khan U. Facial reconstruction using a skull and foam training model. Journal of plastic, reconstructive & aesthetic surgery : JPRAS. 2014;67(1):126–7. doi:10.1016/j.bjps.2013.07.024.
22. Villafane O, Southern SJ, Foo IT. Simulated interactive local flaps: operating room models for surgeon and patient alike. British journal of plastic surgery. 1999;52(3):241.
23. Sanfey HA, Saalwachter-Schulman AR, Nyhof-Young JM, Eidelson B, Mann BD. Influences on medical student career choice: gender or generation? Arch Surg. 2006;141(11):1086–94. doi:10.1001/archsurg.141.11.1086. discussion 94.
24. Erzurum VZ, Obermeyer RJ, Fecher A, Thyagarajan P, Tan P, Koler AK, et al. What influences medical students' choice of surgical careers. Surgery. 2000;128(2):253–6. doi:10.1067/msy.2000.108214.
25. Goldin SB, Wahi MM, Wiegand LR, Carpenter HL, Borgman HA, Lacivita Nixon L, et al. Perspectives of third-year medical students toward their surgical clerkship and a surgical career. J Surg Res. 2007;142(1):7–12. doi:10.1016/j.jss.2006.10.002.
26. O'Herrin JK, Lewis BJ, Rikkers LF, Chen H. Why do students choose careers in surgery? J Surg Res. 2004;119(2):124–9. doi:10.1016/j.jss.2004.03.009.
27. Mooij SC, Antony P, Ruesseler M, Pfeifer R, Drescher W, Simon M, et al. Gender-specific evaluation of student's career planning during medical study in terms of orthopaedic trauma. Z Orthop Unfall. 2011;149(4):389–94. doi:10.1055/s-0030-1271162.
28. Gillen S, Hofmann A, Friess H, Berberat P. [Curriculum for Practical Surgical Education during Internships - with a Strategy for New Perspectives.]. Zentralbl Chir. 2014. doi:10.1055/s-0033-1360292.

16

Use of porous high-density polyethylene grafts in open rhinoplasty: no infectious complication seen in spreader and dorsal grafts

Shabahang Mohammadi[1†], Mohammad Mohseni[1*†], Masoumeh Eslami[1], Hessein Arabzadeh[1†] and Morteza Eslami[2]

Abstract

Objective: The aim of this study is to use porous high-density polyethylene grafts (Medpor) in open rhinoplasty and then assess complication rate and aesthetic outcomes.

Methods: In a prospective cohort study, we performed open rhinoplasty and employed Medpor as rhinoplasty grafts. Then we compared their complication rate.

Results: In a total of 64 patients, 84 Medpor grafts −38 dorsal grafts, 23 strut grafts, 8 rim grafts, 5 button grafts and 10 spreader grafts – were utilized. Moreover, 5septal perforation repairs with Medpor were performed. The complication rates were 5.3% in dorsal graft (complication in dorsal graft was only movement of implant), 21.7% in strut graft and 25.0% in rim graft. No complication was seen in spreader and button grafts. All 5septal perforation repairs were successfully performed with the same rhinoplasty approach.

Conclusion: Medpor can be used as dorsal and spreader graft in reconstruction of severe nose deformity with lowest complication rate and without infectious complication and extrusion.

Keywords: Medpor complication, Rhinoplasty, Spreader graft, Dorsal graft

Introduction

In 1970s porous high-density polyethylene (PHDPE, Medpor) was introduced by its very important advantage that was minimal foreign body reaction [1]. Medpor are made of biocompatible porous polyethylene material with the interconnecting pore structure allows for fibrovascular in-growth and integration of patient's tissue [2]. Upon introduction, use of these implants in rhinoplasty for reconstruction of a nose with severe deformity was a great success, especially in revision rhinoplasty of saddle and deviated nose [3-5]. However, nowadays this practice is limited, duo to potential complications [6,7].

Plastic surgeons and ENT specialists are always in need of a strong and safe support when dealing with sever nose deformities like deviated and saddle noses. Bone and cartilage grafts both are lacking, as bone grafts

may resorb and cartilage grafts may return the deformity because of cartilage memory [3,8].

It seems study of Medpor grafts and finding the ones with minimum complications after treating severe nose deformities will be helpful. The aim of this study is to use Medpor in open rhinoplasty and then assess complication rate and aesthetic outcomes.

Methods and materials
Ethical approval

This study was a prospective cohort study approved by the institutional review board of the ENT research center of Rasool-e-Akram hospital, Iran University of Medical Sciences (IUMS) and started on 2008. We thoroughly explained all the available grafts, and advantages and disadvantages of each one of them to the patients. Only the patients who gave their content to Medpor were included in the study. Although the patients were aware of possible complications such as extrusion, movement, fistule and infection, most of them selected Medpor because of its rigidity and not having to experience the complications of

---

* Correspondence: mohsenient@yahoo.com
†Equal contributors
[1]Ear Nose Throat (ENT) and Head and Neck Surgery Research Center, Hazrat RasoulAkram Hospital, Iran University of Medical Sciences, Sattarkhan St, Tehran, Iran
Full list of author information is available at the end of the article

donor site. Patients were not charged for Medpor grafts or any revision surgery. any surgical procedures was also included in the consent form signed by patients or their guardians. Also another written informed consent was obtained from the patients for publication of the clinical data and any accompanying images. A copy of the written consent is available for review by the Editor of this journal.

Patients

Patients with deviated or saddle nose, who underwent a previous rhinoplasty and patients with severe pinching in supra-alar region, were admitted in this study. In all of the patients, septal cartilage was insufficient due to prior surgery (septoplasty or rhinoplasty), nasal trauma or septal cartilage damage. Patients with underlying diseases especially vasculitis and other condition that may disrupt blood supply such as smoking, were excluded of the study.

The clinical characteristics included gender, age, types of grafts were used and complications which were entered to a self-designed check list before and after surgery.

Surgical techniques

In our study, we used open rhinoplasty procedure and employed Medpor in all 64 patients. In these patients, we used Medpor as columellar strut, dorsal, spreader, rim and batten grafts.

In case of strut grafts, the plates were fixed with 6–0 nylon to the medial crura of both lower lateral cartilages, to have good projection and rotation in the patients with tip ptosis.

For dorsal grafts, the plates were inserted in dorsum in subperiosteal plane (Figure 1), in suitable size and height (in some patients with severe saddle nose, Medpor was inserted in 2 or 3 layers), and then were fixed to the skin with 5–0 nylon (Figure 2). The sutures were removed one week later. In patients with thin skin we used temporalis fascia and covered Medpor with it.

In case of spreader grafts, the plates were inserted and fixed between upper lateral cartilage and septum with

nylon 5–0 to correct the deviation or ULC (upper lateral cartilage) pinching.

We also used Medpor as rim grafts. We first inserted the plates in pocket caudal to the LLC (Lower Lateral Cartilage) through marginal incision and then sutured the incision. In addition, we put Medpor as batten graft overlay LLC through marginal incision. These techniques were used to augment the cartilage in patients with pinching of LLC or severe cartilage weakness.

In patients with septal perforation, due to trauma or prior septoplasty, we repaired the perforation in the same rhinoplasty procedure. Bilateral mucoperichondrium was elevated completely. Then, the nasal floor mucoperiosteum was elevated up to the inferior turbinate. At last, Medpor of adequate size was inserted between septum and left-sided mucoperichondrium. We tried to close the mucosal defect primarily with 4–0 vicryl on Medpor.

In the surgery procedure, we avoided direct handling of Medpor (Figure 1); and implant irrigated with antibiotic solution (gentamycin) before and after implant insertion. Also in all patients, insertion of implant performed without any tension of overlying skin to minimize the risk of extrusion.

In all patients perioperative infusion of Cefazolin IV performed; followed by oral cefalexin for 1 week.

Follow-up

In this study, the surgeons followed up the patients for 3 years in monthly intervals and checked for extrusion, Infectious symptoms (erythema, fistula, and abscess), implant movement, and aesthetic outcomes. Typically, in patients without complication, digital standard photography was performed 1 year after surgery.

Results

In a total of 64 patients, 84 Medpor grafts – 38 dorsal grafts, 23 strut grafts, 8 rim grafts, 5 button grafts and 10 spreader grafts – were utilized. Moreover, 5 septal

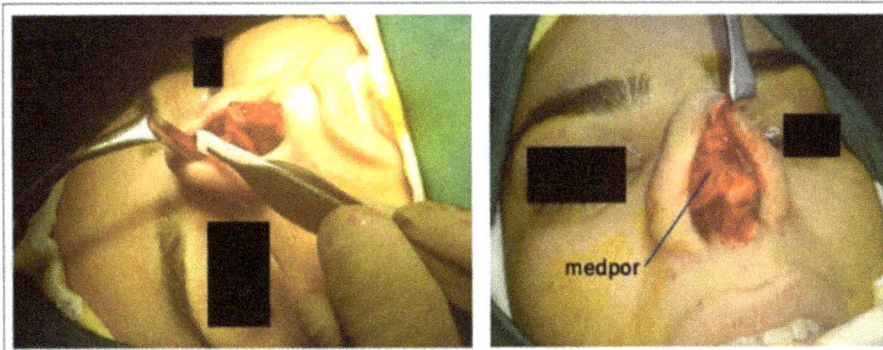

Figure 1 Dorsal Medpor graft insertion. In a patient with saddle nose deformity.

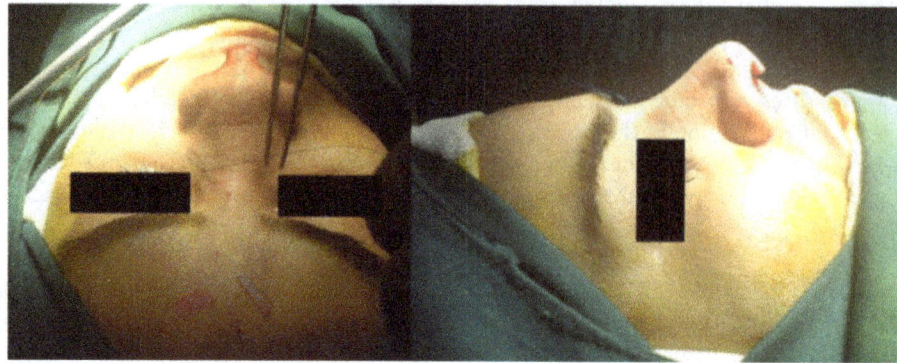

Figure 2 Fixatfion of graft. Medpor were fixed to the skin with 5–0 nylon.

perforations repairs with Medpor were performed (Table 1). Age of the patients ranged from 15 to 58 years with an average of 36 ± 6 years. 39 patients were women and 25 were men.

Among 38 patients with dorsal graft placement, complications (lateral movement of implant) were seen in 2 patients (complication rate = 5.3%), but no infection symptom or extrusion of implant was seen (Figure 3). Revision surgery and graft removal was needed in one of them. However, the other one had deviated nose before surgery, and this movement of implant was acceptable and surgery was not required.

From 23 patients with strut graft insertion, complication was seen in 5 patients, including 3 deviation of implant and tip, and 2 infectious symptoms; 1 fistula formation in culomella and skin thickness and erythema in another without response to antibiotic (complication rate = 21/7%). Revision surgery and implant removal was performed in all 5 patients and replacement with calvarial bone graft or cartilage allograft was performed (Figures 4 and 5).

From 8 patients with rim graft insertion, extrusion was seen in 2patients (complication rate = 25%). In contrast, when Medpor was used as button graft, no complication was seen. Spreader graft insertion was performed in 10 patients and no complication was seen in this group either (Figure 6, Table 2).

In 5 patients who all had previous septoplasty or nasal trauma and saddle nose, septal perforation repair was

done in the same rhinoplasty procedure. Size of the perforations was smaller than 2 centimeters. Follow-up physical exams with nasal endoscopy indicate successful repair of perforations without extrusion and other complication.

The time between surgery and onset of infectious complications and extrusion in patients was 25 to 68 days whit mean 37.2 ± 12 days.

Discussion

Alloplasts and specifically Medpor are used in craniofacial reconstructions for many years [2,9]. Porous high-density polyethylene grafts (Medpor) do not lead to the problems associated with solid and nonporous grafts. Their physical and chemical properties are more compatible and they are less likely to result in complications. Tiny holes with average size of 150 microns allow maximum in-growth in these grafts. This will prevent movement of the graft and formation of dead spaces, which consequently facilitates migration of inflammatory cells and so reduces infection risks [10].

As these implants are artificial, there are no donor site complications associated with them. In contrast, autogenous rib grafts and bone grafts may have complications due to donor site such as pneumothorax in rib graft harvest and increase of operation time. Due to bone grafts' natural proportionate, they may resorb and are difficult to shape. Auricle grafts are not considered an appropriate support as they are weak, thin and non-uniform [8,10].

Medpor can be used as grafts of different size with high biocompatibility to be specifically utilized in reconstruction of deviated noses, saddle deformities and revision surgery rhinoplasty duo to lack of cartilage [3,5]. However, nowadays employment of alloplastic implants especially Medpor has decreased duo to reports of complications such as extrusion and fistula [6,7]. Although most surgeons prefer autologous grafts, selection of graft must be individualized for each patients due to history of prior surgery, associated structural abnormalities and characteristics of the overlying skin and soft tissue [11].

Table 1 A summary of all the implanted grafts

The site of graft	N = grafts	N = complication	N = revision surgery
Dorsal	38	2	1
Strut	23	5	5
Rim	8	2	2
Button	5	0	0
Spreader	10	0	0
Total	84	9	8

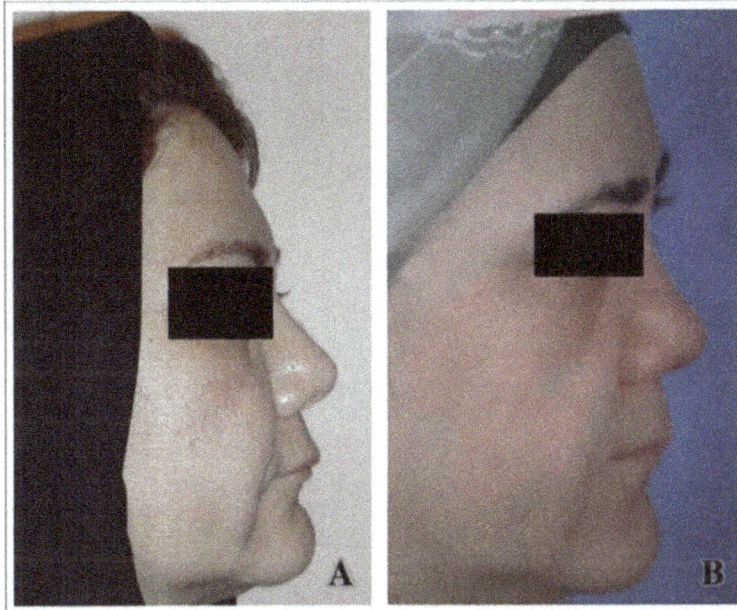

Figure 3 Medpor insertion as dorsal graft for reconstruction of mild saddle nose (supra tip depression). Successful results in a 32-year-old woman one year after surgery (**A** = before surgery, **B** = after surgery).

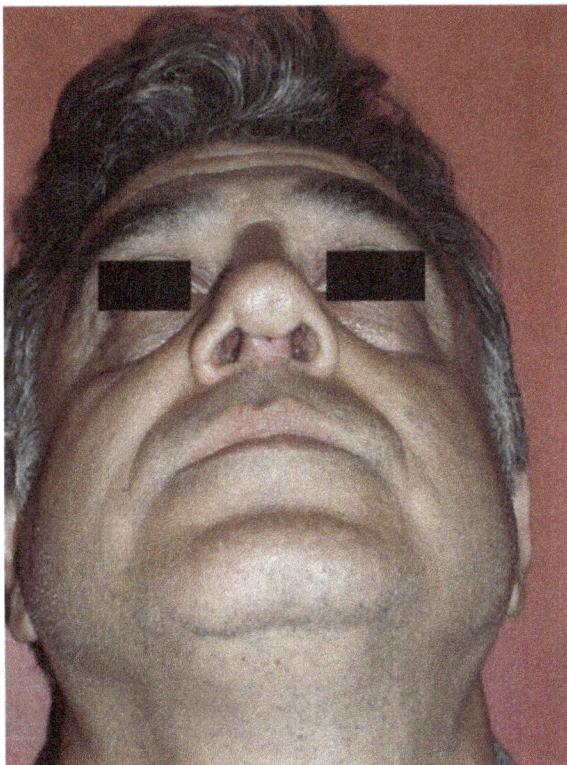

Figure 4 Columella fistula in a 42 years old man with strut Medpor graft. 45 days after surgery.

Many surgical techniques for correction of deviated noses are reported, but recurrence – duo to cartilage memory and scar contracture – is prevalent. Therefore, a stable, strong and permanent support is required to prevent recurrence as well as granting any desirable shape in one or both side of septum. Medpor implants include excellent contouring, increased mechanical stability, decreased risk of implant migration and infection [12]. They improve nose function and can resist to trauma and scar contracture force. They are also superior to cartilage grafts as they are free of cartilage memory problem and do not lead to recurrence [3].

Emsen et al. [3] utilized Medpor as spreader grafts in 18 patients with deviated nose; none of the patients experienced recurrence or extrusion. Two similar studies proved successful performance of Medpor as the spreader graft [13,14]. In Our study, Medpor was used as spreader graft in 10 patients with deviated nose and no complications and recurrences were seen in a two-year follow-up. This agrees with the result of previous studies.

Reconstruction of saddle nose is one the challenges in front of ENT specialists. When nasal septal cartilage is available, it is preferred source [15], but in reconstruction of severe cases of saddle nose, septum and auricle cartilages cannot provide the required augmentation. However, Medpor is useful in these situations and is especially effective in revision rhinoplasty where patient cartilage is not adequate [10,16].

The next option was calvarial bone grafts. Occasionally, patients with calvarial bone grafts do not recognize

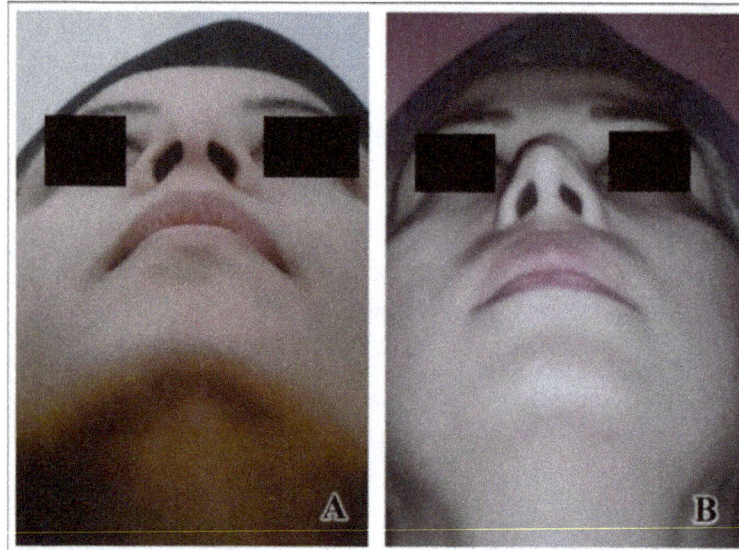

Figure 5 Deviation of strut Medpor graft in a 28-year-old woman. 3 month after surgery (**A** = before surgery, **B** = after surgery).

it as foreign body and they have a better feeling towards it [17]. Nevertheless, most patients reject it because of donor site need [18,19]. Razmpaet al. used a combination of Medpor and irradiated homograft rib cartilage as dorsal grafts in reconstruction of saddle nose. 2 out of 32 patients experienced implant displacement, but no extrusion was reported [16]. Similarly, our study showed successful usage of Medpor as dorsal graft. There was only a single case of implant movement that required revision surgery, but no extrusion was seen.

In our study, most complications occurred in rim grafts, so we do not recommend the use of Medpor as rim grafts. No complication was reported after use of Medpor as button graft, but the data is not sufficient and we cannot recommend its use. After use of Medpor implants as strut graft, 5 patients experienced complications. Therefore, although Medpor provides a strong support for nose tip, it is not recommended to use it as strut graft either.

Complications associated with Medpor could be categorized into implant displacement, infectious (fistula, erythema and abscess formation) complications and extrusion. Our study indicates, 44.5 percent of the cases (4 out of 9) to be infectious complications and extrusion. Use of Medpor implants as dorsal graft resulted in no infectious complication and extrusion. Most infectious complications were recorded strut grafts and most extrusion was seen in rim grafts. It seems insertion of Medpor close to incision site is a risk factor for extrusion.

In addition to implant site, several factors are reported to increase reaction to Medpor and complication rate. For example, anything that disrupts tissue perfusion such as long term cocaine inhalation and underlying vasculitis such as wegner's granulomatosis could lead to implant extrusion [10]. In our study any of patients didn't have these conditions.

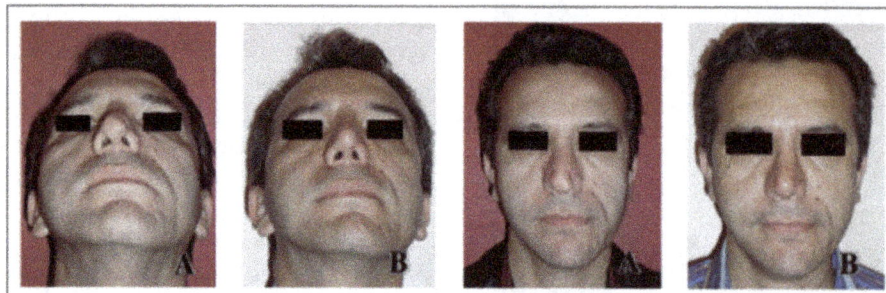

Figure 6 Medpor insertionas left spreader and button graft for deviation and pinching repair. Excellent results in a 45-year-old man one year after surgery (**A** = before surgery, **B** = after surgery).

Table 2 Comparison of complication rates of different rhinoplasty grafts

Grafts	Movement of implant (N)	Infection (N)	Extrusion (N)	Total rate of complication (%)	Rate of rev surgery (due to complication) (%)
Dorsal	2	-	-	5.3	2.6
Strut	3	2	-	21.7	21.7
Rim	-	-	2	20.0	20.0
Spreader	-	-	-	0	0
Button	-	-	-	0	0
Total	**5**	**2**	**2**	**10.7***	**9.5****

*this indicates the overall rate of complication (9 cases in 84 grafts).
**this is the overall percentage of revision surgery (8 cases in 84 grafts).

Findings of this study are consistent with the results of previous studies. Both this study and the previous studies imply that use of Medpor implants as dorsal and spreader grafts is safe, is less prone to complications and has a high success rate. If the implant is used for appropriate patients who have sufficient tissue perfusion, no underlying disease and thick skin for larger tissue support, extrusion and infectious complication risk factor lessens to near zero and Surgeons could use them with more confidence [3,5,13,14,16,17-19]. Although in this study infectious complication and extrusion in dorsal graft was not seen, due to some report of Medpor extrusion in this place in long term follow up [7,20], we can't disregard this late complication. Use of Medpor for dorsal graft can be based on surgeons and patients preference with knowing of this complication that is less frequent in dorsal graft compared with strut or rim graft.

Nasal septal perforation presents a challenging problem to ENT specialists. Different surgical techniques for the repair of septal perforation have been proposed. Kridel et al. [21] popularized an open rhinoplasty approach for septal perforation repair. This approach provides the surgeon with great exposure, andis advantageousin the repair of septal perforation especially in large and posteriorly located perforations and in patients with revision nasal surgery and lack of cartilage. Septal perforation repair can be safely combined with open rhinoplasty. Some of the routine rhinoplasty maneuvers such as medial osteotomies and hump removal could even facilitate septal perforation repair [22,23].

The use of titanium mesh and local pedicled mucoperiosteal flap in repairing septal perforation was first described in 2006 [24]. Because most patients with septal perforation have had previous septal surgeries with removal of cartilage, titanium membrane and Medpor offer another advantage in these situations. These alloplasts also help eliminate the risk of saddle nose deformity that is a long-term complication especially in large high septal perforations [22].

In this study, we used Medpor for septal perforation repair successfully without any complication; all of our patients had small size of perforation (lower than 2 cm).

Conclusion

Minimum complications were reported in use of Medpor implants as dorsal and spreader grafts. Especially in spreader grafts the infectious complication rate was lower. However, most of infectious complications and extrusion were seen after implanting Medpor as strut and rim grafts in our stydy Some complication and extrusion were seen in long term follow up in Medpor dorsal graft in other study and because treatment of infectious complications and skin diseases is complicated, we recommend use of Medpor implants only as spreader graft safely.

Also septal perforation repair with Medpor, can help dorsal augmentation in sever saddle nose deformity and can combine with other graft insertion in open rhinoplasty approach.

Abbreviations
LLC: Lower lateral cartilage; ULC: Upper lateral cartilage; IUMS: Iran University of Medical Sciences.

Competing interests
In the past five years we have not received reimbursements, fees, funding, or salary from an organization that may have any financial gains from the publication of this manuscript, either in now or in future.
We do not hold any stocks or shares in an organization that may in any way gain or lose financially from the publication of this manuscript, either now or in the future.
We do neither hold nor currently applying for any patents relating to the content of the manuscript.
We have not received reimbursements, fees, funding, or salary from an organization that holds or has applied for patents relating to the content of the manuscript.
We have not any financial competing interests. Non-financial competing interests. There are not any non-financial competing interests (political, personal, religious, academic, ideological, intellectual, commercial or any other). The authors declare that they have no competing interests.

Authors' contributions
SM has made substantial contributions to concept design, study design, and acquisition of data; and performed the surgeries (open rhinoplasty). MM has made substantial contributions to concept design, study design, and acquisition of data. ME (corresponding author) has made substantial contributions to concept design, study design, acquisition of data, analysis of data, and writing

the manuscript. She also participated in the surgeries (rhinoplasty). HA participated in coordination of the study; and acquisition and analysis of data. ME participated in coordination of the study; and acquisition and analysis of data. All authors read and approved the final manuscript.

Acknowledgements
We thank ENT department of Rasool e Akram hospital, who provided medical writing services and facilitate performing this research.

Author details
[1]Ear Nose Throat (ENT) and Head and Neck Surgery Research Center, Hazrat RasoulAkram Hospital, Iran University of Medical Sciences, Sattarkhan St, Tehran, Iran. [2]Medical student of Iran University of Medical Sciences, ENT Department of Firouzgar Hospital, Vali Asr Street, Tehran, Iran.

References
1. Mohammadi SH, Ghourchian SH, Izadi F, Daneshi A, Ahmadi A: **Porous high-density polyethylene in facial reconstruction and revision rhinoplasty: a prospective cohort study.** *Head Face Med* 2012, **8:**17. 29 May 2012.
2. Ellis E III, Messo E: **Use of nonresorbable alloplastic implants for internal orbital reconstruction.** *J Oral Maxillofac Surg* 2004, **62:**873–881.
3. Emsen IM: **EM shaped septal encircling with Medpor reconstruction on crooked noses: personal technique and postoperative results.** *J Craniofac Surg* 2008, **19:**216–226.
4. Romo T III, Kwak ES: **Nasal grafts and implants in revision rhinoplasty.** *Facial Plast Surg Clin North Am* 2006, **14:**373–387.
5. Romo T, Sclafani AP, Sabini P: **Reconstruction of the major saddle nose deformity using composite allo-implants.** *Facial Plast Surg* 1998, **14:**151–158.
6. Alonso N, de Pochat VD, de Barros ARG, Tavares LS: **Long-Term Complication after Rhinoplasty using Porous Polyethylene Implant: Cutaneous Fistula of the Forehead.** *J Craniofac Surg* 2013, **24:**2176–2178.
7. Seyhan T, Borman H, Deniz M, Kocer E: **Intranasal porous polyethylene implant extrusion 7 years after insertion in a patient with Hashimoto disease.** *J Craniofac Surg* 2009, **20:**73–74.
8. Uysal A, Kayiran O, Karaaslan Ö, Ulusoy MG, Koçer U, Atalay FÖ, Üstün H: **Evaluation and management of exposed high-density porous polyethylene implants: An experimental study.** *J Craniofac Surg* 2006, **17:**1129–1136.
9. Cenzi R, Farina A, Zuccarino L, Carinci F: **Clinical outcome of 285 Medpor grafts used for craniofacial reconstruction.** *J Craniofac Surg* 2005, **16:**526–530.
10. Choudhury N, Marais J: **Use of Porous Polyethylene Implants in Nasal Reconstruction.** *Intern J Clin Rhinol* 2011, **4:**63–70.
11. Dresner HS, Hilger PA: **An Overview of Nasal Dorsal Augmentation.** *Semin Plast Surg* 2008, **22:**65–73.
12. Sykes JM, Patel KG: **Use of Medpor implants in rhinoplasty surgery.** *Operat Tech Otolaryngol Head Neck Surg* 2008, **19:**273–277.
13. Kim YH, Kim BJ, Jang TY: **Use of porous high-density polyethylene (Medpor) for spreader or extended septal graft in rhinoplasty: aesthetics, functional outcomes, and long-term complications.** *Ann Plast Surg* 2011, **67:**464–468.
14. Reiffel AJ, Cross KJ, Spinelli HM: **Nasal spreader grafts: a comparison of Medpor to autologous tissue reconstruction.** *Ann Plast Surg* 2011, **66:**24–28.
15. Murrell GL: **Dorsal Augmentation with Septal Cartilage.** *Semin Plast Surg* 2008, **22:**124–135.
16. Razmpa E, Saedi B, Mahbobi F: **Augmentation rhinoplasty with combined use of Medpor graft and irradiated homograft rib cartilage in saddle nose deformity.** *Archives of Iranian Medicine* 2012, **15:**235–238.
17. Emsen IM, Benlier E: **Autogenous calvarial bone graft versus reconstruction with alloplastic material in treatment of saddle nose deformities: a two-center comparative study.** *J Craniofac Surg* 2008, **19:**466–475.
18. Gentile P, Bottini DJ, Cervelli V: **Reconstruction of the nasal dorsum with medpor implants.** *J Craniofac Surg* 2007, **18:**1506–1507.
19. Turegun M, Acarturk TO, Ozturk S, Sengezer M: **Aesthetic and functional restoration using dorsal saddle shaped Medpor implant in secondary rhinoplasty.** *Ann Plast Surg* 2008, **60:**600–603.
20. Karnes J, Salisbury M, Schaeferle M, Beckham P, Ersek RA: **Porous High-density Polyethylene Implants (Medpor) for Nasal Dorsum Augmentation.** *Aesthet Surg J* 2000, **20:**26–30.
21. Kridel RW, Foda H, Lunde KC: **Septal perforation repair with acellular human dermal allograft.** *Arch Otolaryngol Head Neck Surg* 1998, **124:**73–78.
22. Daneshi A, Mohammadi S, Javadi M, Hassannia F: **Repair of large nasal septal perforation with titanium membrane: report of 10 cases.** *Am J Otolaryngol* 2010, **31:**387–389.
23. Moor D: **Closure of septal perforations by means of 'external rhinoplasty'.** *Clin Otolaryngol Allied Sci* 1998, **23:**191–191.
24. Deng C, Li R, Yang J, Huang Q, Xu L: **[Repairing large perforation of nasal septum with titanium membrane and local pedicled mucoperiosteum flap].** *J Clin Otorhinolaryngol* 2006, **20:**358–359.

17

Precision of fibula positioning guide in mandibular reconstruction with a fibula graft

Se-Ho Lim[1], Moon-Key Kim[1,2] and Sang-Hoon Kang[1,2]*

Abstract

Background: This study examined the usefulness of the fibula positioning guide for boosting the accuracy of mandible reconstructions.

Methods: Thirty mandibular rapid prototype (RP) models were allocated to experimental ($N = 15$) and control ($N = 15$) groups. For reference, we prepared a reconstructed mandibular RP model with a three-dimensional printer, based on surgical simulation. In the experimental group, a fibula positioning guide template and fibula cutting guide, based on simulation, were used to reconstruct the mandible with a fibula graft. In the control group, only the fibula cutting guide, with reference to the reconstructed RP mandible model, was used to reconstruct the mandible with a fibula graft. The two mandibular reconstructions were compared to the surgical simulation by registering images with the non-surgical right side of the mandible. On the reconstructed side, 3D measurements were compared between the surgical simulation and actual surgery, and the sum of differences was taken as the total error.

Results: The combined use of the fibula cutting and positioning guides produced a smaller total error (mean ± SD: 10.0 ± 7.9 mm) than the fibula cutting guide alone (12.8 ± 8.8 mm; $p = 0.015$). The greatest point error was the vertical error at the mesial point of the anterior fibula segment. The anteroposterior and lateral errors were not significantly different between groups. These results showed that these two methods were not significantly different, except in the total and vertical errors.

Conclusions: Considering the CAD/CAM processes required for creating positioning devices, the benefit provided with a positioning guide justified its use over the fibula cutting guide alone.

Keywords: Computer aided surgery, CAD/CAM, Surgical guide, Mandible reconstruction

Background

The wide distribution of computed tomography (CT) imaging services and advancements in computer technology in recent years have offered surgeons the ability to conduct preoperative surgical simulations. Surgical guides can be manufactured with the use of computer-aided design (CAD) and computer-aided manufacturing (CAM) technologies. These guides help surgeons adhere to surgical simulation plans in actual surgeries for craniofacial reconstructions [1, 2].

The free fibula flap is one of the most commonly-used grafts in mandibular reconstruction. It offers several advantages over other flaps, including a bone length sufficient for mandible reconstruction, a high survival rate, and attached skin for concurrent skin grafting [3]. Mandible reconstruction with a FFF is preceded by surgical simulation to determine the details of the mandibulectomy, which gives preoperative information on the number of fibula bone segments needed and the cutting angles. CAD/CAM techniques are used to manufacture surgical guides to assist in cutting the fibula, according to the preoperative simulation plans. The fibula cutting guide is prepared by converting CT information about the positions of the osteotomy lines and bone segment placements into stereolithography

* Correspondence: omfs1ksh@hanmail.net
[1]Department of Oral and Maxillofacial Surgery, National Health Insurance Service Ilsan Hospital, Goyang, Republic of Korea
[2]Department of Oral and Maxillofacial Surgery, College of Dentistry, Yonsei University, Seoul, Republic of Korea

(STL) data. The guide is designed with a computer, based on data acquired in virtual surgical simulations; then, it is manufactured with a three-dimensional (3D) printer and biocompatible materials [4]. The fibula cutting guide facilitates cutting the fibula bone segments at the correct angles to ensure the segments fit together when placed into the mandible during reconstruction. Thus, using the guide enhances the reconstruction outcomes in the patient [5]. Unfortunately, however, positioning a fibula segment in the mandible is more difficult during an actual reconstruction surgery than it is in the surgical simulation. Methods for placing the fibula bone segments into mandibular reconstruction sites have been reported previously [6, 7]. Fibula segments can be fixed with plates of various sizes and materials, including metal reconstructive plates, mini plates, or resorbable plates. Moreover, a number of methods can be used to guide the fibula bone segments into the reconstructive sites, including methods involving computer imaging techniques (e.g., navigation) [8]. However, few reports have described the use of a fibula positioning guide designed to facilitate the correct placement of fibula segments during mandibular reconstructions.

In the present study, based on CT data, we conducted a surgical simulation of a mandibular reconstruction with a fibula graft. In addition, we used CAD/CAM techniques to manufacture a fibula cutting guide and a fibula positioning guide to facilitate cutting and placing the fibula segments into the correct location during mandible reconstruction, according to the surgical simulation. The results elucidated the usefulness of a fibula positioning guide in boosting the accuracy of mandible reconstructions.

Methods

Rapid prototype models of the mandible and fibula

Based on CT data of 15 mandibles, we prepared computer-assisted 3D-image reconstructions of mandibles with a defect on the left side (Fig. 1a). We then used stereolithographic (STL) data and a three-dimensional (3D) printer (ProJet 360, 3D Systems, Inc, Rock Hill, SC) to manufacture 15 pairs ($N = 30$) of rapid prototype (RP) models of mandibles with partial defects on the left side (Fig. 1b). Each pair of models was separated; one was assigned to the control group ($N = 15$) and the other to the experimental group ($N = 15$).

The CT data for one left fibula were used to prepare a computer-assisted 3D reconstructed image the fibula. Again, the STL data and the same 3D-printer (ProJet 360) were used to manufacture 30 RP models of the fibula. These were assigned to control and experimental groups ($N = 15$ models each).

Surgical simulation for mandibular reconstruction

The surgical simulation process for mandibular reconstruction was as follows: (1) We acquired CT DICOM

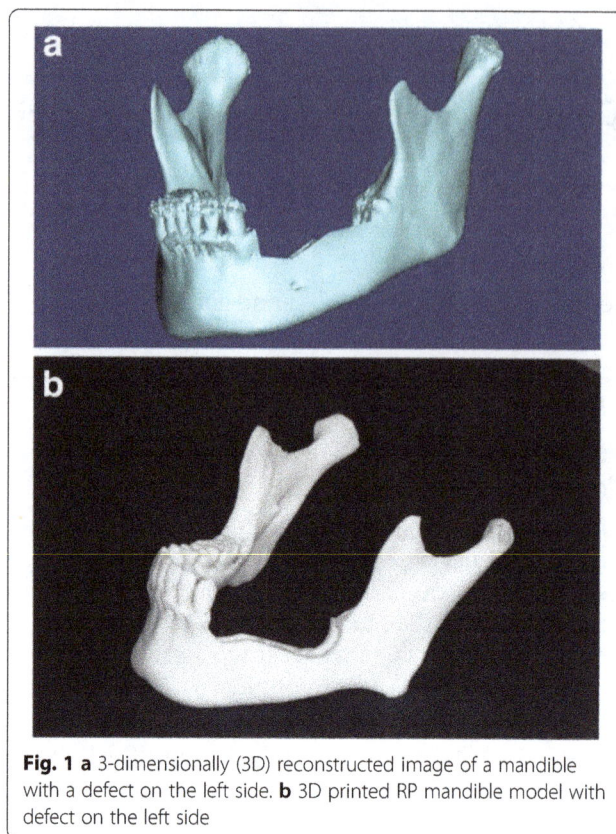

Fig. 1 a 3-dimensionally (3D) reconstructed image of a mandible with a defect on the left side. **b** 3D printed RP mandible model with defect on the left side

data by scanning the mandible and fibula models (1.0 mm slices; Siemens Sensation 64 CT scanner, Siemens AG, Erlangen, Germany). (2) We opened the mandible and fibula DICOM files with Mimics version 14.0 software (Materialise, Leuven, Belgium) to convert them into 3D images. (3) To reconstruct the left mandible (defective area) in the simulation surgery, first we cut the mandible image from the right 1st premolar to the left inferior condylar neck area (Fig. 2a). (4) We placed the 3D fibula image on top of the mandibulectomized area created in the simulated surgery. (5) We then bent the fibula at the canine area and the mandibular angle area to make it fit the curves in the simulated mandible (Fig. 2b). This provided the lengths and angles of three fibula segments. We used the STL file of the left mandible reconstructed with the 3 fibula bony segments (Fig. 3a) and the ProJet 360 3D printer to manufacture the RP reconstructed model (Fig. 3b).

Control group

We manufactured a fibula cutting guide to facilitate cutting the fibula according to the surgical simulation. First, we designed the fibula cutting guide in the Mimics software. We moved the fibula bone fragments that were used to reconstruct the left mandible to their original positions in the intact fibula bone. We rendered planes that would guide cutting, based on the cross sections of

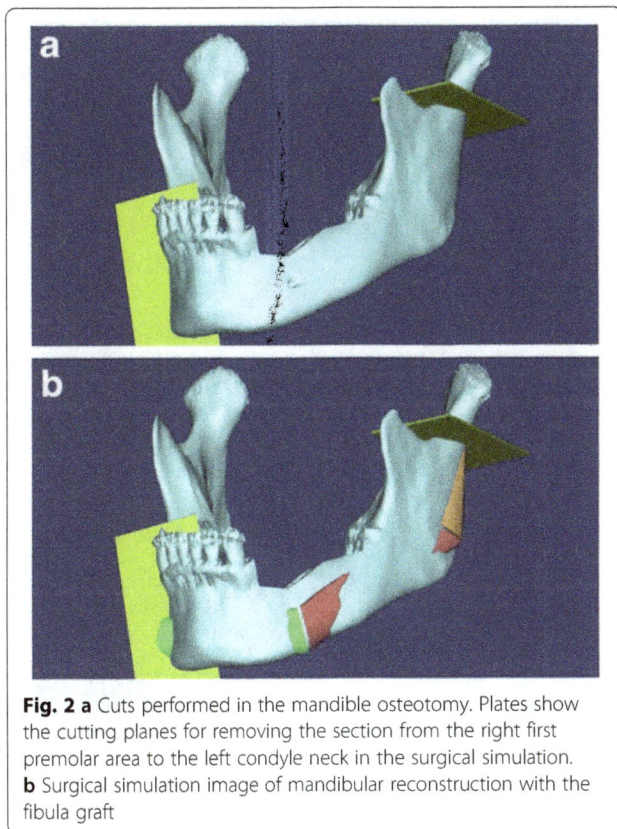

Fig. 2 a Cuts performed in the mandible osteotomy. Plates show the cutting planes for removing the section from the right first premolar area to the left condyle neck in the surgical simulation. **b** Surgical simulation image of mandibular reconstruction with the fibula graft

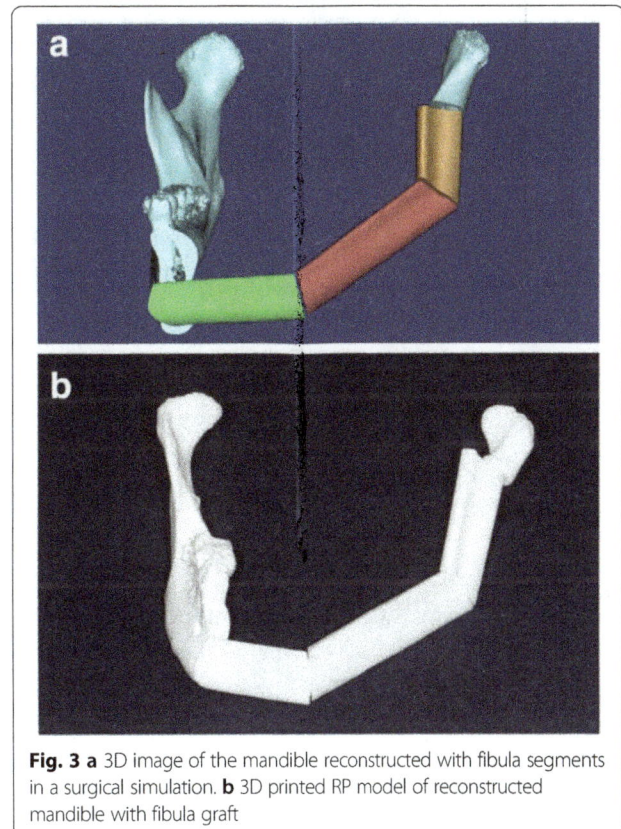

Fig. 3 a 3D image of the mandible reconstructed with fibula segments in a surgical simulation. **b** 3D printed RP model of reconstructed mandible with fibula graft

the fibula fragments (Fig. 4a). We used the STL data of the designed fibula cutting guide to manufacture the fibula cutting guide (Fig. 4b) with the 3D printer (ProJet 3500 HDMax 3D Printer, 3D Systems, Inc, Rock Hill, SC).

For the surgery, we cut the fibula RP model according to the manufactured fibula cutting guide with a fissure bur, an industrial compass saw, and a surgical osteotome. We performed the osteotomy on the RP mandible according to the mandibular surgical simulation, by visually referring to the reconstructed RP model. We used an industrial-grade compass saw to remove the defective left mandibular area, as per the manual. The mandible was cut from the right anterior 1st premolar to the left condylar neck. The cut fibula bony segments were placed with reference to the reconstructed RP model. Then, titanium mini plates (Jaeil, Seoul, Korea) were bent to fix the fibula bony segments (Fig. 5), with two plates at each connection site.

Experimental group

To facilitate placing the fibula segments into the mandible, we designed a fibula positioning guide for each mandible in a reconstruction simulation. The positioning guide comprised five supports that fit onto the remaining right inferior border of the mandible, the three fibula segments, and the left condylar region. These components were stabilized into the correct positions by connecting

them to supporting poles (Fig. 6a). Based on the STL data of this design, the fibula positioning guide was manufactured (Fig. 6b) with the 3D printer (ProJet 3500 HDMax 3D Printer, 3D Systems, Inc, Rock Hill, SC).

For the surgery, in the same manner as in the control group, we first cut the RP mandible, and then we cut the RP fibula model with the fibula cutting guide. Next, we placed the remaining regions of the mandible RP model and the cut RP fibula segments in the positioning guide. Finally, we fixed all the components in the same manner as described above for the control group (Fig. 7).

Superimposed surgical simulation data and actual surgical data for error measurement

We acquired CT images of the RP mandible models after reconstruction surgery. The images were acquired under the same conditions as those used before the experiment. We imported the DICOM file of reconstructed mandible model into the Mimics software to convert it to 3D images, and we exported it in the STL file format. We also exported the surgical simulation data to an STL file. With XOV2 software (INUS Technology, Seoul, Republic of Korea), we superimposed the actual surgical data onto the surgical simulation data and registered them based on the non-operated right mandibular region (Fig. 8).

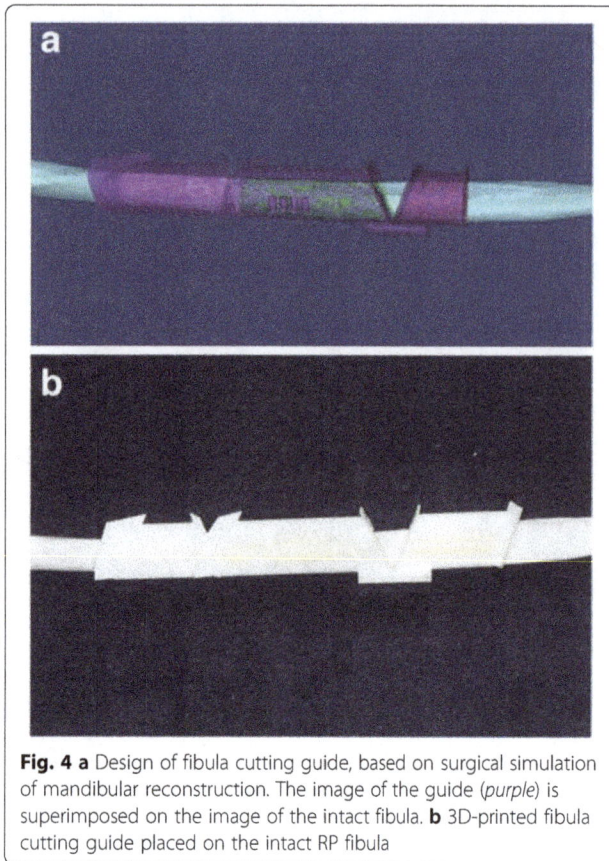

Fig. 4 a Design of fibula cutting guide, based on surgical simulation of mandibular reconstruction. The image of the guide (*purple*) is superimposed on the image of the intact fibula. **b** 3D-printed fibula cutting guide placed on the intact RP fibula

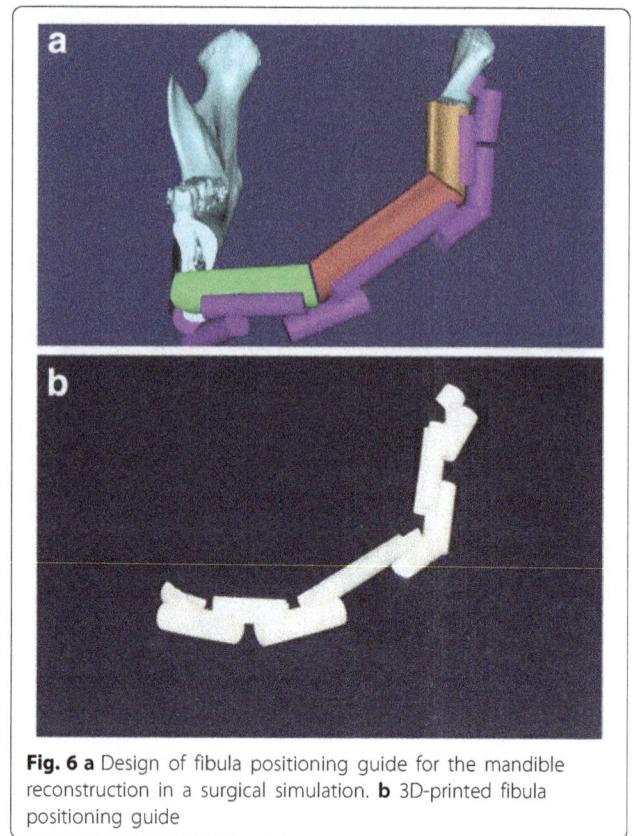

Fig. 6 a Design of fibula positioning guide for the mandible reconstruction in a surgical simulation. **b** 3D-printed fibula positioning guide

Reference planes for error measurement

We opened the superimposed mandible data (surgical simulation and postoperative data) in the Mimics software. We compared the surgical result to the simulation by setting a reference plane in the cranial area and calculating the distances between the plane and several measurement points on the reconstructed mandibles. The error was taken as the difference between the measurements taken at corresponding points on the postoperative model and the surgical simulation. Three reference planes

were established (Fig. 9): the horizontal plane (FH plane for vertical error), the mid-sagittal plane (sagittal plane for lateral error), and the coronal plane (for anteroposterior errors). The FH plane passed through the right orbitale (infraorbital margin) and the two porions (upper external auditory canal areas). The mid-sagittal plane was perpendicular to the FH plane and crossed the nasion and internal occipital crest. The coronal plane was perpendicular to both the FH plane and mid-sagittal plane, and passed through the nasion. Based on these

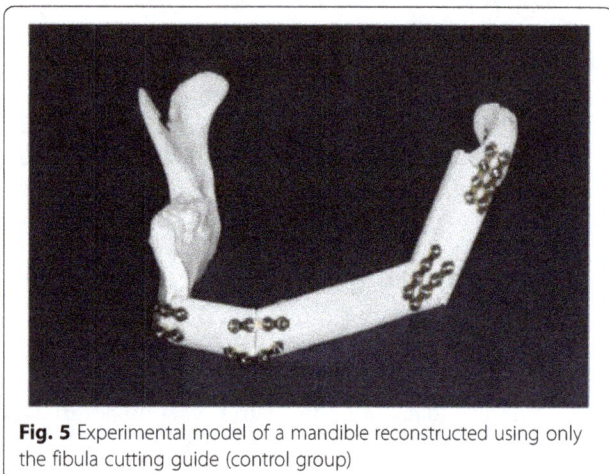

Fig. 5 Experimental model of a mandible reconstructed using only the fibula cutting guide (control group)

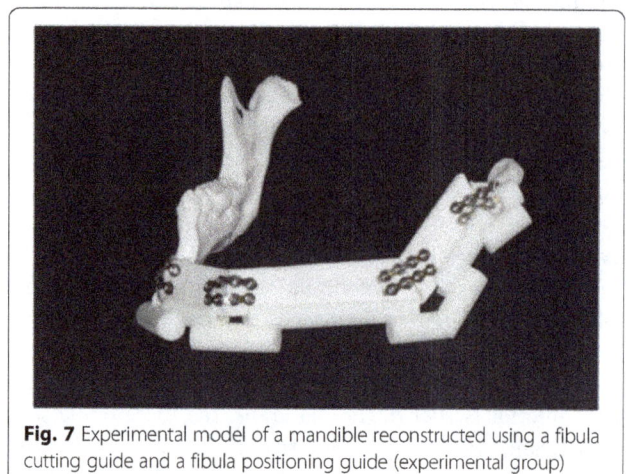

Fig. 7 Experimental model of a mandible reconstructed using a fibula cutting guide and a fibula positioning guide (experimental group)

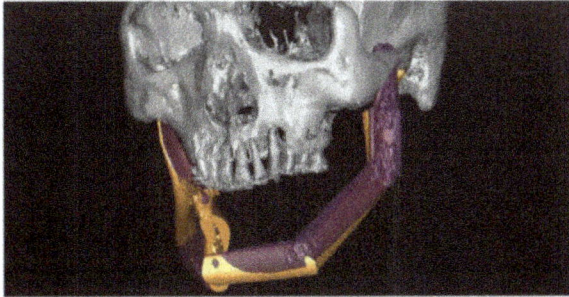

Fig. 8 Superimposition of the surgical simulation image (*orange*) and the postoperative image (*purple*), registered to the right non-surgical mandibular areas to perform measurements of the error

three reference planes, three dimensional (3D) errors were calculated: the vertical error, the anteroposterior error, and the lateral error.

Setting measurement points and measuring errors

Mandibles were measured at the lateral points of each fibula segment and the lateral pole of the left condyle (Fig. 9). One individual performed all the measurements at predetermined points that were set at identical locations in the surgical simulation images and the actual postsurgical model images. The vertical distances (Dv) were measured from the FH reference plane to the measurement point; the vertical error (Ev) was taken as the difference between the distance measured on the simulation (Dvs) and that measured on the postsurgical model (Dvm), as follows: Ev = Dvm−Dvs. The distances in the vertical (Dv), lateral (Dlat), and anteroposterior (Dap) directions were measured from the FH plane, mid-sagittal plane, and coronal plane, respectively, and the errors at each point were evaluated (Ev, Eap, and Elat, respectively). In addition, a line connecting the mesial and distal lateral points of each fibula segment was set as the axis of that segment. The differences in the

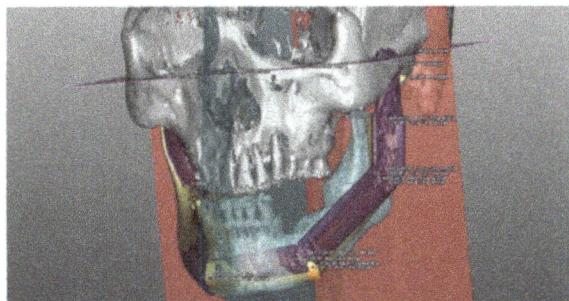

Fig. 9 Reference planes, measurement points, and axes set to measure the errors in mandible reconstruction with fibula bony segments. Distances were measured from the reference planes (FH = *purple*; coronal = *red*; sagittal = *blue*) to the measurement points on the postoperative model (PostOP: *blue points*) and on the surgical simulation (PreOP: *red points*)

angles formed between the axis in the simulation and the corresponding axis in the postsurgical model were measured. The shortest distance between corresponding measurement points on the simulation and postoperative model was considered a 3D distance error. The sum of the 3D distance errors was considered the total 3D error.

Statistical analyses

We evaluated the errors in control and experimental groups to determine whether the fibula positioning guide offered any benefit in the mandibular reconstruction. We used a *t*-test to compare the measurements obtained with the two methods. The significance level was set to 0.05.

To measure the error in placing the measurement points by the surgeon, the surgeon repeatedly (10 times) set a reference point on the left condylar head area; the error was measured by calculating the differences in the reference points.

The error arising from performing the osteotomy without the use of a mandible cutting guide was computed by measuring the distances between the cut right mandibles in the surgery simulation and the postoperative model. The error in superimposing the mandibular images was analyzed by examining the total 3D error in the right mandible reference area.

Results

First, we compared the 3D distance errors (distance between corresponding points on the surgical simulation and the surgical model) between the control and experimental groups (Table 1). When both the fibula cutting and positioning guides were used, the mean (±SD) total 3D distance error was smaller (10.0 ± 7.9 mm) than when only the fibula cutting guide was used (12.8 ± 8.8 mm; $p = 0.015$; Table 1). There was no significant difference between the two groups at any one measurement point, but all the measurement values were larger in the control group, when only the fibula cutting guide was used. The error increased for segments in the more posterior areas of each group; i.e., in both groups, the mean error was greater than 12 mm at all points posterior to the mesial point in the middle fibula segment. The error in the area from the middle fibula segments to the condylar head increased from 12 to 16 mm in the experimental group and from 16 to 19 mm in the control group.

We examined the vertical distances from the previously-established horizontal plane, and calculated the error differences between the surgical simulation and the postoperative data (Table 2). The mean (±SD) vertical distance error at the mesial point of the anterior fibula segment was −0.2 ± 1.1 mm in the experimental group and 1.8 ± 2.0 mm in the control group. Hence, the error was smaller when both the fibula cutting and positioning guides were used ($p = 0.002$). There were no

Table 1 3-d distance errors (mm) for the different surgical guide methods

Measurement point	Fibula cutting guide alone (control group)	Fibula cutting guide & fibula positioning guide (experimental group)	P value
Anterior segment-mesial point (n = 15)	4.3 ± 2.3	3.1 ± 1.5	0.096
Anterior segment-distal point (n = 15)	7.2 ± 3.2	5.7 ± 3.6	0.260
Middle segment-mesial point (n = 15)	7.7 ± 3.5	6.3 ± 3.6	0.290
Middle segment-distal point (n = 15)	16.5 ± 8.1	12.1 ± 7.7	0.147
Posterior segment-mesial point (n = 15)	16.8 ± 7.9	12.0 ± 7.9	0.111
Posterior segment-distal point (n = 15)	18.1 ± 9.8	14.5 ± 8.8	0.304
Condyle lateral point (n = 15)	19.4 ± 8.9	16.2 ± 8.7	0.338
Total (N = 105)	12.8 ± 8.8	10.0 ± 7.9	0.015*

Note: Values represent the mean ± standard deviation. The segment is the fibula segment used to reconstruct the mandible, and the position refers to its placement in the mandible. The condyle is on the left mandible, where it is articulates with the skull
*P < 0.05

significant differences between the groups at any other measurement point, except at the mesial point of the anterior fibula segment. The errors for segments posterior to the distal point on the middle fibula segment ranged from 2 to 5 mm in the experimental group and from 6 to 8 mm in the control group.

The overall mean anteroposterior errors (based on the coronal plane) were not significantly different between the two groups at each measurement point (Table 3). The error for the segments between the distal point on the middle fibula segment and the condylar head ranged from 3 to 4 mm in the experimental group and from –1 to 3 mm in the control group. With the exception of the error at the mesial point on the anterior fibula segment, all errors had positive values in the experimental group, which indicated an anterior displacement after the actual surgery.

There were no significant differences between groups in the lateral errors (based on the sagittal plane) at each measurement point (Table 4). The groups had similar error values at the distal point of the anterior fibula segment (–1.7 mm) and at the mesial point of the middle fibula segment (–2 mm). Negative error values indicated a mesial displacement after surgery. In both groups, the

errors in the segments between the middle fibula segment and the condylar head were positive, indicating a lateral displacement after the actual surgery.

We measured the linear angle of each segment axis compared to the corresponding axis in the simulation, and found no significant angular errors with either method (Table 5). There was an error of about 12° in the posterior segment axis in the control group; but all other errors were under 10°. In the experimental group, errors ranged from 7.8 to 9.1°.

We also calculated the error in cutting the mandible by examining the differences between the surgical simulation and postoperative data. The mean (±SD) total 3D error in the right mandible cut was 1.1 ± 0.6 mm in the experimental group and 0.8 ± 0.5 mm in the control group; thus, the errors were not significantly different between the two groups (p = 0.138).

The mean (±SD) error arising from setting the measurement points by the surgeon was found to be 0.2 ± 0.1 mm.

The mean (±SD) total error in the superimposition of the reference areas (non-surgical right mandible area) of the model and simulation images was 0.009 ± 0.601 mm.

Table 2 Vertical distance errors (mm) for the different surgical guide methods

Measurement point	Fibula cutting guide alone (control group)	Fibula cutting guide & fibula positioning guide (experimental group)	P value
Anterior segment-mesial point	1.8 ± 2.0	−0.2 ± 1.1	0.002*
Anterior segment-distal point	−0.1 ± 5.6	0.1 ± 3.6	0.850
Middle segment-mesial point	−0.1 ± 6.1	0.1 ± 3.7	0.902
Middle segment-distal point	6.0 ± 12.3	2.8 ± 7.6	0.400
Posterior segment-mesial point	6.6 ± 12.3	3.6 ± 7.6	0.432
Posterior segment-distal point	8.5 ± 13.8	5.3 ± 8.7	0.460
Condyle lateral point	7.8 ± 12.9	3.5 ± 7.7	0.287

Note: Values represent the mean ± standard deviation. The segment is the fibula segment used to reconstruct the mandible, and the position refers to its placement in the mandible. The condyle is on the left mandible, where it is articulates with the skull. Negative values indicate that the position of the point in the model was closer to the FH plane than the corresponding point in the simulation
*P < 0.05

Table 3 Anteroposterior errors (mm) for the different surgical guide methods

Measurement point	Fibula cutting guide alone (control group)	Fibula cutting guide & fibula positioning guide (experimental group)	P value
Anterior segment-mesial point	−2.0 ± 3.1	−1.8 ± 1.9	0.854
Anterior segment-distal point	−0.4 ± 5.0	1.0 ± 5.3	0.439
Middle segment-mesial point	−0.6 ± 5.2	0.6 ± 5.8	0.543
Middle segment-distal point	1.2 ± 10.4	4.3 ± 10.3	0.416
Posterior segment-mesial point	0.9 ± 10.6	4.1 ± 10.4	0.408
Posterior segment-distal point	−1.0 ± 11.6	3.0 ± 12.1	0.359
Condyle lateral point	3.2 ± 13.2	4.8 ± 13.9	0.738

Note: Values represent the mean ± standard deviation. The segment is the fibula segment used to reconstruct the mandible, and the position refers to its placement in the mandible. The condyle is on the left mandible, where it is articulates with the skull. Negative values indicate that the position of the point in the model was closer to the coronal plane than the corresponding point in the simulation
*$P < 0.05$

Discussion

This study examined the precision of a fibula positioning guide in mandibular reconstruction with the fibula graft. We found significant errors between reconstructions performed with or without the positioning guide, in the mean total 3D distance and the vertical error at the mesial point in the anterior fibula segment.

In both groups, the 3D distance errors increased from the anterior to the posterior segments. At the points posterior to the middle fibula segment, which are considered the posterior mandible area, both groups showed a mean error greater than 12 mm. When only a fibula cutting guide was used, the error in the condylar head area was about 19 mm. In the present study, the position of the condyle was not fixed; instead, it was held by hand in position within the glenoid fossa to form the temporomandibular joint. Thus, the largest error was observed in the condylar area. This error was believed to be similar to the error associated with movement of the condylar head in the temporomandibular joint. This observation indicated that the condylar head is prone to displaying the greatest error in actual clinical cases.

When only the cutting guide was used, the mean vertical errors in the posterior mandible area were greater than 6 mm. When both the fibula cutting guide and the positioning guide were used, the mean vertical errors for the same region ranged from 2 to 5 mm. This pattern was similar to that observed in the 3D distance errors, and it indicates that the potential for error increased in the posterior direction. Consequently, in actual clinical cases, we can expect a greater potential for error in positioning segments in the posterior mandible.

There were no significant intergroup differences in the anteroposterior error at each measurement point. When a fibula positioning guide was used in the experimental group, the errors were somewhat higher than control group errors at points between the middle fibula and the condylar head areas (range 3 to 4 mm). On the other hand, when only the fibula cutting guide was used (control group), the errors in all measurement areas were ≤3 mm. This suggested that, in real clinical cases, it might be more beneficial to adjust the anteroposterior position of the fibula fragments by referring to the 3D-printed reconstructed model, rather than using a positioning guide.

There were no significant differences in lateral errors between groups at each of the measurement points. In both groups, the errors for the distal point of the anterior fibula segment (−1.7 mm) and the mesial point of the

Table 4 Lateral distance errors (mm) for the different surgical guide methods

Measurement point	Fibula cutting guide alone (control group)	Fibula cutting guide & fibula positioning guide (experimental group)	P value
Anterior segment-mesial point	0.4 ± 2.0	−0.8 ± 1.8	0.080
Anterior segment-distal point	−1.7 ± 2.3	−1.7 ± 1.6	0.997
Middle segment-mesial point	−2.1 ± 2.4	−2.0 ± 1.6	0.883
Middle segment-distal point	0.8 ± 7.3	2.4 ± 4.0	0.478
Posterior segment-mesial point	0.7 ± 7.1	1.7 ± 3.7	0.616
Posterior segment-distal point	4.5 ± 4.6	3.8 ± 5.0	0.694
Condyle lateral point	1.8 ± 6.6	1.6 ± 6.7	0.917

Note: Values represent the mean ± standard deviation. The segment is the fibula segment used to reconstruct the mandible, and the position refers to its placement in the mandible. The condyle is on the left mandible, where it is articulates with the skull. Negative values indicate that the position of the point in the model was closer to the sagittal plane than the corresponding point in the simulation
*$P < 0.05$

Table 5 Axis angles errors (°) for the different surgical guide methods

Measurement line	Fibula cutting guide alone (control group)	Fibula cutting guide & fibula positioning guide (experimental group)	P value
Anterior segment axis	9.9 ± 5.8	8.1 ± 5.3	0.375
Middle segment axis	9.5 ± 4.6	7.8 ± 4.1	0.285
Posterior segment axis	12.8 ± 8.1	9.1 ± 6.8	0.195

Note: Values represent the mean ± standard deviation
*P < 0.05

middle fibula segment (−2 mm) were similar in magnitude. The negative values indicated a medial displacement after surgery. Moreover, in both groups, the errors for the segments between the mid fibula segment and the condylar head were positive, indicating a lateral displacement after surgery. Therefore, in real clinical cases, the segments may change from a medial displacement in the anterior mandible to a lateral displacement in the posterior mandible, indicating an increasing lateral displacement.

There were no significant angular errors in any segments with either method. When only the fibula cutting guide was used, the error was approximately 9° for the anterior and mid fibula segments, and approximate 12° for the posterior segment. When the positioning guide was used, the error ranged from around 7 to 9°. The results of this experiment implied that, in real clinical cases, there may be an axis error of about 10° in each fibula segment.

A mandibular cutting guide may be required for mandibular osteotomy. In the present study, the average error in the right mandible area was about 1.1 mm; the same error was 0.8 mm in the control group. This result may imply that a fibula cutting guide is not required to enhance the precision of the mandibular osteotomy in an actual surgery.

Severe soft tissue damage may accompany mandibular reconstruction. In such cases, the surgeon must consider facial soft tissue in addition to reconstructing the mandible using a fibula. However, the present study only examined whether the fibula bone segment can be placed in the appropriate position, in accordance with the simulation surgery, in mandibular reconstruction. In other words, this study is limited to the reconstruction of hard tissue. Studies with actual clinical cases using fibula positioning devices are needed to examine facial reconstruction involving the fibula and soft tissues.

In this study, the three-dimensional distance error was significantly small when the positioning device was used. There was no statistically significant difference in the anteroposterior error, lateral error, and vertical error from each plane. However, the errors were smaller in general when the positioning device was used. This may be a statistically significant outcome, depending on the numbers included in the experimental and control groups. This study had 15 models for each group, and in such cases, the effect size is 0.94 when α (significance level) is 0.05 and β (test power) is 0.2 according to the statistical power analysis. If the value of n is increased, the effect size will be reduced, which can lead to statistically significant errors in each plane. Therefore, it may be difficult to challenge the usefulness of a positioning device based on this study's results.

This study used a rapid prototyping model. In actual clinical cases, it may be difficult to use a positioning device when a fibula flap with soft tissue is used. However, we believe that if the design is changed to address the positional relationship between the device and the flap, a better surgical device can be manufactured. Depending on its position, the surgical device may interfere when a reconstruction plate is used; although, there should be no problems with the current design if a miniplate is used. Furthermore, the device design can be adjusted if a reconstruction plate is necessary.

Recently, the use of preoperative 3D surgical simulations for the manufacture of surgical guides has been on the rise [9, 10]. The use of surgical guides has also become popular in dental surgeries; in particular, dental implantations in mandibular reconstructions with the fibula can be planned preoperatively with a computer, and relevant surgical equipment can be manufactured for use in actual surgeries [11].

Essentially no clinical studies have described the use of the fibula positioning guide designed in the current study. However, Zheng et al. [12] reported a mandible reconstruction with cadaveric mandibles, where they used a fibular cutting guide and transferring guide, manufactured with preoperative 3D surgical simulation methods. Although a direct comparison with the present study was not possible, they reported an average error of 1.35 mm in the translation of fibular segments and an average error of 3.36° in the angular deviation of fibular segments. In contrast, in the present study, we found an error of about 16 mm in the condylar position, even when a fibula positioning guide was used. This discrepancy may be explained by differences in the experimental designs. Our experiments differed from real clinical cases, because we used models without temporomandibular joints or soft tissues. Moreover, the design of the positioning guide may have contributed to the results; the small supports for each fibula segment in the positioning guide, and the entire right mandibular area may have provided insufficient stability. This would have undermined the stability of the fibula positioning and fixation, which would ultimately generate a large error. Hence, there is a demand for studies that undertake optimizations in the size, position, and shape of the positioning guides to ensure sufficient stability in the mandibular area and fibula segments. This type of optimization could confer better experimental results.

The present study used two mini plates for each connection between fibula segments and between end segments and the mandible. This method for fixing the fibula segments could be modified as reconstruction plate for a better clinical result [13]. Recently, some studies have reported methods for manufacturing CAD/CAM reconstruction plates with 3D printers [14]. Schepers et al. [14] reported an average error of 3.0 mm in the deviation of fibular segments and an average error of 4.2° in the angular deviation of fibular segments in mandible reconstruction, when CAD/CAM reconstruction plates were used. That method enhanced the stabilization of the fibula segments during the positioning. However, for those methods, the metal plates must be manufactured with selective laser sintering and bio-appropriate metals, or it can be milled with a computerized, numerically controlled machine.

In the present study, all surgeries were conducted by a single surgeon. Some error may have been introduced, due to the surgeon's level of proficiency. For instance, small inconsistencies in the contact angles or protrusions in the plating may have altered the abutment between the mandible and anterior fibula segment or between fibula segments. Also, the type of plate and the design of the surgical guides may have introduced errors.

If a reconstruction plate is used, the plate itself can act as a positioning guide for the fibula bone segment through pre-bending. In the present study, the positioning guide was used to secure the bone segment using a miniplate. The miniplate is fixed on the fibular lateral surface, so the positioning guide is presumed to be helpful. If a reconstruction plate is used, the design of the positioning guide can be adjusted to suit the position of the plate. Furthermore, for CAD/CAM reconstruction plates, which are manufactured to guide the position angle of the fibula bone segment according to the simulation outcome, a separate positioning guide may not be necessary.

The present study only sought to determine whether the fibula bone segment can be accurately positioned, according to the surgical simulation results, in cases of mandibular reconstruction using a fibula. The scope of the study is limited to the reconstruction of this hard tissue and the findings are not supported by actual clinical outcomes. If soft tissue is included with the fibula for the mandibular and facial reconstructions, there may be interference when positioning the cutting guide and positioning device on the fibula. Moreover, there may be difficulties in positioning the surgical device on the flap when thick muscle fibers are attached to the lateral surface of the fibula. A cutting guide can assist with accurate angles and positions, even with a small gap in between. However, a positioning device may incur greater error if soft tissues or thick muscles are attached to the fibula because the device is designed based the position of each fibula bone segment. Fixation plates, such as the miniplate or reconstruction plate, and screws limit the region of its placement. The usefulness of a positioning device may be different for each patient, as the fibula flap varies. Thus, CAD/CAM reconstruction plates may be a great alternative because they also guide the fibula bone segment to the accurate position and angle determined by surgical simulation.

Results of actual clinical cases are needed to evaluate the use of fibula positioning devices for facial reconstructions when soft tissues are included in the flap. In an actual surgery, the soft tissues may cause interference, so the positioning device must be designed in consideration of this. The positioning device was manufactured based on the simulation results using the patient's actual CT data, so it is presumed there will be similar clinical outcomes as shown in the present study when only the bone segments are reconstructed using the fibula or when a fibula with little muscle fibers is used. In addition, future designs of the positioning device should be adjusted based on the soft tissue data.

In the present study, the condyle head was not fixed. Therefore, its position and movements may be different in an actual surgery, which is a limitation of this study. This study examined mandible reconstruction with subcondylar osteotomy, not a condylectomy, because mandible reconstruction accompanied by a condylectomy requires the fibula bone segment to be positioned on the glenoid fossa, but this distance and the three-dimensional position was not clearly identified. It is predicted that the error will be different in an actual surgery with condylectomy. Moreover, there may be a long-term error depending on the bone absorption in the distal end of the fibula bone segment, movement at the inner glenoid fossa, and changes in the glenoid fossa. These problems could be examined in an additional study on surgical planning with reference to the long-term prognosis. Although this study could not verify the stability of occlusion, we believe there will be stable occlusion if there is intermaxillary fixation with the side of the mandible that was not osteotomized, there is constant assessment, and implants and prosthetics are used when needed.

In the present study, only one surgeon manually fixed each bone segment, drilled, and inserted the screws simultaneously; therefore, there could have been error during the process of drilling and fixing each segment on the miniplate or in the manual holding of segments.

However, this should not have induced a large experimental error because such errors can also be induced in the actual surgery. The outcomes of an actual surgery are presumed to be similar to that of this study if the condyle head is well fixed on the fossa and is not displaced significantly.

Conclusions

This study aimed to examine the value of using a fibula segment positioning guide in mandibular reconstructions with fibula grafts. We found significant difference in the errors between reconstructions performed with or without the positioning guide, in the mean total 3D distance and the vertical error at the mesial point of the anterior fibula segment. Considering the CAD/CAM processes required for creating positioning devices, the positioning guide provided significant benefit over the use of a fibula cutting guide alone.

Competing interests
The authors declare that they have no competing interests.

Authors' contributions
S-HL, M-KK and S-HK conceived the study design, assembled the data via experimental surgery, and interpretation of result data. S-HL drafted the manuscript. All authors read, edit and approved the final manuscript.

Acknowledgement
This research was supported by Basic Science Research Program through the National Research Foundation of Korea (NRF) funded by the Ministry of Education (2013R1A1A2009251).

References
1. Liu XJ, Gui L, Mao C, Peng X, Yu GY. Applying computer techniques in maxillofacial reconstruction using a fibula flap: a messenger and an evaluation method. J Craniofac Surg. 2009;20:372–7.
2. Lethaus B, Kessler P, Boeckman R, Poort LJ, Tolba R. Reconstruction of a maxillary defect with a fibula graft and titanium mesh using CAD/CAM techniques. Head Face Med. 2010;6:16.
3. Ferri J, Piot B, Ruhin B, Mercier J. Advantages and limitations of the fibula free flap in mandibular reconstruction. J Oral Maxillofac Surg. 1997;55:440–8. discussion 8-9.
4. Foley BD, Thayer WP, Honeybrook A, McKenna S, Press S. Mandibular reconstruction using computer-aided design and computer-aided manufacturing: an analysis of surgical results. J Oral Maxillofac Surg. 2013;71:e111–9.
5. Antony AK, Chen WF, Kolokythas A, Weimer KA, Cohen MN. Use of virtual surgery and stereolithography-guided osteotomy for mandibular reconstruction with the free fibula. Plast Reconstr Surg. 2011;128:1080–4.
6. Mazzoni S, Marchetti C, Sgarzani R, Cipriani R, Scotti R, Ciocca L. Prosthetically guided maxillofacial surgery: evaluation of the accuracy of a surgical guide and custom-made bone plate in oncology patients after mandibular reconstruction. Plast Reconstr Surg. 2013;131:1376–85.
7. Succo G, Berrone M, Battiston B, Tos P, Goia F, Appendino P, et al. Step-by-step surgical technique for mandibular reconstruction with fibular free flap: application of digital technology in virtual surgical planning. Eur Arch Otorhinolaryngol. 2015;272:1491–501.
8. Bell RB, Weimer KA, Dierks EJ, Buehler M, Lubek JE. Computer planning and intraoperative navigation for palatomaxillary and mandibular reconstruction with fibular free flaps. J Oral Maxillofac Surg. 2011;69:724–32.
9. Saad A, Winters R, Wise MW, Dupin CL, St Hilaire H. Virtual surgical planning in complex composite maxillofacial reconstruction. Plast Reconstr Surg. 2013;132:626–33.
10. Matros E, Santamaria E, Cordeiro PG. Standardized templates for shaping the fibula free flap in mandible reconstruction. J Reconstr Microsurg. 2013;29:619–22.
11. Zheng GS, Su YX, Liao GQ, Chen ZF, Wang L, Jiao PF, et al. Mandible reconstruction assisted by preoperative virtual surgical simulation. Oral Surg Oral Med Oral Pathol Oral Radiol. 2012;113:604–11.
12. Zheng GS, Su YX, Liao GQ, Jiao PF, Liang LZ, Zhang SE, et al. Mandible reconstruction assisted by preoperative simulation and transferring templates: cadaveric study of accuracy. J Oral Maxillofac Surg. 2012;70:1480–5.
13. Azuma M, Yanagawa T, Ishibashi-Kanno N, Uchida F, Ito T, Yamagata K, et al. Mandibular reconstruction using plates prebent to fit rapid prototyping 3-dimensional printing models ameliorates contour deformity. Head Face Med. 2014;10:45.
14. Schepers RH, Raghoebar GM, Vissink A, Stenekes MW, Kraeima J, Roodenburg JL, et al. Accuracy of fibula reconstruction using patient-specific CAD/CAM reconstruction plates and dental implants: a new modality for functional reconstruction of mandibular defects. J Craniomaxillofac Surg. 2015;43:649–57.

18

Facial soft tissue response to maxillo-mandibular advancement in obstructive sleep apnea syndrome patients

Julio Cifuentes[1], Christian Teuber[2], Alfredo Gantz[1], Ariel Barrera[1], Gholamreza Danesh[3], Nicolas Yanine[1] and Carsten Lippold[4*] [iD]

Abstract

Background: Facial profile soft tissue changes after orthognathic surgery are crucial for surgery success. This retrospective study evaluated soft tissue changes after maxillo-mandibular Advancement and counter clockwise rotation surgery in obstructive sleep apnea syndrome patients.

Methods: Thirty-seven obstructive sleep apnea syndrome patients (30 male, 7 female, mean age 35.8 years) whose underwent maxillo-mandibular-advancement and counter clockwise rotation surgery were studied after two intervals of time, presurgical, postsurgical and follow up (1–6 months and 1–5 years) using Dolphing Imaging Software. The soft tissue changes that were evaluated included Glabela, nasal projection, Subnasale, superior incisor, superior lip, inferior incisor, inferior lip, soft tissue B' point and soft tissue Pogonion. Points were measured from true vertical line on the horizontal plane according to Arnett soft tissue profile analysis. Wilcoxon test was applied for testing differences between T0 (pre surgical), T1 (1–6 months postsurgical) and T2 (1–5 years postsurgical).

Results: Cephalometric points changed to more aesthetic parameters. The largest advancements took place in the mandible, due to patients' anatomic characteristics and treatment planning, whose were measured at cephalometric points B' (9,05 mm) and Pog' (11,92 mm) at T0–T2. In all patients aesthetics goals were accomplished.

Conclusion: This study showed that maxillo-mandibular advancement and counter clockwise rotation surgery is an effective treatment for OSAS, with good aesthetic results.

Keywords: Obstructive sleep apnoea syndrome, Maxillo-Mandibular Advancement, Facial soft tissue change

Background

Obstructive sleep apnea syndrome (OSAS) is characterized by repetitive episodes of pharyngeal collapse with increased airflow resistance during sleep [1]. Risk factors include obesity, middle aged male gender, advanced age and an anatomically smaller upper-airway [1–7]. Up to 25% of adults represent signs and symptoms of OSAS, and approximately 10% of all adults have a moderate to severe level of OSAS [4, 5]. It is associated with higher rates of cardiovascular and cerebrovascular morbidity and mortality as well. Continuous positive airway pressure (CPAP) therapy has been considered the reference standard treatment for OSAS. However, despite the potential success of CPAP, patient compliance represents a clear problem [8], causing them to seek surgical treatment alternatively. The goal of surgical treatment in OSAS is to enlarge the velo-oropharyngeal airway by anterior/lateral displacement of the soft tissues and musculature by maxillary, mandibular, and possibly genioglossus advancement [2]. From a medical point of view there are two major rationales for surgery that need to be well understood at the time of surgical MMA planning [2]. The first rationale is "behavioral derangement," which is normally due to excessive daytime sleepiness (EDS). Symptoms may include snoring, apneas, morning

* Correspondence: carstenlippold@yahoo.de
[4]Department of Orthodontics, Universitätsklinikum Münster, Albert-Schweitzer-Campus 1, Gebäude W30, Waldeyerstraße 30, 48149 Münster, Germany
Full list of author information is available at the end of the article

headaches, fatigue, day sleepiness, memory loss, irritability or poor work performance [3–5]. The second rationale is "pathophysiologic derangement," which is, in part, cardiorespiratory in nature. Three important well-known physiological processes are involved in OSAS that predispose to these risks: hypoxemia, negative intrathoracic pressure, and disequilibrium of the autonomic nervous system [1–5].

It has been reported in literature that MMA has a high rate of success: beginning in the early 1980s, several studies reported improvement in polysomnographic parameters in patients treated with isolated mandibular advancement surgery [4, 5, 9–11]. However, by the mid-1980s, combined MMA was preferred over mandibular osteotomy alone to treat OSAS patients with normal maxillo- mandibular relationship to preserve the maxillo-mandibular relations, and due to the recognition of the physiologic etiology of OSAS, which is often caused by concomitant mandibular and maxillary deficiencies [12, 13].

Holty and Guillaminault determined in their systematic review and meta-analysis that MMA is an effective treatment for OSAS [5]. The mean apnea hypopnea index (AHI) decreased from 63.9 (severe sleep apnea) to 9.5 (mild sleep apnea) with a pooled surgical success rate of 86%. They also determined univariate predictors for surgical success for young age, lower preoperative AHI, and greater degree of maxillary advancement. To determine the success of performing MMA, Pirkbauer et al.. [14] showed in a systematic review, that MMA therapy has good clinical results, even comparable to ventilation therapy for OSAS patients. Although MMA has been primarily recommended for patients with OSAS and significant maxillo-mandibular deficiency, it could also be advocated for the treatment of OSAS in patients with relatively mild maxillofacial abnormalities. It appeared that, despite the alteration of facial esthetics after MMA, more than 90% of the patients gave positive or neutral responses to their facial appearance after surgery [15].

As a large proportion of OSAS sufferers are mature adult males [4, 15], a number of patients requiring MMA surgery will present with a face showing signs of ageing, in particular skeletal atrophy, a sagging tip of the nose and hollow cheeks. Because MMA brings forward the skeletal structures of the midface and lower face complex and strains cutaneous soft tissues, the procedure can rejuvenate the patient's appearance. Facial changes resulting from MMA are generally well received [14, 15]. Nevertheless, a number of patients find they are less attractive following the procedure. Li et al. found that 10% of their patients thought that they were less attractive [15]. These negative effects, which have also been described by other surgical teams, are nonetheless considered to be of secondary importance by patients compared with the benefits achieved by the surgery [1–5, 9–12].

More research is required into these "aesthetic failures" as a number of patients could refuse surgery to avoid the risk of facial deformity. This is especially true for young subjects with full faces or for women with finer soft tissues, which would not conceal their skeletal contours.

It has been demonstrated that during MMA, the soft tissues follow skeletal displacement to a large extent in the anteroposterior dimension [16–18]. To reduce the convexity of the upper lip, some surgeons systematically incorporate counter-clockwise rotation into the maxillo-mandibular complex during the advancement; but in our surgical team it is used due to the advancement of the mandible.

While soft tissue changes after orthognathic surgery have been studied for many years, little is known about the changes in facial appearance after MMA in patients with OSAS.

In our present retrospective study we performed a cephalometric analysis of soft tissue changes in a typical group of OSAS patients. The hypothesis in this study, was that

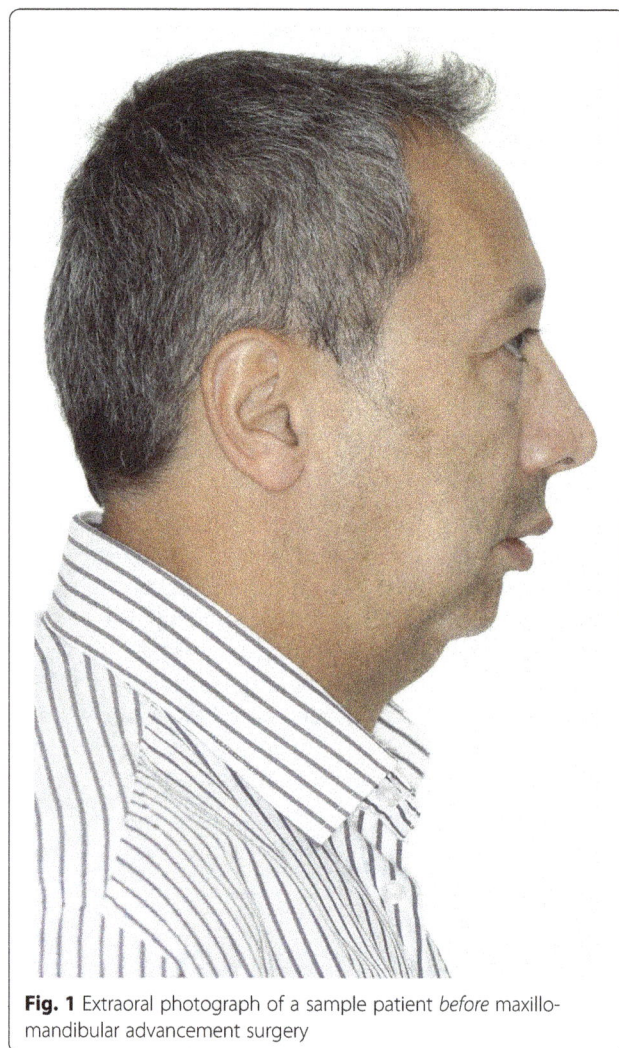

Fig. 1 Extraoral photograph of a sample patient *before* maxillo-mandibular advancement surgery

there are significant differences between the measured values at T0 and T1 and T0 and T2.

Methods

The study sample was compounded of 37 patients (30 males and 7 females) matching the inclusion and exclusion criteria of this retrospective analysis. The patients mean age were 35.8 years. At time of surgery, the youngest patient was 21.1 years old while the oldest patient was 56.2 years old. All OSAS patients were operated on by the same surgical team at the oral and maxillofacial unit (Clínica Alemana, Santiago, Chile) by maxillomandibular advancement and counter clockwise (CCW) rotation (Figs. 1, 2, 3 and 4).

All patients were treated in the same way with regard to preoperative, perioperative and postoperative care. Under general anesthesia a Le Fort I and segmental maxillary osteotomy was performed in addition to a bilateral sagittal osteotomy of the mandibular ramus and a mental osteotomy. The latter osteotomies were performed to allow maxillomandibular and chin advancement. Rigid internal fixation was performed with titanium plates (KLS – Martin and Osteomed). Four "L" miniplates were used in the maxilla, and four "straight" miniplates were used in the bilateral sagittal osteotomy (2.0 mm miniplates, with four 2.0 mm monocortical screws), to give more stability to the mandibular advancement with CCW Rotation. One genioplasty plate, "double Y shape," was used in chin advancement. The movements of the double jaw orthognathic surgery, in addition to chin advancement, were mainly counterclockwise to maxilla-mandibular advancement.

Inclusion criteria were all patients diagnosed with OSAS, skeletal class II, >18 years, who were treated with MMA and CCW rotation. In all patients with these skeletal characteristics we performed MMA with CCW rotation, because we can achieve an improved nasal airway, increased nasopharyngeal and oropharyngeal airway, normal chin projection and facial harmony.

Exclusion criteria included patients previously treated for maxillofacial deformities by other types of orthognathic surgery or orthodontics, facial trauma, systemic diseases and strokes not caused by OSAS.

To assess the soft tissue changes of the surgical procedure cephalometric radiographs were analysed. Radiographs were taken at T0 presurgical, T1 at a mean of 5.2 weeks after surgery, and T2 at a mean of 2.1 years after surgery. They were performed with a standard length marker of 100.0 mm at natural head posture with passive lips as described in the method by Arnett et al. [11], using a Ortophos XG 3D (Sirona, Bensheim, Germany). The imaging proportion used was 1:1, which was digitalized with Dolphin Imaging Version 11.7 Premium (Chatsworth, CA, USA). Based on the cephalometric soft tissue points described by Arnett et al. [11], a cephalometric analysis was performed (Figs. 5 and 6). Nine points (in both hard and soft tissues) were selected in relation to the true vertical line (TVL), which is a perpendicular line that passes through the subnasal point: glabella, nasal

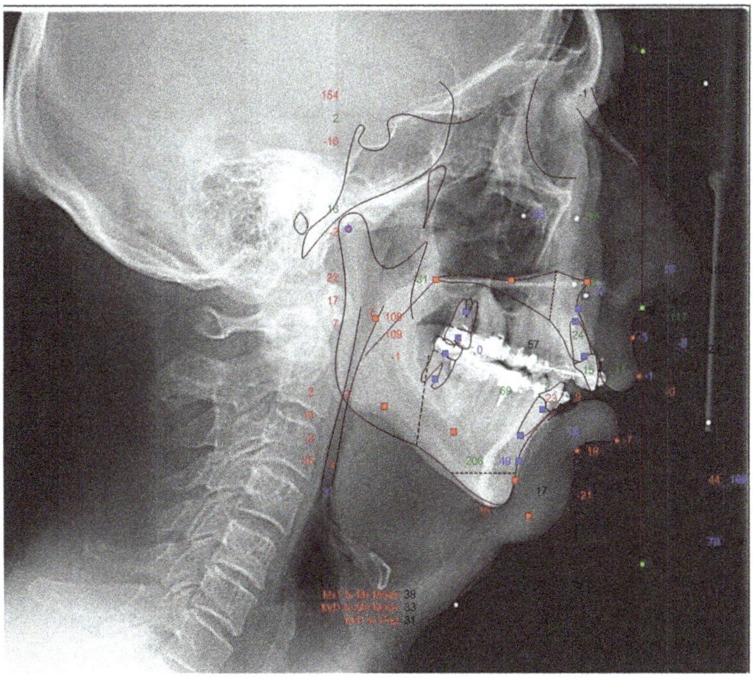

Fig. 2 Lateral cephalograph of a sample patient *before* maxillo-mandibular advancement surgery

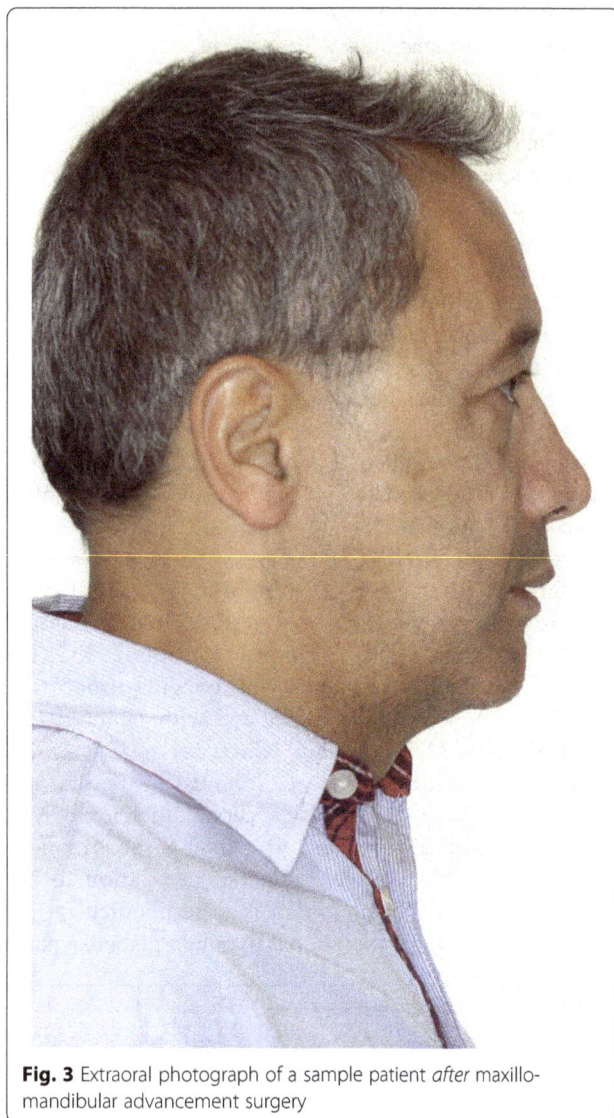

Fig. 3 Extraoral photograph of a sample patient *after* maxillo-mandibular advancement surgery

projection, upper lip anterior, upper incisor, inferior lip, inferior incisor, soft tissue B point, soft tissue pogonion. The distance masurements were carried out between the reference points perpendicular to the TVL. Figure 5 shows the basic principle of this analysis, the corresponding points and the true vertical line. Figure 6 is an example of the analysis. Statistical data analysis was performed with SPSS Version 18.0 statistical software (SPSS Inc., Chicago, IL, USA). Kolmogorov–Smirnov test was used for testing the normal distribution. The samples showed no normal distribution at T0, T1 and at T2. The null hypothesis in this study was, that there are no significant differences between the measured values at T0 and T1 and T0 and T2. To assess differences between T0 and T1 and T0 and T2 the Wilcoxon signed-rank test was applied.

Results

The results of the cephalometric analysis are shown in Table 1 as the mean and the standard deviation minimum and maximum values for T0, T1 and T2. The measurements were obtained in millimeters for each of the points evaluated in relation to the TVL for T0, T1 and T2. Positive values are for a position in front of the TVL, and negative values are for a posterior position. The statistical analysis with Wilcoxon test is shown in Table 2.

Discussion

Skeletal changes upon orthognathic surgery determine the soft tissue facial profile, which is observed by many surgeons as one of the parameters of successful treatment [11–21]. The main objective of MMA for OSAS patients is to cure the disease and decrease AHI values. Although the OSAS can be cured, aesthetics takes a fundamental role in defining a surgical success.

This study assessed the changes in facial profile after skeletal movements observed in patients diagnosed with OSAS. The aim was to describe variations of soft tissues between presurgical (T0) and two postsurgical evaluations (T1 and T2).

The response of the facial soft tissues after orthognathic surgery may be influenced by various factors, such as presurgical, surgical and postsurgical variables. Presurgical variables may include concurrent soft tissue deformities, nasal deformities, a degree of mandibular retrusion, previous trauma or maxillofacial surgeries, and thickness, as well as length and tone of the soft tissue overlying the area. Surgical variables may include a degree of dissection, edema or hematoma formation, an amount of bony resection, an amount of graft procedures, amount and direction of MMA movement, and surgical closure techniques. Postsurgical variables may include degree of bony resorption, weight gain or loss after surgery, relapse of bone segments, resultant soft tissue scaring, postoperative infection, and soft tissue stability [17].

Presurgical variables cannot be controlled; however, surgical and most of the postsurgical variables may be controlled to produce predictable results. Facial tissue changes after MMA and CCW rotation appear to be stable at 6–8 months after surgery [6, 7, 16–18, 20–22]. The evaluation of facial aesthetics must be performed at least 6 months after surgery to obtain reliable results. In this study, we observed patients who had at least 12 months postsurgery.

Upper lip variations shown in Table 1 demonstrate that edema can increase the upper lip's position from TVL up to 66% on the first 4–5 weeks postsurgery, but, as postsurgical time passes, so does the edema, and it finally stabilizes at 15.1% from the TVL, which is 0,22 mm. An inverse pattern occurs at nasal projection,

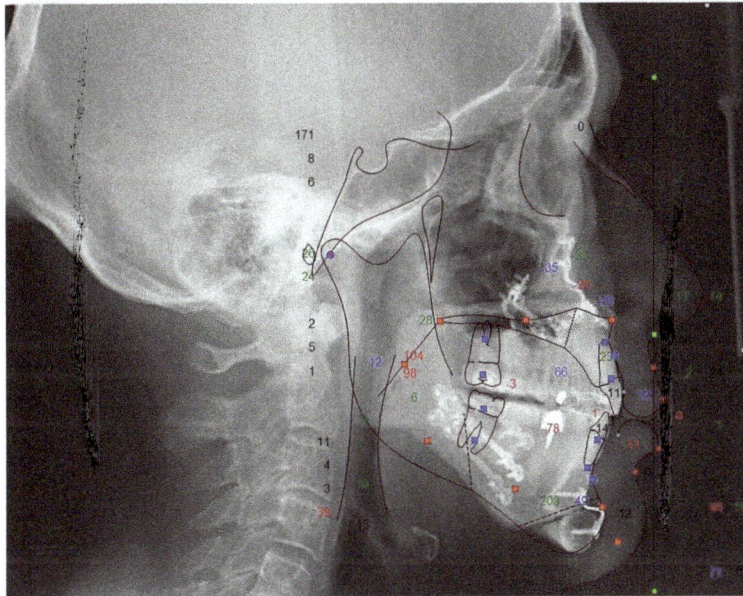

Fig. 4 Lateral cephalograph of a sample patient *after* maxillo-mandibular advancement surgery

where its position decreases –22.6% due to TVL association with edema. Nasal projection finally stabilizes at –11.5% from the TVL, which is –1.97 mm.

Resultant soft tissue scarring of the Le Fort I incision, and if nasolabial muscle reconstruction is performed or not, appear to affect the upper lip's length and thickness.

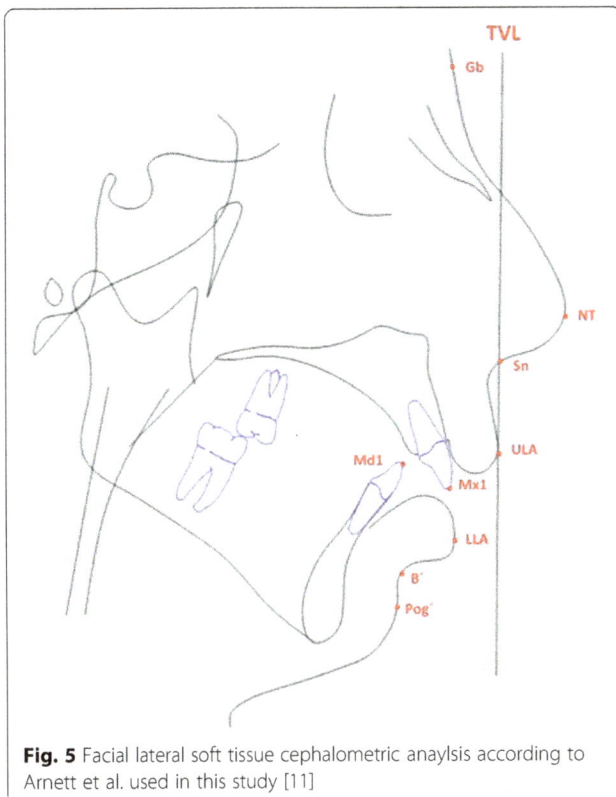

Fig. 5 Facial lateral soft tissue cephalometric anaylsis according to Arnett et al. used in this study [11]

The V-Y closure procedure has been reported to decrease lip thickness by 2 mm. In the same context, an alar base cinch or nasalis muscle suture introduces a surgical variable, which is used to counteract widening of the alar base of the nose that occurs with advancement or superior repositioning of the maxilla [17, 23].

Previous studies have determined that translation or rotation of the maxilla did not lead to a significant volume increase of the nose [16]. However, anterior translation of the maxilla increases lip volume. When no anatomic reorientation of the nasolabial musculature is performed, thin lips follow the maxilla's advancement to a greater degree than do thicker lips [6, 16, 17].

Mandibular soft tissues suffered the highest variations, as expected. All patients were skeletal class II, with a mean presurgical distance at the inferior lip of 5,46 mm, B' of 18,05 and 17,78 mm for Pog'. Variations suffered at the inferior lip, B' and Pog' points from T0 to T2 were 2,70, 9,05 and 11,92 mm, respectively. There was a proportional variation of distance at T0–T1 produced by edema and TVL variation at the subnasal point of 32.2% at the inferior lip, 37.9% at B' and 45.9% at Pog'. Tissues finally stabilized from T0 to T2 with variations of distance of 49,50% at the inferior lip, 50.2% at B' and 67.0% at Pog'. Edema caused tissue enlargement, and it did not stabilize until 6–8 months after surgery.

Conley et al. [6] had similar results, with variations of distance at the inferior lip of 9.5 mm, B' 11.6 mm, and Pog' 15.1 mm. They determined that soft tissue changed by approximately 90% in relation to underlying dental skeletal movements. Several studies [5, 14] have assessed the mean advancement variations of the maxilla (7.4–

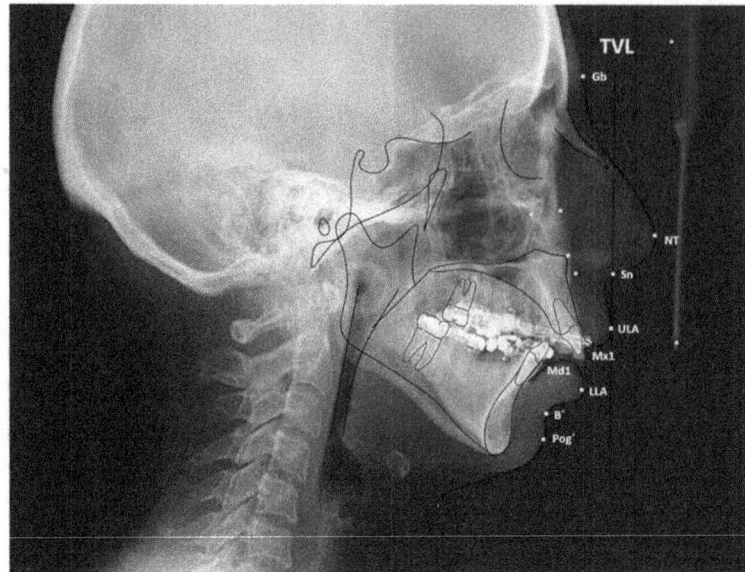

Fig. 6 Sample of a cephamolmetric radiograph of the lateral soft tissue facial analysis

8.7 mm) and the mandible (10.7–11.2 mm), but only a few studies have determined whether the patient truly accepted the aesthetic appearance. The studies of Li et al. [15, 19] revealed that soft tissue changes caused by MMA in their patient population appeared to result in a rejuvenation of the face. Ageing results in soft tissue descent with loss of lips and cheek prominence. MMA leads to skeletal expansion, which increases the soft tissue support with positive aesthetic effect, similar to the facelift procedure. Laxity of soft tissue and the facial thick envelope of the OSAS patients partially mask the effect of the skeletal advancement.

Arnett et al. [8, 24] have described in their studies normal aesthetic cephalometric guidelines, referring to the soft tissue cephalometric diagnosis. Therefore they measured patients in five different but interrelated areas. These areas were dentoskeletal factors, soft tissue structures, TVL Projection, Facial Length and Harmony Values. TVL projections are anteroposterior measurements of soft tissue and represent the sum of the dentoskeletal position plus the soft tissue thickness overlying that hard tissue landmark. The horizontal distance for each individual landmark, measured perpendicular to the TVL, is termed the landmark's absolute value. Although subnasale will frequently be coincident with anteroposterior positioning of the TVL, they are not synonymous. For example, the TVL must be moved forward in cases of maxillary retrusion [8].

The results of the soft tissue cephalometric analysis of Arnett et al. [8] are quite similar to the results of our study. They described aesthetic results for different cephalometric points in females and males. Our study did not describe the cephalometric points by gender due to a

smaller sample size and a small number of 7 female patients in comparison to 30 male patients. If we make a comparison between our results and Arnett et al. [8], they showed that the glabella was measured to be −8.5 mm in females and −8.0 mm in males; our study showed a measurement of −8.3 mm. The nasal projection measured at 16 mm for females and 17.4 mm for males; our study measured the nasal projection at 15.2 mm. The upper lip measurement was 3.7 mm for females and 3.3 mm for males; our study measured the upper lip to be 1.6 mm. The inferior lip measurement was 1.9 mm for females and 1.0 mm for males; our study measurement for the inferior lip was −2.8 mm. The B' point measurement was −5.3 mm for females and −7.1 mm for males; our study measured the B' to be −9 mm. In the same study the Pog' was measured to be −2.6 mm for females and −3.5 mm for males; in our study we measured −5.9 mm. Our aesthetic cephalometric measurements from soft tissues analysis were not as described by Arnett et al. [8], but quite similar. However, we need to consider that these patients had skeletal class II relationships, obstructive sleep apnea syndrome as a severe disease, and an average measure of the B' point and the Pog' of −18.1 mm and −17.8 mm, respectively.

According to the results of our study, there were no disproportionate postsurgery facial features, which otherwise could have affected social relationships and the quality of life.

Conclusions

The results of our study confirm maxillo-mandibular advancement as a valid treatment for obstructive sleep apnea syndrome in patients with normal facial proportions and skelettal class II. An accurate understanding of

Table 1 Descriptive statistics of the patients sample (mean, SD, minimum, maximum)

		Descriptive Statistics				
		N	Mean	SD	Minimum	Maximum
T0	Gb	37	−6.811	3.2900	−15.0	−2.0
	NT	37	17.216	2.0835	11.0	21.0
	Sn	37	0.000	0.0000	0.0	0.0
	ULa	37	1.432	2.2304	−2.0	6.0
	Mx1	37	−12.865	7.2156	−20.0	25.0
	Mn1	37	−5.459	2.9401	−11.0	0.0
	LLa	37	−19.784	3.7575	−26.0	−13.0
	B′	37	−18.054	4.0411	−26.0	−6.0
	Pog′	37	−17.784	5.5183	−30.0	−4.0
T1	Gb	37	−10.000	3.4721	−20.0	−5.0
	NT	37	13.324	1.9868	8.0	18.0
	Sn	37	0.000	0.0000	0.0	0.0
	ULa	37	2.378	2.9660	−4.0	9.0
	Mx1	37	−17.216	3.2586	−25.0	−9.0
	Mn1	37	−3.703	2.7169	−10.0	2.0
	LLa	37	−19.946	3.4637	−29.0	−11.0
	B′	37	−11.216	3.7129	−20.0	0.0
	Pog′	37	−9.622	4.2645	−18.0	3.0
T2	Gb	37	−8.324	4.2495	−22.0	−1.0
	NT	37	15.243	2.0194	10.0	20.0
	Sn	37	0.000	0.0000	0.0	0.0
	ULa	37	1.649	2.7408	−4.0	6.0
	Mx1	37	−12.297	4.7950	−20.0	9.0
	Mn1	37	−2.757	3.2094	−10.0	4.0
	LLa	37	−15.595	3.1838	−22.0	−7.0
	B′	37	−9.000	4.2426	−18.0	−1.0
	Pog′	37	−5.865	4.5532	−17.0	3.0

Mean, standard deviation, minimum and maximum values in millimeters of the measurements for T0 (presurgical), T1 (1–6 months postsurgery) and T2 (6 months to 5 years after surgery) between the cephalometric points and the TVL

Abbreviations: *Gb* Glabella, *NT* Nasal Tip, *Sn* Subnasale, *ULa* Upper Lip Anterior, *Mx1* Upper Central Incisor Edge, *LLa* Lower Lip anterior, *Mn1* Lower Central Incisor Edge, *B′* Soft Tissue B-Point, *Pog′* Pogonion Molle

Table 2 Wilcoxon test at T0–T1 and T0–T2 for the patient sample

Statistics Wilcoxon test									
	Sn–Gb	Sn–NT	Sn–Sn	Sn–ULA	Sn–Mx1	Sn–LLA	Sn–Md1	Sn–B′	Sn–Pog′
T0–T1	−4.31	−5.24	0.000	−1.67	−4.49	−3.05	−0.20	−5.14	−5.15
p-value asymptotic significance (2-sides)	<0.001	<0.001	1.000	0.094	<0.001	0.002	0.837	<0.001	<0.001
T0–T2	−2.31	−4.35	0.000	−0.54	−2.15	−3.94	−4.78	−5.16	−5.24
p-value asymptotic significance (2-sides)	0.021	<0.001	1.000	0.586	0.032	<0.001	<0.001	<0.001	<0.001

The cephalometric points' movement in millimeters (mm) and the proportion of movement (%) between the same points in T0 (presurgical), T1 (1–6 months postsurgery) and T2 (6 months to 5 years after surgery)

the soft tissue response is necessary for treatment planning, prediction and patient education.

Abbreviations
MMA: Maxillo- mandibular advancement; OSAS: Obstructive sleep apnea syndrome; TVL: True vertical line

Acknowledgements
The authors want to thank the Open Publication Fund of the University of Muenster for their support.

Funding
The authors declare, that they received funding from the open acces ublication fond of the University of Münster.

Authors' contributions
JC, CT, AG, NY, GD and CL contributed to the conception, design and coordination of the study. CT, NY and AB made substantial contributions to the acquisition of data. JC, AG, AB and NY performed the operations of the patient sample. GD, CT, AB and CL contributed to the data analysis and made the statistical analysis; CT, NY and JC made the literature research for the study. JC, CT, AG and CL drafted the manuscript. JC, AG and CT created and layouted the figures and tables. All authors read and approved the final manuscript. All authors read and approved the final manuscript and take responsibility for the integrity and accuracy of any part of the study.

Competing interests
The authors declare, that they have no competing interests.

Consent for publication
The patients gave their informed consent for publication. All authors gave their consent for publication.

Author details
[1]Department of Oral and Maxillofacial Surgery, Clinica Alemana, Av Vitacura 5951, Vitacura, Santiago, Chile. [2]Department of Oral and Maxillofacial Surgery, Pontificia Universidad Católica de Chile, Av Libertador Bernardo O'Higgins 340, Santiago, Chile. [3]Department of Orthodontics, Faculty of Health, University Witten/Herdecke, Alfred-Herrhausen-Strasse 44, 58455 Witten, Germany. [4]Department of Orthodontics, Universitätsklinikum Münster, Albert-Schweitzer-Campus 1, Gebäude W30, Waldeyerstraße 30, 48149 Münster, Germany.

References
1. Guilleminault C, Tilkian A, Dement WC. The sleep apnea syndromes. Annu Rev Med. 1976;27:465–84.
2. Schendel S, Powell N, Jacobson R. Maxillary, mandibular, and chin advancement: treatment planning based on airway anatomy in obstructive sleep apnea. J Oral Maxillofac Surg. 2011;69:663–76.
3. National Commission on Sleep Disorders Research. Report of the National Commission on Sleep Disorders Research. Superintendent of Documents, US Government Printing Office, Washington, DC; 1992 (Department of Health and Human Services Publication 92).
4. Caples SM, Rowley JA, Prinsell JR, Pallanch JF, Elamin MB, Katz SG, et al. Surgical modifications of the upper airway for obstructive sleep apnea in adults: a systematic review and meta-analysis. Sleep Med Rev. 2010;33:1396–407.
5. Holty JE, Guilleminault C. Maxillomandibular advancement for the treatment of obstructive sleep apnea: a systematic review and meta-analysis. Sleep Med Rev. 2010;14:287–97.
6. Conley RS, Boyd SB. Facial soft tissue changes following maxillomandibular advancement for treatment of obstructive sleep apnea. J Oral Maxillofac Surg. 2007;65:1332–40.
7. Gerbino G, Bianchi FA, Verzé L, Ramieri G. Soft tissue changes after maxillo-mandibular advancement in OSAS patients: A three-dimensional study. J Craniomaxillofac Surg. 2014;42:66–72.
8. Arnett GW, Jelic JS, Kim J, Cummings DR. Soft tissue cephalometric analysis: diagnosis and treatment planning of dentofacial deformity. Am J Orthod Dentofac Orthop. 1999;116:239–53.
9. Bear S, Priest J. Sleep apnea syndrome: correction with surgical advancement of the mandible. J Oral Surg. 1980;38:543–9.
10. Spire J, Kuo P, Campbell N. Maxillo-facial surgical approach: an introduction and review of mandibular advancement. Bull Eur Physiopathol Respir. 1983; 19:604–6.
11. Powell N, Guilleminault C, Riley R, Smith L. Mandibular advancement and obstructive sleep apnea syndrome. Bull Eur Physiopathol Respir. 1983;19: 607–10.
12. Riley RW, Powell NB, Guilleminault C, Nino-Murcia G. Maxillary, mandibular, and hyoid advancement: an alternative to tracheostomy in obstructive sleep apnea syndrome. Otolaryngol Head Neck Surg. 1986;94:584–8.
13. Jamieson A, Guilleminault C, Partinen M, Quera-Salva MA. Obstructive sleep apneic patients have craniomandibular abnormalities. Sleep Med. 1986;9: 469–77.
14. Pirklbauer K, Russmueller G, Stiebellehner L, Nell C, Sinko K, Millesi G, et al. Maxillomandibular advancement for treatment of obstructive sleep apnea syndrome: A Systematic Review. J Oral Maxillofac Surg. 2011;69:165–76.
15. Li KK, Riley RW, Powell NB, Guilleminault C. Patient's perception of the facial appereance after maxillomandibular advancement for obstructive sleep apnea syndrome. J Oral Maxillofac Surg. 2001;69:165–76.
16. Van Loon B, Van Heerbeek N, Bierenbroodspot F, Verhamme L, Xi T, de Koning J, et al. Three-dimensional changes in nose and upper lip volume after orthognathic surgery. Int J Oral Maxillofac Surg. 2015;44:83–9.
17. Louis PJ, Austin RB, Waite PD, Mathews CS. Soft tissue changes of the upper lip associated with maxillary advancement in obstructive sleep apnea patients. J Oral Maxillofac Surg. 2001;59:151–6.
18. Maal TJ, de Koning MJ, Plooij JM, Verhamme LM, Rangel FA, Bergé SJ, et al. One year postoperative hard and soft tissue volumetric changes after a BSSO mandibular advancement. Int J Oral Maxillofac Surg. 2012;41:1137–45.
19. Li KK. Maxillomandibular advancement for obstructive sleep apnea. J Oral Maxillofac Surg. 2011;69:687–94.
20. Broadbent BH. A new X-ray technique and its application to orthodontia. Angle Orthod. 1931;1:45–66.
21. Kuvat SV, Güven E, Hocaoglu E, Basaran K, Marsan G, Cura N, et al. Body fat composition and weight changes after double-jaw osteotomy. J Craniofac Surg. 2010;21:1516–8.
22. Schendel SA, Williamson LW. Muscle reorientation following superior repositioning of the maxilla. J Oral Maxillofac Surg. 1983;41:235–40.
23. Rosen HM. Lip-nasal aesthetics following Le Fort I osteotomy. Plast Reconstr Surg. 1988;81:171–82.
24. Arnett GW, Bergman RT. Facial keys to orthodontic diagnosis and treatment planning—part II. Am J Orthod Dentofac Orthop. 1993;103:395–411.

19

Normal orbit skeletal changes in adolescents as determined through cone-beam computed tomography

B. Lee[1], C. Flores-Mir[1] and M. O. Lagravère[1,2]*

Abstract

Background: To determine three-dimensional spatial orbit skeletal changes in adolescents over a 19 to 24 months observation period assessed through cone-beam computed tomography (CBCT).

Methods: The sample consisted of 50 adolescents aged 11 to 17. All were orthodontic patients who had two CBCTs taken with an interval of 19 to 24 months between images. The CBCTs were analyzed using the third-party software Avizo. Sixteen anatomical landmarks resulting in 24 distances were used to measure spatial structural changes of both orbits. Reliability and measurement error of all landmarks were calculated using ten CBCTs. Descriptive and *t*-test statistical analyses were used to determine the overall changes in the orbits.

Results: All landmarks showed excellent reliability with the largest measurement error being the Y-coordinate of the left most medial point of the temporalis grooves at 0.95 mm. The mean differences of orbital changes between time 1 and time 2 in the transverse, antero-posterior and vertical directions were 0.97, 0.36 and 0.33 mm respectively. Right to left most antero-inferior superior orbital rim distance had the greatest overall transverse change of 4.37 mm. Right most posterior point of lacrimal crest to right most postero-lateral point of the superior orbital fissure had the greatest overall antero-posterior change of 0.52 mm. Lastly, left most antero-inferior superior orbital rim to left most antero-superior inferior orbital rim had the greatest overall vertical change of 0.63 mm.

Conclusions: The orbit skeletal changes in a period of 19–24 months in a sample of 11–17 year olds were statistically significant, but are not considered to be clinically significant. The overall average changes of orbit measurements were less than 1 mm.

Keywords: Orbit, Cone-beam computed tomography, Growth, Orthodontics

Background

The orbit is a complex structure composed of seven bones. These bones include the frontal, lacrimal, ethmoidal, maxillary, zygomatic, sphenoid and palatine bones [1]. The orbit itself is considered to be a four-walled unit where each wall has its own clinically important structures [2]. Due to the orbit's association with the eye globe and surrounding structures, proper understanding of orbital growth can be beneficial to different fields of medicine and dentistry. Applications include preoperative planning for orbit reconstruction, orbital rehabilitation to promote normal orbital growth, forensic identification and orthodontic diagnosis and treatment planning [3–5]. The latter because of the concept that intraorbital measurements are presumed to be stable after 8 years of life and can be used as reference structures when assessing craniofacial changes.

Escaravage and Dutton have previously done computed tomography (CT) analyses of the orbit and have determined that orbital growth is highly influenced by globe growth [4]. Their findings suggested that orbital growth occurs more significantly during the first 2 years of life and especially during the first year of life [4]. Furthermore, their findings suggested a steady pace that carries on until growth parameters reach 85–90 % of their adult size around 8 years of life [4]. Since the pace

* Correspondence: manuel@ualberta.ca
[1]Department of Dentistry, University of Alberta, Edmonton, Canada
[2]Department of Medicine and Dentistry, School of Dentistry, University of Alberta, 5524 Edmonton Clinic Health Academy, 11405-87 Ave, Edmonton T6G 1C9, Canada

of orbital growth slows past 8 years of life, further growth analyses would be beneficial to determine the stability of the orbits in later years for orthodontic diagnosis and treatment planning as mentioned before.

Imaging is a necessary diagnostic tool in the practice of orthodontics. Traditionally, most intra-oral and extra-oral radiographic imaging was done by means of two-dimensional (2D) radiography until the recent introduction of cone-beam computed tomography (CBCT). The use of CBCT in orthodontic practices have been made possible due to the low radiation doses compared to medical CT, short image acquisition times, low cost and relatively high image quality [6]. Furthermore, three-dimensional (3D) radiography has advantages over 2D radiography as it is not limited by distortion, magnification, superimposition and misrepresentation of structures experienced with 2D projections [7]. With this type of imaging, clinicians and researchers are able to analyze the orbit structural change and stability over time in 3D. This would help clinicians identify if the orbit still presents changes during the adolescent and adult years. Therefore, the purpose of this study was to determine 3D spatial orbit skeletal changes in adolescents over a 19 to 24 months observation period assessed through CBCT.

Methods

This study was approved by an institutional review board. Images used were obtained retrospectively from a previous clinical trial where CBCT scans were used to measure three-dimensional changes produced by normal growth and orthodontic treatment changes. The sample was taken from 50 patients aged 11 to 17. All individuals were developmentally normal and no gross anatomical abnormalities were identified. Each patient had CBCTs taken within a time interval of 19–24 months. The inclusion criteria for the participants were to have full permanent dentition, non-syndromic characteristics nor previous craniofacial surgery. Patients should all be present in the age range of 11–17 years of age. Any patient not following the previous criteria was excluded.

CBCT scans were taken using the ICat New Generation (Imaging Sciences International, Hatfield, USA) machine at 0.3 mm voxel size and 8.9 s (Large field of view 16cmx13.3 cm, 120kVp, 18.54mAs) and converted into DICOM format. AVIZO software (Visualization Sciences Group, Massachusetts, USA) was used to analyze the DICOM format images. Sagittal (YZ-plane), coronal (XZ-plane), and axial (XY-plane) volumetric slices, as well as 3D reconstructions of the images were used to determine 16 landmarks located in the cranial base and skeletal orbits. The analysis was done by the main researcher (BL) having been trained

previously by ML who has extensive experience and publications in terms of CBCT landmarking.

Each landmark was recorded as a point with X, Y and Z values in the Cartesian coordinate system. The investigator was blind to the patient's age and time when the CBCT was taken. Landmarks were located using both 3D reconstructions and 2D slices. Definitions of the landmarks located are listed in Fig. 1.

By using these landmarks, 24 distances were used to assess changes of the orbits through comparison of two time-deferred data sets of each patient. These distances (Table 1) assessed growth of the orbits through measuring transverse, antero-posterior and vertical spatial and structural changes of the orbits. Linear distances (d) between landmarks were analyzed using the XYZ coordinates in the following equation.

$$d = \sqrt{(X_1 - X_2)^2 + (Y_1 - Y_2)^2 + (Z_1 - Z_2)^2}$$

To test examiner reliability in terms of consistent landmarking, a reliability trial was performed separate from the study trials. The 16 landmarks were identified from each image on three occasions at different times, for ten randomly selected images from ten different individuals. Intra-examiner reliability values were determined using intraclass correlation coefficients (ICCs). Landmark definitions and procedures were the same as those used in the study.

Twenty-four linear distances were obtained for each CBCT image. Distances were selected to cover all possible orientations and dimensions without being repetitive. Descriptive statistics were calculated for all distances and for the differences between corresponding distances at the two time points. Sex and age distribution are shown in Table 2. All distances were then analyzed using paired t-test to verify statistical significance ($P < 0.05$). Distances were also grouped dependent on their orientation and a univariate analysis of variance followed by Bonferroni post-hoc test was done to verify any statistical significance between dimensional changes.

Results

Overall measurement errors of all landmarks in the study were determined by analyzing ten CBCT data sets that were chosen randomly. The largest measurement error was in the Y-coordinate of the left most medial point of the temporalis grooves at 0.95 mm. The smallest measurement error was the x-coordinates of both the right most antero-inferior point of the superior orbital rim and left most antero-inferior point of the superior orbital rim at <0.01 mm. The lowest ICC value was from the right most antero-inferior point of the superior orbital rim and the left most antero-inferior point of the superior orbital rim with ICC values of 0.99

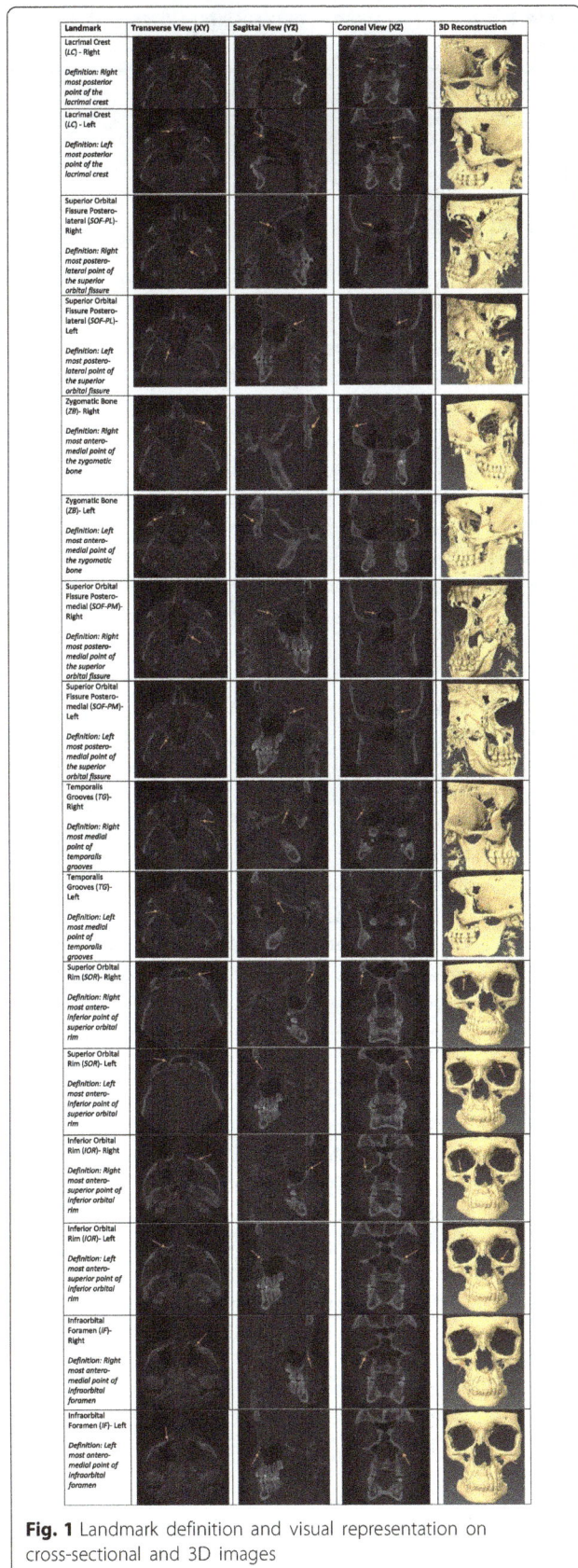

Fig. 1 Landmark definition and visual representation on cross-sectional and 3D images

Table 1 Overall change of the distances between T1 and T2 in the transverse, antero-posterior and vertical dimensions

Distances (mm)	Greatest overall change	
	Mean	Std. deviation
Transverse		
Right *LC* to Left *LC*	0.37	1.76
Right *SOF-PL* to Left *SOF-PL*	0.80	0.92
Right *ZB* to Left *ZB*	1.13	2.54
Right *SOF-PM* to Left *SOF-PM*	0.53	0.96
Right *TG* to Left *TG*	0.91	2.47
Right *SOR* to Left *SOR*	4.37	2.48
Right *IOR* to Left *IOR*	4.35	2.42
Right *IF* to Left *IF*	0.83	0.96
Right *LC* to Right *ZB*	0.39	2.14
Left *LC* to Left *ZB*	0.41	2.30
Right *SOF-PL* to Right *SOF-PM*	0.14	0.81
Left *SOF-PL* to Left *SOF-PM*	0.13	1.12
Antero-posterior		
Right *LC* to Right *SOF-PL*	0.52	1.32
Left *LC* to Left *SOF-PL*	0.45	1.38
Right *ZB* to Right *SOF-PM*	0.46	1.08
Left *ZB* to Left *SOF-PM*	0.50	1.27
Right *ZB* to Right *TG*	0.50	2.01
Left *ZB* to Left *TG*	0.13	1.98
Right *TG* to Right *SOF-PM*	0.03	1.67
Left *TG* to Left *SOF-PM*	0.27	1.69
Vertical		
Right *SOR* to Right *IOR*	0.42	1.79
Left *SOR* to Left *IOR*	0.63	1.78
Right *IOR* to Right *IF*	0.17	2.55
Left *IOR* to Left *IF*	0.38	2.02

(C/I 0.96–1.00). Given the smallest and largest measurement errors, all landmarks have excellent reliability. Table 3 shows all the landmarks and their respective measurement errors.

By using the 24 distances obtained from the 16 landmarks, we calculated the differences between time 1 and time 2 and correlated the changes to transverse, antero-posterior and vertical directions. After applying a multivariate analysis, age and sex did not have a statistical significant effect on the measurement changes obtained.

Table 2 Sex and age distribution

Category	Average age (Years)
Males (18)	13.6 +− 2.7
Females (32)	14.7 +− 2.5
Total (50)	14.2 +− 2.5

Table 3 Mean X, Y, Z coordinate measurement errors for each landmark

Landmark		Mean	Std. deviation
Lacrimal Crest (LC)- Right	X	.3091	.43438
	Y	.4303	.43550
	Z	.0909	.10445
Lacrimal Crest (LC)- Left	X	.1758	.27370
	Y	.3576	.44649
	Z	.0909	.10445
Superior Orbital Fissure Postero-lateral (SOF-PL)- Right	X	.3576	.43642
	Y	.3091	.33236
	Z	.0909	.10445
Superior Orbital Fissure Postero-lateral (SOF-PL)- Left	X	.5770	.25629
	Y	.1515	.39787
	Z	.1030	.12424
Zygomatic Bone (ZB)- Right	X	.3394	.32722
	Y	.2121	.29936
	Z	.0909	.10445
Zygomatic Bone (ZB)- Left	X	.4121	.38852
	Y	.1152	.22329
	Z	.0909	.10445
Superior Orbital Fissure Postero-medial (SOF-PM)- Right	X	.3879	.45978
	Y	.3758	.33635
	Z	.0909	.10445
Superior Orbital Fissure Postero-medial (SOF-PM)- Left	X	.1412	.26373
	Y	.3212	.44703
	Z	.0909	.10445
Temporali s Grooves (TG)- Right	X	.2061	.30178
	Y	.7939	.77198
	Z	.0909	.10445
Temporalis Grooves (TG)- Left	X	.2667	.32249
	Y	.9515	.75548
	Z	.0909	.10445
Superior Orbital Rim (SOR)- Right	X	0.0000	0.00000
	Y	.0333	.04714
	Z	.4667	.56569
Superior Orbital Rim (SOR)- Left	X	0.0000	0.00000
	Y	.3000	.42426
	Z	.3000	.14142
Inferior Orbital Rim (IOR)- Right	X	.1000	.14142
	Y	.1000	.14142
	Z	.2000	.18856
Inferior Orbital Rim (IOR)- Left	X	.1000	.14142
	Y	.4667	.28284
	Z	.4667	.18856

Table 3 Mean X, Y, Z coordinate measurement errors for each landmark (Continued)

Infraorbital Foramen (IF)- Right	X	.2606	.32449
	Y	.0909	.20715
	Z	.0545	.09342
Infraorbital Foramen (IF)- Left	X	.3733	.32933
	Y	.0667	.16600
	Z	.0545	.09342

Therefore those variables were not further considered in the follow up statistical analysis. When applying the univariate analysis of variance, the orientation of the distances did present a statistical significant difference in terms of change ($P < 0.05$). When applying the Bonferroni post-hoc test, the transverse dimension showed to be statistically significantly different to the other dimensions ($P < 0.05$). Table 4 shows the mean differences of orbital changes between T1 and T2 in the transverse, antero-posterior and vertical directions as 0.97 mm ($P < 0.05$), 0.36 mm ($P < 0.05$) and 0.33 mm ($P > 0.05$) respectively. As a result, the transverse and antero-posterior changes are statistically significant. Given that the changes were less than 1 mm for the transverse, antero-posterior and vertical directions, the changes should not necessarily be considered clinically significant. The greatest overall transverse change was 4.37 mm which occurred with the right to left most antero-inferior superior orbital rim distance. The greatest overall antero-posterior change was 0.52 mm which was observed with the right most posterior lacrimal crest to right most postero-lateral superior orbital fissure. Lastly, the greatest overall vertical change was 0.63 mm and was from the left most antero-inferior superior orbital rim to left most antero-superior inferior orbital rim.

Discussion

CBCT imaging has been gaining wide acceptance in recent years due to its low radiation exposure, low imaging costs and high spatial resolution [6]. Given its recent acceptance in the field of dentistry, research in the area of CBCT has not been as vast as compared to CT. This is largely due to the fact that CT scanners were invented in 1972 by Hounsfield and Cormack, while the first commercial CBCT dental unit was not introduced

Table 4 Mean difference of orbital change between T1 and T2 in the transverse, antero-posterior and vertical dimensions

Direction (mm)	Paired differences		
	Mean	Std. deviation	Sig. (2-tailed)
Transverse	0.97205	2.24565	0.000
Antero-posterior	0.35879	1.54073	0.000
Vertical	0.32636	2.04374	0.071

to Europe until 1999 [8]. One disadvantage present of CBCT vs. CT is the distinction between soft tissues having CT presenting a higher contrast [8, 9]. In terms of orbit growth, selecting the landmarks to be used to measure changes in the orbit can be difficult. Escaravage and Dutton's study [4] based on CT analyses of the orbit largely influenced our study. Landmarks such as the most posterior point of the lacrimal crest, most antero-medial points of the zygomatic bone and the most medial points of the temporalis grooves were also analyzed in our study. With our 16 landmarks and corresponding 24 distances, we were able to comprehensively analyze 3D spatial orbit skeletal changes in adolescents through CBCT imaging.

It is worth noting that landmark identification is a major source of measurement error. These errors arise in the process of identifying specific landmarks with factors including sharpness of the radiographic images, landmark definition, human error and procedural errors [10, 11]. Three-dimensional imaging has been shown to greatly reduce projection errors compared to traditional two-dimensional imaging. Thus, in the process of selecting adequate landmarks, all these possible errors should be taken into account [12].

To better analyze the results of our study, we decided that grouping the landmark distances in terms of their dimensional orientation, on a three-space plane orientation, could allow us to better visualize growth patterns. Given the fact that we were unable to find other publications as references which tried this measurement approach, we hypothesized that assessed distances in the transverse, antero-posterior and vertical measurements present the most logical sequence. Our interpretations included twelve, eight and four distance measurements for the transverse, antero-posterior and vertical dimensions respectively (Fig. 2). The mean differences of orbital changes between T1 and T2 in the transverse, antero-posterior and vertical dimensions were 0.972, 0.359 and 0.326 mm respectively.

The greatest overall change of all the distances was found to be the right to left most antero-inferior superior orbital rim and antero-superior inferior orbital rim at 4.37 and 4.35 mm respectively. Given that changes in all other distances were less than 1 mm, it could be hypothesized that these landmarks were influenced by normal growth. The right to left most antero-inferior and antero-superior orbital rim were closely located to where the frontal sinus ends. Since the ICC values showed that these landmarks are reliable, it is possible that the frontal sinus is not entirely stable during adolescent growth. It has been previously reported that the frontal sinus undergoes significant growth changes well into adolescence. This is supported by Ruf and Pancherz's study [13] which showed that frontal sinus growth velocity has a large variation intra- and inter-individually. Pubertal peaks were determined to exist at a mean of 1.9 mm/year and cessation of frontal sinus growth could not be determined as sinus growth has been seen to finish at the end of pubertal growth while in other cases growth exceeded the skeletal maturity stage. Another study [14] reported that frontal sinus development is completed by age 18 with increased expansion mostly in length until age 8 and between years 12 to 14 were not statistically associated with the study findings.

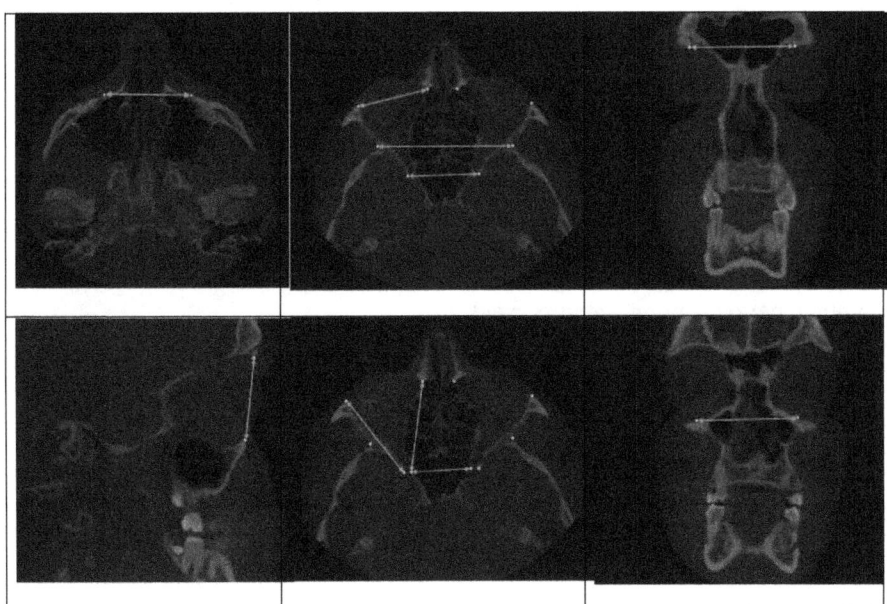

Fig. 2 Diagrams illustrating some of the distances used to assess Transverse, Antero-posterior and Vertical Dimensions

Limitations

The small study sample size can be considered a limitation and our results can be interpreted as preliminary findings.

Additional limitations revolve around the difficulty of determining landmarks due to the quality of some of the CBCT data sets in terms of noise and slice orientation. Landmarks of particular difficulty in terms of identification and pinpointing were the posterior lacrimal crest, infraorbital foramens, superior and inferior orbital rim. Due to the quality of certain CBCT data sets, omissions occurred for some landmarks due to the inability to accurately define them in the given data sets. Furthermore, since slice angulations were based off of the individual's positioning while taking the CBCT, some CBCT data sets were not used in cases where the slice orientations were heavily skewed in order to limit inaccuracies.

A change in the CBCT machine (from NewTom 3G - Aperio Services, Verona, Italy at 110 kV, 6.19mAs and 8 mm aluminum filtration, voxel size of 0.3 mm) used in the graduate orthodontic program also occurred between some T1 and T2 data sets and should be considered as a potential limitation to consistency. This occurred in only three of the cases so the real impact is likely unimportant.

Another limitation was the fact that although we grouped the distances in terms of dimensional orientation, the distances are not entirely in 2D of transverse, anteroposterior or vertical as they contain 3D coordinates. These limitations need to be addressed in the future direction of our study along with the inclusion of additional angular measurements and volumetric changes of the orbit based off of the existing landmarks.

Conclusion

The orbit skeletal and spatial changes were statistically significant, but should not normally be considered clinically significant. The overall average orbit dimensional changes were less than 1 mm. Our results show that the orbits should be considered a good structure to be used for superimposition since in this sample there were minimal, but not clinically relevant, changes during the 19 to 24 months observation period among patients aged between 11 and 19 years.

Abbreviations

2D: Two-dimensional; 3D: Three-dimensional; CBCT: Cone-beam computed tomography; CT: Computed tomography; ICC: Intraclass correlation coefficients

Acknowledgements

Not applicable.

Funding

There is no source of funding for the research reported.

Authors' contributions

BL collected the data, analyzed and interpreted the results and wrote the manuscript. CF and ML mentored BL and participated in planning the study, analyzing the data, and writing the manuscript. All authors read and approved the final manuscript.

Competing interests

The authors declare that they have no competing interests.

Consent for publication

Not applicable.

References

1. Hatcher DC. CT & CBCT imaging assessment of the orbits. Oral Maxillofac Surg Clin North Am. 2012;24:537–43.
2. Rontal E, Rontal M, Guilford FT. Surgical anatomy of the orbit. Ann Otol Rhinol Laryngol. 1979;88:382–6.
3. Zizelmann C, Gellrich NC, Metzger MC, Schoen R, Schmelzeisen R, Schramm A. Computer-assisted reconstruction of orbital floor based on cone beam tomography. Br J Oral Maxillofac Surg. 2007;45:79–80.
4. Escaravage Jr GK, Dutton JJ. Age-related changes in the pediatric human orbit on CT. Ophthal Plast Reconstr Surg. 2013;29:150–6.
5. Sforza C, Elamin F, Tomassi DG, Dolci C, Ferrario VF. Morphometry of the soft tissues of the orbital region in Northern Sudanese persons. Forensic Sci Int. 2013;228:180.e1–11.
6. White SC. Cone-beam imaging in dentistry. Health Phys. 2008;95:628–37.
7. Scarfe WC, Farman AG. What is cone-beam CT and how does it work? Dent Clin North Am. 2008;52:707–30.
8. Angelopoulos C, Scarfe WC, Farman AG. A comparison of maxillofacial CBCT and medical CT. Atlas Oral Maxillofac Surg Clin North Am. 2012;20:1–17.
9. Yilmaz HG, Ayali A. Evaluation of the neurovascular bundle position at the palate with cone beam computed tomography: an observational study. Head Face Med. 2015;11:39.
10. Athanasiou AE. Orthodontic cephalometry. London; Baltimore: Mosby-Wolfe; 1995.
11. Major PW, Johnson DE, Hesse KL, Glover KE. Landmark identification error in posterior anterior cephalometrics. Angle Orthod. 1994;64:447–54.
12. Oz U, Orhan K, Abe N. Comparison of linear and angular measurements using two-dimensional conventional methods and three-dimensional cone beam CT images reconstructed from a volumetric rendering program in vivo. Dentomaxillofac Radiol. 2011;40:492–500.
13. Ruf S, Pancherz H. Development of the frontal sinus in relation to somatic and skeletal maturity. A cephalometric roentgenographic study at puberty. Eur J Orthod. 1996;18:491–7.
14. Spaeth J, Krügelstein U, Schlöndorff G. The paranasal sinuses in CT-imaging: development from birth to age 25. Int J Pediatr Otorhinolaryngol. 1997;39:25–40.

20

Parotidectomy using the Harmonic scalpel: ten years of experience at a rural academic health center

Marc A. Polacco[1,2]*, Andrew M. Pintea[1], Benoit J. Gosselin[1] and Joseph A. Paydarfar[1]

Abstract

Background: Parotidectomy is one of the most commonly performed procedures by otorhinolaryngologists. Traditionally dissection is performed with a combination of a steel scalpel and bipolar cautery; however, starting in the early 2000s, the Harmonic scalpel has provided an alternative method for dissection and hemostasis. The purpose of this study is to compare operative time, blood loss, complications, and cost between the Harmonic scalpel and steel scalpel plus bipolar cautery for superficial and total parotidectomy.

Methods: Retrospective cohort of patients who underwent superficial or total parotidectomy with the Harmonic or cold steel between 2000 and 2015. Across 255 patients, comparison between operative time, blood loss, complications, and cost was performed.

Results: Superficial parotidectomy was performed on 120 patients with the Harmonic and 54 with steel scalpel. Total parotidectomy was performed on 59 patients using the Harmonic and 22 patients with cold steel. For superficial parotidectomy, the Harmonic reduced operative time (216 ± 42 vs. 234 ± 54 min, $p = 0.03$) and decreased blood loss (28 ± 19 vs. 76 ± 52 mls, $p < 0.05$). With total parotidectomy the Harmonic decreased operative time (240 ± 42 vs. 288 ± 78 min, $p = 0.01$) and reduced blood loss (38 ± 21 mls vs. 85 ± 55 mls, $p < 0.05$). There were no differences in complication rates between groups. Harmonic use was associated with surgical cost reduction secondary to reduced operative times.

Conclusions: The Harmonic scalpel decreases blood loss and operating time for superficial and total parotidectomy. Shorter operative times may decrease the overall cost of parotidectomy.

Keywords: Parotidectomy, Harmonic, Blood loss, Operative time, Cost

Background

The incidence of salivary gland neoplasm has been reported to be 1 – 1.4 per 100,000 people annually [1]. Relatively rare, salivary gland tumors account for 5% of all head and neck tumors, the majority of which occur in the parotid gland [2, 3]. Patients who are diagnosed with a parotid gland tumor often undergo parotidectomy. While commonly performed, the procedure is technically challenging and time-consuming as it requires careful dissection of the facial nerve in a region with high vascularity.

The Harmonic scalpel (HS) (Ethicon, Somerville, NJ), an instrument which utilizes ultrasonic vibrations to induce cutting and immediate coagulation of tissue, was introduced in the early 1990s. A low power setting allows for greater hemostasis and slower cutting, while a high power setting offers less hemostasis but faster cutting ability. Since its introduction, the HS has been shown to reduce operative time and intra-operative blood loss across a range of otolaryngologic procedures including thyroidectomy, parotidectomy, glossectomy, and neck dissection [4–7].

The HS reduces bleeding and prevents thermal injury to surrounding tissues greater than 2–3 mm

* Correspondence: Marc.A.Polacco@hitchcock.org

The data within this manuscript were presented at the 9th International Conference on Head and Neck Cancer 2016 Seattle WA.

[1]Department of Otolaryngology, Dartmouth-Hitchcock Medical Center, Lebanon, NH, USA

[2]Dartmouth-Hitchcock Medical Center, One Medical Center Drive, Lebanon, NH 03766, USA

distance, making it an ideal instrument for procedures requiring fine dissection [8, 9]. Prior studies have shown that the HS is useful for reducing blood loss and operative time in superficial and total parotidectomy procedures when compared to using a steel scalpel and bipolar cautery; however, most have contained relatively small cohorts over brief study periods [10–12]. To our knowledge, this is the largest study comparing parotidectomy outcomes between the HS and steel scalpels plus bipolar cautery (SB), and the first to report superficial and total parotidectomy outcomes separately (Table 1). Moreover, this study reports the effect HS use has on the overall cost of performing a parotidectomy.

Methods
The medical records of all patients who underwent superficial or total parotidectomy at Dartmouth-Hitchcock Medical Center from 2000–2015 were retrospectively reviewed after gaining approval from the institutional review board. A total of 424 cases were identified. Cases were excluded if the patient had history of prior parotid surgery, radiation, a bleeding disorder, prior facial nerve disorder, was lost in follow up, or if they underwent a combination of procedures such as parotidectomy with neck dissection. This resulted in exclusion of 148 cases. An additional 21 cases were excluded as they were performed by two surgeons who did not routinely perform parotidectomies, defined as less than five parotidectomies per year (Fig. 1).

All included cases were performed by two surgeons (Table 2). For both surgeons, cases prior to 2006 were performed with a combination of steel scalpels and bipolar cautery, while most cases after 2006 were performed with the Harmonic scalpel. A resident surgeon was present in 81% of cases.

In addition to categorizing cases according to superficial and total parotidectomy with or without use of the HS, cases meeting inclusion criteria were assessed for patient age, sex, operative time, blood loss, postoperative drain output, length of follow up, and complications. Complications assessed included hematoma, seroma, Frey's syndrome, facial nerve weakness, auricular numbness, keloid, and first bite syndrome. The cost of each procedure was calculated using the reported operating room cost per minute for superficial and total parotidectomy multiplied by total minutes to procedure completion. If the HS was opened, the cost of the instrument was added to the cost of the surgical case. The percentage of cost reduction was calculated by taking the ratio of cost of parotidectomy with HS to that of SB, averaged across all procedures. Statistical analyses were conducted using unpaired t-tests for contiguous data and Fisher's exact test for categorical data (Microsoft Excel 2013, Redmond, WA).

Table 1 Literature comparing parotidectomy outcomes

Surgery	Instrument	No.	OR Time (min)	Blood Loss (ml)	Drain Output (ml)
Superficial parotid					
Muhanna et al. 2014 [12]	SB	32	163.12 ± 21.8	NR[a]	73.5 ± 38.2
	HS	26	137.3 ± 18.6	NR[a]	68 ± 22.3
Blankenship et al. 2004 [11]	SB	21	195.5 ± 37.5	60.0 ± 37.1	48.7 ± 33.8
	HS	19	167.5 ± 42.6	37.5 ± 25.8	48.0 ± 22.7
Jackson et al. 2005 [10]	SB	37	NR[a]	68 ± 12	NR[a]
	HS	35	NR[a]	38 ± 4.23	NR[a]
Polacco et al.	SB	54	234 ± 54	76 ± 52	43 ± 36
	HS	120	216 ± 42	28 ± 19	24 ± 15
Total parotid					
Jackson et al. 2005 [10]	SB	4	NR[a]	NR[a]	NR[a]
	HS	9	NR[a]	NR[a]	NR[a]
Polacco et al.	SB	22	288 ± 42	85 ± 55	33 ± 20
	HS	59	240 ± 78	38 ± 21	35 ± 30
Superficial and Total parotid					
Deganello et al. 2014 [5]	SB	63	151.6 ± 54.1	NR[a]	78 ± 81
	HS	67	146.9 ± 39.9	NR[a]	69 ± 52
Jackson et al. 2005 [10]	SB	41	200.5 ± 41.43	66.0 ± 10.8	NR[a]
	HS	44	183.88 ± 58.17	38.0 ± 3.6	NR[a]

[a]*NR* not reported

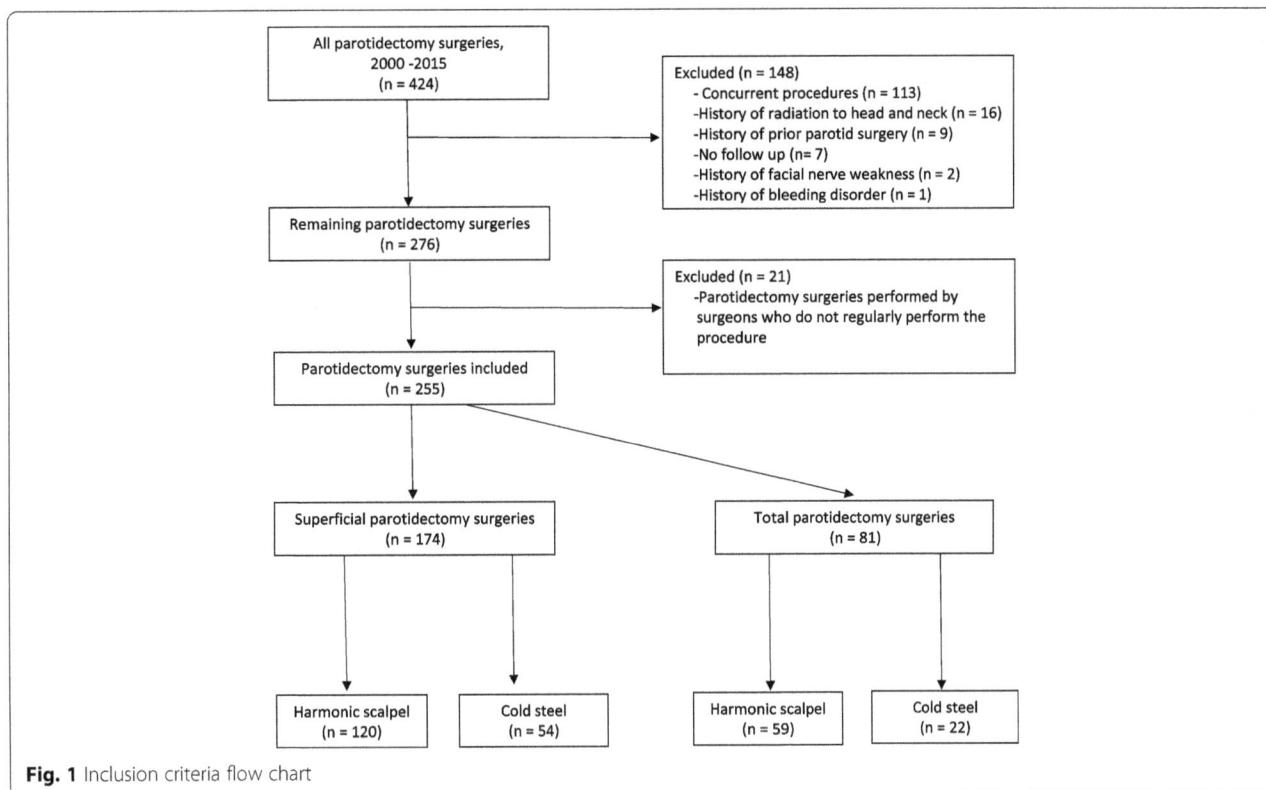

Fig. 1 Inclusion criteria flow chart

Results

Superficial parotidectomy

A total of 174 patients underwent superficial parotidectomy, 120 with the HS and 54 with SB. There was no significant difference for patient age, sex, and mean follow up duration between groups. Use of the HS compared with SB resulted in shorter duration of surgery (216 ± 42 vs. 234 ± 54 min, $p = 0.03$) and less blood loss (28 ± 19 mls vs. 76 ± 52 mls, p < 0.05), but no significant difference in post-operative drain output (24 ± 15 mls vs. 43 ± 36 mls, $p = 0.09$) or complications (Table 3). Taking the cost of the HS into account, there was a 5.6% average reduction in cost for superficial parotidectomy procedures when the HS was used.

Total parotidectomy

In the total parotidectomy group, there were a total of 81 patients who met inclusion criteria, 59 of whom

Table 2 Cases per surgeon

Parotidectomy	Surgeon 1	Surgeon 2
Superficial (SB)[a]	21	33
Superficial (HS)[a]	64	56
Total (SB)[a]	13	9
Total (HS)[a]	28	31
Sum Total Cases	126	129

[a]SB steel scalpel plus bipolar cautery, HS Harmonic scalpel

underwent surgery using the HS and 22 with SB. There was no significant difference in regard to patient age, sex, and mean follow up duration between groups. With total parotidectomy, use of the HS compared with SB resulted in shorter duration of surgery (240 ± 42 vs. 288 ± 78 min, $p = 0.01$) and less blood loss (38 ± 21 mls vs. 85 ± 55 mls, $p < 0.05$), but no significant difference in post-operative drain output (35 ± 30 mls vs. 33 ± 20 mls, $p = 0.78$) or complications. HS use resulted in a 15% average cost reduction of total parotidectomy.

Discussion

The HS utilizes ultrasonic vibration to denature proteins, forming a coagulum for hemostasis while also limiting thermal injury to surrounding tissue. Since the introduction of the HS, it has been shown to be effective in decreasing operative blood loss across a variety of procedures, from total colectomy to hepatectomy [13, 14]. In the otolaryngology literature, the HS has been shown to decrease blood loss and operative times for thyroidectomies, parotidectomies, and neck dissections [10, 15, 16].

This study is the largest to date comparing the Harmonic Scalpel to cold steel in parotidectomy. Our results corroborate prior parotidectomy studies on the HS, showing both a reduction in blood loss and decrease in operating room time when compared to SB (see Table 1). The benefit of using the HS in total parotidectomy procedures is even more compelling as the differences in blood

Table 3 Patient characteristics and outcomes

Variables	Superficial (n = 174)			Total (n = 81)		
	HS (n = 120)	SB (n = 54)	P value	HS (n = 59)	SB (n = 22)	P Value
Mean age (years)	59 ± 14	56 ± 15	0.19	56 ± 15	55 ± 14	0.75
Sex						
Male	56 (47%)	24 (43%)	0.87	31 (53%)	10 (45%)	0.62
Female	64 (53%)	30 (56%)		28 (47%)	12 (55%)	
Blood Loss (ml)	28 ± 19	76 ± 52	<0.05	38 ± 21	85 ± 55	< .05
Drain Output (ml)	24 ± 15	43 ± 36	0.09	35 ± 30	33 ± 20	0.78
OR Time (min)	216 ± 42	234 ± 54	0.03	240 ± 42	288 ± 78	0.01
Length of Follow Up (mo)	7 ± 12	7 ± 7	0.13	9 ± 6	13 ± 12	0.17
Complications						
Auricular Numbness	7 (5%)	2 (4%)	0.72	5 (8%)	3 (14%)	0.68
Transient facial paresis	1 (0.8%)	2 (4%)	0.23	1 (1.6%)	1 (4.5%)	1
Permanent facial paresis	0	0	1	1 (1.6%)	0	1
Facial paralysis	0	0	1	0	0	1
Hematoma	0	0	1	0	0	1
Seroma	1 (0.8%)	0	1	0	0	1
Keloid	1 (0.8%)	0	1	0	0	1
Frey's syndrome	0	0	1	0	1 (4.5%)	1
First Bite	1 (0.8%)	0	1	0	0	1
Average Cost (including cost of Harmonic Scalpel)	$23,190	$24,570		$25,710	$30,240	

loss and operative time between groups was greater. While the difference in blood loss between groups in this study was significant statistically, it is unlikely that the volume of blood saved using the HS is clinically significant.

For both the superficial and total parotidectomy groups, there was a significant difference in operative time between the use of the HS and SB dissection. For the superficial group, the amount of time saved using the HS equated to 18 min, while this difference increased to 48 min in the total parotidectomy group. At our institution the amount of operating room time saved, even in the superficial parotidectomy group, translates into a cost reduction greater than the cost of the HS, resulting in a $1381 (5.6%) and a $4530 (15%) decrease in cost of performing superficial and total parotidectomy respectively. We expect the percentage of cost reduction to be relatively consistent across institutions, whereas the monetary value could be highly variable depending on operating room utilization cost per institution. These data are compelling as healthcare costs continue to soar in the United States and cost reduction efforts become increasingly important. In 2014, 17.1% of the gross domestic product was allocated for health-care, and the Congressional Budget Office estimates this figure to increase to 25% by 2025 should the rate of increasing expenditures remain constant [17]. Being at the forefront of health-care

expenditure, physicians have an obligation to create efforts to control cost in order to continue to provide accessible quality health-care [18].

Moreover, with a decrease in operative time there is also a realized reduction in opportunity cost. Opportunity cost is traditionally defined as the value of a rejected opportunity or alternative [19]. By reducing the overall operative time allocated to performing a parotidectomy, particularly total resections, time resources may be redistributed to endeavors such as additional cases, research, or education. Additionally, this reduction in opportunity cost could translate to increased patient access to providers.

A weakness of this study is that there is no method to determine the degree of resident involvement in the 81% of cases in which there was a resident present. While it could be presumed that junior residents would operate at a slower rate than senior residents, the amount of actual operating time for each resident is likely highly variable as senior residents are granted more autonomy while there is traditionally more attending physician involvement when a junior resident is operating. While one of two attending physicians were present for all cases reported, it is possible that surgeons operating without a resident may not experience a significant difference in blood loss, operating time, or cost.

Conclusion

Use of the HS for superficial and total parotidectomy is associated with a significantly shorter duration of surgery and less blood loss when compared to use of SB. Shorter operative times were great enough to generate cost savings to offset the cost of the HS and decrease the overall cost of parotidectomy.

Acknowledgements
None.

Funding
This research did not receive any specific grant from funding agencies in the public, commercial, or not-for-profit sectors.

Author contributions
MP, JP, Study concept and design. MP, AP, BG, JP, Acquisition, analysis, or data interpretation. MP, AP, BG, JP, Drafting of manuscript. MP, AP, BG, JP, Critical revision for important intellectual content. MP, AP, Statistical analysis. BG, JP, Study supervision. All authors read and approved the final manuscript.

Competing interests
The authors declare that they have no competing interests.

Consent for publication
Not applicable.

References

1. Kimberly H, Lin H, Ann D, Chu P, Yen Y. An overview of the rare parotid gland cancer. Head Neck Oncol. 2011;3(9):40.
2. Laurie S, Licitra L. Systemic therapy in the palliative management of advanced salivary gland cancers. J Clin Oncol. 2006;24(17):2673–8.
3. O'Brien C, Soong S, Herrera G, Urist M, Maddox W. Malignant salivary tumors-analysis of prognostic factors and survival. Head Neck Surg. 1986;9(2):82–92.
4. Koh Y, Park J, Lee S, Choi E. The harmonic scalpel technique without supplementary ligation in total thyroidectomy with central neck dissection: a prospective randomized study. Ann Surg. 2008;247(6):945–9.
5. Deganello A, Meccariello G, Busoni M, Parrinello G, Bertolai R, Gallo O. Dissection with harmonic scalpel versus cold instruments in parotid surgery. B-ENT. 2014;10(3):175–8.
6. Pons Y, Gauthier J, Clement P, Conessa C. Ultrasonic partial glossectomy. Head Neck Oncol. 2009;6(1):21.
7. Dean A, Alamillos F, Centella I, Garcia-Alvarez S. Neck dissection with the Harmonic scalpel in patients with squamous cell carcinoma of the oral cavity. J Craniomaxillofac Surg. 2014;42(1):84–7.
8. Koch C, Friedrich T, Metternich F, Tannapfel A, Reimann H, Eichfeld U. Determination of temperature elevation in tissue during the application of the harmonic scalpel. Ultrasound Med Biol. 2003;29(2):301–9.
9. Tirelli G, Camilot D, Bonini P, Del Piero G, Biasotto M, Quatela E. Harmonic scalpel and electrothermal bipolar vessel sealing system in head and neck surgery: a prospective study on tissue heating and histological damage on nerves. Ann Otol Rhinol Laryngol. 2015;124(11):852–8.
10. Jackson L, Gourin C, et al. Use of the harmonic scalpel in Superficial and total parotidectomy for benign and malignant disease. Laryngoscope. 2005;115:1070–3.
11. Blankenship D, Gourin C, Porubsky E, et al. Harmonic scalpel versus cold knife dissection in superficial parotidectomy. Otolaryngol Head Neck Surg. 2004;131(4):397–400.
12. Muhanna N, Peleg U, Schwartz Y, Shaul H, Perez R, Sichel J. Harmonic scalpel assisted superficial parotidectomy. Ann Otol Rhinol Laryngol. 2014; 123(9):636–40.
13. Bodzin A, Leiby B, Ramirez C, Frank A, Doria C. Liver resection using cavitron ultrasonic surgical aspirator (CUSA) versus harmonic scalpel: a retrospective cohort study. Int J Surg. 2014;12(5):500–3.
14. Rimonda R, Arezzo A, Garrone C, Allaix M, Giraudo G, Morino M. Electrothermal bipolar vessel sealing system vs. harmonic scalpel in colorectal laparoscopic surgery: a prospective, randomized study. Dis Colon Rectum. 2009;52(4):657–61.
15. Da Silva F, Limoeiro A, Del Bianco J, et al. Impact of the use of vessel sealing or harmonic scalpel on intra-hospital outcomes and the cost of thyroidectomy procedures. Einstein. 2012;10(3):354–9.
16. Shin Y, Koh Y, Kim S, Choi E. The efficacy of the Harmonic scalpel in neck dissection: a prospective randomized study. Laryngoscope. 2013;123(4):904–9.
17. The World Bank. Health expenditure, total (% of GDP). http://data. worldbank.org/indicator/SH.XPD.TOTL.ZS?year_high_desc=true. Accessed 24 May 2016.
18. Bosco J, Iorio R, Barber T, Barron C, Caplan A. Ethics of the physician's role in health-care cost control: AOA critical issues. J Bone Joint Surg Am. 2016; 98(14):e58.
19. Spiller S. Opportunity cost consideration. J Consum Res. 2011;38(12):595–610.

Clinical and radiographic evaluation of pulpectomy in primary teeth

Xiaoxian Chen[1], Xinggang Liu[2*] and Jie Zhong[1]

Abstract

Background: To avoid untoward changes when primary teeth are replaced by permanent teeth, resorption of the material used in primary teeth root canal filling should occur at the same rate as root resorption. The Aim of this study was to compare the success rates of a mixed primary root canal filling (MPRCF, ingredients: zinc oxide–eugenol [ZOE], iodoform, calcium hydroxide) to those of ZOE and Vitapex in pulpectomised primary molars.

Methods: One hundred and sixty primary molars from 155 children (average age 5.88 ± 1.27 years) underwent two-visit pulpectomy using one of the three materials. The clinical and radiographic findings at 6, 12 and 18 months were assessed.

Results: At 6 and 12 months, the MPRCF and ZOE success rates were 100%. The Vitapex group showed clinical success rate and radiographic success rate of 100 and 94.5% at 6 months, and 80.4 and 60.7% at 12 months. The 18-month clinical success rates of the MPRCF, ZOE and Vitapex were 96.2, 92.2 and 71.4% and radiographic success rates were 92. 5, 88.2 and 53.6%, respectively. There was a statistically significant difference in the success rates between MPRCF and Vitapex and no significant differences between MPRCF and ZOE. More MPRCF were resorbed at same rate with roots than ZOE and Vitapex. Early resorption of root filling resulted in more failure.

Conclusions: The mixture of ZOE, iodoform and calcium hydroxide can be considered an effective root canal filling material in pulp involved primary teeth and had no adverse effect on tooth replacement.

Keywords: Pulpectomy, Primary teeth, Zinc Oxide-Eugenol, Iodoform, Calcium hydroxide

Background

According to the report of the third national oral health epidemiology investigation of China in 2005, 5-year-old children suffered from caries prevalence rate as high as 67% and the dmft index was 3.59 [1]. Endodontic treatment is considered the last option for keeping a primary tooth that has irreversibly affected pulp tissue due to caries in a child. The aim of pulpectomy is to preserve teeth in a symptom free state until they are replaced by their successor naturally during the transition from primary to permanent dentition, thus avoiding extraction. The adequate

restoration of the involved teeth may preserve the arch length, reestablish the masticatory function and esthetics and prevent harmful tongue habits and speech alterations due to anterior teeth decay. The rationale includes the chemical and mechanical removal of irreversibly inflamed or necrotic radicular pulp tissue, followed by root canal filling with a material that can resorb at the same rate as the primary tooth and be eliminated rapidly if accidentally extruded through the apex [2].

Zinc oxide–eugenol (ZOE) was reported to more successfully manage those hyperemic primary pulp teeth than iodoform containing $Ca(OH)_2$ pastes [3]. Nevertheless it has been reported to have a possibility to alter the path of eruption of the succedaneous tooth when it extrudes beyond the apex of the tooth because of forming a hard mass [4]. As far as resorption rate was concerned,

* Correspondence: iceworlds0033@126.com
[2]Department of Prosthodontics, Beijing Stomatological Hospital&School of Stomatology, Capital Medical University, 4 Tian Tan Xi Li, Beijing 100050, People's Republic of China
Full list of author information is available at the end of the article

ZOE often showed characteristic of slower rate than that of the primary teeth root resorption [5, 6].

Various clinical and radiographic success rates (65–100%) of iodoform have been reported [4, 7, 8]. However, Moskovitz et al. found that root resorption of primary molars is accelerated following pulpectomy with iodoform filling material in comparison with teeth without endodontic treatment [9].

The success rate with calcium hydroxide varied between 86.7 and 100% [10, 11]. Its main disadvantage is when used in primary teeth with hyperemic pulp, calcium hydroxide can come in contact with some vital pulp tissue remnants and can trigger the cascade of inflammatory root resorption [12].

Vitapex, which mainly contains calcium hydroxide and iodoform, were also discovered the early intraradicular resorption of the material, which means that the resorption rate is faster than that of the primary teeth root resorption [5, 13]. Though Nurko et al. found Vitapex was resorbed extraradicularly and intraradicularly without apparent ill effect, whether this affects the prognosis of pulpectomised teeth requires confirmation by further studies [14].

These root canal filling materials for primary teeth available at present do not fully meet the ideal requirements of primary teeth root canal treatment. The failure of root canal therapy in many primary teeth is due to inappropriate degradation of the material. The hypothesis of the study was adding the more resorbable materials (iodoform and calcium hydroxide) into ZOE would get favourable absorbability results of the mixture and improve the success rate of treatment. In this prospective study, a modified primary root canal filling (MPRCF), a mixture of ZOE, iodoform, and calcium hydroxide, was made and used in pulpectomies of primary molars in clinic. The aim of this paper is to evaluate the success rate of MPRCF, ZOE and Vitapex, which were the popular choose of dentists, as primary molar root canal filling materials and to compare the resorption rates.

Methods
Preparation of MPRCF
In an in vitro study, the preparation of MPRCF was tested. The proportions of ZOE and iodoform were determined by the consistency of the paste and manufacturers guidance, approximately 1:1 in volume. Five different weight of calcium hydroxide, 0.01 g, 0.02 g, 0.03 g, 0.04 g and 0.05 g, was added and the applicable setting time of mixture was recorded. Calcium hydroxide could accelerate the setting process and the more calcium hydroxide added, the shorter the setting time. The final amount of calcium hydroxide was determined in as low as 0.01 g. The eventual proportion of ZOE: iodoform: calcium hydroxide in the MPRCF was 0.28 g: 0.18 g: 0.01 g. The working time was 6 min and 50 s and setting time was 31 min, which was suitable for clinical use. The pH of MPRCF was 9.8. Zinc oxide, eugenol, iodoform and calcium hydroxide were provided by hospital preparation workroom. The schematic figure about the advantage of MPRCF compared with ZOE was showed in Fig. 1.

Subjects
The present study was a double blind randomized controlled trail. The participants were collected in Department of Pediatric Dentistry, First Dental Center, Peking University School and Hospital of Stomatology. The name of trial registry was Chinese clinical trial registry and the registration number was ChiCTR-TRC-14004938. The Ethics Committee of Peking University School and Hospital of Stomatology approved this study. The parents/guardians of the participants signed individual informed consent forms containing information about the aim of the study and the treatment procedures.

Children between the ages of 4 and 9 were recruited and data concerning clinical and radiographic evaluation were collected in 6, 12 and 18 months or longer follow-up thereafter. The criteria for case selection were irreversible pulpitis, necrotic pulp or periodontitis as follow [15]:

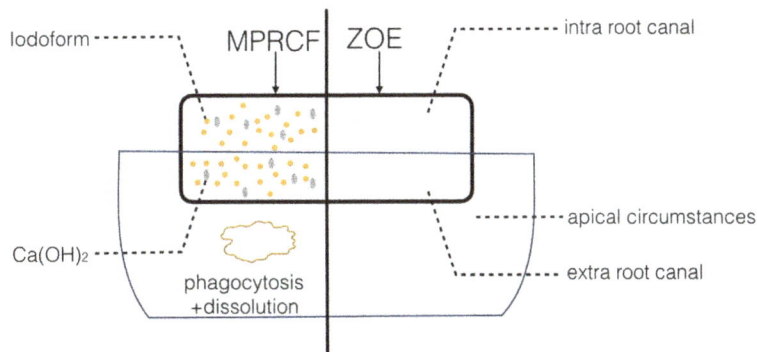

Fig. 1 Schematic figure of MPRCF and ZOE. High solubility of calcium hydroxide, strength of chelation was lower and filling mass become porous when contacting with tissue fluid create the favourable resorb ability

1. Clinical characteristics, defined as spontaneous pain and the presence of a deep carious lesion with pulp exposure and bleeding that did not halt within five minutes following removal of the coronal pulp tissue. Gingival abscesses or fistula openings were absent or present. Abnormal mobility was requested.

2. Radiographic evaluation revealing that the molar had no internal resorption, with or without furcal or periapical radiolucencies and that physiological root resorption was less than 1/3.

Candidates were excluded if their molar could not be restored or if they had pathologic root resorption.

The sample size was calculated using the sample size formula in order to estimate a proportion. The clinical success rate in centre of ZOE was 85.7% reported by Gupta [13]. The desired accuracy of 10% and the significance level of 5% were considered. The sample size found was 47 children. Therefore, the sample of 51 children in each group used allowed a safety margin of 10% to account for possible losses to follow-up.

Treatment, radiography, and follow-up

One dentist treated each molar involved in two visits. At the first appointment, the molar was isolated with a rubber dam following local anaesthesia. The pulp chamber was accessed after removal of all carious tooth structures. Pulpal debris was removed with barbed broaches. The working length was determined by superimposing an endodontic instrument over the preoperative radiograph and keeping it 1–2 mm short of the radiographic apex. Cleaning and shaping of the root canals was carried out using Mani k files (MANI Inc., Tochigi, Japan). The files were used sequentially in a pullback direction up to a maximum size of 35–40. Continuous irrigation with 2.5% sodium hypochlorite was carried out throughout the procedure.

Sterile paper points were used to dry the root canals. Calcium hydroxide (Multi-Cal, Pulpdent Corporation, Watertown, MA, USA) was injected into the root canal and a sterile cotton ball was placed in the pulp chamber and sealed with Cavit (3M ESPE, St. Paul, MN, USA) as temporary sealing material. At the second visit, which was typically two weeks later, the root canal was irrigated with 2.5% sodium hypochlorite and dried with sterile paper points. The prepared molars were allocated to ZOE, Vitapex (Neo Dental Chemical Products Co. Ltd., Tokyo, Japan), or MPRCF groups by random number table. The list was annexed in opaque covers and maintained the confidentiality of allocation until the time of obturation.

ZOE

Root canals were filled with ZOE paste (0.42 g zinc oxide, 0.14 g eugenol) mixed to medium consistency and delivered using lentulo spirals (MANI Inc.).

Vitapex

A syringe was inserted into the root canal near the apex and the material was extruded using moderate pressure. The syringe was then slowly withdrawn and the paste injected until it flowed back from the root canal into the pulp chamber.

MPRCF

We weighed 0.21 g zinc oxide (44.7%), 0.07 g eugenol (14.9%), 0.18 g iodoform (38.3%), and 0.01 g calcium hydroxide (2.1%) using an electronic scale, then combined them in sequence to medium consistency, packed it into the root canal using lentulo spirals.

Radiographs were obtained to determine whether the root canals were completely filled. The root canal fillings were categorised with regard to length in relation to the radiographic apex: underfilled (longer than 2 mm), adequate (0–2 mm), or overfilled (over apex). A tooth was categorized as overfilled even if other roots were filled short or adequate [16]. The pulp chambers of all molars were restored with GIC (Lime-Lite Light Cure Cavity Liner, Pulpdent Corporation) and cavities were restored with composite resin (Filtek Z250 Universal Restorative, 3M ESPE) or 3M stainless steel crown.

Molars were evaluated clinically and radiographically at 6, 12 and 18 months later by two investigators blinded to the type of filling material used for each molar. The patients and their guardians also didn't know which group they allocated in. The teeth would be refilled if any recurrent caries present to ensure no leakage. The intra-examiner reliability of the first and second co-investigator was calculated by Cohen's kappa statistic (0.85 and 0.95, respectively). The evaluations of the two co-investigators were calibrated and standardised to determine inter-examiner reliability by independently analysing the radiographs of 20 primary molars. Cohen's kappa statistic indicated excellent reproducibility between the two co-investigators with a measurement agreement of 0.85.

Clinical and radiographic success criteria

The criteria for clinical success were that patients were completely free of clinical signs and symptoms including pain, gingival abscesses, fistula openings, and abnormal mobility [17, 18].

The criteria for radiographic success were no pathologic external root resorption and no radiographic lesions [7, 19].

The radiographic examination also included resorption of excess extraradicularly extruded materials and filling material in the root canal, and direction of the successor permanent molars. The overfilled material was described as non-resorbed, partly resorbed, or completely resorbed. The state of filling material in the root canal were divided into five levels: both root and filling no change; root no change but filling resorbed; root began resorption, filling resorbed at faster rate; root began resorption, filling resorbed at same rate (the distance from the apex in the radiograph to the bottom of the filling being less than 1 mm); root began resorption, filling resorbed at slower rate [20].

Statistical analysis

Statistical analysis was performed using SPSS 17.0. The Chi-square Test was used to compare the distribution and success rate difference between the three groups. Relationship of faster resorption of materials in the root canals and radiographic success in Vitapex group at 18 months was determined with Fisher's exact test. Comparison of resorption of overfilled material between ZOE and MPRCF group used Mann–Whitney U test. A P-value <0.05 was considered statistically significant.

Results

The final sample of the clinical trial consisted of 155 children (average age 5.88 ± 1.27 years), 160 molars in

total. The loss of follow up rate was 1.84%. The participant CONSORT flow diagram was shown in Fig. 2. The distribution of the 160 primary molars at baseline is equilibrium in age, gender, first or second molars and maxillary or mandibular between groups.

Clinical and radiographic success rates of ZOE, Vitapex, and MPRCF root canal treatment at 6,12 and 18 months were showed in Table 1. No molar in the ZOE and MPRCF groups failed the 6- and 12-month clinical and radiographic evaluations. At 18-month evaluation six molars in ZOE group and four molars in MPRCF groups showed radiologically failed compared with 26 molars failure (46.4%) in Vitapex group. There was a significant difference in clinical and radiographic success rate between the ZOE and Vitapex groups ($P = 0.01$) and between the MPRCF and Vitapex groups ($P = 0.01$) at 12 months and 18 months. There were no significant differences between MPRCF and ZOE group at any time-point.

More teeth filled with MPRCT showed the same resorption rate between the root filling material and roots. In the MPRCF group, when roots had begun physiological resorption, the filling material was resorbed at the same rate in 87.1% molars at 18 months (Fig. 3). During the roots were in stable stage, the MPRCF filling inner the roots kept intact synchronously (Figs. 4, 5 and 6). ZOE was resorbed slowly than roots in 39.2% teeth at 18 months (Fig. 7). The Chi-square test showed that at

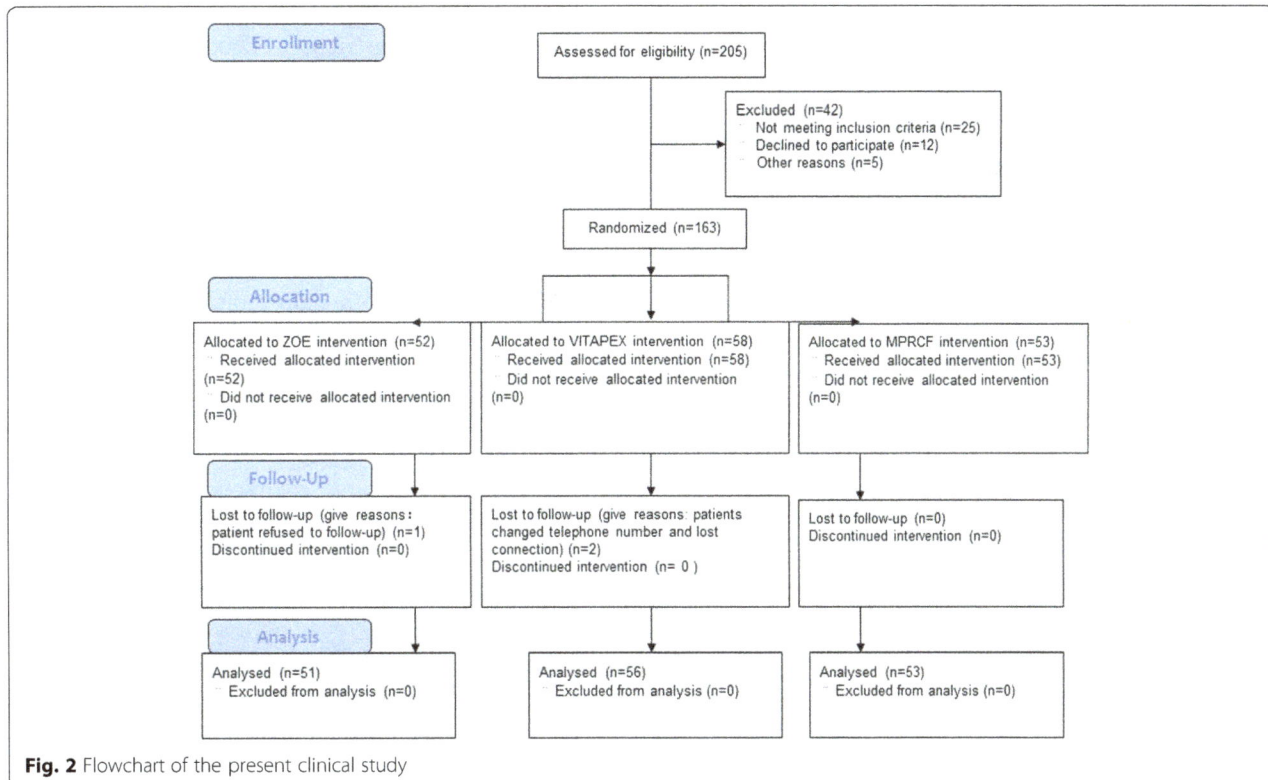

Fig. 2 Flowchart of the present clinical study

Table 1 Clinical and radiographic success rates of ZOE, Vitapex, and MPRCF root canal treatment at 6,12 and 18 months

	Clinical success						Radiographic success					
	6 months		12 months		18 months		6 months		12 months		18 months	
	N	%	N	%	N	%	N	%	N	%	N	%
ZOE	51	100	51	100[a]	47	92.2[a]	51	100	51	100[a]	45	88.2[a]
Vitapex	56	100	45	80.4[ab]	40	71.4[ab]	53	94.5	34	60.7[ab]	30	53.6[ab]
MPRCF	53	100	53	100[b]	51	96.2[b]	53	100	53	100[b]	49	92.5[b]

[a]mean the success rate were significantlly different between ZOE group and Vitapex group
[b]mean the success rate were significantlly different between Vitapex group and MPRCF group

18 months there was a significant difference of the proportions of resorption at same rate between the MPRCF and ZOE ($P = 0.001$) and the MPRCF and Vitapex groups ($P = 0.01$) (Table 2).

At 18 months, the proportion of molars in which Vitapex was resorbed faster than the root was 84% and 26 molars of them failed in radiographic evaluation. Fisher's exact test showed the situation of Vitapex was resorbted faster than root resulted in more failure pulpectomy than non-resorbed condition, at least in radiographic evaluation (Table 3).

The resorption of overfilled materials wsa showed in Table 4. Extruded Vitapex was resorbed completely at 6-month follow-up. Two-thirds extruded ZOE was not resorbed at 12 months and about one-thirds at 18 months. Extruded MPRCF was completely resorbed in 72.7% of cases at 12 months and 100% at 18 months. There were significant difference of the resorption of overfilled material between ZOE and MPRCF group.

Discussion

Clinical studies have shown the success rate of ZOE paste used alone to range from 54 to 100% [6, 19–21] and there is no difference between the success rates of ZOE, calcium hydroxide, or iodoform paste [19, 21]. The bacterial leakage test model of Sisodia R et al. indicated that Zinc Oxide Eugenol showed no bacterial leakage and better resistance to bacterial leakage than Apexit plus (a calcium hydroxide based root canal sealer paste) [22]. ZOE showed better inhibitory activity against most of the organisms isolated than Vitapex, Calcium

hydroxide and Metapex, which proved by Harini PM et al. [23]. These characteristics may be the cause of good clinical manifestations of ZOE, and was also the reason why the present study chooses the ZOE as the main component of the mixed paste.

However, particles of extruded material remained evident after 18 months in most cases in the ZOE group, which was consistent with the findings of previous studies [4–6, 24]. Several researchers found that ZOE extruded extraradicularly was resorbed slowly and might need several months or even years [5, 25, 26]. Allen explained the reason might be the ability of ZOE to resist phagocytising macrophages [27]. With respect to the negative effect of extruded ZOE, Ozalp et al. and other investigators observed that ZOE caused the permanent tooth germ to erupt abnormally [6, 26].

The relatively high number of overfilled molars for the ZOE (41.2%) and MPRCF (41.5%) groups was caused by the use of lentulo spirals and the consistency of pastes. There is no apical constriction of root in primary teeth and measuring the working length in primary teeth is relatively difficult also contributed to the extrusion of material.

In this study, patients with Vitapex that extruded beyond the apex all exhibited complete resorption within six months, which consisted with other researchers' findings [14, 28, 29]. Vitapex had been used as root filling material in primary tooth pulpectomies for many years until rescently researchers have observed that Vitapex resorption was faster than root canal in follow-up period [6, 21, 29]. Ramar reported 56.6% of Vitapex treated

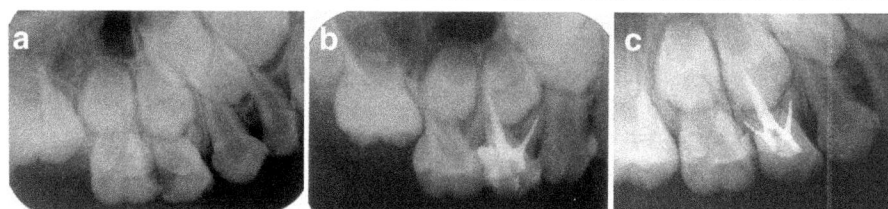

Fig. 3 Eighteen months follow-up of MPRCF. **a** Pre–operative radiograph of 54 considered for root canal treatment with MPRCF. **b** Radiograph taken immediately postoperatively showing adequate filled. **c** Radiograph 18 months postoperatively showing the fillings were resorbed at the similar rate with palatal root

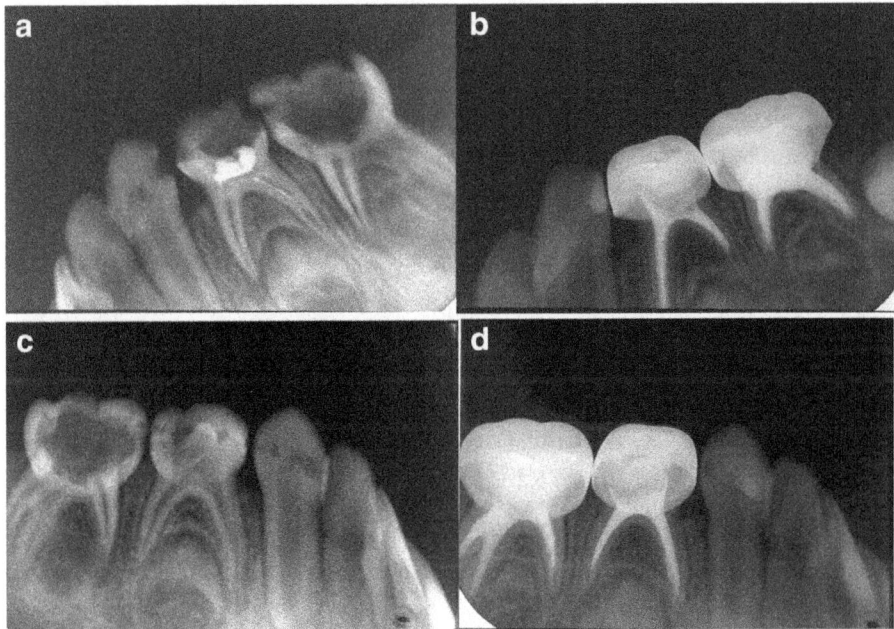

Fig. 4 Eighteen months follow-up of MPRCF. **a, c** Pre–operative Radiograph of *right* and *left* mandibular first and second primary molar considered for root canal treatment with MPRCF. **b, d** Radiograph 18 months postoperatively showing the MPRCF fillings were stable and intact

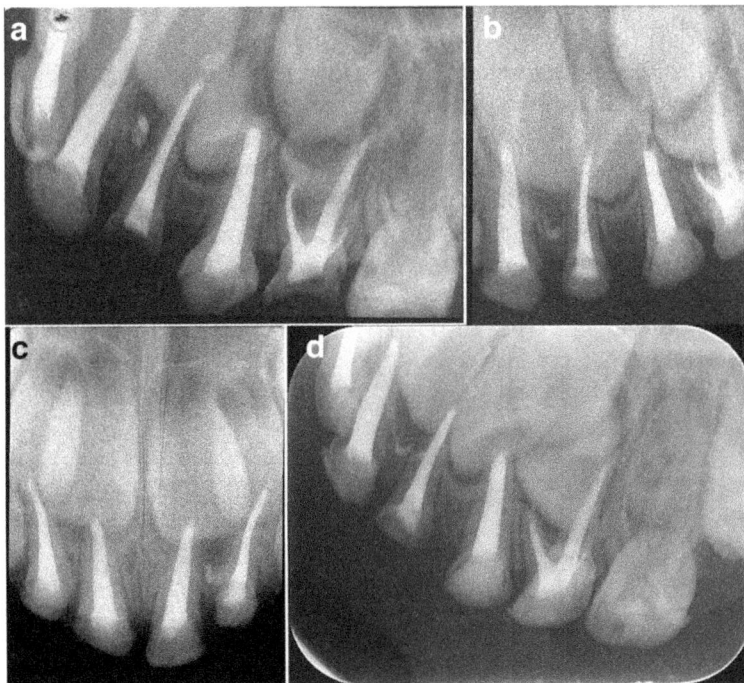

Fig. 5 Twenty-four months follow-up of MPRCF. **a** Radiograph of 52–64 treated with MPRCF taken 6 months postoperatively. **b, c** Radiograph taken 18 months postoperatively showing partly resorption of overfilled materials in 62. **d** Radiograph taken 24 months postoperatively showing intact filling

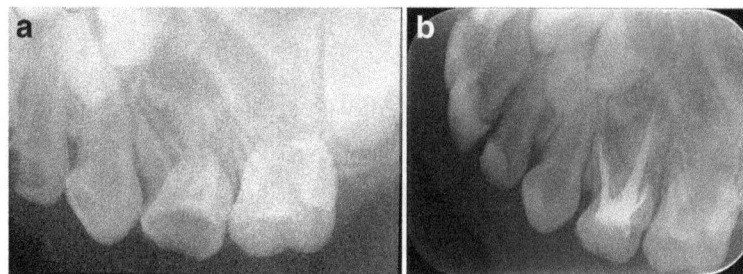

Fig. 6 Eighteen months follow-up of MPRCF. **a** Pre–operative radiograph of maxillary first left primary molar of a 3-year-old girl considered for root canal treatment with MPRCF **b** Radiograph taken 18 months postoperatively showing no resorption of materials in all roots canal

teeth showed material resorption ahead of the roots in 9 months [30]. In the present study, when Vitapex was resorbed faster than roots, 55% teeth failed in radiographic evaluation and 61% the radiographic-failed cases exhibited clinical signs and symptoms. Our study confirmed that the excessive resorption rate of root canal filling affected both clinical and radiographic success rate. Though Nurko et al. found Vitapex was resorbed faster than roots without apparent ill effect [14], the authors mentioned a longer follow-up is recommended to evaluate if there is any effect on the permanent succedaneous tooth. Actually the early resorption of Vitapex may form a narrow channel for bacterial growth and cause reinfection in the root canal [5]. Nakornchai and Banditsing also revealed the clinical success rate of Vitapex could as high as 96%, but the 6- and 12-month radiographic success rates were 80 and 56% respectively; their findings were similar to ours [16].

Root canal filling material of primary teeth should be resorbed at an identical rate, or as similarly as possible, to that of physiological root resorption. This study used a modified paste comprising a mixture of ZOE, iodoform, and calcium hydroxide as root canal filling material in primary molars. Our results indicated that the modified paste with a success rate of 92.5% is a much better material compared with Vitapex and had better absorbability compared with ZOE alone. The possible reason was that the mixture does not set into a hard mass. The potential mechanism lied in two aspects.

Firstly, the essence of formation of ZOE is the reaction of eugenol and bivalent zinc ions to form insoluble chelation, wrapping remanent zinc oxide in it and forming a solid mass. Because calcium ion dissolves more easily than zinc ions, adding calcium hydroxide forms divalent metal chelate salt containing mainly eugenol calcium. Owing to the high solubility of calcium hydroxide, the reaction time is shorter, but strength of chelation was slightly low, thus degrade more quickly. Secondly, iodoform dissolves easily upon contact with solutions and tissue fluid, changing the structure of the filling mass to a porous and loose state that might be resorbed more easily [14].

Interestingly, Endoflas, produced in South America, also comprising of triiodomethane, zinc oxide eugenol, calcium hydroxide, has been reported having the resorption limited to the excess material [17] and resorbs at the same pace as the physiological resorption of root [15]. The antimicrobial efficacy in-vitro study showed Endoflas had good antimicrobial potential against eight microbial strains including E. faecalis compared to other primary root canal filling materials [31, 32]. Specifically, MPRCF had the advantage of resorption that was limited to the material extruded extraradicularly without intraradicular early resorption. As the property of resorption, the MPRCF fulfilled the basic requirement of an ideal root canal filling material for primary molars more compared with ZOE. However, further in-depth study is need to complete the in-vitro antibacterial effects of this

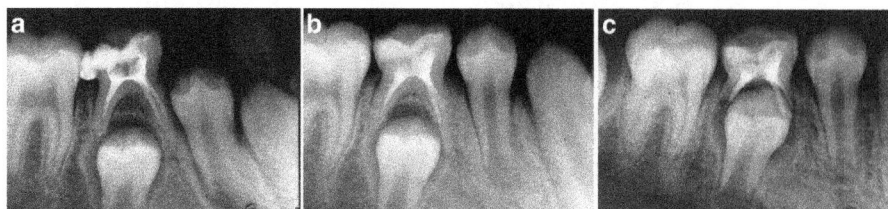

Fig. 7 Twelve months follow-up of ZOE. **a** Radiograph of 84 treated with ZOE taken immediately postoperatively showing adequate filled. **b** Radiograph taken 6 months postoperatively showing slower resorption rate of filling material than roots. **c** Radiograph taken 12 months postoperatively showing remaining of filling material

Table 2 Relationship of resorption rates of materials in the root canals and roots

	ZOE		Vitapex		MPRCF	
	N	%	N	%	N	%
6 months						
A	48	94.1	23	41.1	32	68.2
B	0	0	27	48.2	0	0
C	0	0	2	3.6	0	0
D	2	3.9 [a]	4	7.1 [b]	21	31.8 [ab]
E	1	2.0	0	0	0	0
12 months						
A	32	62.7	10	17.9	26	49.1
B	0	0	14	25	0	0
C	0	0	28	50	3	5.7
D	3	5.9[a]	4	7.1[b]	24	45.2[ab]
E	16	31.4	0	0	0	0
18 months						
A	25	49.0	7	12.5	20	37.7
B	0	0	16	28.6	2	3.6
C	0	0	31	55.4	4	7.5
D	6	11.8[a]	2	3.5[b]	27	50.9[ab]
E	20	39.2	0	0	0	0
Total	51	100	56	100	53	100

A: both no changes, B: root no change but filling resorbed, C: root began resorption, filling resorbed at faster rate, D: root began resorption, filling resorbed at same rate, E: root began resorption, filling resorbed at slower rate
[a]mean the proportions of resorption at same rate were significantlly different between ZOE group and MPRCF group
[b]mean the proportions of resorption at same rate were significantlly different between Vitapex group and MPRCF group

combination and understanding the degradation mechanism of this mixed root filling material and longitudinal study involving a larger sample size is necessary to evaluate the success and resorpsion rate until the teeth' eventual exfoliation.

Conclusion

Endodontic treatment using a mixture of ZOE, iodoform, and calcium hydroxide in primary teeth has shown better clinical and radiographic success than Vitapex at 12 and 18 months and had similar success rate with ZOE. The MPRCF can be considered an effective root canal filling material in primary teeth due to its better resorbable characteristics.

Table 3 Relationship of faster resorption of materials in the root canals and radiographic success in Vitapex group at 18 months

	Faster filling resorption		
	+	−	P
Success	21	9	
Fail	26	0	0.0001

Table 4 Comparison of resorption of overfilled material between ZOE and MPRCF group

	ZOE		MPRCF		P
	N	%	N	%	
6 months					
Non resorb	15	71.4	0	0	
Partly resorb	5	23.8	12	54.5	
Completely resorb	1	4.8	10	45.5	0.000
12 months					
Non resorb	14	66.7	0	0	
Partly resorb	4	19.0	6	27.3	
Completely resorb	3	14.3	16	72.7	0.000
18 months					
Non resorb	8	66.7	0	0	
Partly resorb	8	19.0	0	0	
Completely resorb	5	14.3	22	100	0.000
Total	21	100	22	100	

Abbreviations
MPRCF: Mixed primary root canal filling; ZOE: Zinc oxide–eugenol

Acknowledgements
The authors would like to thank all the residents and the nursing staff at the Department of Pediatric Dentistry, First Dental Center, Peking University School and Hospital of Stomatology who were involved in the management and care of our patients.

Funding
This research received grant from the Funds Program for New Clinical Techniques and Therapies of Peking University School and Hospital of Stomatology.

Authors' contributions
XC contributed to the implementation of the study, analysis and writing of this manuscript. XL supervised the development of the manuscript and participated in the design of the study and performed the statistical analysis. JZ contributed to the study design, initiated the study, and provided comments on the manuscript. All authors read and approved the final manuscript.

Competing interests
The authors declare that they have no competing interests.

Consent for publication
Written informed consent was obtained from the patient's legal guardian(s) for publication of this article and any accompanying images.

Author details
[1]Department of Pediatric Dentistry, First clinical Division, Peking University School and Hospital of Stomatology, Beijing, China. [2]Department of Prosthodontics, Beijing Stomatological Hospital&School of Stomatology, Capital Medical University, 4 Tian Tan Xi Li, Beijing 100050, People's Republic of China.

References
1. Xiaoqiu Q. Report of the third national oral health epidemiology investigation [J]. Beijing: People's Medical Publishing House; 2008. p. 60.
2. Machida Y. Root canal obturation in primary teeth: a review. Jap Dent Assoc J. 1983;36:796–802. www.aapd.org/assets/1/25/Goerig-05-01.pdf
3. Walia T. Pulpectomy in hyperemic pulp and accelerated root resorption in primary teeth: a review with associated case report. J Indian Soc Pedod Prev Dent. 2014;32(3):255–61. http://dx.doi.org/10.4103/0970-4388.135844. PMid:25001448
4. Coll JA, Sadrian R. Predicting pulpectomy success and its relationship to exfoliation and succedaneous dentition. Pediatr Dent. 1996;18:57–63. PMid: 8668572
5. Mortazavi M, Mesbahi M. Comparison of zinc oxide and eugenol, and Vitapex for root canal treatment of necrotic primary teeth. Int J Paediatr Dent. 2004;14:417–24. http://dx.doi.org/10.1111/j.1365-263X.2004.00544.x. PMid:15525310
6. Ozalp N. Sarog¨lu I, Sönmez H. Evaluation of various root canal filling materials in primary molar pulpectomies: an in vivo study. Am J Dent. 2005; 18:347–50. PMid:16433405
7. Garcia-Godoy F. Evaluation of an iodoform paste in root canal therapy for infected primary teeth. J Dent Child. 1987;54:30–4. PMid:3468139
8. Primosch RE, Glomb TA, Jerrell RG. Primary tooth pulp therapy as taught in predoctoral pediatric dental programs in the United States. Pediatr Dent. 1997;19:118–22. PMid:9106874
9. Moskovitz M, Tickotsky N, Ashkar H, Holan G. Degree of root resorption after root canal treatment with iodoform containing filling material in primary molars. Quintessence Int. 2012;43:361–8. PMid:22536587
10. Chawla HS, Mani SA, Tewari A, Goyal A. Calcium hydroxide as a root canal filling material in primary teeth—a pilot study. J Indian Soc Pedod Prev Dent. 1998;16:90–2. PMid:10635131
11. Nadkarni U, Damle SG. Comparative evaluation of calcium hydroxide and zinc oxide eugenol as root canal filling materials for primary molars: a clinical and radiographic study. J Indian Soc Pedod Prev Dent. 2000;18:1–10. PMid:11323998
12. Ravi GA, Subramanyam RV. Calcium hydroxide – induced resorption of deciduous teeth: a possible explanation. Dent Hypotheses. 2012;3:90–4. http://dx.doi.org/10.4103/2155-8213.103910
13. Gupta S, Das G. Clinical and radiographic evaluation of zinc oxide eugenol and metapex in root canal treatment of primary teeth. J Indian Soc Pedod Prev Dent. 2011;29:222–8. http://dx.doi.org/10.4103/0970-4388.85829. PMid: 21985878
14. Nurko C, Ranly DM, García-Godoy F, Lakshmyya KN. Resorption of a calcium hydroxide/iodoform paste (Vitapex) in root canal therapy for primary teeth: a case report. Pediatr Dent. 2000;22:517–20. PMid:11132515
15. Santamaria RM, Innes NPT, Machiulskiene V, Evans DJP, Splieth CH. Caries management strategies for primary molars: 1-yr randomized control trial results. J Dent res. 2014;93(11):1062–9. http://dx.doi.org/10.1177/0022034514550717. PMid:25216660 PMCid:PMC4293767
16. Nakornchai S, Banditsing P, Visetratana N. Clinical evaluation of 3Mix and Vitapex as treatment options for pulpally involved primary molars. Int J Paediatr Dent. 2010;20:214–21. http://dx.doi.org/10.1111/j.1365-263X.2010.01044.x. PMid:20409203
17. Fuks AB, Eidelman E, Pauker N. Root fillings with Endoflas in primary teeth: a retrospective study. J Clin Pediatr Dent. 2002;27:41–6. http://dx.doi.org/10.17796/jcpd.27.1.pp237453707386m1. PMid:12413171
18. Payne RG, Kenny DJ, Johnston DH, Judd PL. Two-year outcome study of zinc oxide-eugenol root canal treatment for vital primary teeth. J Can Dent Assoc. 1993;59:528–30. 533-6. PMid:8513418
19. Holan G, Fuks AB. Root canal treatment with ZOE and KRI paste in primary molars: a retrospective study. Pediatr Dent. 1993;15:403–7. PMid:8153002
20. Rewal N, Thakur A, Sachdev V, Mahajan N. Comparison of Endoflas and zinc oxide Eugenol as root canal filling materials in primary dentition. J Indian Soc Pedod Prev Dent. 2014;32:317–6. http://dx.doi.org/10.4103/0970-4388.140958. PMid:25231040
21. Trairatvorakul C, Chunlasikaiwan S. Success of pulpectomy with zinc oxide-eugenol vs calcium hydroxide/ iodoform paste in primary molars: a clinical study. Pediatr Dent. 2008;30:303–8. PMid:18767509
22. Sisodia R, Ravi KS, Shashikiran ND, Singla S, Kulkarni V. Bacterial penetration along different root canal fillings in the presence or absence of smear layer in primary teeth. J Clin Pediatr Dent. 2014;38:229–34. http://dx.doi.org/10.17796/jcpd.38.3.q8w63111t2354786. PMid:25095317
23. Harini PM, Bhat SS, Sundeep HK. Comparative evaluation of bactericidal potential of four root canal filling materials against microflora of infected non-vital primary teeth. J Clin Pediatr Dent. 2010;35(1):23–9. http://dx.doi.org/10.17796/jcpd.35.1.u57p4500360g2752
24. Bawazir OA, Salama FS. Clinical evaluation of root canal obturation methods in primary teeth. Pediatr Dent. 2006;28:39–47. PMid:16615374
25. Sadrian R, Coll JA. A long-term followup on the retention rate of zinc oxide eugenol filler after primary tooth pulpectomy. Pediatr Dent. 1993;15:249–53. PMid:8247898
26. Reddy VV, Fernandes. Clinical and radiological evaluation of zinc oxide-eugenol and Maisto's paste as obturating materials in infected primary teeth–nine months study. J Indian Soc Pedod Prev Dent. 1996;14:39–44. PMid:9522755
27. Allen KR. Endodontic treatment of primary teeth. Aust Dent J. 1979;24:347–51. http://dx.doi.org/10.1111/j.1834-7819.1979.tb05807.x. PMid:294240
28. Ranly DM, Garic-Godoy F. Reviewing pulp treatment for primary teeth. J am Dent Assoc. 1991;122:83–5. http://dx.doi.org/10.14219/jada.archive.1991.0263. PMid:1918674
29. Kawakami T, Nakamura C, Eda S. Effects of the penetration of a root canal filling material into the mandibular canal. 1. Tissue reaction to the material. Endod Dent Traumatol. 1991;7:36–41. http://dx.doi.org/10.1111/j.1600-9657.1991.tb00180.x. PMid:1915124
30. Ramar K, Mungara J. Clinical and radiographic evaluation of pulpectomies using three root canal filling materials: an in-vivo study. J Indian Soc Pedod Prev Dent. 2010;28:25–9. http://dx.doi.org/10.4103/0970-4388.60481. PMid:20215668
31. Navit S, Jaiswal N, Khan SA, Malhotra S, Sharma A, Mukesh, et al. Antimicrobial efficacy of contemporary Obturating materials used in primary teeth- an in-vitro study. J Clin Diagn res. 2016;10(9):ZC09–12. PMid:27790570
32. Hegde S, Lala PK, Dinesh RB, Shubha AB. An in vitro evaluation of antimicrobial efficacy of primary root canal filling materials. J Clin Pediatr Dent. 2012;37(1):59–64. PMid: 23342568

22

Dentin abrasivity of various desensitizing toothpastes

W. H. Arnold[1*], Ch. Gröger[1], M. Bizhang[2] and E. A. Naumova[1]

Abstract

Background: The aim of this study was to compare the abrasivity of various commercially available toothpastes that claim to reduce dentin hypersensitivity.

Methods: Dentin discs were prepared from 70 human extracted molars. The discs were etched with lemon juice for 5 min, and one half of the discs were covered with aluminum tape. Following this, they were brushed with 6 different toothpastes, simulating a total brushing time of 6 months. As a negative control, discs were brushed with tap water only. The toothpastes contained pro-arginine and calcium carbonate, strontium acetate, stannous fluoride, zinc carbonate and hydroxyapatite, new silica, or tetrapotassium pyrophosphate and hydroxyapatite. After brushing, the height differences between the control halves and the brushed halves were determined with a profilometer and statistically compared using a Mann–Whitney U test for independent variables.

Results: A significant difference ($p < 0.001$) in height difference between the controls and the toothpaste-treated samples was found in all cases, except for the stannous fluoride-containing toothpaste ($p = 0.583$). The highest abrasion was found in the toothpaste containing zinc carbonate and hydroxyapatite, and the lowest was found in the toothpaste containing pro-arginine and calcium carbonate.

Conclusions: Desensitizing toothpastes with different desensitizing ingredients have different levels of abrasivity, which may have a negative effect on their desensitizing abilities over a long period of time.

Keywords: Toothpaste, Dentin, Dentin tubules, Root dentin, Hypersensitivity

Background

The prevalence of dentin hypersensitivity has been increasing over the past decades [1], and there is a need for adequate treatment of this condition. The causes of dentin hypersensitivity include open dentin tubules due to gingival recession and subsequent cervical dentin erosion [2]. Dentin erosion occurs for a variety of reasons. Amongst them are erosive foods and beverages, as well as esophageal reflux or eating disorders [3]. Another reason for dentin erosion may be the use of toothpastes and toothbrushes [4]. Various strategies have been developed to handle this problem. They range from home-use dental products, such as desensitizing toothpastes [5–10], to in-office treatments, such as sealing dentin tubules either with a varnish [11–13] or with a dentin adhesive [14, 15]. The first choice treatment of dentin hypersensitivity is home-use dental products, mainly desensitizing toothpastes.

Desensitizing toothpastes are divided into two groups with different mechanisms of action. The first group comprises toothpastes that block pulp nerve responses, whereas the second group comprises toothpastes that occlude dentin tubules [16]. All desensitizing toothpastes have different ingredients, which have different effects on the ability to occlude dentin tubules [5]. All of these toothpastes are similar in that they have certain levels of abrasivity within a relative-dentin-abrasion (RDA) value range between 20 and 120. In a recent study, it was shown that toothpastes with high RDA values resulted in greater losses of dentin [4] after tooth brushing. The abrasivity of desensitizing toothpastes may have an adverse effect on the occlusion of dentin tubules because the tubules might be reopened during the brushing procedure.

Therefore, the aim of this study was to compare the abrasivity of various desensitizing toothpastes quantitatively.

* Correspondence: wolfgang.arnold@uni-wh.de
[1]Department of Biological and Material Sciences in Dentistry, School of Dentistry, Witten/Herdecke University, Witten, Germany
Full list of author information is available at the end of the article

The null hypothesis stated that there is no difference in the abrasivity of the different included toothpastes.

Methods

Seventy caries-free extracted human molars were used for this experimental study. The collection of the teeth was approved by the ethical committee of Witten/Herdecke University (116/2013). Informed verbal consent was obtained from the patients before the use of their teeth. The teeth were stored in 0.9 % NaCl containing 0.1 % thymol until use.

Experimental design

From the 70 teeth, 3-mm-thick dentin discs were prepared using a saw microtome (Leica 1600, Leitz Wetzlar, Germany). The discs were randomly divided into 7 groups of 10 discs each and etched with lemon juice (Hitchcock, Mönchen Gladbach, Germany) for 5 min, and one half of each disc were covered with aluminum tape. Following this, the discs were placed into a tooth-brushing machine, and a tooth brushing time of 6 months was simulated. The brushing time was calculated as follows: 28 teeth per oral cavity assuming a vestibular and an oral surface = 56 surfaces. A recommended brushing time of 360 s per day results in a brushing time of 6.4 s per tooth surface. This is multiplied by 182.5 days (6 months) and results in a total brushing time per tooth surface of 19 min 33 s. The used toothbrush has an active brushing field of 28 mm length which would cover two tooth surfaces at one time in the oral cavity, therefore, the brushing time was again doubled and resulted in a total bushing time per surface of 39 min and 6 s. As toothbrush the American Dental Association Standard Toothbrush was used. The toothbrush load was 2 N. The standard toothbrush of the American Dental Association was used with 120 linear strokes per min. The toothpastes and the active ingredients that were used are summarized in Table 1. One group served as a negative control and was brushed with tap water only. After tooth brushing, the aluminum tape was removed, and the height differences between the covered halves and the brushed halves of the discs were determined using an optical profilometer (Infinite focus G3,

Alicona, Germany). Twenty measurements per disc were made, and the mean value was calculated for each disc.

Statistical analysis

Sample size calculation was carried out (Axum 7, Mathsoft, Cambridge, Massachusetts, USA) with data obtained in a preliminary experiment with a power of 0.8 and a significance level of $\alpha < 0.05$, revealing a minimum number of 8 specimens per group. The mean values of the height differences were compared between the different toothpastes and the negative controls using a Wilcoxon-Mann–Whitney test for independent variables and post hoc Bonferroni adjustment, which resulted in a final p value of 0.0083. The correlation between abrasivity and RDA value was calculated with the nonparametric Spearman-Rho test. Descriptive statistics are presented as boxplots. All calculations were performed with SPSS (IBM Corporation, Armonk, NY, USA; Rel. 21) statistical software.

Results

The statistical evaluation showed significant differences ($p < 0.001$) between the negative control and toothpastes 1–5 (Fig. 1). The difference between toothpaste 6 with tetrapotassium pyrophosphate, hydroxyapatite and the negative control was not significant ($p = 0.583$). The exact descriptive data are summarized in Table 2. The highest abrasion was found in the toothpaste containing zinc carbonate and hydroxyapatite carbonate (toothpaste #1). A significant correlation ($p < 0.001$) between the height difference on the dentin discs and RDA value with a correlation coefficient of $r = 0.568$ was found. The graphic representation demonstrated a rather mild correlation (Fig. 2)

Discussion

Erosion of the tooth surface in the cervical area results in a loss of covering cementum and an opening of dentin tubules, which in turn leads to dentin hypersensitivity. The use of desensitizing toothpastes is always the first recommendation for the treatment of dentin hypersensitivity [6]. The mechanism of action of the majority of desensitizing toothpastes is an effect on dentin tubule occlusion [5, 16]. The cleaning effect of toothpastes is due to their RDA values and other abrasive components

Table 1 Summary of toothpastes used

Product name	Active ingredient	RDA value[a]	Company
BioRepair (#1)	Zinc carbonate hydroxyapatite	69	Dr. K. Wolff, Bielefeld, Germany
Elmex Sensitive Professional (#2)	Pro-arginine, calcium carbonate	30	CP-GABA, Hamburg, Germany
Elmex (#3)	Amine fluoride	77	CP-GABA, Hamburg, Germany
Sensodyne Rapid (#4)	Strontium acetate	70	GlaxoSmithKline, Brentford, UK
Sensodyne Repair (#5)	Stannous fluoride	119	GlaxoSmithKline, Brentford, UK
Dontodent Sensitive (#6)	Tetrapotassium pyrophosphate, hydroxyapatite	20	DM Dogeriemarkt, Karlsruhe, Germany

[a]RDA values were obtained from the manufacturer

Comparison of the dentin abrasiveness in µm

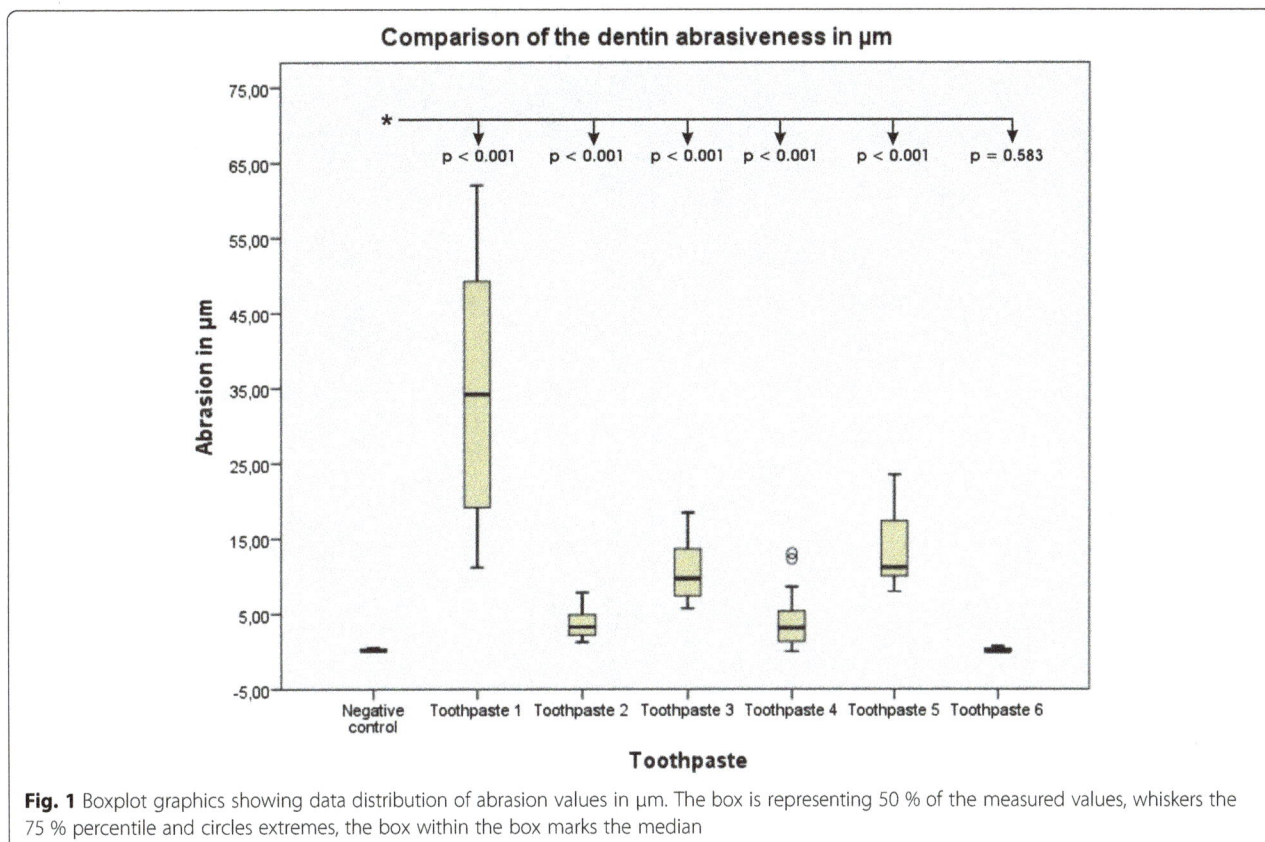

Fig. 1 Boxplot graphics showing data distribution of abrasion values in µm. The box is representing 50 % of the measured values, whiskers the 75 % percentile and circles extremes, the box within the box marks the median

such as nanoparticles. A high RDA value results in a large amount of dentin abrasion, which then might reopen occluded tubules and diminish the sensitizing effect.

The results of this study demonstrated large differences in the abrasivity of the various investigated desensitizing toothpastes. The abrasivity of toothpaste is dependent on numerous factors. The main factor is the content of abrasives [17]. All toothpastes used in this study employed silica as an abrasive substance. However, other ingredients, such as $CaCO_3$, hydroxyapatite, and other nanoparticles, may also contribute to the abrasivity of toothpaste [17]. All toothpastes contain a variety of different ingredients, which makes it almost impossible to determine the influence of a certain substance on the abrasivity of

a toothpaste. This is emphasized by the results of this investigation. Especially toothpaste 6 demonstrated no abrasiveness compared to water but does contain tetrapotassium pyrophosphate, hydroxyapatite as active ingredient. It remains speculative weather the hydroxyapatite particles are too small for being abrasive. The influence of the RDA on the loss of hard dental tissue has been discussed widely in the literature [4, 17–20]. In this study, a correlation between RDA value and amount of dentin loss was also found. Although the correlation was significant ($p < 0.001$), the correlation coefficient was not very strong ($r = 0.568$), and the graphic representation did not show a clear linear correlation between increasing RDA value and amount of substance loss. This finding is in accordance with the results of another study, which did not find a correlation between RDA value and dentin abrasivity [21]. The reason for this mild correlation might be the relatively low number of investigated specimens.

There is still an ongoing debate as to whether toothpastes are contributing to dentine hypersensitivity [18, 22]. Desensitizing toothpastes should remove the smear layer on dentin and leave deposits of particles, which occlude dentin tubules [2, 23]. Another study showed that desensitizing toothpastes partly occlude dentin tubules [5], but the abrasivity of toothpastes was not investigated. In this study, it could be shown that under experimental conditions and

Table 2 Descriptive data of abrasion values

Toothpaste #	Median	Minimum	Maximum	Interquartile range
1	34.20	11.22	61.98	50.76
2	32.66	1.25	7.84	6.59
3	9.73	5.72	18.47	12.75
4	3.11	0.00	13.04	13.04
5	11.21	7.96	23.52	15.55
6	0.00	0.00	0.67	0.67
tape water	0.02	0.00	0.49	0.49

All values are in µm

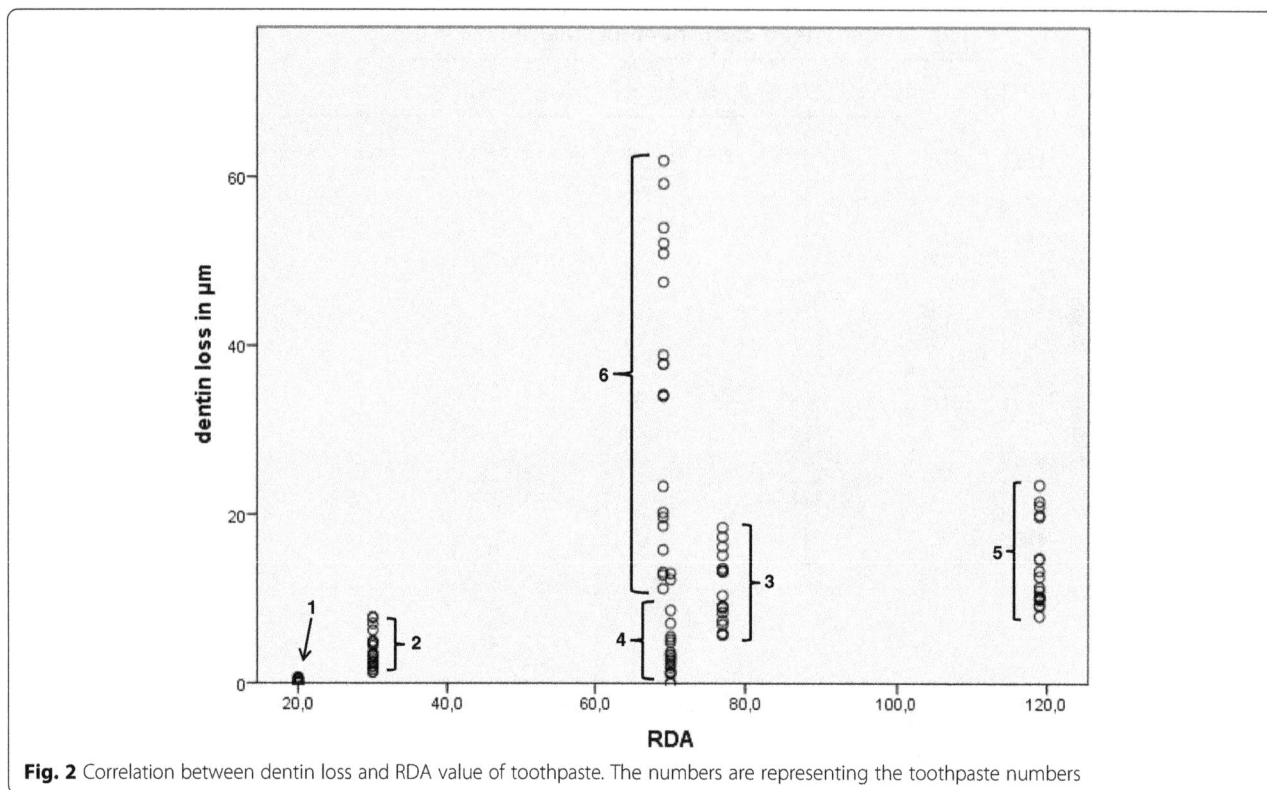

Fig. 2 Correlation between dentin loss and RDA value of toothpaste. The numbers are representing the toothpaste numbers

after dentin erosion a maximum of 61.98 µm dentin was removed. Therefore, it is very likely that dentine tubules were not occluded in these cases.

Conclusions

Within the limitations of an in vitro study, it can be concluded that different desensitizing toothpastes have different abrasivity regardless of their content of active desensitizing ingredients. Abrasivity of toothpastes may hamper their desensitizing effects.

Competing interests
The authors declare that they have no competing interests.

Author contributions
WHA: wrote the manuscript, calculated the statistics. CG: conduced the experiments. MB: planning the experiments, clinical advice. EAN: responsible for final correction of the manuscript, supervising the project. All authors read and approved the final manuscript.

Acknowledgements
The authors would like to thank Mrs. Susanne Haussman for her technical assistance in preparing the dentin discs and Mr. Christin Greune for assistance with the brushing machine.
CP-GABA, Hamburg provided the Elmex toothpastes.

Author details
[1]Department of Biological and Material Sciences in Dentistry, School of Dentistry, Witten/Herdecke University, Witten, Germany. [2]Department of Preventive and Operative Dentistry, School of Dentistry, Witten/Herdecke University, Witten, Germany.

References
1. Cummins D. Dentin hypersensitivity: from diagnosis to a breakthrough therapy for everyday sensitivity relief. The Journal of clinical dentistry. 2009;20(1):1–9.
2. West NX. Dentine hypersensitivity. Monographs in oral science. 2006;20: 173–89. doi:10.1159/000093362.
3. Milosevic A, Bardsley PF, Taylor S. Epidemiological studies of tooth wear and dental erosion in 14-year old children in North West England. Part 2: The association of diet and habits. Br Dent J. 2004;197(8):479–83. doi:10.1038/sj. bdj.4811747. discussion 3; quiz 505.
4. Bizhang M, Riemer K, Arnold, WH, Domin J, Zimmer, S. Influence of Bristle Stiffness of Manual Toothbrushes on Eroded and Sound Human Dentin - an In Vitro Study. Plos ONE (in press).
5. Arnold WH, Prange M, Naumova EA. Effectiveness of various toothpastes on dentine tubule occlusion. J Dent. 2015;43(4):440–9. doi:10.1016/j.jdent.2015.01.014.
6. Canadian Advisory Board . Consensus-based recommendations for the diagnosis and management of dentin hypersensitivity. J Can Dent Assoc. 2003;69(4):221–6.
7. Cummins D. Advances in the clinical management of dentin hypersensitivity: a review of recent evidence for the efficacy of dentifrices in providing instant and lasting relief. The Journal of clinical dentistry. 2011; 22(4):100–7.
8. Gillam DG, Newman HN, Davies EH, Bulman JS. Clinical efficacy of a low abrasive dentifrice for the relief of cervical dentinal hypersensitivity. Journal of clinical periodontology. 1992;19(3):197–201.
9. Markowitz K, Pashley DH. Discovering new treatments for sensitive teeth: the long path from biology to therapy. Journal of oral rehabilitation. 2008; 35(4):300–15. doi:10.1111/J.1365-2842.2007.01798.x.
10. Petrou I, Heu R, Stranick M, Lavender S, Zaidel L, Cummins D, et al. A breakthrough therapy for dentin hypersensitivity: how dental products containing 8 % arginine and calcium carbonate work to deliver effective relief of sensitive teeth. The Journal of clinical dentistry. 2009;20(1):23–31.
11. Baysan A, Lynch E. Treatment of cervical sensitivity with a root sealant. American journal of dentistry. 2003;16(2):135–8.
12. Duran I, Sengun A. The long-term effectiveness of five current desensitizing products on cervical dentine sensitivity. Journal of oral rehabilitation. 2004; 31(4):351–6. doi:10.1046/j.1365-2842.2003.01241.x.

13. Kielbassa AM, Attin T, Hellwig E, Schade-Brittinger C. In vivo study on the effectiveness of a lacquer containing CaF2/NaF in treating dentine hypersensitivity. Clinical oral investigations. 1997;1(2):95–9.

14. Panduric V, Knezevic A, Tarle Z, Sutalo J. The efficiency of dentine adhesives in treating non-caries cervical lesions. Journal of oral rehabilitation. 2001; 28(12):1168–74.

15. Trowbridge HO, Silver DR. A review of current approaches to in-office management of tooth hypersensitivity. Dental clinics of North America. 1990;34(3):561–81.

16. Addy M, West NX. The role of toothpaste in the aetiology and treatment of dentine hypersensitivity. Monographs in oral science. 2013;23:75–87. doi:10. 1159/000350477.

17. Moore C, Addy M. Wear of dentine in vitro by toothpaste abrasives and detergents alone and combined. Journal of clinical periodontology. 2005; 32(12):1242–6. doi:10.1111/j.1600-051X.2005.00857.x.

18. Addy M. Tooth brushing, tooth wear and dentine hypersensitivity–are they associated? International dental journal. 2005;55(4 Suppl 1):261–7.

19. Addy M, Hughes J, Pickles MJ, Joiner A, Huntington E. Development of a method in situ to study toothpaste abrasion of dentine. Comparison of 2 products. Journal of clinical periodontology. 2002;29(10):896–900.

20. Turssi CP, Messias DC, de Menezes M, Hara AT, Serra MC. Role of dentifrices on abrasion of enamel exposed to an acidic drink. American journal of dentistry. 2005;18(4):251–5.

21. Aykut-Yetkiner A, Attin T, Wiegand A. Prevention of dentine erosion by brushing with anti-erosive toothpastes. Journal of dentistry. 2014. doi:10. 1016/j.jdent.2014.03.011.

22. West N, Addy M, Hughes J. Dentine hypersensitivity: the effects of brushing desensitizing toothpastes, their solid and liquid phases, and detergents on dentine and acrylic: studies in vitro. Journal of oral rehabilitation. 1998; 25(12):885–95.

23. West NX, Addy M, Jackson RJ, Ridge DB. Dentine hypersensitivity and the placebo response. A comparison of the effect of strontium acetate, potassium nitrate and fluoride toothpastes. Journal of clinical periodontology. 1997;24(4):209–15.

23

Quality of life and problems associated with obturators of patients with maxillectomies

Marwa Mohammed Ali[1], Nadia Khalifa[1,2] and Mohammed Nasser Alhajj[1,3*]

Abstract

Background: Maxillary defects predispose patients to different undesirable effects. The aim of this study was to assess the quality of life (QoL) of patients with maxillary defects (acquired/congenital) wearing obturators.

Methods: The study comprised 30 patients aged between 16 and 78 years. Interviews were conducted to collect information pertaining to patients; sociodemographic, self-reported function of obturator using Obturator Functioning Scale (OFS), self-evaluation of general health using Visual Analogue Scale (VAS), radiotherapy treatment, salivary gland removal, reconstructive surgery, neck dissection and length of time obturators were worn. Clinical examination included type of maxillectomy, Aramany classification of the defect, and evaluation of obturator function using the Kapur retention and stability scoring system.

Result: Quality of life was affected significantly by marital status ($P = 0.026$). Married patients had better quality of life 61.3%, followed by divorced patients 38.8%, widowed 37.3% and the least QoL was detected in single patients 36.5%. Significant association between the type of maxillectomy and QoL was detected ($P = 0.002$). Retention of obturator prosthesis had a highly significant association with QoL ($P < 0.001$). Type of maxillectomy had a significant relation with obturator retention ($P = 0.005$). Stability had a significant correlation with QoL ($P = 0.022$). Obturator wearers who were treated with radiotherapy had lower QoL than those who were not treated with radiotherapy.

Conclusion: Rehabilitation of patients with maxillary defects using obturator prosthesis is an appropriate and not invasive treatment modality. Results support that good obturators contribute to a better life quality.

Keywords: Quality of life, Obturators, Maxillectomy, Obturator functioning scale

Background

One of the most important structures in the midface is the maxilla, which separates the oral, antral, and orbital cavities, and provides support to the eyeballs, lower eyelids, cheeks, lips, and nose. Furthermore, the maxilla plays a critical role in speech, swallowing, and mastication. Therefore, reconstruction of maxillectomy defects are particularly challenging for head and neck reconstructive surgeons [1]. Probably the most common of all intraoral defects are in the maxilla, and can be divided into defects resulting from congenital malformations and acquired defects resulting

from surgery to remove oral neoplasms. Post-surgical maxillary defects predispose the patient to hypernasal speech, leakage of fluid into the nasal cavity, and impaired masticatory function [2].

The most frequent treatment modality for patients diagnosed with a maxillary malignancy is surgical removal of the tumour. This very often leaves an oronasal and/or oroantral defect, resulting in severe functional problems concerning mastication, deglutition, and speech. Therefore, an appropriate substitute for the tissue lost is inevitably necessary to restore function and regain quality of life (QoL) [3, 4]. Maxillofacial defects are usually complex, involving skin, bone, muscle, cartilage, and multiple layers of mucosa, so reconstruction of such defects is often challenging. A multidisciplinary approach is needed to rehabilitate such patients [5]. The

* Correspondence: m.n.alhajj@hotmail.com
[1]Department of Oral Rehabilitation, Faculty of Dentistry, University of Khartoum, Khartoum, Sudan
[3]Department of Prosthodontics, Faculty of Dentistry, Thamar University, Dhamar, Yemen
Full list of author information is available at the end of the article

maxillofacial prosthodontist has two primary objectives in the total rehabilitation of the maxillectomy patient, i.e., to restore the functions of mastication, deglutition, and speech and to achieve a normal orofacial appearance [6–8].

The benefit of prosthodontic rehabilitation of maxillectomy over autogenous tissue reconstruction is that it simplifies oncological surveillance [1]. The surgical site can be easily examined after removing the obturator prosthesis and tumour recurrence may be detected at that time [9]. A prosthesis used to close a palatal defect in a dentate or edentulous mouth is called an obturator [10] (from the Latin word *obturare*, meaning "to close up") and is a disc or plate, natural or artificial, that closes an opening or defect of the maxilla as a result of a cleft palate or partial or total removal of the maxilla because of a tumour [8]. According to the Glossary of Prosthodontics Terms, an obturator is a prosthesis used to close a congenital or an acquired tissue opening, primarily of the hard palate and/or contiguous alveolar structures [11].

Individuals who require a maxillectomy often ask about the QoL they should expect following surgery. A well-constructed obturator can have a positive effect on individual's QoL [12–15]. It is important for patients to be able to return to a normal life after maxillectomy without functional impairment or psychological trauma.

There is a lack of information pertaining to the relationship between subjective and objective assessment methods among patients with maxillectomy who are rehabilitated with obturator prostheses. The aim of this study was to evaluate subjectively functions such as mastication, swallowing, and speech along with aesthetics and psychological status in patients with maxillary obturators and to assess objectively the retention and stability of obturators. The subjective and objective assessment methods were then compared.

Methods

This cross-sectional study was conducted at the Prosthodontic Department, Faculty of Dentistry, University of Khartoum, Sudan. The study population comprised patients with a maxillary defect who attended the Prosthodontic Department between April 2010 and October 2014. Patients were enrolled consecutively using the following inclusion criteria: adult of either sex, a maxillary defect, and wearing of an interim or definitive obturator for at least 1 month. The exclusion criteria were: recurrent disease and physical or mental instability. The patients were interviewed by the principal investigator (M.M.A.) and the collected data were entered in a spread sheet. The data collection sheet consisted of four parts as follows.

Section A: sociodemographic information

Sociodemographic information included age, sex, marital status, level of education, and employment status. Patients were also asked about how long they have been wearing an obturator and whether they had received radiotherapy. Individuals with a new removable prosthesis were evaluated 1 month later to allow for the stimulatory effect on the oral cavity (foreign body) to subside [16].

Section B: obturator functioning scale

The Obturator Functioning Scale (OFS) was developed at Memorial Sloan Kettering Cancer Center (New York, NY, USA) as a means of assessing self-reported functioning of an obturator. It was designed by Kornblith et al. [14] to assess eating ability, speech, and cosmetic satisfaction. To rate the items with higher scores (reflecting greater difficulty with obturator function), a 5-point Likert scale was used ("not at all", "a little difficult", "somewhat difficult", "very difficult", "extremely difficult"). One item, i.e., "difficulty talking on the phone", was added to the scale to assess communication difficulties in the absence of visual cues [14]. For analysis, the responses were coded from 1 ("not at all") to 5 ("extremely difficult"). The total score was then calculated by summing the responses "not at all"/"a little difficult", and responses of "very difficult"/"extremely difficult" reflecting the mean score of the scale's items, with higher scores reflecting greater difficulty.

An Arabic version of the OFS (OFS-Ar) was developed and adapted according to the translation guidelines using a forward-backward approach as follows. First, for the forward translation, an English version was translated by two separate teams of bilingual doctors. Both teams then worked together to create one combined translation. Second, for the backward translation, two independent bilingual translators produced two separate backward translations from the combined forward translation. Neither of the translators looked at the original English version of the questionnaire. A final version of the questionnaire was then produced by a team consisting of two Arabic linguistic experts and forward translators who revised all the translations and merged them into a final Arabic version [17]. The questionnaire was then pilot-tested on five patients. To check for the accuracy of the Arabic translation, each participant was interviewed after completing the questionnaire to make sure that the meaning of each part of it was clear and understandable. The typical question format was as follows: "Have you had (impact item) because of problems with your maxillary obturator?"

Section C: visual analogue scale

This is a vertically graded scale that is numbered every 10 mm. The scale is similar to that on a thermometer and helps people to describe how well or bad they feel their health status to be. The subjects are instructed to put a mark on the scale that best reflected the intensity of their symptoms. The results are expressed in millimeters from zero (worst possible symptom severity) to 100 (no symptoms) [18–20].

Section D: clinical examination

The clinical examination included recording type of maxillectomy, Aramany classification of the defect, presence of reconstructive surgery, surgical removal of salivary gland, and neck dissection. Obturator retention and stability were evaluated using the scoring system described by Kapur [21, 22].

Statistical analysis

The data were analysed using descriptive statistics in terms of frequency distributions, means, and the standard deviation. The contingency coefficient was used for the association between selected variables and the retention and stability of obturators. Pearson coefficient was applied to test for a correlation between the OFS-Ar and the VAS. The independent-samples t-test (two groups) and analysis of variance (more than two groups) were used to compare QoL according to patient characteristics. A P-value <0.05 considered to be statistically significant. The Statistical Package For the Social Sciences version 17.0 (SPSS Inc., Chicago, IL, USA) and Microsoft Excel 2007 (Microsoft, Bothell, WA, USA) were used to enter and analyze the data.

The study protocol was approved in writing by the Ethical Committee of the University of Khartoum (Faculty of Dentistry). Written informed consent was obtained from all study participants after they had received a detailed explanation of the aims of the study.

Pilot study

Five patients were investigated in a pilot study. These patients had maxillary obturators fabricated by MSc students under the supervision of prosthodontic specialists in the prosthodontic clinics. This preliminary study was performed to help assess the intelligibility of the questionnaire and the scales used, the feasibility of clinical evaluation of obturators, and construction of dummy tables.

Results

Section A: sociodemographic data

The sample consisted of an equal number of male ($n = 15$) and female ($n = 15$) patients. The mean patient age was 45.10 ± 19.03 years with a minimum age of 16 years. For statistical analysis, the variable of age was divided into groups as shown in Table 1. The majority of patients were in the age group of 40–59 years and the smallest number of patients were in the age group of 60–69 years.

Table 1 Characteristics of the participating patients

Variable		Percentage
Gender	Male	50.0
	Female	50.0
Age of patients	<20	13.3
	20–39	20.0
	40–59	40.0
	60–69	6.7
	≥70	20.0
Marital status	Single	30.0
	Married	53.3
	Divorced	13.3
	Widow	3.3
Education	Preschool education	30.0
	Primary school	30.0
	Secondary school	23.3
	University and above	16.7
Occupation	Professional	13.3
	Private business	13.3
	Labor	13.3
	Not employed	13.3
	housewives	33.3
	Retired	13.3
Radiotherapy treatment	Yes	26.7
	No	73.3
Duration of obturator wearing	Mean ± SD	24.47 ± 69.65

Fifty-three percent of the patients were married, 30% were single, 13.3% were divorced, and 3.3% were widowed. Thirty percent of respondents were not educated or had only received preschool education ('khalwa' or kindergarten), another 30% of respondents had completed primary school, 23.3% had completed secondary school, and 16.7% were educated at college, university, and postgraduate qualifications. Most of the patients were housewives (33.3%) and other occupation groups were equal in percentage (13.3%). The mean time that an obturator had been worn was 24.47 months (median 9.00 months, standard deviation 69.65 months, minimum 1 month, and a maximum of 384 months). Twenty-six percent of patients had received radiotherapy.

Section B: obturator functioning scale

As shown in Table 2, 50% of subjects reported no or little difficulty chewing. Similarly, 50% had no or little leakage when swallowing food. The majority (80%) of respondents reported not having any difficulty with their voice before surgery. This is in contrast to after surgery, when four (13.3%) respondents reported extreme difficulty talking in public (although 70% reported no or little

Table 2 Subjects' responses to the Arabic version of Functional Obturator Scale

Variables		Not at all	A little	Somewhat	Very much	Extremely
Difficulty in chewing foods	Count	13	2	4	3	8
	%	43.3	6.7	13.3	10.0	26.7
Leakage when swallowing foods	Count	10	5	5	3	7
	%	33.3	16.7	16.7	10.0	23.3
Voice different from before surgery	Count	18	6	2	2	2
	%	60.0	20.0	6.7	6.7	6.7
Difficulty talking in public	Count	13	8	4	1	4
	%	43.3	26.7	13.3	3.3	13.3
Speech is nasal	Count	18	5	2	2	3
	%	60.0	16.7	6.7	6.7	10.0
Difficulty pronouncing words	Count	22	4	2	1	1
	%	73.3	13.3	6.7	3.3	3.3
Speech is difficult to understand	Count	22	4	1	0	3
	%	72.4	13.8	3.4	.0	10.3
Difficulty talking on the phone	Count	21	6	0	0	3
	%	70.0	20.0	0	.0	10.0
Mouth feels dry	Count	15	5	1	7	2
	%	50.0	16.7	3.3	23.3	6.7
Dissatisfaction with looks	Count	17	6	1	2	4
	%	56.7	20.0	3.3	6.7	13.3
Clasp on front teeth noticeable	Count	16	7	2	4	1
	%	53.3	23.3	6.7	13.3	3.3
Any area feels numb	Count	21	2	0	5	2
	%	70.0	6.7	0	16.7	6.7
Avoidance of family or social events	Count	13	6	3	4	4
	%	43.3	20.0	10.0	13.3	13.3
Difficulty to insert or remove obturator	Count	23	2	2	0	3
	%	76.7	6.7	6.7	.0	10.0
Upper lip looks funny	Count	11	6	5	3	5
	%	36.7	20.0	16.7	10.0	16.7

difficulty). More than 75% felt they had no or little nasal speech. Pronunciation of words was not a problem for more than 85% of respondents. About 86.2% (26 respondents) felt that their speech was not or a little difficult to understand, and 10% (three respondents) reported extremely difficulty when talking on the telephone. Dry mouth was reported as absent or slight by 66.7% (20 respondents) and two (6.7%) reported severe dryness. Four respondents (13.3%) were extremely dissatisfied with their appearance but more than 75% were not or a little dissatisfied. The clasps on the anterior teeth were reported to be extremely noticeable by only one patient (3.3%) while more than 75% reported that these clasps were not or a little noticeable. Seventy percent of respondents no numbness and two reported feeling numbness all the time. Avoidance of family or social events was not reported by 43.3% of

subjects, but 20% reported a little avoidance and 13.3% reported avoidance all the time. Insertion and removal of the obturator was not or a little difficult for more than 80% of respondents but was extremely difficult for three (10%). More than half of the respondents (56.7%) felt that their upper lip "looked funny" and only five (16.7%) had no concerns about the appearance of their upper lip.

Section C: visual analogue scale
The mean VAS score for patient health status was 65.83 mm (standard deviation 23.57 mm, median 70.00 mm, minimum 0 mm, and maximum 100 mm).

Section D: clinical examination
The majority of obturator wearers presented with an Aramany class II defect (40%) followed by class I (33%),

class IV (16.7%), class VI (6.7%), and class III (3.3%). Of the patients with an obturator, 73.7% had had a partial maxillectomy, 20% had had a hemi-maxillectomy, and 6.7% had had a subtotal maxillectomy. Only 26% of respondents had received radiotherapy. None had undergone reconstructive or salivary gland surgery. Forty-three percent of obturators presented with good retention, 30% with minimum retention, 13.3% with moderate retention, and 13.3% with no retention. Forty-six percent of obturators were adequately stable, 26.7% had some stability, and 26.7% were not stable (Table 3).

Chi-squared test for the association between type of maxillectomy and Aramany classification with retention and stability of the obturator revealed significant association between type of maxillectomy and retention of the obturator. However, the other associations were not significant (Table 4). The influence of patients' characteristics on the quality of life is presented in Table 5. The effect was significant for type of maxillectomy, retention of the obturator, and presence of radiotherapy. No any other significant effect was found.

Discussion

Even though a large number of studies have investigated QoL after treatment for cancer [23–26], only a few articles have focused on patients using an obturator prosthesis

Table 3 Clinical examination of the participating subjects

Variable		Percentage
Aramany classification	Class I	33
	Class II	40
	Class III	3.3
	Class IV	16.7
	Class VI	6.7
Type of Maxillectomy	Partial	73.3
	Subtotal	6.7
	Hemi-maxillectomy	20
Neck Dissection	Yes	6.7
	No	93.3
Presence of reconstructive surgery	No	100
	Yes	0
Previous surgery for Salivary Gland	No	100
	Yes	0
Retention	No retention	13.3
	Minimum retention	30
	Moderate retention	13.3
	Good retention	43.3
Stability	No stability	26.7
	some stability	26.7
	Sufficient stability	46.6

Table 4 Association between type of maxillectomy and Aramany classification with retention and stability

	Contingency Coefficient	P-value
Type of maxillectomy and retention	0.621	0.005
Type of maxillectomy and stability	0.430	0.146
Aramany classification and retention	0.352	0.979
Aramany classification and stability	0.439	0.519

after maxillectomy [9]. The present study investigated QoL after rehabilitation with an obturator prosthesis in Sudanese patients who had undergone maxillectomy. The study was conducted at the Faculty of Dentistry and Khartoum Dental Teaching Hospital of the University of Khartoum because these facilities are considered to be the main providers of dental care for patients who have undergone maxillectomy in the country.

In this study, 30 individuals with maxillary defects (irrespective of cause) and wearing maxillary obturators were investigated to determine their QoL at least 1 month after insertion of the obturator [16]. The sample size in this study was small because maxillary cancer is a rare tumour with high mortality. In fact, the number of samples in our study is within the range of 10–42 patients in other studies investigating patients who have undergone maxillectomy [12, 14, 23, 27–29]. The fact that the proportions of male and female patients in this study were equal may in part be attributable to the small sample size. Arigbede et al. [30] reported a similar sex distribution in their study, whereas others have reported a female [12, 13] or male [9, 14] predominance.

The mean patient age was approximately 45 years. The majority of patients were aged 40–59 years, which is similar to the finding by Riaz et al. [9] and most respondents were married (53%), which corresponds to the observations of other researchers [9, 12–14]. Most patients were not educated or had just received primary school education, which again is similar to findings by Khalifa et al. [31], and necessitates the use of simple questionnaires or scales that can be understood by these patients and yield more valid results. About a third of the patients were housewives (33%) and the remaining occupational groups were represented in equal percentages. The median time that the obturators had been worn was more than 10 months, which corresponds to the findings of Riger et al. [32].

The OFS has been used in numerous investigations [9, 13, 14, 27, 32], allowing comparisons to be made more easily. Half of the respondents reported little or no problems with leakage and chewing difficulties were noticed in the group investigated in this study. This may be attributable to the fact that nearly three quarters of the patients had undergone partial maxillectomy. This is in agreement with Irish et al. [13].

Table 5 Characteristics of patients and their influence on quality of life

Item scale	N	Quality of life% Mean ± SD	Test statistic	P- value
Gender				
Male	15	38.8 ± 12.03	T = 0.598	0.585
Female	15	42.2 ± 18.47		
Age (years)				
<20	4	35.44 ± 8.49	F = 1.420	0.256
20–39	6	38.44 ± 16.33		
40–59	12	39.67 ± 16.12		
60–69	2	47.33 ± 7.72		
70+	6	58.67 ± 49.02		
Marital status				
Single	9	36.5 ± 10.2	F = 3.620	0.026
Married	16	61.3 ± 10.9		
Widowed	1	37.3		
Divorced	4	38.8 ± 15.3		
Education				
No education/ Khalwa/ kindergarden	9	37.63 ± 11.75	F = 0.595	0.625
Primary	9	39.67 ± 16.12		
Secondary	7	41.87 ± 15.62		
University +	5	45.78 ± 18.99		
Occupation				
Employed	12	35.22 ± 12.33	T = 1.581	0.125
Non employed	18	44.07 ± 16.54		
Duration (months)				
1–5	10	36.17 ± 11.26	F = 0.362	0.781
6–11	7	39.80 ± 9.96		
12–17	8	41.87 ± 17.17		
18 and above	5	43.87 ± 20.95		
Aramany classification				
Class 1	10	37.60 ± 12.80	F = 1.272	0.307
Class 2	12	41.33 ± 11.22		
Class 3	1	26.67		
Class 4	5	51.73 ± 26.72		
Class 6	2	29.33 ± 1.89		
Type of maxillectomy				
Partial Maxillectomy	22	74.67 ± 26.39	F = 7.847	0.002
Hemimaxillectomy	6	40.22 ± 13.24		
Sub-total maxillectomy	2	37.52 ± 11.50		
Retention				
No retention	4	30.56 ± 7.93	F = 8.602	<0.001
Minimum retention	9	40.74 ± 8.95		
Moderate retention	4	53.0 ± 10.46		
Good retention	13	60.0 ± 24.02		

Table 5 Characteristics of patients and their influence on quality of life (Continued)

Item scale	N	Quality of life% Mean ± SD	Test statistic	P- value
Stability				
No stability	8	32.57 ± 10.7	F = 4.426	0.022
Some stability	8	46.0 ± 10.8		
Sufficient stability	14	49.0 ± 20.28		
Neck Dissection				
Yes	2	40.14 ± 15.66	T = 0.513	0.612
No	28	46.0 ± 14.14		
Radiotherapy				
Yes	8	35.27 ± 11.09	T = 3.727	0.001
No	22	55.0 ± 16.98		

Patients in the present study reported having little difficulty with speech intelligibility or manipulating the obturator (e.g., insertion, removing, and cleaning) which is consistent with the observations of Kornblith et al. and Irish et al. [13, 14] Again, most patients were satisfied with their appearance and reported few or no aesthetic problems, similar to the previous observations of Irish et al. [13]. Nearly a quarter of individuals reported extreme difficulty accepting their appearance and thought that their upper lip looked peculiar. Kornblith et al. reported a higher percentage of patients with aesthetic problems [14]. Thirty percent of respondents felt that their mouth was very dry, which is comparable with the report by Irish et al. [13], but higher than the percentages in other studies [9, 12, 14]. This may be attributable to the fact that nearly a quarter of respondents had received radiotherapy. It is worth mentioning that no patient in the present study underwent any form of reconstructive surgery. As reported by Irish et al. [13], most of our respondents did not complain of numbness. More than a quarter of the study population avoided family and social events, which was less than the figures reported by other authors [13, 14].

The importance of using both general and disease-specific QoL measures has been emphasized by several authors [13, 14, 27, 33] because they each contribute unique information about QoL and can help to validate each other. In the current study, the VAS was used as a general QoL measure. Most of the patients rated their general health status as relatively good. The majority of obturator wearers presented with an Armany class II defect, similar to the findings of Arigbede et al. but different from those of Kumar et al. [29, 30].

Obturator retention and stability were evaluated using the scoring system described by Kapur, which is simple, applicable, and does not need any special instruments. The results using the Kapur scoring system revealed that the majority of obturators had good retention and stability. No statistically significant correlation was found between results for the OFS and the VAS. This was unexpected and not in agreement with previous studies in which OFS usually correlated significantly with other QoL measurements [13, 14, 27, 32]. Again, the small sample size in the current study could have partly contributed to this finding. It must also be remembered that difficulties in acceptance of a maxillary obturator are complex, and other factors that were not included in the present study may have had an effect on QoL. Female patients rated their QoL better than male patients. This could be because women are more self-motivated and more likely to attend for review visits. These observations are similar to those of Riaz et al. and Depprich et al. [9, 12].

In the current study, younger patients presented with worse QoL scores when compared with the older age groups. These findings are in agreement with those of Kumar et al. [29]. This may be explained by better acceptance of age-related health problems by elderly individuals and might also explain why they experience less distress related to cancer than their younger counterparts, who feel that their life span has been shortened and their QoL impaired because of the disease [29]. Married respondents evaluated their QoL better than single and widowed respondents. This was not surprising, and corresponds to observations by other investigators who have reported that the presence of loved ones helped people with cancer to enjoy a good QoL [12, 13].

This study revealed that patients with the highest level of education rated their QoL better than those with minimal education. This could be because of better awareness and understanding of instructions, manipulation methods, and limitations of maxillary obturators. Some of the previous studies support this finding [9, 12], while others have reported that level of education was not related to QoL [13]. Our patients with an obturator who were employed rated their QoL much lower than those who were not employed. This is not surprising given that some authors have commented that socioeconomic advantages, valued activities, and interests helped people with cancer enjoy a better QoL [13]. As expected, the longer a patient has worn the obturator the better the QoL, which corresponds to findings by Rieger et al. [32]. Further, as anticipated, individuals who had had a smaller area of palate resected (less than one quarter) had more retentive and stable obturators as well as better QoL than those who had more than one quarter of their palate resected. Again this is similar to the results reported by other authors [14, 34].

As expected, the retention and stability of obturators and QoL was better in our dentulous and partially dentulous patients than in those who were edentulous. This is consistent with the findings of Komaya et al., who reported that the presence of teeth in the maxillary dentition and different types of defect configuration had a significant correlation with the masticatory function score [34]. However, our results are different from those of Irish et al., who reported finding no difference in QoL between dentulous and edentulous individuals [13]. It was not surprising to find that good obturator function correlated with better QoL, as many previous studies have reported the same finding [9, 13, 14, 23, 27]. In addition to the small sample size, the type of analysis tools used may have contributed to the lack of statistically significant results when we examined the relationships between the study variables.

Whilst the Aramany classification system of maxillectomy defects has been widely used by prosthodontists, it is not the most commonly used by surgeons. This because Aramany classification system provides classification after healing has occurred and after the loss of any opportunity of immediate surgical reconstruction [35, 36]. On the other side, surgeons' perspective of classification depends on the surgical resection [37, 38]. Hence, several maxillectomy classification systems have been proposed but, till now, no consensus has been reached [35–39].

It is important to encourage surgeons to keep the resection site as small as possible, because this is associated with better retention and stability of an obturator, which in turn leads to better QoL for wearer. Although free microvascularized flaps or pedicled flaps can be used as surgical means to repair maxillofacial defects, these flaps might be not suitable for large resections or defects. Instead, maxillofacial prostheses can be used effectively to obturate these defects. Several advantages can be achieved with obturators such as: replacing teeth as well as soft and hard tissues, allowing approximately normal speaking and swallowing for the patient. In addition, it prevent fluids leakage and communication between nasal and oral cavities. Moreover, it enhances the facial appearance as it provides support for the face tissues. Another benefit of the obturator is that it permits clear vision and may be early detection of tumor recurrence [2, 40, 41]. It would be useful to conduct studies using larger sample sizes to investigate QoL in patients using maxillary obturators further and to determine why certain individuals (female, married, unemployed and educated) have better QoL than others.

Conclusion

Within the limitations of the current study, the following conclusions could be drawn: different variables can affect the patient's response to a QoL questionnaire; the Arabic version of the OFS seems to be a valid instrument and can be used effectively in Arabic-speaking patients; there is no association between defect classification and patient QoL; a good obturator contributes to better QoL; and rehabilitation of patients with maxillary defects using well-designed obturator prostheses can be an appropriate and non-invasive means of treatment.

Abbreviations
Ar: Arabic; OFS: Obturator functioning scale; QoL: Quality of life; VAS: Visual analogue scale

Funding
Not applicable.

Authors' contributions
MMA participated in the data collection and in the design of the study. NK participated in the design of the study and drafted the manuscript. MNA participated in the statistical analysis and drafted the manuscript. All authors read and approved the final manuscript.

Consent for publication
Not applicable.

Competing interests
The authors declare that they have no competing interests.

Author details
[1]Department of Oral Rehabilitation, Faculty of Dentistry, University of Khartoum, Khartoum, Sudan. [2]Department of Preventive and Restorative Dentistry, Faculty of Dental Medicine, University of Sharjah, Sharjah, United Arab Emirates. [3]Department of Prosthodontics, Faculty of Dentistry, Thamar University, Dhamar, Yemen.

References

1. Moreno MA, Skoracki RJ, Hanna EY, et al. Microvascular free flap reconstruction versus palatal obturation for maxillectomy defects. Head Neck. 2010;32:860–8.
2. Keyf F. Obturator prostheses for hemimaxillectomy patients. J Oral Rehabil. 2001;28:821–9.
3. Newton JT, Fiske J, Foote O, et al. Preliminary study of the impact of loss of part of the face and its prosthetic restoration. J Prosthet Dent. 1999;82:585–90.
4. Lethaus B, Lie N, de Beer F, et al. Surgical and prosthetic reconsiderations in patients with maxillectomy. J Oral Rehabil. 2010;37:138–42.
5. Metha S, Kohli D, Solanki K, et al. Prosthodontic rehabilitation of hemimaxillectomy patient with permanent silicon based obturator. JADCH. 2011;2:55–8.
6. de Carvalho-Teles V, Pegoraro-Krook MI, Lauris JR. Speech evaluation with and without palatal obturator in patients submitted to maxillectomy. J Appl Oral Sci. 2006;14:421–6.
7. Okay DJ, Genden E, Buchbinder D, et al. Prosthodontic guidelines for surgical reconstruction of the maxilla: a classification system of defects. J Prosthet Dent. 2001;86:352–63.
8. Garhnayak M, Garhnayak L, Kumar Kar A, et al. Prosthetic rehabilitation of a unilateral maxillary defect with an intermediate Obturator. IJDA. 2002;2:378–82.
9. Riaz N, Warriach RA. Quality of life in patients with obturator prostheses. J Ayub Med Coll Abbottabad. 2010;22:121–5.
10. Singh M, Bhushan A, Kumar N, et al. Obturator prosthesis for hemimaxillectomy patients. Natl J Maxillofac Surg. 2013;4:117–20.
11. The Glossary of Prosthodontic Terms. Ninth edition. J Prosthet Dent. 2017; 117:e1–e105.
12. Depprich R, Naujoks C, Lind D, et al. Evaluation of the quality of life of patients with maxillofacial defects after prosthodontic therapy with obturator prostheses. Int J Oral Maxillofac Surg. 2011;40:71–9.
13. Irish J, Sandhu N, Simpson C, et al. Quality of life in patients with maxillectomy prostheses. Head Neck. 2009;31:813–21.
14. Kornblith AB, Zlotolow IM, Gooen J, et al. Quality of life of maxillectomy patients using an obturator prosthesis. Head Neck. 1996;18:323–34.
15. Ono T, Kohda H, Hori K, et al. Masticatory performance in postmaxillectomy patients with edentulous maxillae fitted with obturator prostheses. Int J Prosthodont. 2007;20:145–50.
16. Jacob RF, Weber RS, King GE. Whole salivary flow rates following submandibular gland resection. Head Neck. 1996;18:242–7.
17. Khalifa N, Allen PH, Abu-bakr NH, et al. Psychometric properties and performance of the oral helth impact profile (OHIP-14-ar) among Sudanese adults. J Oral Sci. 2013;55:1–10.
18. McCormack HM, Horne DJ, Sheather S. Clinical applications of visual analogue scales: a critical review. Psychol Med. 1988;18:1007–19.
19. Kind P, Dolan P, Gudex C, et al. Variations in population health status: results from a United Kingdom national questionnaire survey. BMJ. 1998;316:736–41.
20. Paul-Dauphin A, Guillemin F, Virion JM, et al. Bias and precision in visual analogue scales: a randomized controlled trial. Am J Epidemiol. 1999;150:1117–27.
21. Burns DR, Unger JW, Elswick RK Jr, et al. Prospective clinical evaluation of mandibular implant overdentures: part I–retention, stability, and tissue response. J Prosthet Dent. 1995;73:354–63.
22. Gehan FM. Clinical evaluation of the efficacy of soft acrylic denture compared to conventional one when restoring severely resorbed edentulous ridge. CDJ. 2008;24:313–33.
23. Hertrampf K, Wenz HJ, Lehmann KM, et al. Quality of life of patients with maxillofacial defects after treatment for malignancy. Int J Prosthodont. 2004; 17:657–65.
24. Fang FM, Tsai WL, Chien CY, et al. Health-related quality of life outcome for oral cancer survivors after surgery and postoperative radiotherapy. Jpn J Clin Oncol. 2004;34:641–6.
25. Terrell JE, Fisher SG, Wolf GT. Long-term quality of life after treatment of laryngeal cancer. The veterans affairs laryngeal cancer study group. Arch Otolaryngol Head Neck Surg. 1998;124:964–71.
26. Wan Leung S, Lee TF, Chien CY, et al. Health-related quality of life in 640 head and neck cancer survivors after radiotherapy using EORTC QLQ-C30 and QLQ-H&N35 questionnaires. BMC Cancer. 2011;11:128.
27. Rogers SN, Lowe D, McNally D, et al. Health-related quality of life after maxillectomy: a comparison between prosthetic obturation and free flap. J Oral Maxillofac Surg. 2003;61:174–81.
28. Matsuyama M, Tsukiyama Y, Tomioka M, et al. Clinical assessment of chewing function of obturator prosthesis wearers by objective measurement of masticatory performance and maximum occlusal force. Int J Prosthodont. 2006;19:253–7.
29. Kumar P, Alvi HA, Rao J, et al. Assessment of the quality of life in maxillectomy patients: a longitudinal study. J Adv Prosthodont. 2013; 5:29–35.
30. Arigbede AO, Dosumu OO, Shaba OP, et al. Evaluation of speech in patients with partial surgically acquired defects: pre and post prosthetic obturation. J Contemp Dent Pract. 2006;7:89–96.
31. Khalifa N, Allen PF, Abu-bakr NH, et al. A survey of oral health in a Sudanese population. BMC Oral Health. 2012;12:5.
32. Rieger JM, Wolfaardt JF, Jha N, et al. Maxillary obturators: the relationship between patient satisfaction and speech outcome. Head Neck. 2003;25:895–903.
33. D'Antonio LL, Zimmerman GJ, Cella DF, et al. Quality of life and functional status measures in patients with head and neck cancer. Arch Otolaryngol Head Neck Surg. 1996;122:482–7.
34. Koyama S, Sasaki K, Inai T, et al. Effects of defect configuration, size, and remaining teeth on masticatory function in post-maxillectomy patients. J Oral Rehabil. 2005;32:635–41.
35. Aramany MA. Basic principles of obturator design for partially edentulous patients. Part I: classification. J Prosthet Dent. 1978;40:554–7.
36. Umino S, Masuda G, Ono S, et al. Speech intelligibility following maxillectomy with and without a prosthesis: an analysis of 54 cases. J Oral Rehabil. 1998;25:153–8.
37. Wells MD, Luce EA. Reconstruction of midfacial defects after surgical resection of malignancies. Clin Plast Surg. 1995;22:79–89.
38. Spiro RH, Strong EW, Shah JP. Maxillectomy and its classification. Head Neck. 1997;19:309–14.
39. Bidra AS, Jacob RF, Taylor TD. Classification of maxillectomy defects: a systematic review and criteria necessary for a universal description. J Prosthet Dent. 2012;107:261–70.
40. Alhajj MN, Ismail IA, Khalifa N. Maxillary obturator prosthesis for a hemimaxillectomy patient: a clinical case report. Saudi. J Dent Res. 2016;7:153–9.
41. Ali A, Fardy MJ, Patton DW. Maxillectomy–to reconstruct or obturate? Results of a UK survey of oral and maxillofacial surgeons. Br J Oral Maxillofac Surg. 1995;33:207–10.

24

Comparative evaluation of insertion torque and mechanical stability for self-tapping and self-drilling orthodontic miniscrews –an in vitro study

Michele Tepedino* ⓘ, Francesco Masedu and Claudio Chimenti

Abstract

Background: The aim of the present study was to evaluate the relationship between insertion torque and stability of miniscrews in terms of resistance against dislocation, then comparing a self-tapping screw with a self-drilling one.

Methods: Insertion torque was measured during placement of 30 self-drilling and 31 self-tapping stainless steel miniscrews (Leone SpA, Sesto Fiorentino, Italy) in synthetic bone blocks. Then, an increasing pulling force was applied at an angle of 90° and 45°, and the displacement of the miniscrews was recorded.

Results: The statistical analysis showed a statistically significant difference between the mean Maximum Insertion Torque (MIT) observed in the two groups and showed that force angulation and MIT have a statistically significant effect on miniscrews stability. For both the miniscrews, an angle of 90° between miniscrew and loading force is preferable in terms of stability.

Conclusions: The tested self-drilling orthodontic miniscrews showed higher MIT and greater resistance against dislocation than the self-tapping ones.

Keywords: Miniscrew, Implant design, Orthodontic mini-implant, Insertion torque, Stability

Background

Anchorage management is often an issue in orthodontic treatment, and many devices and solutions are offered to deal with different clinical situations. In some cases an "absolute anchorage" is needed to dissipate all unwanted reaction forces: such a task can be afforded by orthodontic miniscrews.

Orthodontic miniscrews (also known as microscrews, micro/mini-implants, orthodontic implants or TADs —temporary anchorage devices) are devices specially designed to be placed within the maxillofacial bones with the aim of providing anchorage for an orthodontic appliance [1]. They can have different diameters and lengths, body designs and thread shapes, and can be made of different alloys (basically grade 5 titanium alloy or stainless steel). Depending on the insertion technique, orthodontic miniscrews can be divided into self-drilling screws (which have a cutting tip that determines a drill-like action during placement) and self-tapping ones (which have a non-cutting tip and require pre-drilling of the surgical site to create a pilot hole).

Orthodontic miniscrews can be helpful in many situations: when patient compliance is an issue, when teeth are insufficient to assure appropriate biomechanics, or when anchorage management is critical [1].

Orthodontic miniscrews are designed for temporary usage, so in most cases osseointegration of the screw is unwanted in order to facilitate its removal, and only a primary stability is pursued [2]. Such devices are widely used in orthodontic practice and their success rate is reported to be between 37% and 94% [3–5]: many factors affect success rate, like miniscrew design, intra-oral position, surgical technique and loading. According to Melsen and

* Correspondence: m.tepedino@hotmail.it
Department of Biotechnological and Applied Clinical Sciences, University of L'Aquila, Viale S.Salvatore, Edificio Delta 6, 67100 L'Aquila, Italy

Costa [6], primary stability is one of the key factors for clinical success. Stability is a variable that can be evaluated with quantitative methods, such as periotest, resonance frequency analysis, pullout test or insertion/removal torque recording [7]. During the placement of miniscrews, it is necessary to have a certain amount of insertion torque to achieve good primary stability [7, 8]: however, an excessive torque can lead to fractures in the cortical bone and bone resorption, hence to failure of the miniscrew [9]. Values of Maximum Insertion Torque (MIT, the maximum value of insertion torque registered during the insertion of the miniscrew) ranging from 5 to 10 N·cm have been presented as a reference in many articles [7–10]. A systematic review of the literature has been conducted to assess the correlation between insertion torque and success of miniscrews [7]: only non-randomized studies were judged eligible for the revision, and no evidence was found indicating the ideal insertion torque for achieving clinical success. Moreover the authors concluded that further high quality studies are required, and that there is the need to analyse individually each factor that can affect maximum insertion torque, starting from laboratory models.

The aim of the present work was to evaluate the relationship between insertion torque and stability of miniscrews in terms of resistance against a dislocating force applied at different angulations, then comparing the behaviour of a self-tapping miniscrew with a self-drilling one.

Methods

Sixty-one stainless steel orthodontic miniscrews (Leone SpA, Sesto Fiorentino, Italy) were used, 30 self-drilling (Fig. 1) and 31 self-tapping (Fig. 2). Both types of miniscrew had inner diameter of 1.3 mm, pitch of 0.8 mm, cylindrical trunk shape, length of 8 mm and high head (worse biomechanical condition). Self-tapping mini-implants had an outer diameter of 2 mm, while self-drilling ones had an outer diameter of 1.75 mm.

Synthetic bony blocks made of rigid polyurethane foam (Sawbones, Pacific Research Laboratories Inc., Vashon, WA, USA) were used. Each bone block was composed of a cortical layer with a density of 0.64 g/cm^3 (40 pcf) and a thickness of 2 mm, and a cancellous bone layer with a density of 0.32 g/cm^3 (20 pcf). Such a configuration was chosen to simulate the bone quality of a maxillary premolar region, as reported by other authors [2].

The synthetic bone blocks were placed over a digital torque gauge (MGT12E, Mark-10, New York, USA) (Fig. 3) and the miniscrews were positioned, in order to measure the maximum insertion torque (MIT). Care was taken to ensure that the insertion site of the screw was aligned with the centre of the platform. The torque gauge was calibrated before each measurement.

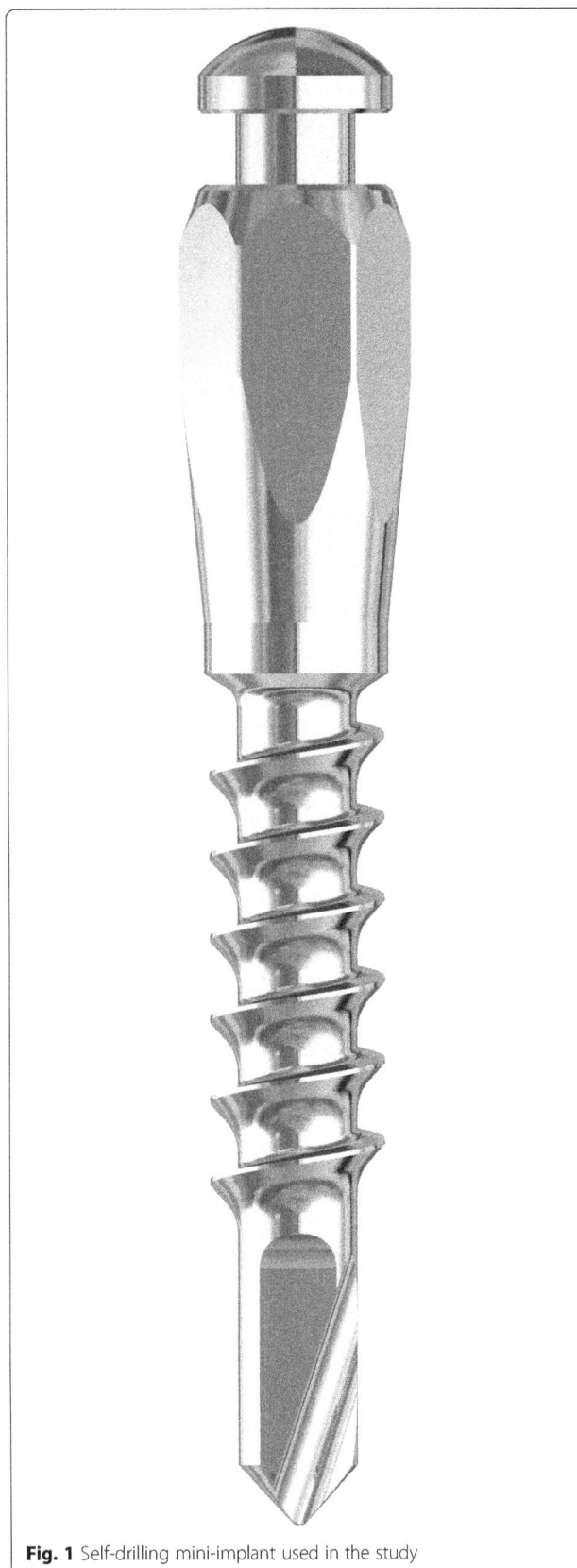

Fig. 1 Self-drilling mini-implant used in the study

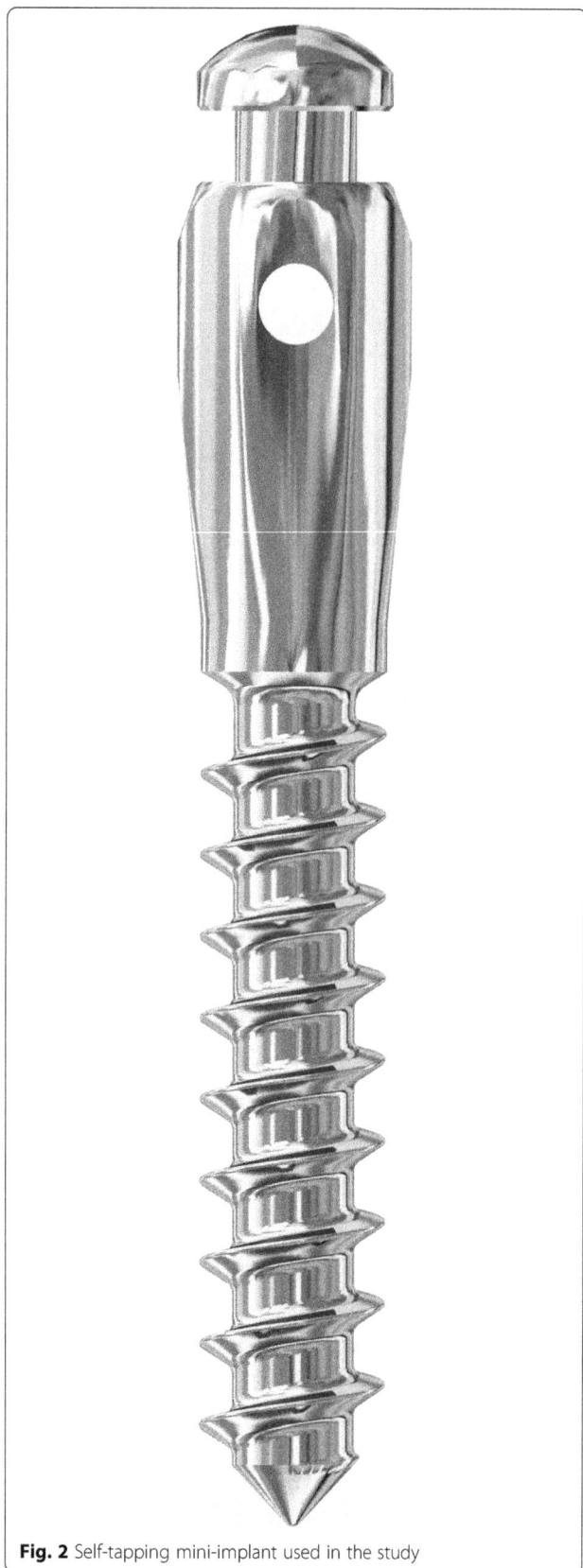

Fig. 2 Self-tapping mini-implant used in the study

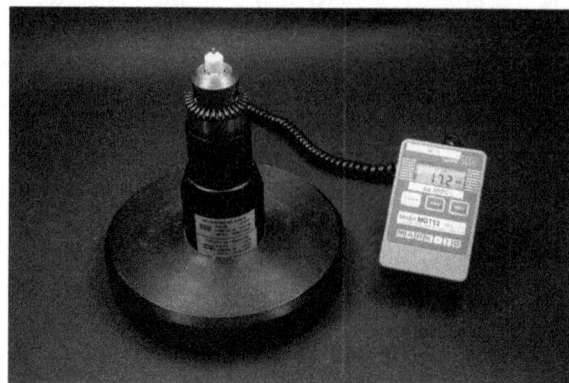

Fig. 3 Digital torque gauge

Both types of miniscrew were positioned in a block with a 30:1 contra-angle mounted over a surgical engine (ChiroPro 980, Bien-Air Dental, Bienne, Switzerland) at a rotating speed of 15 rpm, taking care to place the screw tilted at an angle of 90° with respect to the surface of the block and fully inserting the miniscrew till the end of the threaded portion. The insertion of the self-tapping screws, however, required site preparation using a 1.5-mm-diameter pilot drill with a rotational speed of 300 rpm.

In order to apply the displacing force and then measure the miniscrew displacement, an Instron® mechanical testing machine (3365 Series, Instron®, Norwood, USA) with a loading cell of 100 N was used (Fig. 4). The specimens were secured to the testing machine and connected to the loading cell through a 0.12 in. stainless steel orthodontic ligature (Leone SpA, Sesto Fiorentino, Italy) by the same operator (MT) in such a way that force was applied either at an angle of 90° (Fig. 5) or 45° in the opposite direction of the pulling force. All the specimens were tested in both configurations.

The loading cell was set to run for a maximum distance of 1 mm, with an increasing force. When the applied force reached the value of 20 N, the distance covered by the loading cell was measured and stored: such a distance corresponds to the sum of the mini-implant's displacement and of the wire ligature's elongation. The loading cell was calibrated before each measurement.

Preliminary tests had been performed to evaluate the elongation of the stainless steel wire used for the testing of dislocation and to test the reproducibility of the operator who made the wire ligatures: the elastic deformation of the orthodontic wire was subtracted from the total loading cell displacement, thus obtaining the pure displacement of the miniscrews.

Statistical analysis

A statistical analysis of the data was performed. Descriptive statistics, mean values and standard deviations of

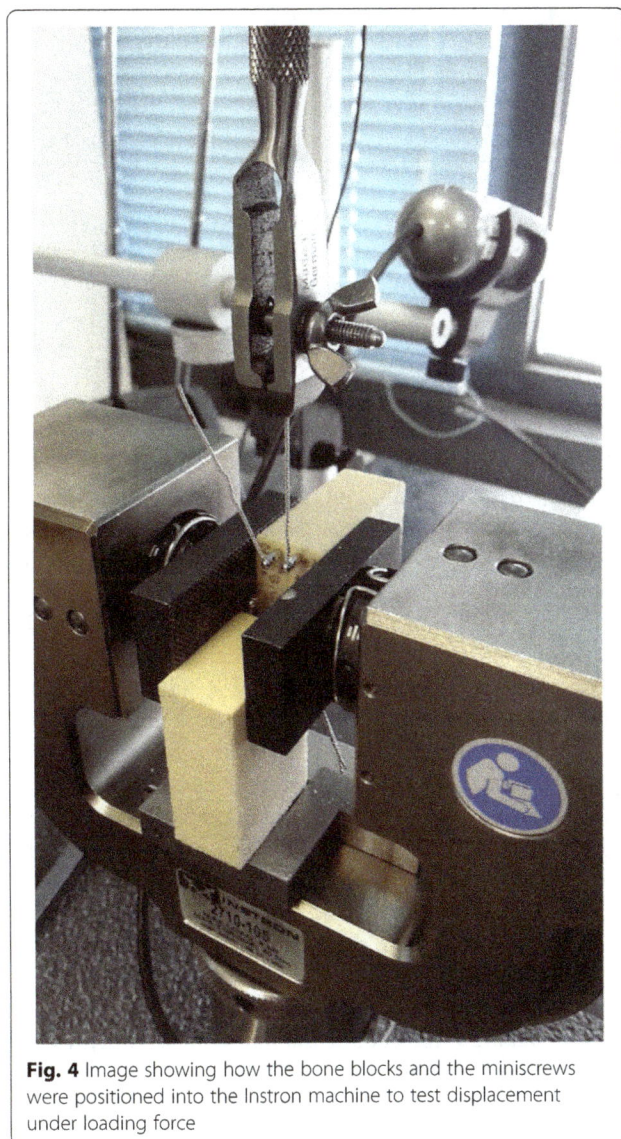

Fig. 4 Image showing how the bone blocks and the miniscrews were positioned into the Instron machine to test displacement under loading force

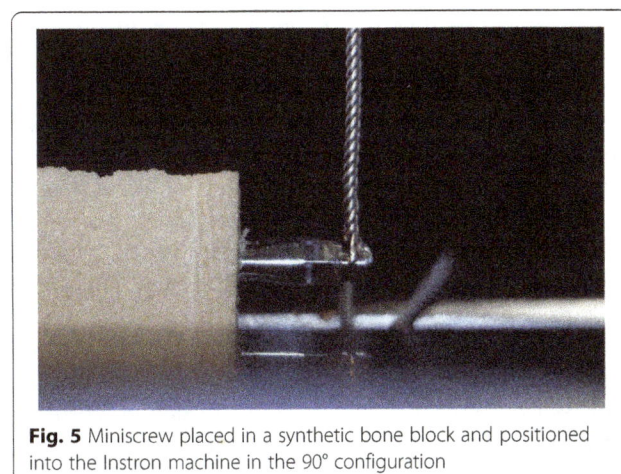

Fig. 5 Miniscrew placed in a synthetic bone block and positioned into the Instron machine in the 90° configuration

the variables considered were computed. First type error was set at 0.05.

A preliminary Hotelling test was carried out to assess any overall difference between MIT and the screw displacement with respect to miniscrew type.

The effect of the miniscrew type on the variable MIT was assessed and estimated by a linear regression model, and likewise a linear regression model was used to address the behaviour of the screw displacement with respect to force angulation and insertion torque.

Model fitting was estimated by F test. The analysis was carried out by STATA software version 13 (StataCorp LP, Texas, USA).

Results

Descriptive statistics are reported (Tables 1 and 2). Mean values for MIT were higher for self-drilling screws (6.43 ± 2.09 N·cm), while self-tapping ones showed higher mean values for each screw displacement (0.37 ± 0.08 mm). Miniscrews positioned at an angle of 45° in the opposite direction of applied force had higher mean values of displacement (0.38 ± 0.06 mm) than those placed at 90°.

The statistical analysis showed a statistically significant difference between the mean MIT observed in the groups with different screws, yielding an average difference between self-drilling and self-tapping screws of 2.31 ± 0.43 N·cm ($p < 0.05$) (Table 3).

After regressing the screw displacement with respect to miniscrew type, force angulation and MIT, a statistically significant effect of force angulation (0.06 ± 0.02) and MIT (-0.01 ± 0.02) regressors was detected (Table 4). No effects of miniscrew type were observed (0.02 ± 0.02, $p = 0.236$).

Discussion

Primary stability is defined as the mechanical stability in the bone immediately after miniscrew insertion. It is a function of the screw diameter and length, the number and design of the threads, the cortical thickness and the cortical bone density. It can be subjectively assessed by a clinician or evaluated by means of different quantitative methods (periotest, resonance frequency analysis, pullout test or insertion/removal torque recording) [7]. Many authors used insertion torque as a method to evaluate mechanical stability of miniscrews in an indirect way [1, 11–13], either with mechanical torque gauges and digital torque sensors.

Table 1 Mean values and standard deviations (SD) for maximum insertion torque (MIT) divided by miniscrew's type

	Self-drilling		Self-tapping	
	Mean	SD	Mean	SD
MIT (N·cm)	6.43	2.09	4.12	1.21

Table 2 Mean values and standard deviations (SD) for miniscrew displacement at a force of 20 N, divided by miniscrew's type and angulation of force applied

	Self-drilling				Self-tapping			
	90°		45°		90°		45°	
	Mean	SD	Mean	SD	Mean	SD	Mean	SD
Displacement (mm)	0.30	0.04	0.36	0.04	0.35	0.09	0.40	0.08

In the present study, a digital torque sensor was used, as this type of instruments offers greater precision compared to other clinical devices, which are subject to errors related to axial loads, position and posture of the clinician and can be damaged over time [14]. Also, a displacing force was applied either at 90° or 45° to directly measure the dislocation of the miniscrews and then evaluate their stability under loading conditions. It was decided to apply a dislocating force with such angulations, instead of a pull-out test with the force applied along the miniscrew's long axis, to mimic the orthodontic forces that are used in a clinical environment, which are usually applied perpendicular to the miniscrew's long axis at various angulations. The amount of elastic deformation of the orthodontic wire had been pre-determined and eliminated. Even if the wire ligatures were tied manually, they were made by the same calibrated operator thus reducing variability in wire tightening. In addition, to evaluate the behavior of miniscrew under orthodontic loading, the presence of an elastic tie should be considered, since it is the way they are employed clinically. Concerning this matter, it is worth underlining that the purpose of the present study was not to assess absolute values of displacement, but to analyze comparatively the different behavior of two different miniscrew types under the same experimental conditions.

According to Motoyoshi et al. [8], an ideal insertion torque should be in a range between 5 and 10 N·cm in order to achieve higher success rate. However, a systematic review [7] revealed that no evidence exists to support this statement, and to recommend any value of insertion torque as more efficient. Heidemann et al. [15] found that, when pre-drilling of the implant site is performed, the pilot hole should not have a diameter greater than 80% of

Table 3 Linear regression model for maximum insertion torque (MIT) by miniscrew's type

MIT vs Miniscrew type Linear Model*

Covariates	$\hat{\beta}_i$	$\hat{\sigma}_i$	t	p_i	Conf. Interval (95%)	
Type	−2.31	0.43	−5.32	0.00	−3.18	−1.44
Constant	6.43	0.31	20.74	0.00	50.81	7.05

*$F_{(1, 59)} = 28.32$; $p = 0.00$, Adjusted $R^2 = 0.21$

Table 4 Linear regression model for miniscrew's displacement (mm) at a force of 20 N by maximum insertion torque (MIT) and angulation of applied force

Miniscrew Displacement Linear Model**

Covariates	$\hat{\beta}_i$	$\hat{\sigma}_i$	t	p_i	Conf. Interval (95%)	
Angulation	0.06	0.02	3.33	0.00	0.02	0.09
MIT	−0.01	0.00	−3.14	0.00	−0.02	0.00
Constant	0.39	0.02	16.60	0.00	0.35	0.44

**$F_{(2, 58)} = 9.17$; $p = 0.00$, Adjusted $R^2 = 0.21$

that of the screw in order to maintain good primary stability and an ideal insertion torque. In this study, the mean MIT value for self-tapping screws (4.12 ± 1.21 N·cm) was smaller than the mean MIT value for self-drilling screws (6.43 ± 2.09 N·cm); with regards to self-tapping miniscrews the diameter of the pilot drill was equal to 75% of the mini-implant's one.

The two used miniscrew types differed —except for the shape of the tip— only for the outer diameter (2 mm for self-tapping miniscrews, 1.75 mm for self-drilling ones, whilst both miniscrew types had the same inner diameter of 1.3 mm, therefore the self-tapping miniscrews had greater threads' depth). The different outer diameter is a consequence of different design requirements (self-drilling miniscrews bore themselves into the bone without any pre-drilling, whilst self-tapping ones advance into a pre-drilled pilot hole). Even if in case of comparison among miniscrews of the same design this could be considered a confounding factor [16], the present study was aimed to compare the behavior of self-drilling and self-tapping miniscrews, taking into account the differences related to the design of each device.

Regarding the definition of bone-like supports, several considerations were taken into account: human cadaver bone or fresh animal bone suffer quality modifications over time, and selecting various bone blocks of the same quality represents a highly variable operation. To avoid any possible bias due to differences in bone quality, synthetic bony blocks made of rigid polyurethane foam were used instead of fresh bone [2, 17–19]. According to international standards [20] the uniformity and consistent properties of rigid polyurethane foam make it an ideal material for comparative testing of bone screws and other medical devices and instruments.

Although orthodontic forces usually range between 0.3 and 4.0 N [1, 21], the value of 20 N was chosen to be representative of the general behaviour of the screw under loading conditions: in fact the goal of the present study was to evaluate differences between self-tapping and self-drilling miniscrews, not to define absolute properties. The orthodontic forces clinically used to load miniscrews are not sufficient to provoke their immediate displacement, while forces measured during pullout tests are usually above 100 N and don't have a clinical meaning, but are used to describe absolute mechanical properties [17–19].

According to our results, there is a strong correlation between MIT and miniscrew type, probably due to the mini-implant design [17] as well as to the insertion technique, since the use of a pilot drill reduces the insertion torque [15]. Interestingly, while according to literature the greater outer diameter and deeper threads should provide greater MIT and stability [17, 22, 23], in the present experimental setup the self-tapping screws that had an outer diameter of 2.0 mm and an inner diameter of 1.3 mm showed lower MIT values compared to the self-drilling screws having an outer diameter of 1.75 mm and an inner diameter of 1.3 mm. Therefore, the main reason for the MIT values measured can be probably ascribed to the insertion technique.

When evaluating the stability of the screw by applying a displacing force, self-drilling screws showed a better behaviour (0.30 ± 0.04 mm at an angle of 90°) than self-tapping ones (0.35 ± 0.09 mm at an angle of 90°), and this difference was statistically significant ($p < 0.05$). Both miniscrew types showed better performances at an angle of 90° than at 45° in the opposite direction of the applied force, and this result was similar to those obtained by other authors [2]. Although statistically significant, the differences between the two groups were relatively small. Therefore, further clinical studies are needed to evaluate the impact of such different performances in a clinical environment.

On the basis of these results self-drilling screws look as preferable since they can be placed with higher insertion torque and therefore have greater primary stability. However, while this is true for this in vitro experimental set, in a clinical situation more variables have to be taken into account when pursuing an optimal primary stability and clinical success. The quality of the cortical bone is critical for miniscrew success [24, 25], but when inserting a screw in a thick or dense cortical layer micro-cracks or heat-damage can occur and cause bone resorption, which leads to a failure of the screw [26–29]: in these cases, for example, pre-drilling of the insertion site may be useful. In two clinical studies comparing self-drilling and self-tapping orthodontic miniscrews [10, 30], no statistically significant difference was found between them in terms of success/failure rate.

However, the use of a drill increases the risk of root or nerve damage, and self-drilling screws are simpler to manage (decrease in operative time, little bone debris, lower morbidity, and minimal patient discomfort as pre-drilling is not required).

According to the results of this study, it is possible to say that the tested self-drilling screws can achieve higher primary stability. However, self-drilling screws cannot be considered as absolutely preferable: a higher MIT is not always desirable, and the choice of the device depends on bone quality and quantity and the specific clinical situation.

Conclusions

Force angulation and MIT have a statistically significant effect on miniscrews stability. An angle of 90° between miniscrew and loading force is preferable. Under the same conditions of bone-like support and same inner diameter, the tested self-drilling orthodontic miniscrews showed higher MIT and greater resistance against dislocation than the self-tapping ones.

Abbreviations
MIT: maximum insertion torque; TAD: temporary anchorage device

Acknowledgement
We would like to thank Gabriele Scommegna, Giulio Taddei, Lorenzo Lorenzini and the Technical Department of Leone SpA (Sesto Fiorentino, Firenze, Italy) for authorizing the use of their laboratory and technical equipment.

Funding
No funding were given for the realization of this study, and the authors declare no conflicts of interest.

Authors' contributions
MT performed all the measurements, and wrote the manuscript. FM performed the statistical analysis and helped with interpretation of data. CC is supervisor of the study and helped to draft the manuscript. All authors read and approved the final manuscript.

Competing interests
The authors declare that they have no competing interests.

Consent for publication
Not applicable.

References
1. Elias CN, de Oliveira Ruellas AC, Fernandes DJ. Orthodontic implants: concepts for the orthodontic practitioner. Int J Dent. 2012;2012:1–7.
2. Petrey JS, Saunders MM, Kluemper GT, Cunningham LL, Beeman CS. Temporary anchorage device insertion variables: effects on retention. Angle Orthod. 2010;80:446–53.
3. Moon C-H, Lee D-G, Lee H-S, Im J-S, Baek S-H. Factors associated with the success rate of orthodontic miniscrews placed in the upper and lower posterior buccal region. Angle Orthod. 2008;78:101–6.
4. Miyawaki S, Koyama I, Inoue M, Mishima K, Sugahara T, Takano-Yamamoto T. Factors associated with the stability of titanium screws placed in the posterior region for orthodontic anchorage. Am J Orthod Dentofac Orthop. 2003;124:373–8.
5. Park H-S, Jeong S-H, Kwon O-W. Factors affecting the clinical success of screw implants used as orthodontic anchorage. Am J Orthod Dentofac Orthop. 2006;130:18–25.
6. Melsen B, Costa A. Immediate loading of implants used for orthodontic anchorage. Clin Orthod Res. 2000;3:23–8.
7. Meursinge Reynders RA, Ronchi L, Ladu L, van Etten-Jamaludin F, Bipat S. Insertion torque and success of orthodontic mini-implants: a systematic review. Am J Orthod Dentofac Orthop. 2012;142:596–614.e5.
8. Motoyoshi M, Hirabayashi M, Uemura M, Shimizu N. Recommended placement torque when tightening an orthodontic mini-implant. Clin Oral Implants Res. 2006;17:109–14.

9.   Lee N-K, Baek S-H. Effects of the diameter and shape of orthodontic mini-implants on microdamage to the cortical bone. Am J Orthod Dentofac Orthop. 2010;138:8.e1–8.

10. Son S, Motoyoshi M, Uchida Y, Shimizu N. Comparative study of the primary stability of self-drilling and self-tapping orthodontic miniscrews. Am J Orthod Dentofac Orthop. 2014;145:480–5.

11. da Cunha HA, Francischone CE, Filho HN, de Oliveira RCG. A comparison between cutting torque and resonance frequency in the assessment of primary stability and final torque capacity of standard and TiUnite single-tooth implants under immediate loading. Int J Oral Maxillofac Implants. 2004;19:578–85.

12. Inoue M, Kuroda S, Yasue A, Horiuchi S, Kyung H-M, Tanaka E. Torque ratio as a predictable factor on primary stability of orthodontic miniscrew implants. Implant Dent. 2014;23:576–81.

13. Suzuki EY, Suzuki B. Placement and removal torque values of orthodontic miniscrew implants. Am J Orthod Dentofac Orthop. 2011;139:669–78.

14. Kim S-H, Lee S-J, Cho I-S, Kim S-K, Kim T-W. Rotational resistance of surface-treated mini-implants. Angle Orthod. 2009;79:899–907.

15. Heidemann W, Gerlach KL, Grobel K, Kollner H. Influence of different pilot hole sizes on torque measurements and pullout analysis of osteosynthesis screws. J Craniomaxillofac Surg. 1998;26:50–5.

16. Katic V, Kamenar E, Blazevic D, Spalj S. Geometrical design characteristics of orthodontic mini-implants predicting maximum insertion torque. Korean J Orthod. 2014;44:177–83.

17. Gracco A, Giagnorio C, Incerti Parenti S, Alessandri Bonetti G, Siciliani G. Effects of thread shape on the pullout strength of miniscrews. Am J Orthod Dentofac Orthop. 2012;142:186–90.

18. Carano A, Lonardo P, Velo S, Incorvati C. Mechanical properties of three different commercially available miniscrews for skeletal anchorage. Prog Orthod. 2005;6:82–97.

19. Shah AH, Behrents RG, Kim KB, Kyung H-M, Buschang PH. Effects of screw and host factors on insertion torque and pullout strength. Angle Orthod. 2012;82:603–10.

20. ASTM. F1839–08(2012), standard specification for rigid polyurethane foam for use as a standard material for testing Orthopaedic devices and instruments. West Conshohocken, PA: ASTM International; 2012.

21. Burstone CR. Deep overbite correction by intrusion. Am J Orthod Dentofac Orthop. 1977;72:1–22.

22. Brinley CL, Behrents R, Kim KB, Condoor S, Kyung H-M, Buschang PH. Pitch and longitudinal fluting effects on the primary stability of miniscrew implants. Angle Orthod. 2009;79:1156–61.

23. Migliorati M, Signori A, Silvestrini BA. Temporary anchorage device stability: an evaluation of thread shape factor. Eur J Orthod. 2012;34:582–6.

24. Baumgaertel S, Hans MG. Buccal cortical bone thickness for mini-implant placement. Am J Orthod Dentofac Orthop. 2009;136:230–5.

25. Baumgaertel S. Quantitative investigation of palatal bone depth and cortical bone thickness for mini-implant placement in adults. Am J Orthod Dentofac Orthop. 2009;136:104–8.

26. O'Sullivan D, Sennerby L, Meredith N. Influence of implant taper on the primary and secondary stability of osseointegrated titanium implants. Clin Oral Implants Res. 2004;15:474–80.

27. Meredith N. Assessment of implant stability as a prognostic determinant. Int J Prosthodont. 1998;11:491–501.

28. Ueda M, Matsuki M, Jacobsson M, Tjellström A. Relationship between insertion torque and removal torque analyzed in fresh temporal bone. Int J Oral Maxillofac Implants. 1991;6:442–7.

29. Huiskes R, Nunamaker D. Local stresses and bone adaption around orthopedic implants. Calcif Tissue Int. 1984;36(Suppl 1):S110–7.

30. Gupta N, Kotrashetti SM, Naik V. A comparitive clinical study between self tapping and drill free screws as a source of rigid orthodontic anchorage. J Maxillofac Oral Surg. 2012;11:29–33.

25

Orthokeratinized odontogenic cysts: a Spanish tertiary care centre study based on HPV DNA detection

Beatriz Vera-Sirera[1], Luis Rubio-Martínez[2], Leopoldo Forner-Navarro[1] and Francisco Vera-Sempere[3*] (iD)

Abstract

Background: The role of human papillomavirus (HPV) in orthokeratinized odontogenic cysts (OOCs) has rarely been studied. The objective is to describe the clinicopathological findings in a series of OOCs from a Spanish population that were investigated in relation to the possible presence of HPV.

Methods: A clinicopathological retrospective analysis followed by a molecular analysis of 28 high- and low-risk HPV genotypes was performed in OOC samples of patients seen during the last 15-years in a Spanish tertiary care center.

Results: Of 115 odontogenic cysts with keratinization, 16 cases of OOCs were confirmed and evaluated. OOCs occurred predominantly in the mandible of males (mean age 36.06 ± 13.16 years). Swelling of the jaw followed by pain were the most common clinical symptoms, and 56.5% of the OOC cases were associated with an unerupted tooth. After a mean post-cystectomy follow-up of 3.8 years, only one recurrent case was observed, resulting in a verrucous cystic lesion that was considered premalignant after immunohistological examination. DNA extraction was successful from 14 of the 16 OOC cases. None of the primary OCCs or the single recurrent OOC were positive for HPV in the molecular analysis.

Conclusions: OOCs show a very limited potential for recurrence. Our results suggest that neither high- or low-risk HPV subtypes are likely to play a role in the etiology or neoplastic transformation of OOC, at least in the Spanish population.

Keywords: Orthokeratinized odontogenic cyst, Recurrence, HPV, High- and low-risk

Background

Orthokeratinized odontogenic cyst (OOC) is a rare intraosseous cyst characterized by an orthokeratinized epithelial lining and minimal clinical aggressiveness [1]. OOCs were first described in 1927 by Schultz [2] as a variant of odontogenic keratocysts, now known as keratocystic odontogenic tumours (KCOTs) [3]. It was not until 1981 that Wright [4] described their clinicopathological aspects, indicating that OOCs are a distinct entity from odontogenic keratocysts. Several series of OOCs have been reported, confirming that their distinctive clinical, histopathological and biological features differ substantially from those of odontogenic keratocysts, as well as demonstrating a better prognosis and lower recurrence rates [1, 5, 6].

Nonetheless, rare cases of bilateral [7], multiple [8] and recurrent [9] OOCs have been reported, and although OOCs are considered clinically to be minimally aggressive, both dysplastic and malignant transformation have been reported [10]. OOCs sometimes transform into an uncommon type of well-differentiated squamous carcinoma known as carcinoma cuniculatum [11].

Over the last two decades, keratinizing cysts from various sites have been evaluated to assess a possible role of human papillomavirus (HPV) in their development and malignant transformation [12]. Reports are also available on odontogenic keratocysts [13] as well as carcinoma

* Correspondence: fco.jose.vera@uv.es
[3]Department of Pathology, Faculty of Medicine and Dentistry, La Fe University Hospital, University of Valencia, Torre A, 2° planta, Avda. Fernando Abril Martorell 106, 46026 Valencia, Comunidad Valenciana, Spain
Full list of author information is available at the end of the article

cuniculatum [14], in which specific HPV subtypes have been detected.

In this study, we evaluated the clinicopathological profile of OOCs seen at our institution over the last 15 years and analysed the possible presence of HPV.

Methods

This study was approved by our institutional Ethics Committee for Biomedical Research (protocol no. 2013/0045). Files of the Department of Pathology at La Fe University Hospital (Valencia, Spain) from 2000 to 2015 were reviewed. A retrospective search of a pathological diagnosis database (Pat Win® v4.6.0), employing the search terms "keratocyst", "primordial cyst", "keratocystic odontogenic tumor", "orthokeratinized odontogenic cyst", and "keratinized cyst", to reflect changes in terminology over time, identified 115 odontogenic cysts with keratinization.

Histological and clinical revision

Following a histological review of these 115 cases, 16 cases of OOC were selected based on the morphological criteria established by Wright [4]. Lesions in which all or a predominant portion of the epithelial lining showed non-corrugated orthokeratinization, with the presence of a granular layer, were included in this series. The presence of this orthokeratinization on the epithelial surface as well as of a granular layer in the thickness of the epithelium was clearly demonstrated with PAS staining in all selected cases. Likewise, we also included lesions in which basal and parabasal cells were not prominent and did not palisade or polarize. Cystic lesions containing only focal OOC areas or various skin appendages (i.e. hair follicles and sebaceous and sweat glands) were excluded.

Clinical data, including age, sex, lesion location (maxilla or mandible) (anterior, premolar or molar regions), radiologic features, surgical procedures, and information on recurrence (including optical and immunohistochemical data obtained from the recurrent OOC samples), were reviewed.

Immunohistochemistry

Our immunohistochemical study, performed on recurrent OOC samples included the analysis of two well-known markers (p53 and Ki67), both of which are implicated in tumorigenesis and cell proliferation [6]. Briefly, 5-μm sections were cut from the original paraffin-embedded blocks and mounted on poly-L-lysine-coated glass slides prior to immunohistochemical staining, performed using monoclonal antibodies: mouse antihuman p53 (clone DO-7, dilution 1:50, Dako®, Glostrup, Denmark) and antihuman Ki67 (clone MIB-1, dilution 1:100, Dako®, Glostrup, Denmark). Immunostaining was visualized using the

high-pH EnVision FLEX system (Dako®, Glostrup, Denmark); hematoxylin was used for counterstaining and for both techniques tonsil sections with oropharyngeal epithelium were employed as positive staining controls and the negative controls were mock-stained test sections (the primary antibody was replaced with PBS).

Amplification and detection of HPV DNA

After histological and clinical revision, formalin-fixed, paraffin embedded (FFPE) blocks of all selected OOC cases, including the one recurrent OOC, were retrieved from the archives of the Department of Pathology. The FFPE blocks were cut into three 5-μm sections, and DNA extraction was performed using a MagCore® Super HF16 automated nucleic acid extractor (RBC Bioscience Corp., New Taipei City, Taiwan).

For HPV detection and genotyping, an Anyplex II HPV28 (CE-IVD) kit (Seegene, Seoul, South Korea) was used to identify 14 high-risk and 14 low-risk HPV genotypes in two PCR reactions: mixture A (types 16, 18, 31, 33, 35, 39, 45, 51, 52, 56, 58, 59, 66 and 68) and mixture B (types 6, 11, 26, 40, 42, 43, 44, 53, 54, 61, 69, 70, 73 and 82), respectively. This semi-quantitative multiplex real-time PCR Anyplex II HPV28 system uses both dual priming oligonucleotides and tagging oligonucleotide cleavage and extension technology that combines five dyes and seven different melting-curve temperatures to distinguish the 28 HPV genotypes. PCR reactions were performed on a CFX96 real-time thermocycler (Bio-Rad Laboratories, Hercules, CA, USA) using 5 μL DNA for both mixtures A and B.

As internal control, the L1 gene of HPV DNA was simultaneously co-amplified with the human beta-globin housekeeping gene in the same PCR reaction tube. In addition, two positive controls (high-risk and low-risk HPV genotypes) were included in each PCR run along with two negative controls (non-template control) from the DNA extraction step and PCR experiment. Finally, all data from the PCR runs were interpreted using Seegene viewer software supplied by the manufacturer (Seegene, Seoul, South Korea).

Results

Clinicopathological data

The histological review of 115 keratinizing jaw cysts detected only 16 OOCs (13.91%). The cases were accepted for inclusion as OOC if they fulfilled the criterion of a complete or predominant epithelial lining with non-corrugated orthokeratinization and the presence of a granular layer. Of these 16 patients, 10 were male and 6 were female (male-to-female ratio, 1.66:1). Age at diagnosis ranged from 13 to 65 years (average 36.06 ± 13.16 years), with a clear predilection for the fourth decade of life (50%) in both sexes (Fig. 1). The mandible was affected in 12 cases (75%) and the maxilla in 4

(25%). Molars (65%) and premolars (16%) were the most commonly affected regions. Only one case showed bilateral involvement of two mandibular cystic lesions, which were diagnosed simultaneously. Of the 16 OOCs, 9 (56.5%) were associated with an impacted tooth, of which 6 were interpreted clinically as dentigerous cysts.

Jaw swelling was the most common symptom (12 cases; 75%). Four (25%) patients also complained of pain. The evolution of the symptoms ranged from 20 days to 5 years (mean, 9 months), with 7 patients (43.75%) having an evolution of less than 3 months. Interestingly, a maxillary OOC manifesting with odontogenic sinusitis was initially considered clinically and radiologically to be a periapical inflammatory cyst.

Enucleation, with or without curettage, was performed in 13 of the OOC cases; 1 case required marsupialization followed by enucleation, and the remaining 2 cases underwent a peripheral ostectomy because of their relatively large size. Related follow-up data were available for all patients. The follow-up period ranged from 12 to 120 months, average 31.12 months, during which only one case (1/16; 6.25%) recurred. We describe this case in detail below.

The only recurrence in our series was a teenage male (13 years old) who presented with a left mandibular radiolucent lesion measuring 30 mm, which displaced the roots of neighbouring molars without paresthesia, pain, or tooth mobility. Initially, an intra-oral double exodontia with cystectomy was performed. Histological examination revealed an odontogenic cyst lined by a stratified epithelium showing orthokeratotic keratiniza tion on its surface as well as the presence of an evident layer of granular cells (Fig. 2a-c). Eight months after the cystectomy, the patient reported a painful swelling at the site of the operation. Panoramic radiography showed an increased radiolucent mandibular area with a poorly defined lower edge; new and wider curettage of the lesion was performed. Histological examination of the recurrent lesion revealed an OOC with features of verrucous hyperplasia. Distinct endophytic and "pushing" invasion together with a well-differentiated pattern of verrucous appearance showing dysplastic features with mild cellular atypia was observed, although there was no rupture of the basement membrane. Proliferative cellular activity (positive for Ki67) was not restricted to basal cells, and p53 expression was observed in all cell nuclei in the immunohistochemical analysis (Fig. 3a-f). These morphological changes were interpreted as early signs of malignization, although there was no evidence of invasive growth based on basement membrane integrity. After surgery, clinical and radiological long-term follow-up of the patient was planned. After 2 years of quarterly visits, there was no evidence of growth or new recurrence.

Amplification and detection of HPV DNA

In total, 38 FFPE blocks from the 16 OOC cases (including the recurrent case 13) were used for DNA extraction. Two of the 16 OOCs (cases 5 and 7) were invalid for the Anyplex II HPV28 test due to lack of beta-globin amplification and were excluded from the study (see Table 1). For the remaining 14 cases, we performed HPV analysis in 32 FFPE blocks with good DNA quality, but observed no HPV positivity in any of the primary OOCs or the recurrent lesion.

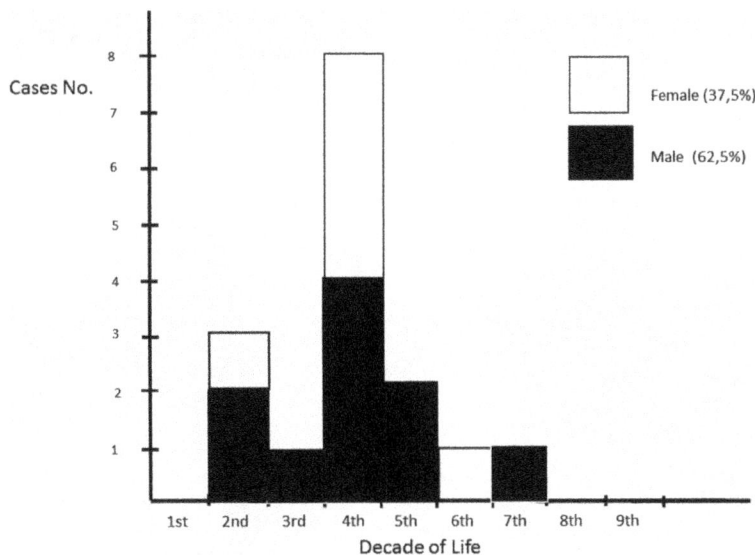

Fig. 1 Distribution of OOC cases by sex and age

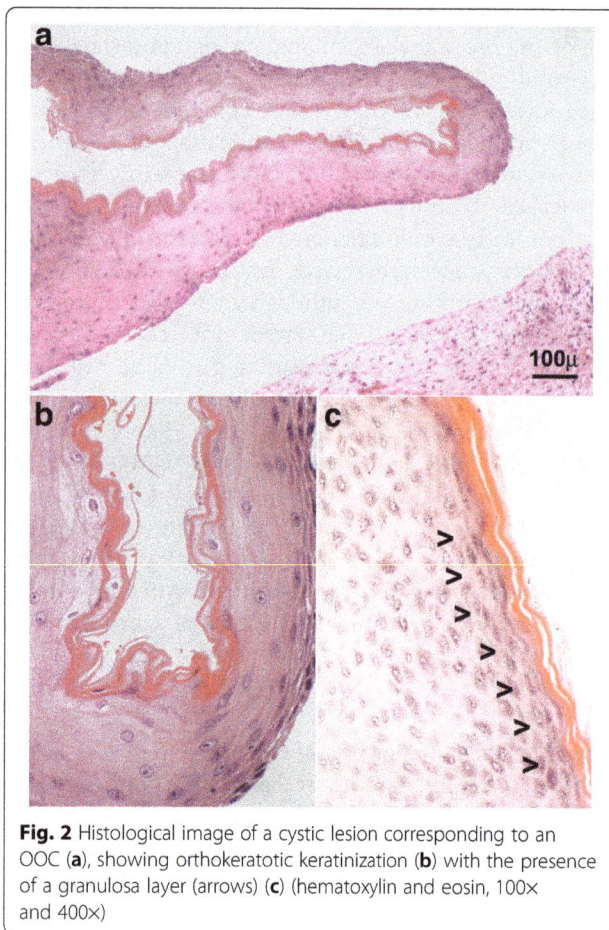

Fig. 2 Histological image of a cystic lesion corresponding to an OOC (**a**), showing orthokeratotic keratinization (**b**) with the presence of a granulosa layer (arrows) (**c**) (hematoxylin and eosin, 100× and 400×)

Discussion

This study, complemented by molecular detection of HPV DNA, examined the largest series of OOCs affecting a Spanish population reported to date.

Of our odontogenic cysts with keratinization, 13.91% were identified as OOCs. This incidence agrees with those previously reported for OOCs (range 5.2–16.8%) among cases previously coded as KCOT [1, 5].

The average age at diagnosis of our patients was 36.06 ± 13.16 years with a tendency to occur during the fourth decade (50%). There was a male predominance, which is consistent with most published series [1, 4, 5, 9]. More than half our OOC cases were radiographically associated with an impacted tooth, a characteristic observed at varying rates in previous reports, with an average incidence of approximately 60.8% [1]. Of note in our series, a maxillary OOC that manifested clinically as odontogenic sinusitis was radiologically considered a periapical inflammatory cyst. Thus indicating that OOC should be included in the differential diagnosis of radiolucencies in the periapical region, especially considering that up to seven cases of an OOC resembling a radicular cyst have been described previously [15].

Regarding the evolution of OOCs, our study confirmed the low rate of recurrence of these cysts, with only one recurrence observed among 16 patients who were followed up after surgery for 12–120 months (average 31.12 months). This low recurrence rate is somewhat higher than the reported mean of 4%, based on pooled data from OOC series with adequate follow-up [9]; however, it is less than the overall rate reported for KCOTs (12–60%) [1]. This difference in the recurrence rate is important, since the morphological distinction of

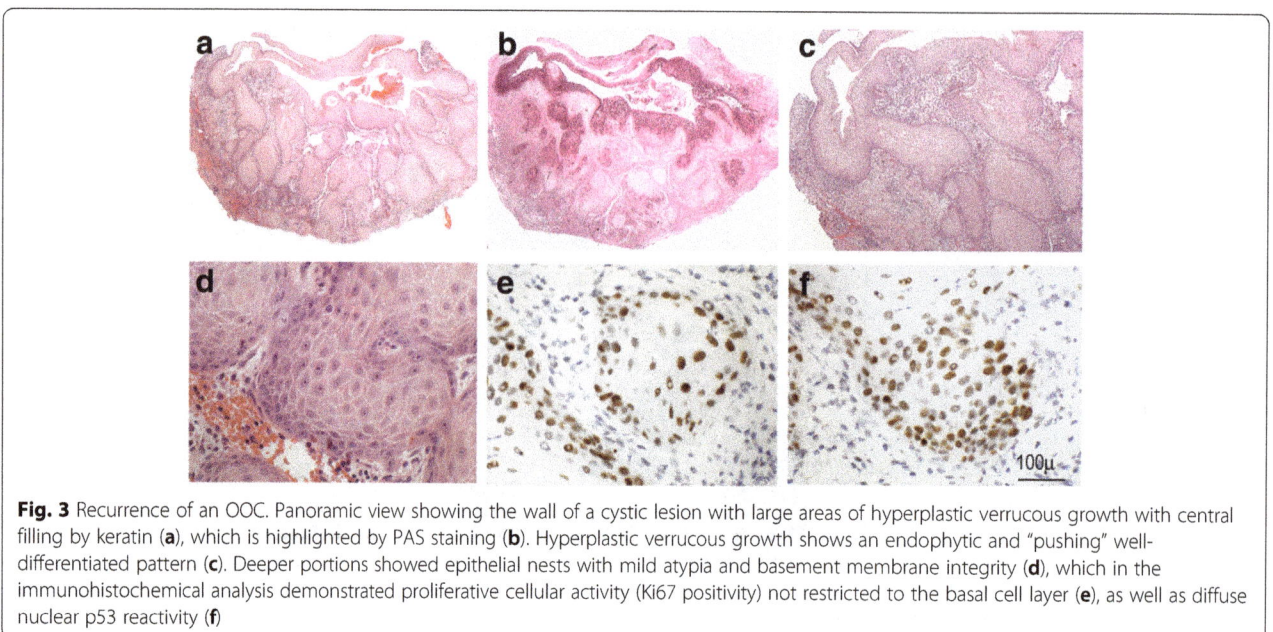

Fig. 3 Recurrence of an OOC. Panoramic view showing the wall of a cystic lesion with large areas of hyperplastic verrucous growth with central filling by keratin (**a**), which is highlighted by PAS staining (**b**). Hyperplastic verrucous growth shows an endophytic and "pushing" well-differentiated pattern (**c**). Deeper portions showed epithelial nests with mild atypia and basement membrane integrity (**d**), which in the immunohistochemical analysis demonstrated proliferative cellular activity (Ki67 positivity) not restricted to the basal cell layer (**e**), as well as diffuse nuclear p53 reactivity (**f**)

Table 1 Clinicopathological characteristics and HPV genotyping results

Case	Age	Gender	Location	Primary/Recurrence	# FFPE	year	HPV 28	IC[a]
1	38	Female	Mandible	P	1	2007	negative	1
2	34	Female	Maxilla	P	2	2002	negative	1
3	39	Male	Mandible	P	3	2004	negative	3
4	37	Female	Mandible	P	1	2006	negative	1
5	18	Female	Mandible	P	1	2007	ND	0
6	42	Male	Mandible	P	2	2006	negative	2
7	25	Male	Mandible	P	1	2007	ND	0
8	36	Female	Mandible	P	1	2011	negative	1
9	38	Male	Mandible	P	2	2006	negative	2
10	19	Male	Mandible	P	6	2001	negative	5
11	35	Male	Mandible	P	2	2014	negative	2
12	45	Male	Mandible	P	2	2014	negative	2
13	14	Male	Mandible	P&R	4 & 5	2015 / 2016	negative	4 & 5
14	39	Male	Mandible	P	1	2016	negative	1
14	45	Male	Mandible	P	3	2014	negative	2
16	65	Male	Maxilla	P	1	2013	negative	1

IC[a]: DNA Internal Control (number of the FFPE bloks showing a positive beta-globin gene amplification)

OOCs from KCOTs is supported mainly by studies that indicated a significantly lower rate of OOC recurrence following surgery [1, 4, 5].

Although rare, recurrence of OOC is possible, and may be indicative of malignant transformation. In our series, there was one recurrence observing hyperplastic verrucous changes in the lining of the OOC. These findings were histopathologically interpreted as atypical based on the overexpression of p53 as well as by the presence of proliferative activity in suprabasal cells. This case is unusual considering the young age of the patient, existence of a prior OOC, and the short period from the original OOC to recurrence; this supports the importance of performing additional microscopic studies of all resected cystic lesions in the jaws and the need for careful follow-up after their removal [10].

Previous studies have reported the appearance of verrucous proliferation in OOCs [16], as well as the possible emergence of squamous cell carcinomas (SCCs) from pre-existing OOCs [17]. Cysts with keratinization have a higher incidence of malignization than other OOCs [18], often presenting as highly differentiated SCCs [17], including cases of verrucous [19] or cuniculatum carcinoma [20], with some well-documented cases arising from OOCs [20–23]. Thus, although OOCs are considered clinically less aggressive lesions than KCOTs, the epithelial lining of OOCs may have neoplastic potential [21].

The pathogenesis of malignant transformation of OOC epithelia remains unclear [17]. Different hypotheses, such as long-standing chronic inflammation [17], genetic mutations in exon 6 of the *TP53* gene [23] or oncogenic viral effects [13] have been suggested as predisposing factors, but the specific underlying mechanisms of this carcinogenesis remain unclear. It is thought that HPV may be associated with the pathogenesis of keratinizing OOC [13] and carcinoma cuniculatum [14], as well as some other carcinomas arising from epidermal cysts [12]. In addition, HPV may play a role in the development of verrucous proliferation in various sites, including oral locations [16, 24, 25]; however, this remains controversial [26].

In agreement with previous reports [16, 24, 27], we did not detect HPV genotypes in our molecular analysis of atypical verrucous hyperplasia in the recurrent case, suggesting that neither high- or low-risk HPV subtypes are likely to play a role in the pathogenesis of atypical verrucous changes that may develop into OOC recurrence. Moreover, molecular analysis did not detect HPV involvement in our series of primary OOC samples with successful DNA extraction. Thus, it is unlikely that HPV plays a role in the pathogenesis of OOCs, at least in the Spanish population. However, we cannot completely exclude that HPV is involved in OOCs in patients from other geographic areas, as commonly occurs in other virus-related disorders [28]. Additional epidemiological and molecular investigations in a large series of patients with OOCs of different ethnicities using molecular analysis of a broad spectrum of HPV types are required to confirm our results.

Conclusions

OOCs are a rare type of odontogenic cyst that show minimal clinical aggressiveness. Nonetheless, although very rare, recurrence is possible and can be a source of malignant transformation. Neither high- or low-risk HPV subtypes are likely to play a role, at least in the Spanish population, in the etiology of an OOC or in its neoplastic transformation.

Abbreviations
FFPE: Formalin-fixed, paraffin embedded; HPV: Human papillomavirus; KCOT: Keratocystic odontogenic tumour; OOC: Orthokeratinized odontogenic cyst; PCR: Polymerase chain reaction; SCC: Squamous cell carcinomas

Funding
The authors of this article did not receive funding from any source for the design and realization of this study.

Authors' contributions
FVS conceived the project, reviewed the process and drafted the manuscript. LFN made substantial contributions to the acquisition of clinical data. BVS and FVS performed the histological and immunohistochemical examination. LRM performed the HPV molecular analysis. LFN, LRM and BVS critically revised the manuscript. All authors read and approved the final manuscript.

Competing interest
The authors declares that they have no competing interests.

Consent for publication
Not applicable

Author details
[1]Department of Stomatology, Faculty of Medicine and Dentistry, University of Valencia, Valencia, Comunidad Valenciana, Spain. [2]Molecular Pathology Unit, Department of Pathology, La Fe University Hospital, University of Valencia, Valencia, Comunidad Valenciana, Spain. [3]Department of Pathology, Faculty of Medicine and Dentistry, La Fe University Hospital, University of Valencia, Torre A, 2° planta, Avda. Fernando Abril Martorell 106, 46026 Valencia, Comunidad Valenciana, Spain.

References
1. Dong Q, Pan S, Sun L-S, Li T-J. Orthokeratinized odontogenic cyst. A clinicopathologic study of 61 cases. Arch Pathol Lab Med. 2010;134:271–5.
2. Schultz L. Cysts of the maxillae and mandible. J Am Dent Assoc. 1927;14:1395–402.
3. Philipsen HP. Keratocystic odontogenic tumour in pathology and genetics of head and neck tumours. In: Barnes EL, Eveson JW, Reichart P, Sidransky D, editors. World Health Organization classification of Tumours. Lyon, France: IARC press; 2005. p. 306–7.
4. Wright JM. The odontogenic keratocyst: orthokeratinized variant. Oral Surg Oral Med Oral Pathol. 1981;51:609–18.
5. Crowley TE, Kaugars GE, Gunsolley JC. Odontogenic keratocysts: a clinical and histologic comparison of the parakeratin and orthokeratin variants. J Oral Maxillofac Surg. 1992;50:22–6.
6. Da Silva MJ, de Sousa SOM, Correa L, Carvalhosa AA, De Araujo VC. Immunohistochemical study of the orthokeratinized odontogenic cyst: a comparison with the odontogenic keratocyst. Oral Surg Oral Med Oral Pathol Radiol Endod. 2002;94:732–7.
7. Pimpalkar RD, Barpande SR, Bhavthankar JD, Mandale M. Bilateral orthokeratinized odontogenic cyst: a rare case report and review. Oral Maxillofac Pathol. 2014;18:262–6.
8. Cheng Y-SL, Liang H, Wright J, Teenier T. Multiple orthokeratinized odontogenic cysts. A case report. Head Neck Pathol. 2015;9:153–7.
9. MacDonald-Jankowski DS. Orthokeratinized odontogenic cyst: a systematic review. Dentomaxilloofacial Radiol. 2010;39:455–67.
10. Yoshida H, Onizawa R, Yusa H. Squamous cell carcinoma arising in association with an orthokeratinized odontogenic keratocyst. Report of a case. J Oral Maxillofac Surg. 1996;54:647–51.
11. Allon D, Kaplan I, Manor R, Calderon S. Carcinoma cuniculatum of the jaw: a rare variant of oral carcinoma. Oral Surg Oral Med Oral Pathol Radiol Endod. 2002;94:601–8.
12. Pusiol T, Zorzi MG, Piscioli F. Squamous cell carcinoma arising in epidermal and human papillomavirus associated cysts: report of three cases. Pathologica. 2010;102:88–92.
13. Cox M, Eveson J, Scully C. Human papillomavirus type 16 DNA in an odontogenic keratocyst. J Oral Pathol Med. 1991;20:143–5.
14. Knobler RM, Schneider S, Neumann RA, Bodemer W, Radlwimmer B, Aberer E, Söltz-Szöts J, Gebhart W. DNA dot-blot hybridization implicates human papillomavirus type 11-DNA in epithelioma cuniculatum. J Med Virol. 1989;29:33–7.
15. Servato JPS, Cardoso SV, Da Silva MCP, Cordeiro MS, Faria PR, Loyola AM. Orthokeratinized odontogenic cysts presenting as a periapical lesion: report of a case and literature review. J Endod. 2014;40:455–8.
16. Aldred MJ, Talacko AA, Allan PG, Shear M. Odontogenic cyst with verrucous proliferation. J Oral Pathol Med. 2002;31:500–3.
17. Bodner L, Manor E, Shear M, van der Waal I. Primary intraosseous squamous cell carcinoma arising in an odontogenic cyst – a clinicopathologic analysis of 116 reported cases. J Oral Pathol Med. 2011;40:733–8.
18. Brown RM, Gough NG. Malignant change in the epithelium lining odontogenic cysts. Cancer. 1972;29:1199–207.
19. Chaisuparat R, Coletti D, Kolokythas A, Ord RA, Nikitakis NG. Primary intraosseous odontogenic carcinoma arising in an odontogenic cyst or de novo: a clinicopathological study of six new cases. Oral Surg Oral Med Oral Pathol Radiol Endod. 2006;101:194–200.
20. Fonseca FP, Pontes HAR, Pontes FSC, Carvalho PL, Sena-Filho M, Jorge J, Santos-Silva AR, De Almeida OP. Oral carcinoma cuniculatum: two cases illustrative of a diagnostic challenge. Oral Surg Oral Med Oral Pathol Oral Radiol. 2013;116:457–63.
21. Shiar CH, Ng KH. Squamous cell carcinoma in an orthokeratinised odontogenic keratocyst. Int J Oral Maxillofac Surg. 1987;16:95–8.
22. Yoshida H, Onizawa K, Yusa H. Squamous cell carcinoma arising in association with an orthokeratinized odontogenic keratocyst. J Oral Maxillofac Surg. 1996;54:647–51.
23. Cox DP. P53 expression and mutation analysis of odontogenic cysts with and without dysplasia. Oral Surg Oral Med Oral Pathol Oral Radiol. 2012;113:90–8.
24. Argyris PP, Nelson AC, Koutlas IG. Keratinizing odontogenic cyst with verrucous pattern featuring negative human papillomavirus status by polymerase chain reaction. Oral Surg Oral Med Oral Pathol Oral Radiol. 2015; 119:e233–40.
25. Samman M, Wood H, Conway C, Berri S, Pentenero M, Gandolfo S, Cassenti A, Cassoni P, Al Ajlan A, Barrett AW, Chengot P, MacLennan K, High AS, Rabbitts P. Next-generation sequencing analysis for detecting human papillomavirus in oral verrucous carcinoma. Oral Surg Oral Med Oral Pathol Oral Radiol. 2014;118:117–25.
26. Del Pino M, Bleeker MC, Quint WG, Snijders PJ, Meijer CJ, Steenbergen RD. Comprehensive analysis of human papillomavirus prevalence and the potential role of low-risk types in verrucous carcinoma. Mod Pathol. 2012;10:1354–63.
27. Lalla K, Mahomed F, Meer S. Keratinizing odontogenic cysts with a spectrum of verrucous morphology: investigation of a potential role of human papillomavirus. Oral Surg Oral Med Oral Pathol Oral Radiol. 2016;122:625–30.
28. Hauck F, Oliveira-Silva M, Dreyer JH, Perrusi VJ, Arcuri RA, Hassan R, Bonvicino CR, Barros MH, Niedobitek G. Prevalence of HPV infection in head and neck carcinomas shows geographical variability: a comparative study from Brazil and Germany. Virchows Arch. 2015;466:685–93.

26

Ectopic third molars in the sigmoid notch: etiology, diagnostic imaging and treatment options

Marcel Hanisch[*], Leopold F. Fröhlich and Johannes Kleinheinz

Abstract

Background: The etiology of ectopic third molars located in the sigmoid notch of the mandible is unclear. Only a few cases have been reported. The aim of this article is to discuss the etiology as well as treatment options and diagnostic imaging techniques.

Methods: A PubMed and Medline search of the literature from 1965 to 2015 to ectopic third molars in the mandibular notch was performed. Furthermore, a clinical case provided by the authors is reported.

Results: Among the eight reviewed cases, two male and six female patients were affected that ranged from 25 to 62 years of age (mean 48.4). Pain and swelling in the preauricular region or trismus but also the absence of symptoms was reported. Only in two of the summarized articles an extra-oral access for the removal of the tooth was used. The etiology seems to be individually different, however dentigerous cysts and chronic inflammation seem to play an important role in their appearance. While previous diagnostic reports described two-dimensional diagnostic imaging, currently the three-dimensional imaging is common for preoperative surgical planning with respect to removing ectopic molars.

Conclusions: Ectopic third molars in the mandible are a rare condition. The etiology seems to be individually different. Nowadays, three-dimensional imaging is common for preoperative surgical planning.

Keywords: Dentigerous cyst, Ectopic third molar, Ectopic tooth, Mandibular notch, Sigmoid notch

Background

Ectopic molars in the mandible are rare cases and the etiology of this condition is still unclear [1]. Ectopic third molars of the mandible have been described in the condylar region, the coronoid process, the ascending ramus and the sigmoid notch. A review by Wang et al. indicated only 13 reported cases in the literature depicting ectopic molars in the ramus region during a period of 30 years [2]. The surgical excision of third molars is one of the most common outpatient surgeries [3], whereas the removal of ectopic molars seem to be an unusual surgical intervention. Preoperative diagnosis is based on clinical findings and diagnostic X-ray examination [4]. In the present paper, we review the literature of all cases describing ectopic third molars found in the mandibular sigmoid notch region, which have been reported over a period of 50 years from 1965 to 2015. Subsequently, we add to this summary our own experience by presenting a new case with an ectopic third molar in the sigmoid notch.

Methods

A clinical case provided by the authors is reported. Furthermore, a literature search in PubMed and Medline databases was achieved by using the following MeSH terms: "sigmoid notch" OR "mandibular notch" AND "ectopic tooth" OR "third molar". Inclusion criteria were international cases of ectopic third molars in the sigmoid notch, which have been reported in English or native language from 1965 to 2015.

* Correspondence: marcel.hanisch@ukmuenster.de
Department of Cranio-Maxillofacial Surgery, University Hospital Münster,
Albert-Schweitzer-Campus 1, Gebäude W 30, Münster D-48149, Germany

Results

From 1965 to 2015 only eight cases with ectopic third molars that occurred in the sigmoid notch of the mandible have been reported. In addition to six case reports which were written in English language [5–10], two cases that were presented in native language by an Italian and a Japanese group [11, 12], respectively, were also included. Clinical and radiological features of these eight cases are summarized in Table 1.

Gender and age prevalence

Six female patients and two male patients were diagnosed with ectopic molars in the sigmoid notch. The age ranged from 25 to 62, with an average age of 48.4 years.

Clinical symptoms

As clinical symptoms the eight reported cases describes pain [8], swelling [7], trismus [5], discomfort of the mucosa [10] as well as combinations of these symptoms [11, 12] or no symptoms [6, 9]. The clinical features of the eight reported cases are summarized in Table 2.

Treatment

Treatment was described in all cases except one [8]. Granite et al. reported periodic radiographic examination [6], Giordano et al. indicated denied treatment by the patient [11] whereas three authors referred their patients to intraoral access and extraction of the ectopic molar under general anesthesia [7, 9, 10]. Only two cases described extra-oral surgical access for the extraction of the ectopic molar [5, 12]. In detail, submandibular access was selected in both reports.

Association with cystic lesions

Cystic lesions were described in four cases [5, 7, 9, 12]. Giordano et al. described encircling radiolucency [11].

Adachi et al. also reported encircling radiolucency which was diagnosed pathologically as granulation tissue [10]. One report referred to an area of sclerotic bone surrounding the tooth [6] whereas Balan did not describe any cystic lesion or other abnormalities which could be detected in the radiologic image [8].

Diagnostic imaging

Diagnostic imaging techniques reports from 1992 to 1965 described lateral oblique radiographs [7, 8, 11, 12], a panoramic radiograph [6], or posteroranterior and lateral jaw projection [5, 11, 12]. Diagnostic imaging by three-dimensional methods, in addition to a two-dimensional panoramic radiograph, was only reported by Fidink et al. and Adachi et al. in 2015 [9, 10].

Case presentation

A 51 year-old male was referred to our Clinic of Cranio-Maxillofacial Surgery by his dentist. The patient described pain in the preauricular region for a few days. The panoramic radiograph revealed lower right third molar being dislocated in the sigmoid notch associated with a radioluscent lesion (Fig. 1). In addition, the panoramic radiograph offered generalized periodontitis and an impacted third molar surrounded with a radioluscent lesion on the left side of the mandible. Unfortunately, no earlier radiographic images of the patient were available for comparing the development of the ectopic molar. Clinical intra- and extraoral inspection disclosed no further inflammation signs like swelling, trismus, fever or redness. Also signs of chronic inflammation like fistula did not appear. Cone beam scans (CT) showed the impacted tooth with cranial-dorsal directed roots and bone apposition in the sigmoid notch (Figs. 2, 3, 4). A radiolucent cystic lesion was extending from the pericoronary region of the tooth to the dental arch. The

Table 1 Clinical and radiological features of ectopic molars in the sigmoid notch reported from 1965 to 2015

Author	Gender	Age	Symptoms	Surgical access	Radiology
Traiger J. et al. 1965 [5]	female	47	firm, hard swelling of the side of the face	extraoral, general anesthetic	posteroanterior and lateral jaw projection; encircling radiolucency
Giardino et al. 1966 [11] (Article in Italian)	female	62	trismus, sporadic pain praeauricular	none	posteroranterior roentgenogram, lateral oblique radiograph; encircling radiolucency
Nishijima et al. 1976 [12] (Article in Japanese)	female	60	trismus, pain and swelling in preauricular region	extraoral, general anesthetic	posteroranterior roentgenogram, lateral oblique radiograph; encircling radiolucency
Granite EL et al. 1985 [6]	female	60	none	none	panoramic radiograph; area of sclerotic bone
Metha DS et al. 1986 [7]	male	25	slowly growing swelling since 2 years	intraoral, general anesthetic	lateral oblique radiograph; radiolucent lesion
Balan N. 1992 [8]	female	30	pain in preauricular region	not specified	lateral oblique radiograph
Fidink Y et al. 2015 [9]	male	45	none	intraoral, general anesthetic	CT, panoramic radiograph; radiolucent lesion
Adachi M. et al. 2015 [10]	female	58	discomfort in the left buccal mucosa	intraoral, general anesthetic	CT, panoramic radiograph; radiolucent lesion

Table 2 Clinical Symptoms described in eight reported cases

Clinical Symptoms described in the eight reported cases	
Symptom	Author
Firm hard swelling with complete trismus	Traiger J. et al. 1965 [5]
Trismus and sporadic pain preauricularly	Giardino et al. 1966 [11] (Article in Italian)
Trismus, pain and swelling in preauricular region	Nishijima et al. 1976 [12] (Article in Japanese)
No symptoms	Granite EL et al. 1985 [6]
Slowly growing swelling for two years	Metha DS et al. 1986 [7]
Pain in the preauricular region	Balan N. 1992 [8]
No symptoms	Fidink Y et al. 2015 [9]
Discomfort in the left buccal mucosa	Adachi M. et al. 2015 [10]

mandibular canal was compressed but covered by a small sclerotic bone (Fig. 1). Under endotracheal general anesthesia, an intraoral access was selected by incising the anterior edge of the mandibular ramus. In order to expose the sigmoid notch, a subperiosteal dissection was done lingually. Because the tooth was completely osseously covered, bone was removed and the tooth was separated with a surgical drill. The cystic lesion was enucleated and sent routinely for pathological analysis to the Department of Pathology, University Hospital Muenster. Microscopic analysis of the specimen showed stratified epithelium, fibrous tissue with lymphocytic-, plasma cell- and granulocytic infiltration of neutrophilic type and chronic inflammation (Fig. 5). Furthermore, all second molars and the third molar on the left mandible have also been removed. No complications occurred in the postoperative phase. Antibiotics were not given during the entire therapy. Subsequently, periodontal therapy will be performed by the patient's dentist.

Discussion

Up to now, only a few reports of ectopic third molars located in the mandible were recorded in the literature. The etiology of this condition is still unclear but several causes were discussed. Capelli described a correlation between the lack of space between second molar and the ramus mandibulae leading to an ectopic position of the

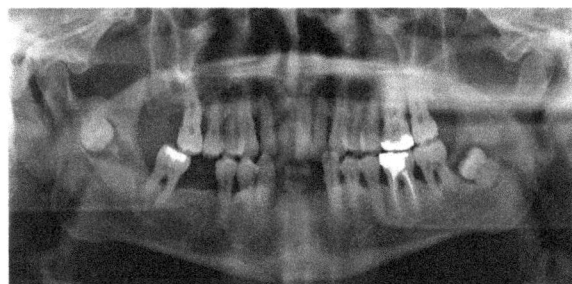
Fig. 1 Panoramic radiograph showing the ectopic third right molar

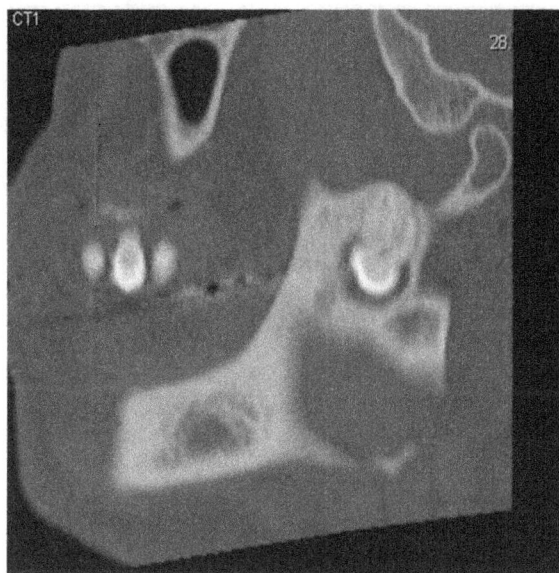
Fig. 2 Sagital cone beam scan showing the impacted tooth with cranial-dorsal directed roots and bone apposition in the *right* sigmoid notch

impacted third molar [13]. Also a relationship involving the growth of the coronoid process and the ectopic position was suspected whenever the base of the ectopic third molar was embedded in the bony-growth tissue of the coronoid process [14]. Moreover, deviant eruption patterns were also assumed as a primordial deviance of the germ leading to ectopic teeth [15]. These theories may apply to be causative for the individual ectopic molars illustrated in the case reports which were summarized in this review. For the case presented in this article, the theory reported by Thoma in 1958 [16] and several other authors like Stafne [17] seems to apply for the identified ectopic molar. Thoma suspected that the pressure of the cystic fluid was responsible for the

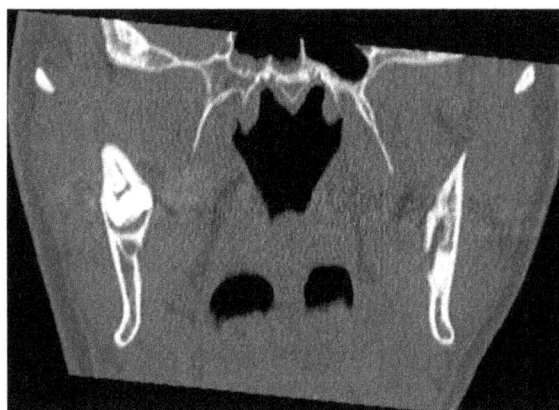
Fig. 3 Coronal cone beam scan showing the impacted tooth with radiolucent cystic lesion superior the inferior alveolar nerve

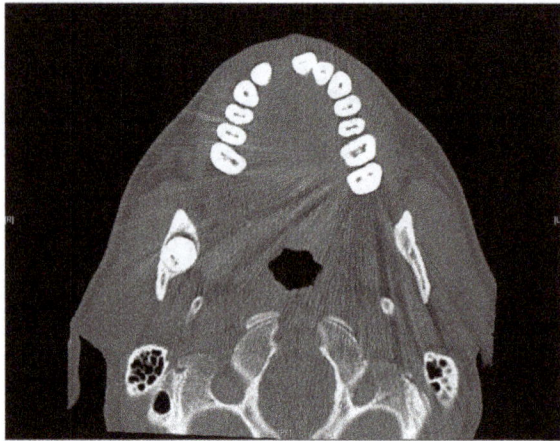

Fig. 4 Axial cone beam scan showing the impacted tooth in the right sigmoid notch

migration of the tooth. In our reported patient, a dentigerous cyst surrounds the crown. In the panoramic radiograph a radiolucent area similar to a "path" that extended from the dental arch to the ectopic molar in the sigmoid notch, appeared. Possibly, this "path" represents the route of migration starting at the dental arch and ending at the sigmoid notch. As inflammations are known to be supporting the expansion of cysts, the periodontitis determined in our patient could serve as an additional factor for the expansion of the cyst, leading to migration of the tooth. The same theory was reported by Adachi et al. which describes "granulation tissue with chronic inflammation around the crown" being etiological to the process of retrograde migration and forcing up the tooth into an ectopic position [10].

In symptomatic patients surgical removal, after a careful preoperative planning, is the recommended treatment [18]. In the past, diagnostic X-ray examinations were mainly implemented by two-dimensional diagnostic

imaging techniques like panoramic radiograph or lateral jaw projection. Reports about complications during or after the removal of ectopic molars in the sigmoid notch like nerve injury, damage of the mandibular joint, bleeding or infections were not described in the reviewed literature. Ghaeminia et al. illustrated in their study that three-dimensional diagnostic imaging, compared to panoramic radiography, can contribute to optimal risk assessment and, as a consequence, allow better surgical planning [19]. Currently, three-dimensional diagnostic imaging techniques are established and can be beneficial in identifying position of the tooth, associated pathology and identifying the position of neurovascular structures [20]. Thus, preoperatively, the appropriate surgical method can be chosen [2].

Conclusions

Ectopic third molars in the sigmoid notch of the mandible are a rare condition with higher prevalence in women. The etiology seems to be individually different, however dentigerous cysts and chronic inflammation seem to play an important role in their appearance. For planning the surgical entryway, which is mostly selected from intraoral as well as the assessment of operative-risks, three-dimensional diagnostic imaging techniques should be a preoperative standard in diagnostics.

Acknowledgements
We acknowledge support by Open Access Publication Fund of University of Muenster.

Funding
This research did not receive any specific grant from funding agencies in the public, commercial or not-for-profit sectors.

Authors' contributions
MH conceived the study. LFF and JK helped in the acquisition and interpretation of data. MH, LFF and JK participated in literature review, design and drafting of the manuscript. All authors read and approved the final manuscript.

Competing interests
The authors declare that they have no competing interests.

Consent for publication
Written informed consent was obtained from the patient for publication. A copy of the written consent is available for review by the Editor-in-Chief of this journal.

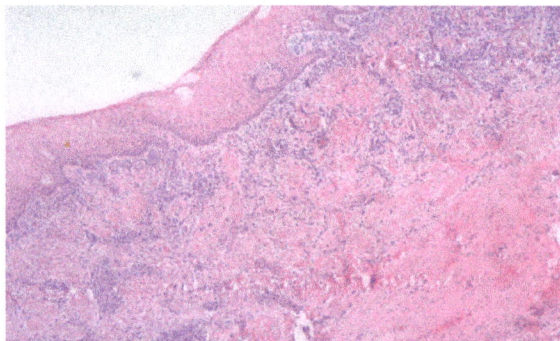

Fig. 5 Microscopic image of the stratified epithelium demonstrating fibrous tissue with lymphocytic-, plasma cell- and neutrophilic granulocyte infiltration, as well as chronic inflammation (PAS, magnification: 100)

References

1. Iglesias-Martin F, Infante-Cossio P, Torres-Carranza E, Prats-Golczer VE, Garcia-Perla-Garcia A. Ectopic third molar in the mandibular condyle: a review of the literature. Med Oral Patol Oral Cir Bucal. 2012;17(6):1013–7.
2. Wang CC, Kok SH, Hou LT, Yang PJ, Lee JJ, Cheng SJ, Kuo RC, Chang HH. Ectopic mandibular third molar in the ramus region: report of a case and literature review. Oral Surg Oral Med Oral Pathol Oral Radiol Endod. 2008; 105(2):155–61.
3. Eklund SA, Pittman JL. Third-molar removal patterns in an insured population. J Am Dent Assoc. 2001;132(4):469–75.
4. Salmerón JI, del Amo A, Plasencia J, Pujol R, Vila CN. Ectopic third molar in condylar region. Int J Oral Maxillofac Surg. 2008;37(4):398–400.
5. Traiger J, Koral K, Catania AJ, Nathan AS. Impacted third molar and dentigerous cyst of the sigmoid notch of the mandible. Report of a case. Oral Surg Oral Med Oral Pathol. 1965;19:459–61.
6. Granite EL, Isaacs M, Kross JF. Asymptomatic impacted mandibular third molar in the subcondylar-sigmoid notch region associated with extensive sclerotic bone. J Oral Med. 1985;40(2):91–2.
7. Mehta DS, Mehta MJ, Murugesh SB. Impacted mandibular third molar in the sigmoid notch region associated with dentigerous cyst-a case report. J Indian Dent Assoc. 1986;58(12):545–7.
8. Balan N. Tooth in the sigmoid notch. Oral Surg Oral Med Oral Pathol. 1992; 73(6):767.
9. Fındık Y, Baykul T. Ectopic third molar in the mandibular sigmoid notch: Report of a case and literature review. J Clin Exp Dent. 2015;7(1):133–7.
10. Adachi M, Motohashi M, Nakashima M, Ehara Y, Azuma M, Muramatsu Y. Ectopic Third Molar Tooth at the Mandibular Notch. J Craniofac Surg. 2015; 26(5):455–6.
11. Giardino C, Valletta G. Heterotopia of the lover 3d molar on the level of the sigmoid notch. Clinical case. Arch Stomatol (Napoli). 1966;7(4):323–7.
12. Nishijima K, Kishi K, Komai M, Maeda K, Wake K. A case of impacted third molar and dentigerous cyst located below the sigmoid notch of the mandible. Nihon Koku Geka Gakkai Zasshi. 1976;22(3):391–5.
13. Capelli Jr J. Mandibular growth and third molar impaction in extraction cases. Angle Orthod. 1991;61(3):223–9.
14. Keros J, Susić M. Heterotopia of the mandibular third molar: a case report. Quintessence Int. 1997;28(11):753–4.
15. Toranzo Fernandez M, Terrones Meraz MA. Infected cyst in the coronoid process. Oral Surg Oral Med Oral Pathol. 1992;73(6):768.
16. Thoma KH. Oral Surgery. 3rd ed. St. Louis: C.V. Mosby Co; 1958. p. 538.
17. Stafne EC. Oral Roentgenographic Diagnosis. 4th ed. Philadelphia: W.B. Saunders Co; 1958. p. 51–5.
18. Procacci P, Albanese M, Sancassani G, Turra M, Morandini B, Bertossi D. Ectopic mandibular third molar: report of two cases by intraoral and extraoral access. Minerva Stomatol. 2011;60(7–8):383–90.
19. Ghaeminia H, Meijer GJ, Soehardi A, Borstlap WA, Mulder J, Vlijmen OJ, Bergé SJ, Maal TJ. The use of cone beam CT for the removal of wisdom teeth changes the surgical approach compared with panoramic radiography: a pilot study. Int J Oral Maxillofac Surg. 2011;40(8):834–9.
20. Okuyama K, Sakamoto Y, Naruse T, Kawakita A, Yanamoto S, Furukawa K, Umeda M. Intraoral extraction of an ectopic mandibular third molar detected in the subcondylar region without a pathological cause: A case report and literature review. Cranio. 2016;3:1–5.

27

Use of modified lateral upper arm free flap for reconstruction of soft tissue defect after resection of oral cancer

Xu-Dong Yang[†], Su-Feng Zhao[†], Qian Zhang, Yu-Xin Wang, Wei Li, Xiao-Wei Hong and Qin-Gang Hu[*]

Abstract

Background: To evaluate the suitability of a modified lateral upper arm free flap (LAFF) for reconstruction of soft tissue defects after resection of oral cancer.

Methods: Eighteen cases of soft tissue defect repair performed between January 2011 and December 2013 using a modified LAFF after resection of oral cancer were reviewed. The design and harvest of the LAFF, the reconstruction procedure, and postoperative morbidity were reviewed and evaluated over a follow-up period of at least 12 months.

Results: The overall flap survival was 94.4 % (17/18 patients). A broad scar at the donor site was the most common morbidity, but patients did not report dissatisfaction with the scar because they could easily cover it. All wounds at the donor site achieved primary recovery. One case of flap loss was repaired with a radial forearm free flap. One case complicated by diabetes mellitus involved infection of the flap with one-third of the flap becoming necrotic. This flap survived after removal of the necrotic tissue. In one other case, fat liquefactive necrosis (1.5 × 1.0 cm) occurred in the flap on the tip of the tongue, and this flap survived after debridement. Overall, the shape and function of the reconstructed tissues were well restored, and there was no severe morbidity at the donor site in any case.

Conclusion: The modified LAFF was safe and reliable for the reconstruction of soft tissue defects after resection of oral cancer.

Keywords: Extended lateral upper arm free flap, Oral cancer, Soft tissue defect, Repair, Anastomosis

Background

Oral cancer is the 11th most common cancer type worldwide, with a still increasing incidence, and it is typically associated with squamous cell carcinoma and a high risk of metastases to lymph nodes in the neck [1, 2]. Surgical resection is an appropriate treatment strategy for oral cancer [3, 4]. However, tissue defects that are created by resection of oral cancer can severely affect speech and swallowing as well as disturb the aesthetic appearance of the oral cavity. A variety of free tissue flaps have been researched and then widely used in the reconstruction of tumor-related defects in the oral cavity [5], with the most common flaps included the anterolateral tight flap and the

pectoralis major and latissimus dorsi muocutaneous flap. Unfortunately, these flaps are bulky and not always suitable for restoring the function of the delicate oral anatomy [5]. In 1982, Song et al. [6] introduced the lateral upper arm free flap (LAFF), which has since been used in a variety of anatomical reconstruction procedures for areas including the head and neck because it is a thin, soft, and sensory tissue flap that offers a suitable amount of tissue and color for reconstruction as well as low morbidity at the donor site [5–8]. However, the utility of the LAFF in the repair of oral defects following resection of oral cancer has not been established in the literature. Therefore, in the present study, we report the outcomes of 18 cases in which the modified LAFF was applied to reconstruct a tissue defect after radical resection of oral cancer.

* Correspondence: njkqyywk@163.com
[†]Equal contributors
Department of Oral and Maxillofacial Surgery, Nanjing Stomatological Hospital, Medical School of Nanjing University, No. 30 Zhong Yang Rd, Nanjing 210008, People's Republic of China

Methods

Clinical data

From January 2011 to December 2013, 18 patients with cancer of the oral cavity first underwent radical resection of the cancer and then intraoral reconstruction using a modified LAFF in the Department of Oral and Maxillofacial Surgery, Affiliated Stomatological Hospital, Nanjing University Medical School. The preoperative assessment included clinical examination of the donor site by an experienced surgeon. The study was approved by Ethical institutional review board of Stomatological Hospital of Nanjing University School of Medicine (NO. LC 2010-17/1).

LAFF anatomy

The conventional LAFF is situated on the lower lateral aspect of upper arm immediate above the medial condyle of humerus and is a typical intermuscular septum flap. The posterior radial collateral artery (PRCA) as well as the deep brachial artery and its branches are the main feeding vessels of the LAFF, according to the intermuscular septum of the lateral arm. The deep brachial artery originates from the proximal lateral segment of the branchial artery and runs close to the radial nerve in a spiral groove and then bifurcates into the PRCA and anterior radial collateral artery. The PRCA runs in the septum between the triceps, brachialis, and brachioradialis, and a number of branches extending from the PRCA feed the lateral head of the triceps. Upon harvesting the LAFF, the terminal of the PRCA was anastomosed with the terminal of arteria radialis recurrens around the humeral lateral epicondyle, which composed the vascular network around the humeral lateral epicondyle. The range of blood supply could extend 8 cm distally. These features are the anatomic basis for the harvest and modification of the LAFF.

LAFF harvesting

A color ultrasonic Doppler blood flow survey meter was used to examine the left upper arm to exclude variations in the septocutaneous perforators preoperatively while all patients were under general anesthesia. A line was marked between the deltoid insertion and the lateral condyle, and 1 cm behind which indicated the lateral intermuscular septum and PRCA. The flap had the shape of an ellipse and a width of no more than 6 cm (Fig. 1a). The free flaps were harvested with the combination of anterograde and retrograde tracing without blood evacuation (Fig. 1b). First, the vascular pedicle was isolated. The front of the lateral triceps head was

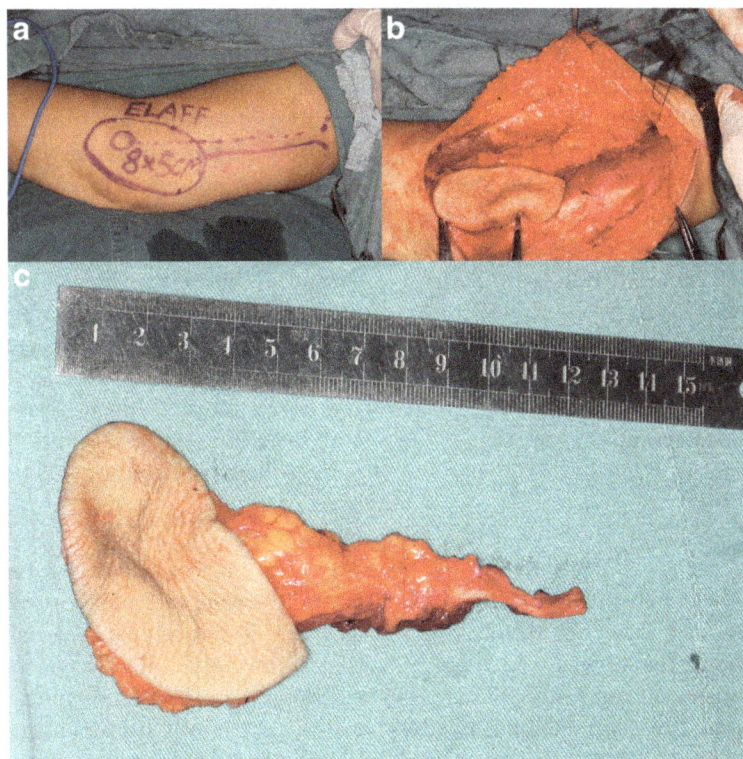

Fig. 1 a Representative image showing the LAFF design with the lateral intermuscular septum as the central axis and the lateral condyle at the inferior trisection point of flap. The flap had the shape of an ellipse with a width of no more than 6 cm. **b** Representative image during harvesting of the LAFF showing both the anterograde and retrograde anatomy. **c** Representative image of a free cutaneous flap with a 10.2-cm vascular pedicle isolated at the junctional part of the deltoid muscle and triceps muscle after the skin and subcutaneous tissue were dissected at the base of the line. Next, the muscle was pulled back and the vascular pedicle was carefully isolated proximally before the radial collateral artery was isolated to the extendible portion of the deep brachial artery. Because the radial nerve might be touched during the procedure, the vascular was isolated precisely by lifting with moderate tension of a rubber band, which could avoid injury to the radial nerve. The anterior radial collateral artery was ligatured, and then the flap was isolated until the posterior radial collateral artery and the parallel vein of the vascular pedicle. Secondly, the posterior incision was made, and the skin, subcutaneous tissue, and triceps fascia were cut. Then the tracing proceeded along the muscle surface to the lateral intermuscular septum. Then, the septocutaneous perforators in the intermuscular septum were identified, and close attention was paid to protecting these from injury. The main vascular pedicle of the flap PRCA and its parallel vein were preserved by continuing to isolate the intermuscular septum to its bottom. The front and distal ends of the flap were cut as deep as the brachioradialis and brachial muscle fascia after the vascular pedicle was isolated to its deep surface, and then the front of the lateral intermuscular septum was identified after isolation along the muscular belly. The flap was designed with the lateral intermuscular septum as the central vascular axis and the lateral condyle located at the inferior third point. The flap then extended below the lateral condyle by approximately 3–4 cm and extended to the upper part of the forearm. Finally, the flap was well prepared after isolation with the vascular retrograde anatomy directed upward to the upper part. The vascular pedicles for reconstruction were at least 6 cm in length. The muscle tissue of the lateral triceps head could be included in the flap when a complex lateral arm flap was needed (Fig. 1c).

Defect reconstruction and postoperative evaluation
The follow-up period was at least 12 months in all patients.

Results
This study included 16 male patients (88.9 %) and 2 female patients (11.1 %) with a mean age of 54.8 years (range, 30–72 years). Among the 18 cases analyzed in this study, there were 17 cases of squamous cell carcinoma and 1 case of adenoid cystic carcinoma, and the cancers were located on the tongue (10 cases), pars buccalis (6 cases), and palate (2 cases). The mean LAFF size was 6.7 × 5.1 cm, and the mean length of the vascular pedicle was 9.5 cm. The thickness of the

skin and subcutaneous tissue ranged from 7–15 mm (mean, 10.7 mm), and the perforators were present with no variation between flaps. Seven patients received adjuvant radiotherapy early in the postoperative period after the surgical wound had healed completely. The purpose of this delay was to ensure that poor functional outcomes could be correlated with postoperative adjuvant radiotherapy.

The mean surgery time was 7.4 h, and the mean blood loss was 550 ml. The overall survival rate of the transferred flaps was 94.4 % (17/18). One patient experienced total loss of the flap and underwent a reparative procedure using a radial forearm free flap. In one other case complicated by diabetes mellitus, the flap became infected with *Staphylococcus aureus* β and one-third of the flap became necrotic. However, the flap survived after pruning of the necrotic front end. In one case, fat liquefactive necrosis (1.5 × 1.0 cm) was observed in the flap on the tip of the tongue, and the flap survived after debridement. Figure 2a, b, c shows representative images of reconstructed defects 6 months after resection of tongue cancer, buccal carcinoma, and carcinoma of the palate.

The artery was end-to-end anastomosed to the external maxillary artery in 7 cases and with the superior thyroid artery in 11 cases. The parallel vein was end-to-side anastomosed to the internal jugular vein in all cases. An additional second vein was added in 7 cases, including the common facial vein in 5 cases and the external jugular vein in 2 cases. The ratio of vein-to-vein to artery-to-artery anastomosis was 1.39 to 1. In addition, in three patients with tongue cancer, the flap carried the posterior brachial cutaneous nerve, which was anastomosed to the stump of the lingual nerve.

As shown in the representative image in Fig. 3, the wound at the donor site in all cases achieved primary healing with no arm dysfunction, no necrosis of the skin and muscle tissue, and no severe scarring. Five cases experienced sensory disturbance at the proximal end of the lateral forearm (hypoesthesia in 2, paresthesia in 1, and hyperesthesia in 2), and two cases reported mild pain at the lateral condyle.

Discussion
The ideal flap for soft tissue reconstruction in the oral cavity following oral cancer resection must not only offer aesthetically acceptable repaired tissue but also be able to restore speech and swallowing functions. Specifically, the donor site should provide a sufficient amount of tissue to permit easy harvest of the flap. The pedicle must be long enough to reach recipient vessels, and the vessels should long enough and large sufficiently for easy anastomosis. Closure of the donor site should be easy, with minimal morbidity after harvesting of the flap. The

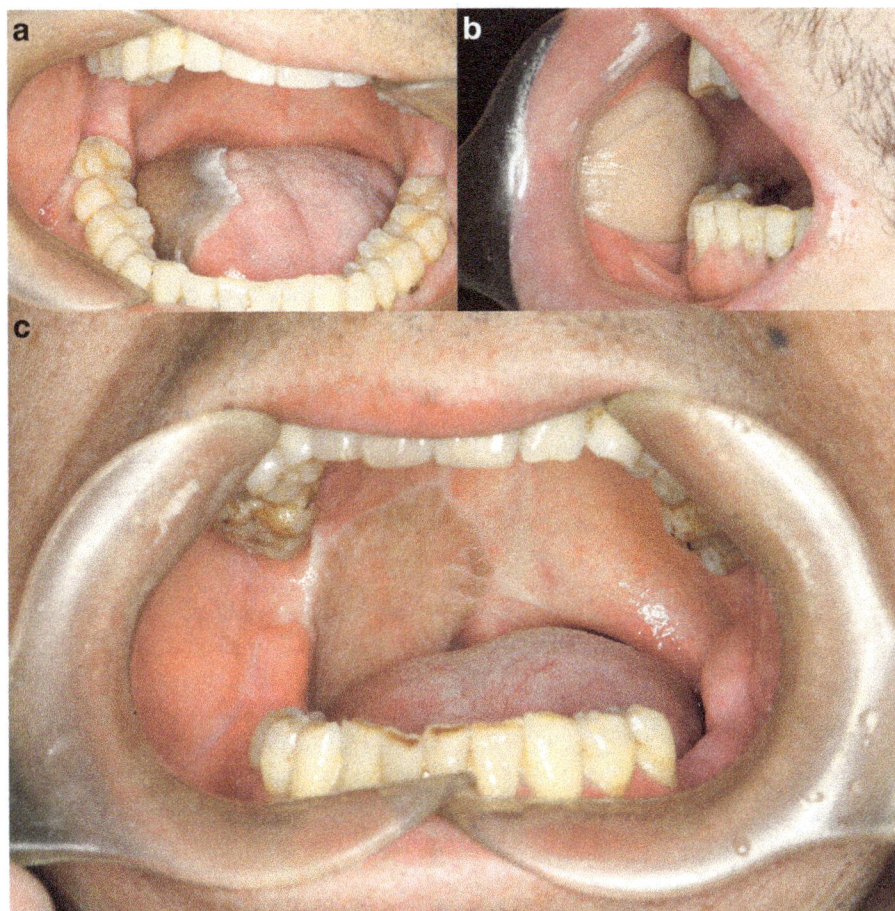

Fig. 2 a Image of a LAFF transferred to the tongue of a patient at 6 months postoperatively, showing the soft texture and appropriate shape of the flap in a patient who recovered near-normal tongue movement. **b** Image of the transferred flap at 6 months postoperatively, showing the soft texture and clear dermatoglyph. **c** Image of the oral cavity of a patient at 6 months after transfer of a LAFF that healed well and provided good recovery of speech and swallowing functions

availability of a sensory cutaneous nerve is beneficial when reinnervation is required for functional recovery, and last but not least, the donor site should be in a location that would allow for simultaneous harvesting of tissue to repair head and neck defects [5, 9]. Based on these extensive requirements of the perfect donor site and flap for soft tissue reconstruction in the oral cavity, reconstructive surgeons have had difficulty choosing the most appropriate donor site and flap [9] and evaluating flaps against the criteria for an ideal flap.

A variety of tissue flaps have been applied to soft tissue repair after resection of oral cancer, including a forearm flap, the anterolateral tight flap, and the latissimus pectoris flap [10]. Each of these flaps meets some criteria for an ideal flap, but typically at the expense of other criteria. Thus, none of them can meet all of the criteria. Harvesting of the forearm flap requires severing the radial artery, which is the main feeding artery of the forearm. Moreover, with the use of this flap, the sense and motor function of hand as well as the appearance of the

operative wound have not been satisfactory. The anterolateral tight flap and latissimus pectoris flap include too much fat tissue, making them rather bulky for most medium-size defects.

The use of the LAFF was introduced first by Song et al. [6] and then further described by Katsoros et al. [11]. The LAFF has been applied in the reconstruction of not only defects in the oral cavity [5, 12–14], but also defects in the pharyngeal cavity, lateral defects of temporal bone [15], lateral defects at the skull base [16], and defects resulting from parotidectomy [17], and these studies reported advantages of low morbidity at the donor site, moderate thickness of the flap, and excellent plasticity. However, the application of the conventional LAFF was limited due to the short pedicle and small vessel size. These disadvantages were overcome by application of the extended lateral upper arm free flap (ELAFF) introduced by Kuek and Chuan [18], which extended the inferior margin of the conventional LAFF to the upper part of the forearm by designing the

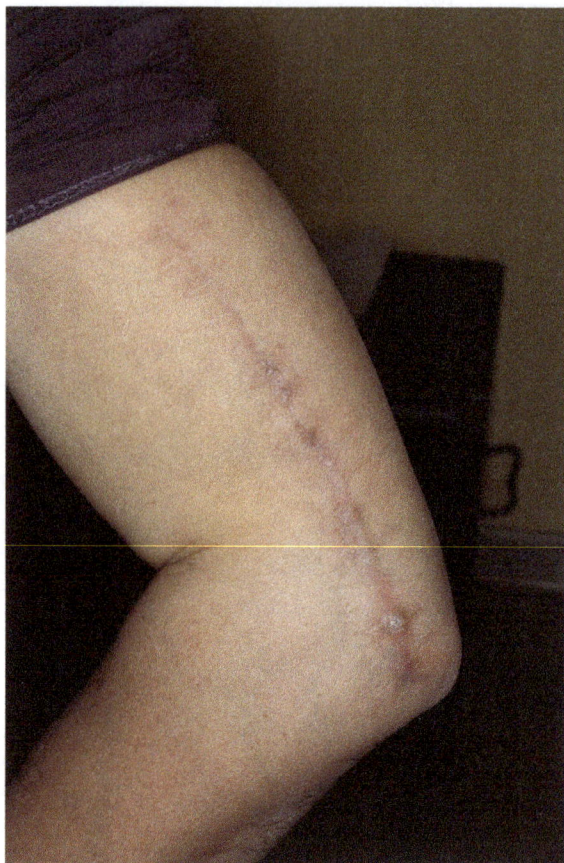

Fig. 3 Representative image of the donor site at 6 months postoperatively, showing the absence of severe morbidity in a patient who experienced only mild hypoesthesia

inferior margin of the modified LAFF to be located at the attachment point of the deltoid. Compared with the conventional LAFF, the ELAFF offers enhanced texture, a longer vascular pedicle, and similar flexibility in the forearm. A previous study demonstrated that the ELAFF can meet most of the criteria for an ideal flap for soft tissue reconstruction in defects of the head and neck [9].

In the cases described in this study, we modified the conventional procedure for harvesting the ELAFF that was reported previously [19, 20]. In the modified design of the LAFF used in our study, the flap was extended distally below the lateral condyle, making the modified LAFF 3–4 cm longer than the conventional LAFF. A position too distal might leave a conspicuous scar, but a previous systematic review demonstrated that scar formation did not cause much patient dissatisfaction [7]. In our study, the linear scar at the donor site could be covered with appropriate dressing. The vascular pedicle was usually 7–9 cm when it was cut off at the terminus of the deltoid. Therefore, there was no need to extend the vascular pedicle, because it was already long enough, which served to simplify the operative procedure. The

width of the modified LAFF was no larger than 6 cm, which permitted direct suturing and facilitated primary recovery of the donor site in all cases. Moreover, additional incisions could be applied if the donor site cannot be closed directly due to high tension. The proximal vascular pedicle was isolated first because it was not under excessive tensile stress, which could reduce injury to the vasculature in the flap. A previous study [21] demonstrated that sensory disturbance was the most common morbidity (61.4 %) at the LAFF donor site, and we speculated that this may be related to nerve injury. Therefore, harvesting of the modified LAFF was performed in the absence of a tourniquet, which avoided squeeze-induced injury to the radial nerve. To further avoid injury to the radial nerve, the vascular pedicle was isolated precisely under the moderate tensile force of a rubber band. One study showed that numbness and hypoesthesia can occur even when the posterior arm or forearm cutaneous nerve was preserved, but that these symptoms would resolve gradually [22]. The patients in our study who reported pain at the lateral epicondyle and hypoesthesia at the lateral aspect of the proximal forearm also reported that these symptoms gradually resolved. Finally, the use of LAFFs containing a vascularized posterior brachial cutaneous nerve as a sensory flap to reconstruct hemi-tongue defects and an anterior brachial cutaneous nerve of the LAFF anastomosed with a facial nerve for reconstruction of soft tissue defect after the resection of parotid carcinoma was reported previously. In three cases, the posterior brachial cutaneous nerve was anastomosed to the stump of the lingual nerve, but the effectiveness of this approach remains to be determined. The majority of soft tissue defects in the oral cavity need to be repaired with a composite flap including a portion of the muscle of the lateral head of the triceps, because the defects usually involve defects in both the muscle tissue and mucosa.

In the repair of tongue defects, the thin distal part of the modified LAFF (forearm part) was used to repair defects on the front-end of the tongue, while triceps muscle flaps were used to repair muscle defects at the floor of the mouth and the base of the tongue. Also, the proximal part of the modified LAFF was used to cover defects at the floor of the mouth and the base of the tongue. Liquefactive necrosis at the tip of tongue occurred in one female patient, which might be related to the bulk of the flap and the high tensile stress at the tip of the tongue. In another case complicated by diabetes mellitus, the flap became infected but recovered completely after resection of the forepart of the flap. In this case, the symptoms of itching, sensory disturbance, and cold intolerance at the upper arm were considered to be related to hyperglycemia.

Although the modified LAFF offers plenty of advantages, the available volume of tissue and the vessels available for anastomosis were reported to be major limitations to its widespread application [20]. The vessels of the LAFF are certainly smaller than those of a forearm flap, and the PRCA, which is a terminal branch of the deep brachial artery, is the main feeding vessel of the LAFF. Two main venous systems are present in this flap area: the deep venous system that travels along the PRCA and the subcutaneous network that is not involved in draining the flap. The diameters of the artery and vein of the upper arm are similar at 1.1 mm (range, 0.8–1.4 mm) and 1.2 mm (range, 0.9–1.5 mm) on average, respectively [23]. Thus, the artery and vein must be labeled during flap harvest. The external maxillary artery was isolated to the submandibular gland, to harvest the artery which diameter is similar with the PRCA. Considering that the diameter of the superior thyroid artery becomes gradually smaller, we recommend the superior thyroid artery as the first choice.

Moreover, sufficient blood supply at the donor site was achieved after PRCA anastomosis. The diameter of the vein that ran with the PRCA was much smaller than that of the superior thyroid vein or external maxillary vein. Thus, end-to-side anastomosis with the internal jugular vein was applied and a second vein anastomosis was added in some cases, which offered a more reliable and effective approach. The Allen test was not used to detect the PRCA because it was not main feeding vessel of the flap, and only a color ultrasonic Doppler blood flow survey meter was used to detect the PCRA and its branches and exclude variation.

Specific limitations of the present study include the lack of explicit inclusion and exclusion criteria for patients. Generally, the volume of the LAFF varies by gender, age, and weight. Flaps harvested from females are superior to those from males in terms of color, but flaps from female patients have more cutaneous fat [5]. Although flaps from female patients may better match the donor site, they may be less suitable for transfer in older patients, who might have thinner subcutaneous tissue and less hair compared to young patients [5]. Based on such expected variations in flap characteristics, we cannot draw decisive conclusions regarding the use of the modified LAFF for reconstructing soft tissue defects in the oral cavity, and further studies need to be performed.

Conclusion

In summary, the modified ELAFF was found to be safe and suitable for the reconstruction of soft tissue defects after resection of oral cancer, especially for medium size defects, and therefore, we propose that the modified ELAFF provides a well-vascularized and reliable donor flap for this purpose.

Competing interests

The authors declare that they have no competing interests.

Authors' contributions

HQG is the corresponding author and he contributed to the conception of the study. YXD and ZSF are co-first author, contributed significantly to analysis and manuscript preparation; ZQ, LW performed the data analyses and wrote the manuscript; HXW helped perform the analysis with constructive discussions. All authors read and approved the final manuscript.

Acknowledgement

This study is supported by National Key Clinical Specialty Construction Project (2011); Technology Specialty of Clinical Medicine in Jiangsu Province; BL2012012, BL2013005; Nanjing Tumor Clinical Medicine Center We thank Medjaden Bioscience Limited for assisting in the preparation of this manuscript.

References

1. Kelner N, Vartanian JG, Pinto CAL, Coutinho-Camillo CM, Kowalski LP. Does elective neck dissection in T1/T2 carcinoma of the oral tongue and floor of the mouth influence recurrence and survival rates? Brit J Oral Maxillofac Surg. 2014;52(7):590–7. doi:10.1016/j.bjoms.2014.03.020.
2. Wang YY, Tail YH, Wang WC, Chen CY, Kao YH, Chen YK, et al. Malignant transformation in 5071 southern Taiwanese patients with potentially malignant oral mucosal disorders. BMC Oral Health. 2014;14:99. doi:10.1186/1472-6831-14-99.
3. Tesseroli MA, Calabrese L, Carvalho AL, Kowalski LP, Chiesa F. Discontinuous vs. in-continuity neck dissection in carcinoma of the oral cavity. Experience of two oncologic hospitals. Acta Otorhinolaryngol Ital. 2006;26(6):350–5.
4. Liu J, Wu H, Zhu Z, Wu X, Tan H, Wang K. Free anterolateral thigh myocutaneous flap for reconstruction of soft tissue defects following en block resection of tongue cancer. Zhongguo Xiu Fu Chong Jian Wai Ke Za Zhi. 2010;24(1):82–6.
5. Song XM, Yuan Y, Tao ZJ, Wu HM, Yuan H, Wu YN. Application of lateral arm free flap in oral and maxillofacial reconstruction following tumor surgery. Med Princ Pract. 2007;16(5):394–8. doi:10.1159/000104815.
6. Song R, Song Y, Yu Y, Song Y. The upper arm free flap. Clin Plast Surg. 1982; 9(1):27–35.
7. Thankappan K, Kuriakose MA, Chatni SS, Sharan R, Trivedi NP, Vijayaraghavan S, et al. Lateral arm free flap for oral tongue reconstruction: an analysis of surgical details, morbidity, and functional and aesthetic outcome. Ann Plast Surg. 2011;66(3):261–6. doi:10.1097/SAP.0b013e3181d50e9e.
8. Agostini T, Lazzeri D, Spinelli G. Anterolateral thigh flap: systematic literature review of specific donor-site complications and their management. J Craniomaxillofac Surg. 2013;41(1):15–21. doi:10.1016/j.jcms.2012.05.003.
9. Ross DA, Thomson JG, Restifo R, Tarro JM, Sasaki CT. The extended lateral arm free flap for head and neck reconstruction: the Yale experience. Laryngoscope. 1996;106(1 Pt 1):14–8.
10. Schusterman MA, Miller MJ, Reece GP, Kroll SS, Marchi M, Goepfert H. A single center's experience with 308 free flaps for repair of head and neck cancer defects. Plast Reconstr Surg. 1994;93(3):472–8. discussion 9–80.
11. Katsaros J, Schusterman M, Beppu M, Banis Jr JC, Acland RD. The lateral upper arm flap: anatomy and clinical applications. Ann Plast Surg. 1984; 12(6):489–500.
12. Haas F, Seibert FJ, Koch H, Hubmer M, Moshammer HE, Pierer G, et al. Reconstruction of combined defects of the Achilles tendon and the overlying soft tissue with a fascia lata graft and a free fasciocutaneous lateral arm flap. Ann Plast Surg. 2003;51(4):376–82. doi:10.1097/01.sap.0000068080.76814.D7.
13. Gellrich NC, Kwon TG, Lauer G, Fakler O, Gutwald R, Otten JE, et al. The lateral upper arm free flap for intraoral reconstruction. Int J Oral Maxillofac Surg. 2000;29(2):104–11.
14. Vico PG, Coessens BC. The distally based lateral arm flap for intraoral soft tissue reconstruction. Head Neck. 1997;19(1):33–6.
15. Moncrieff MD, Hamilton SA, Lamberty GH, Malata CM, Hardy DG, Macfarlane R, et al. Reconstructive options after temporal bone resection for squamous

cell carcinoma. J Plast Reconstr Aesthet Surg. 2007;60(6):607–14. doi:10.1016/j.bjps.2006.11.005.

16. Malata CM, Tehrani H, Kumiponjera D, Hardy DG, Moffat DA. Use of anterolateral thigh and lateral arm fasciocutaneous free flaps in lateral skull base reconstruction. Ann Plast Surg. 2006;57(2):169–75. doi:10.1097/01.sap.0000218490.16921.c2. discussion 76.

17. Teknos TN, Nussenbaum B, Bradford CR, Prince ME, El-Kashlan H, Chepeha DB. Reconstruction of complex parotidectomy defects using the lateral arm free tissue transfer. Otolaryngol Head Neck Surg. 2003;129(3):183–91.

18. Kuek LB, Chuan TL. The extended lateral arm flap: a new modification. J Reconstr Microsurg. 1991;7(3):167–73. doi:10.1055/s-2007-1006775.

19. Sieg P, Hakim SG, Bierwolf S, Hermes D. Subcutaneous fat layer in different donor regions used for harvesting microvascular soft tissue flaps in slender and adipose patients. Int J Oral Maxillofac Surg. 2003;32(5):544–7.

20. Reinert S. The free revascularized lateral upper arm flap in maxillofacial reconstruction following ablative tumour surgery. J Craniomaxillofac Surg. 2000;28(2):69–73. doi:10.1054/jcms.2000.0118.

21. Gellrich NC, Schramm A, Hara I, Gutwald R, Duker J, Schmelzeisen R. Versatility and donor site morbidity of the lateral upper arm flap in intraoral reconstruction. Otolaryngol Head Neck Surg. 2001;124(5):549–55. doi:10.1067/mhn.2001.115522.

22. Depner C, Erba P, Rieger UM, Iten F, Schaefer DJ, Haug M. Donor-site morbidity of the sensate extended lateral arm flap. J Reconstr Microsurg. 2012;28(2):133–8. doi:10.1055/s-0031-1289165.

23. Yu AX, Chen ZG, Yu GR. Applied anatomy of distal humerus pe-riosteo-cutaneous flap pedicled with collater-alis radialis vessels. Chin J Exp Surg. 1995;12(6):368-9.

28

Assessing the effect of multibracket appliance treatment on tooth color by using electronic measurement

Anja Ratzmann[1*], Christan Schwahn[2], Anja Treichel[3], Andreas Faltermeier[4] and Alexander Welk[5]

Abstract

Background: The purpose of this study was to investigate how tooth color is affected by multibracket appliance (MBA) treatment.

Methods: The color of teeth #14 to #24 of 15 patients with MBA was measured on body and gingival tooth segments using the spectrophotometer Shade Inspector™. Colors of both segments were recorded before start of MBA treatment (baseline T_0), end of MBA treatment (T_1; 2 years ±0.3), and 3 months after T_1 (T_2). A 2D color system and a 3D system served as reference systems.
Multilevel models were used to analyze color change within segments and to compare the difference in color change between segments (treatment effect).

Results: 2D system. Changes within tooth segments from T_0 to T_2 were at worst 2.0 units (ΔE in the gingival segment), which is less than the threshold of 2.7 units for a clinically meaningful difference. Confidence intervals for the treatment effect indicated no clinically important differences in color change between body and gingival segments.
3D system. Changes within tooth segments from T_0 to T_2 were at worst 2.3 units (ΔE in the body segment), which is less than the threshold of 2.7 units for a clinically meaningful difference. Confidence intervals for the treatment effect indicated no clinically important differences in color change between body and gingival segments.
Thus, MBA treatment did not lead to clinically relevant changes in tooth color.

Conclusion: Within the limitation of this study the MBA treatment can be seen as a safe method with respect to tooth color.

Background

Changes in tooth color may be caused by several factors, for instance, by extrinsic (external) and intrinsic (internal) discolorations, or by aging [1]. Further causes of color changes are dental treatments, including bleaching or restorative therapy [2]. In addition, tooth color can be changed by the acid-etching process used for bonding orthodontic brackets [3]. Formation of white spots and irreversible penetration of resin tags that remain in the enamel as the two main causes have been reported [4–7]. Therefore, multibracket treatment (MBA) may be

associated with enamel discoloration due to changes in the enamel by tooth cleaning, enamel conditioning procedures (etching), and the debonding and subsequent polishing processes [8, 9].

Association between tooth color changes due to bonding and debonding procedure and multibracket treatment (MBA) is discussed controversial. Some studies [4, 10, 11] have shown that enamel color variables were significantly affected by bonding and debonding procedures, other investigations [3, 12–14] did not find clinically important influence of this procedures on the enamel discolorations.

The purpose of this in vivo study was to investigate how tooth color is affected by multibracket appliance (MBA) treatment, especially whether: (1) the change in tooth color during MBA treatment is clinically important; (2) the color change differs by bracket (body) and

---
* Correspondence: anja.ratzmann@uni-greifswald.de
[1]Department of Orthodontics and Department of Dental Propaedeutics/Community Dentistry, Dental School, University Medicine, Walther-Rathenau Straße 42a, 17475 Greifswald, Germany
Full list of author information is available at the end of the article

non-bracket (gingival) tooth segments; and (3) the change is substantially the same for the conventionally used 2D system and the scientifically favorable 3D system.

Methods
Subjects and clinical examination procedure
All subjects expecting MBA treatment were regular patients of the orthodontic department and participated on a voluntary basis. All measurements were performed during regular visits. All procedures performed in this study were in accordance with the ethical standards of the institutional research committee Ärztekammer Mecklenburg-Vorpommern (Reg. Nr.III UV 15/08). Informed consent was obtained from the patients and parents before start of the study. Initially, 26 patients were included. The inclusion criteria were good oral hygiene, non-carious and restoration-free permanent teeth, and

no white spots. The multibracket appliances had been present in situ for 2.0 (SD $\pm$ 0.3) years (individual study period of each patient). The entire period of study data collection lasted from 2005 to 2009. Time points of measurements were start of MBA treatment (baseline - T_0), end of MBA treatment (2 years SD $\pm$ 0.3 - T_1), and 3-month after end of MBA treatment (T_2) (Fig. 1). The complete clinical procedure was performed by an experienced orthodontist under standardized conditions (color neutral such as same room and light conditions, patient was covered by a drape, tooth surfaces were always saliva-wet) according to the standardized bonding protocol of the orthodontic department. Enamel was etched with 35% orthoposphoric acid (Scotchbond, 3 M Unitek) for 10 s, rinsed with air-water spray for 20 s and dried for 10 s. Transbond XT™ Ligth Cure Primer (3 M, Unitek) was used in conjunction with Transbond XT™ Ligth Cure Adhesive (3 M Unitek) according to the manufacturer's

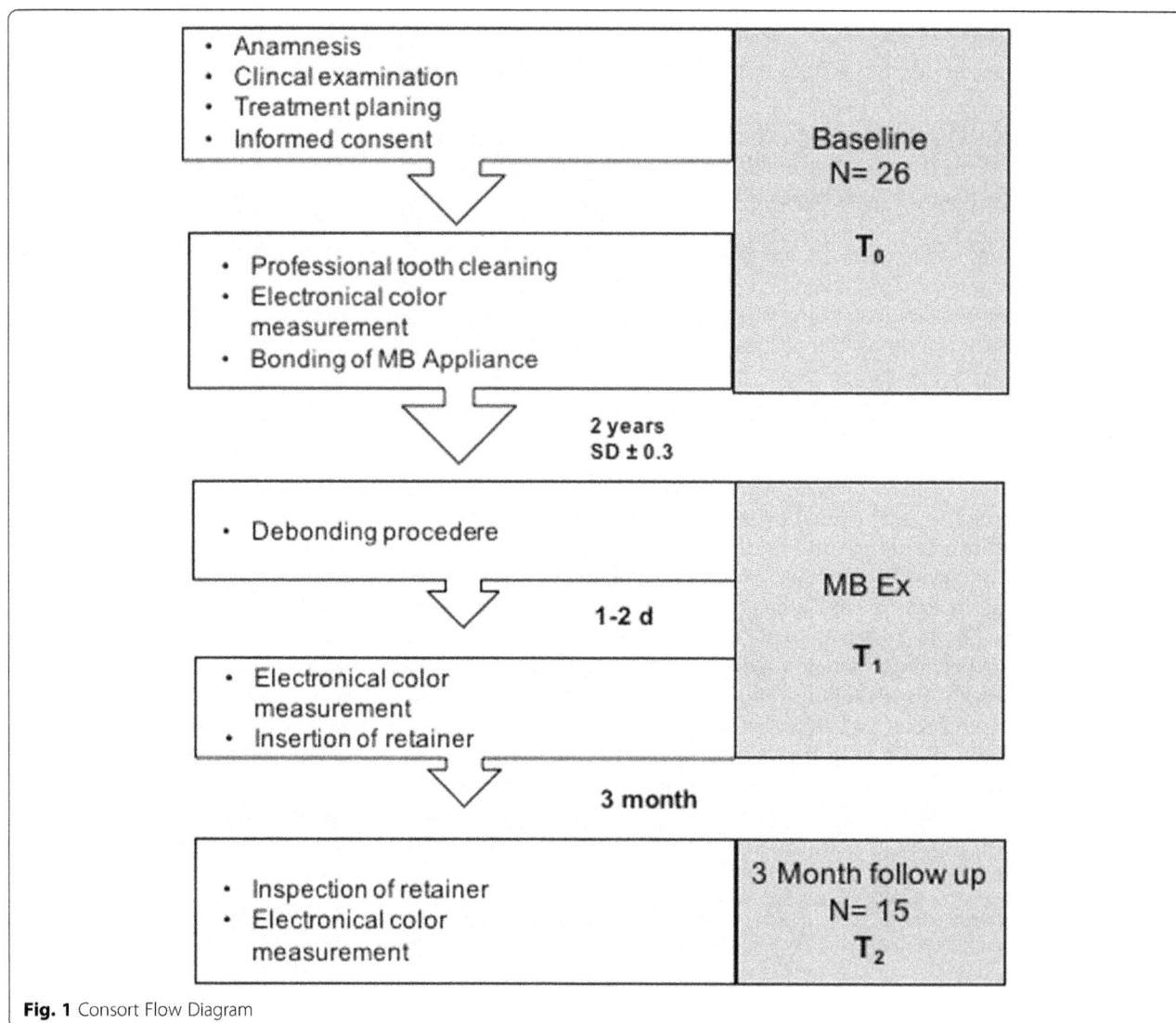

Fig. 1 Consort Flow Diagram

instructions for bonding Mini-Mono – .022 Roth Technique Stainless Steel Brackets (Forestadent, Germany). After that the bracket was pressed firmly on the enamel surface and the excess adhesive resin was removed with a probe. Light curing was performed with LED source Starlight Pro (Mectron, Germany) for 10 s. For study purposes, the protocol was slightly modified by the additional advice "avoiding etching of the gingival segment". Each tooth was categorized into the gingival (S_1), the body (S_2), and the incisal (S_3) segment (Fig. 2). For standardization of the measurements, we used the facial axis point (FA point) for placing the bracket determined with a Dental Bracket Placement Gauge accordingly the MBT™-technique for the middle segment S_2 and for gingival segment S_1 we placed the tip of the measuring probe perpendicularly 1 mm above of the middle point of the gingival line of the corresponding tooth (Fig. 3). The probe was moved slightly around the defined measurement points measuring automatically four times giving an overall value of these measurements at the end. The incisal segment S_3 was not included into analysis because of its transparency. All measurements were performed by a calibrated examiner from a pilot study [15].

During the entire study period we lost 11 patients. Drop out reasons were lack of oral hygiene with breakup of fixed orthodontic treatment, move, repeated schedule failure and withdrawal of informed consent.

Electronic color measurement

Tooth color was measured electronically with the spectrophotometer Shade Inspector™ (Schuetz Dental, Rosbach, Germany- presently not available). The tooth color measuring device operates independently of light on the principle of spectral photometry. For color determination, the color data of the test specimen are compared with manufacturer-furnished color

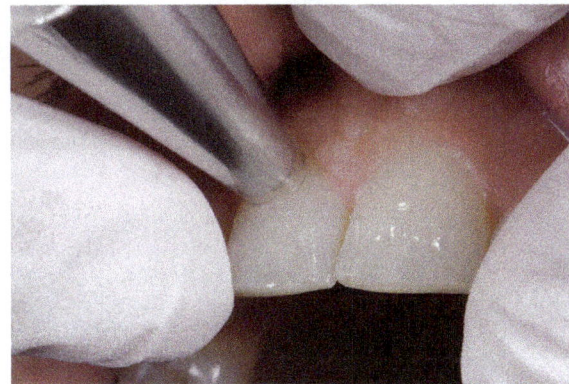

Fig. 3 Shade Inspector™ - Measurement of the gingival segment (S_1)

rings. The tested spectrophotometer is calibrated with a factory-provided selection of industrially fabricated color reference scale VITAPAN Classical® and VITA 3D-Master® by the company (*Schuetz Dental, Rosbach, Germany*). In the present study, the color references VITAPAN Classical® and VITA SYSTEM 3D-Master® were selected from the device software. The *VITAPAN® Classical* Color System has a two-dimensional structure that enables the description of *hue* (category A to D) and *lightness* including *chroma* (group 1 to 4) [16, 17]. It serves as standard shade guide for visual color assessment in dental praxis. The *VITA 3D-Master®* Color System has a three-dimensional structure that enables the separate description of *lightness* (1 to 5 and 0 for bleaching), *chroma* (1 to 3, including half points), and *hue* (M, L, R) [18]. It was developed to obtain a method for systematic and ordered color determination and a better hit rate. The examiners were provided with device operating instructions to ensure observance of the manufacturer's specifications and calibrated in a pilot study [15]. Within a 1 mm measurement range diameter, the probe measures 26 standard colors and three bleaching colors from the VITA 3D–Master® color ring as well as 16 standard colors and 48 intermediate colors (calculated) from the VITA Classical® color ring. The measuring probe was protected by a detachable hygiene cap. During the measurements the probe was placed vertically to the tooth surface (Fig. 3).

Statistical methods

As the 3D-system (*VITA 3D-Master*) is "a more ordered shade guide" than the 2D-system (*VITAPAN® Classical*) [16], we considered the 3D-system as the primary outcome [19, 20].

Besides *lightness* and *chroma*, we analyzed color distributions in terms of L^* (CIE lightness) and C^*_{ab} (CIE chroma) after having assigned *VITA 3D-Master®* shades to values given in Table 1 in Ahn et al. [21] via data

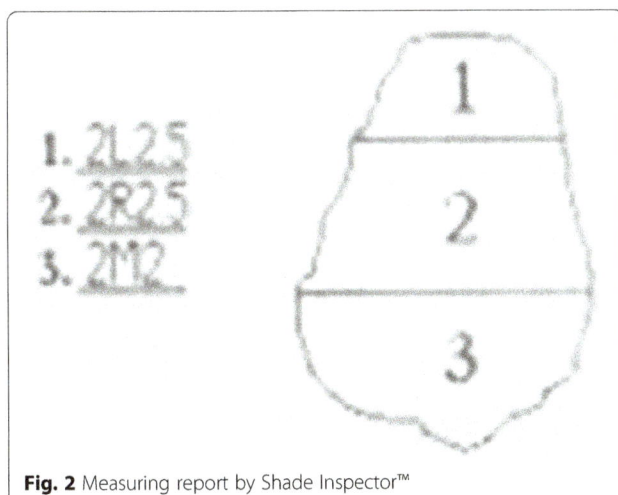

Fig. 2 Measuring report by Shade Inspector™

Table 1 Description of color distributions on tooth level ($n = 120$)

	Time point	Gingival (S_1)			Body (S_2)			P value
		Mean	Gmd	Median (1st – 3rd quartile)	Mean	Gmd	Median (1st – 3rd quartile)	
3D system								
Lightness[a]	T_0	1.93	0.72	2 (1–2)	1.84	0.75	2 (1–2)	0.170
	T_1	2.02	0.83	2 (2–2)	1.96	0.94	2 (1–2)	
	T_2	2.06	0.73	2 (2–2)	1.98	0.73	2 (2–2)	
Chroma[b]	T_0	2.45	0.40	2.5 (2.0–2.5)	2.38	0.35	2.5 (2.0–2.5)	0.018
	T_1	2.48	0.39	2.5 (2.0–2.5)	2.39	0.38	2.5 (2.0–2.5)	
	T_2	2.54	0.39	2.5 (2.5–3.0)	2.48	0.39	2.5 (2.0–2.5)	
L^*	T_0	61.8	2.6	61.7 (61.3–65.0)	62.0	2.7	61.8 (61.3–65.0)	0.388
	T_1	61.5	3.0	61.6 (61.3–61.8)	61.6	3.3	61.6 (61.3–65.0)	
	T_2	61.4	2.5	61.6 (61.3–61.8)	61.6	2.5	61.6 (61.3–61.8)	
C^*_{ab}	T_0	12.1	2.1	11.8 (8.7–14.3)	11.7	2.6	11.8 (8.7–13.5)	0.042
	T_1	12.3	2.0	13.5 (10.1–14.3)	11.9	2.1	12.6 (8.7–14.3)	
	T_2	12.7	1.7	13.5 (11.8–14.3)	12.2	1.9	11.8 (10.1–14.3)	
ΔE	$T_0 - T_1$	2.10	2.57	0.90 (0.00–4.22)	2.46	2.82	1.88 (0.00–4.42)	
	$T_1 - T_2$	2.15	2.54	1.88 (0.00–4.36)	2.35	2.50	1.88 (0.00–4.36)	
	$T_0 - T_2$	1.80	2.21	0.90 (0.00–3.48)	1.86	2.17	1.01 (0.00–3.60)	
d(OM1)	T_0	13.9	3.8	13.7 (9.2–15.8)	13.5	3.9	13.7 (9.2–15.4)	0.038
	T_1	14.3	4.1	15.3 (12.5–15.8)	13.9	4.5	15.3 (9.2–15.8)	
	T_2	14.6	3.7	15.3 (13.7–15.8)	14.1	3.8	14.5 (12.5–15.8)	
2D system[c]								
L^*	T_0	58.1	2.1	58.4 (56.8–59.7)	58.4	2.1	58.4 (57.1–59.7)	0.004
	T_1	57.8	2.4	58.4 (55.8–59.7)	58.1	2.4	58.4 (57.1–59.7)	
	T_2	57.7	2.3	57.1 (55.8–59.7)	58.1	2.0	58.4 (57.1–59.7)	
C^*_{ab}	T_0	12.4	2.1	12.3 (11.0–13.6)	12.2	2.1	12.3 (11.0–13.6)	0.031
	T_1	12.7	2.4	12.3 (11.0–14.9)	12.4	2.6	12.3 (11.0–13.6)	
	T_2	12.9	2.0	13.6 (11.0–14.9)	12.5	2.3	12.3 (11.0–13.6)	
ΔE	$T_0 - T_1$	1.63	1.79	1.81 (0.00–1.87)	1.74	1.78	1.87 (0.00–1.87)	
	$T_1 - T_2$	1.45	1.65	1.81 (0.00–1.87)	1.65	1.80	1.87 (0.00–1.91)	
	$T_0 - T_2$	1.61	1.62	1.87 (0.00–1.87)	1.39	1.42	1.84 (0.00–1.87)	

[a]3D lightness values were assessed on a six-point integer scale from 0 to 5
[b]3D chroma values were assessed on a three-point scale from 1 to 3 at half points
[c]2D second shade designation numbers were assessed on a five-point scale at quarter points
Gmd denotes Gini's mean difference (see statistical methods)

analysis syntax. Additionally to L^*, values for a^* and b^* were calculated from values of C^*_{ab} and h degrees as given in Ahn et al. and were then used to calculate ΔE (defined [22] [as square root of $[(\Delta L^*)^2 + (\Delta a^*)^2 + (\Delta b^*)^2]$]). For example, the change from 1 M2 to 2 L2.5 was calculated in two steps. First, a^* and b^* values were calculated ($a^*_{1M2} = 8.7^*\cos(89.4^*2^*\pi/360) = 0.09$; $b^*_{1M2} = 8.7^*\sin(89.4^*2^*\pi/360)$); then the square root of $[(65.0-61.3)^2 + (0.09-0.82)^2 + (8.70-13.5)^2] = 6.1$ was calculated, which can also be found in Table III in Ahn et al. [21]. Because ΔE is restricted to non-negative values, we computed the distance of

each shade to 0 M1 additionally, denoted by d(0 M1). A positive change in d(0 M1) indicates a darker or stronger color; a negative change indicates a lighter or purer color.

In the 2D-system, the shade group B is ordered by C^*_{ab} (CIE chroma), but not by L^* (CIE lightness); for the latter B2 > B1 > B4 > B3) [16]. Therefore, we analyzed color distributions only in terms of L^*, C^*_{ab}, and ΔE after having assigned *VITAPAN® Classical* shades to values given in the D_{65} columns of Table I in *Park* et al. [16] as described for the 3D system. Because the second shade designation numbers of the

2D-system were assessed on a five-point scale at quarter points, extrapolation to five and interpolation to quarter points were applied.

In the 2D-system, the shade group B is ordered by C^*_{ab} (CIE chroma), but not by L^* (CIE lightness); for the latter B2 > B1 > B4 > B3) [16]. Therefore, we analyzed color distributions only in terms of L^*, C^*_{ab}, and ΔE after having assigned *VITAPAN® Classical* shades to values given in the D_{65} columns of Table I in *Park* et al. [16] as described for the 3D system. Because the second shade designation numbers of the 2D-system were assessed on a five-point scale at quarter points, extrapolation to five and interpolation to quarter points were applied.

As the *American Statistical Association* [23] recommends to avoid over-reliance on *p*-values, we estimated and interpreted confidence intervals [24]. Treatment effects were corrected for tooth level and subject level by using multilevel modeling [25], and adjusted for tooth type and quadrant. The group difference in change from baseline was calculated in order to estimate treatment effects. Originally, a difference in shade ≥3.7 CIELAB units had been prespecified as clinically meaningful both for changes within groups and treatment effects [16] which was revised to ≥2.7 [26]. The treatment group difference in change (change in S_1 versus change in S_2) was estimated by linear multilevel models with Kenward-Roger correction for small samples [27] via the procedure "mixed" by Stata software, release 14.2 (Stata Corporation, College Station, TX, USA); changes within groups were computed afterwards using the command "margin". The relative treatment effect of the difference in change was estimated by ordinal logistic multilevel models via Stata's procedure "meologit". Odds ratios in the ordinal logistic regression can be interpreted as those in the binary logistic regression whatever the cutoff point of the ordinal outcome is [28]. Box plots and descriptive statistics, including quantiles and Gini's mean difference (Gmd) as a robust measure of dispersion [28], were generated using R, release 3.3.3 (R Core Team (2017). R: A Language and Environment for Statistical Computing. R Foundation for Statistical Computing. Vienna, Austria. https://www.r-project.org), especially the "ggplot2" package [29].

Results
Subjects, teeth, and observations
The initial study sample consisted of 26 consecutive patients. Eleven patients were excluded from the study for different reasons, including lack of oral hygiene, decalcification, or relocation. The multibracket appliances had been present in situ for 2.0 years (SD ± 0.3). At the end of MBA treatment, data for tooth color of 120 teeth of the upper jaw (#14 to #24) of 12 female and 3 males were available, resulting in a total of 720 observations

for each color system (120 teeth, 2 tooth segments, 3 time points). All patients were Caucasian, aged 11 to 18 years.

Measurements results
2D-system
At baseline, 13 different shades were measured (Fig. 4a). Five shades with a frequency greater than 30 occurred: B2, B2.25, B2.5, B2.75 and B3 (Fig. 4a). Coordinates (CIE L^*, a^*, b^*) of quarter points for the second shade designation number were interpolated to (61.0, 59.7, 58.4, 57.1, and 55.8) for L^* of B2, B2.25, B2.5, B2.75 and B3, respectively, and to (9.8, 11.1, 12.4, 13.6, and 14.9) for C^*_{ab} of B2, B2.25, B2.5, B2.75 and B3, respectively (Fig. 5). Note that B2.25, B2.5, and B2.75 lie in a space not well covered by the 3D-system (Fig. 5). Gingival segments were darker (L^*) and stronger (C^*_{ab}) than body segments ($P = 0.004$ and $P = 0.031$, respectively; Table 1).

Changes within segments S_1 and S_2 from baseline to 3 months after MBA treatment ($T_0 - T_2$) were at worst $1.97 \approx 2.0$ units (ΔE for gingival segment; Table 2), which is less than the threshold of 2.7 units for a clinical meaningful difference (Fig. 6a). Moreover, confidence intervals for the treatment effects in terms of the difference in change indicated no clinically important differences between body and gingival segments (Table 2).

3D-system
At baseline, 13 different shades were measured (Fig. 4b). Four shades with a frequency greater than 30 occurred: 1 M2, 2 L2.5, 2 M3, and 3R2.5 (Fig. 4b). Note that shades 2 L2.5, 2 M3, and 3R2.5 limit a space that is not well covered by the 3D system (Fig. 5; 3R2.5 is nearest neighbor of 3 L2.5). *Chroma* of gingival segments was stronger than that of body segments ($P = 0.018$; Table 1); differences in *lightness* were uncertain ($P = 0.17$; Table 1).

Changes within segments S_1 and S_2 from baseline to 3 months after MBA treatment ($T_0 - T_2$) were at worst $2.28 \approx 2.3$ units (ΔE for body segment; Table 2), which is less than the threshold of 2.7 units for a clinical meaningful difference. Figs. 6b and 7 illustrate that ΔE is prone to information bias (measurement error). The value of $\Delta E = 9.9$ for $T_0 - T_1$ and $T_1 - T_2$ at the gingival segment as shown in Fig. 6b resulted from a change from 1 M2 to 3 L2.5 and back to 1 M2 for T_0, T_1, and T_2, respectively. This change is more appropriately described in terms of d(0 M1): Values of 9.2, 19.0, and 9.2 for T_0, T_1, and T_2, respectively, correspond to a change in d(0 M1) of 9.8, and – 9.8 for $T_0 - T_1$ and $T_1 - T_2$, respectively, because d(0 M1) allows negative values to describe purer or lighter changes. Moreover, confidence intervals for the treatment effects in terms of the difference in change indicated no clinically important differences between body and gingival segments (Table 2).

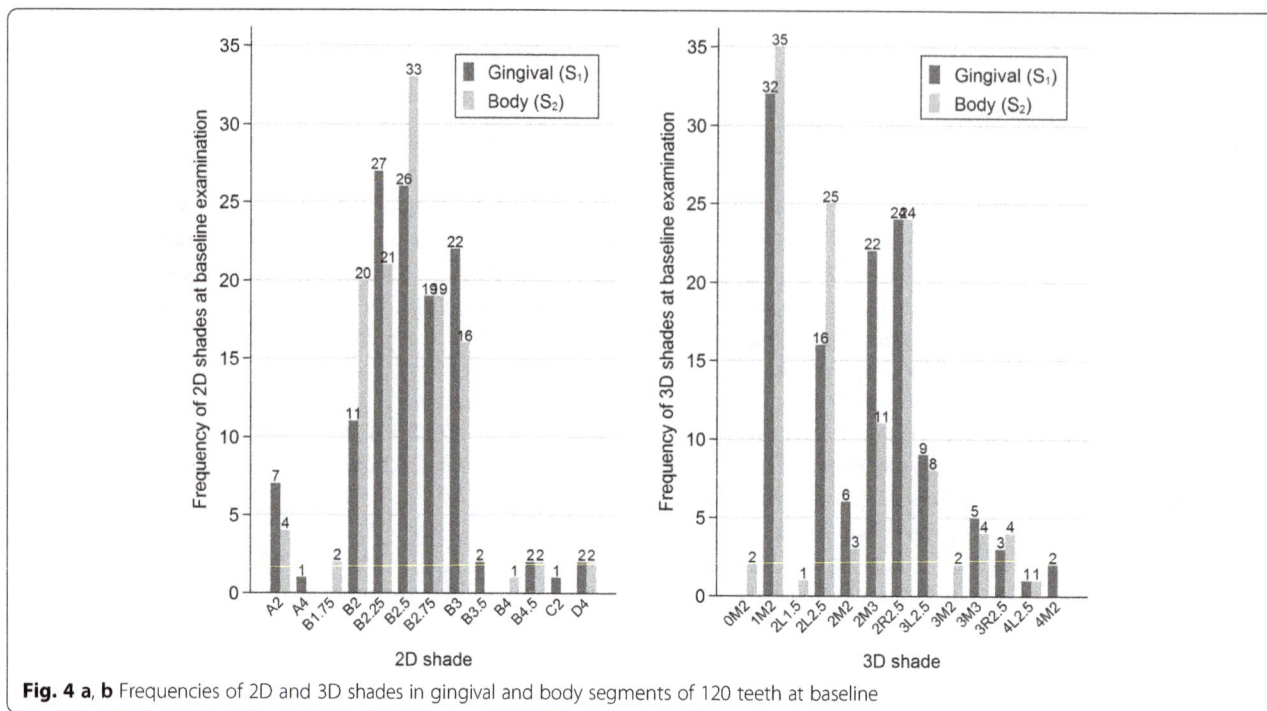

Fig. 4 a, b Frequencies of 2D and 3D shades in gingival and body segments of 120 teeth at baseline

Discussion

During MBA treatment, color changes in bracket (body) and non-bracket (gingival) tooth segments were not clinically relevant. Moreover, body and gingival tooth segments differed in change in tooth color only slightly and possibly by zero. The extent of change in color depended on color metrics (2D, 3D); nevertheless, our findings using different color metrics were sufficiently robust insofar as color change during MBA treatment was not clinically relevant, even if using small thresholds down to 2.3 units for a clinically relevant difference (ΔE).

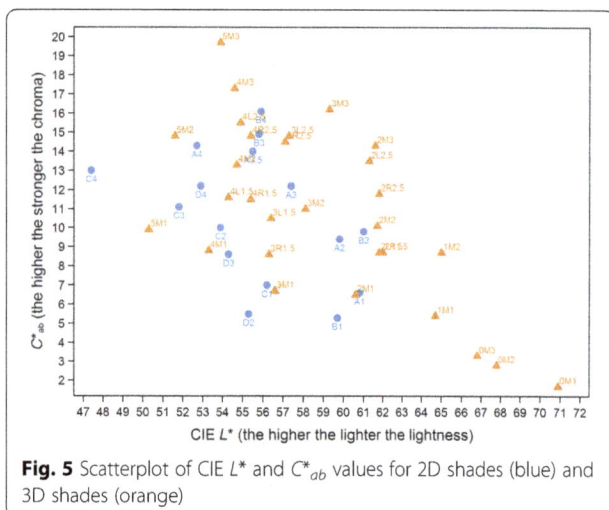

Fig. 5 Scatterplot of CIE L* and C*$_{ab}$ values for 2D shades (blue) and 3D shades (orange)

Methods of the study

In this study, we preferred electronical measurements instead of visual measurements for several reasons. First, it was assumed that problems due to the regression to the mean [30] which is "one of the most important of all phenomena regarding data and estimation" [31] could not have been substantially reduced by repeated visual measurements; the judger will be biased after the first measurement. Second, we aimed to use measurements of two systems (2D and 3D) for which judgers would have introduced bias regarding the second measurement. Third, four measurements as used internally by the electronic device to compute the overall value increased the reliability according to the Spearman-Brown formula. Fourth, by using quarter points, electronic 2D measurements could have been more accurate than visual 2D measurements. Finally, it could be expected that our adolescent patient group (11–18 years) was homogeneous concerning tooth colors, especially in terms of B color shades of the 2D system. Therefore, it could be assumed that a systematic measurement error will be substantially the same in this highly homogeneous group – an assumption which would not be justified in a sample with a wide age range (and more frequent color shades different from B of the 2D system). This is a crucial point because in presence of a constant systematic measurement error the validity of the measurement of change will not be threatened. In short, we looked for a trade-off between reliability and validity issues, including regression to the mean.

Table 2 Treatment effects in terms of the difference in change using linear multilevel models to account for 15 subjects and 120 teeth, and relative treatment effects of the change in terms of the odds ratio of the body segment referred to the gingival segment using ordinal multilevel models

| | | Linear multilevel model (mixed model) | | | | Ordinal multilevel model | |
| | | Change within gingival segment (S_1) | Change within body segment (S_2) | Treatment effect (difference in change) | | Relative treatment effect | |
	Time points	(95% CI)	Change (95% CI)	Coefficient (95% CI)	P value	Odds ratio (95% CI)	P value
3D system							
Lightness	$T_0 - T_1$	0.09 (−0.10–0.28)	0.12 (−0.07–0.31)	0.025 (−0.11–0.16)	0.716	1.08 (0.62–1.90)	0.780
Lightness	$T_1 - T_2$	0.04 (−0.15–0.23)	0.02 (−0.17–0.22)	−0.017 (−0.15–0.12)	0.807	0.95 (0.54–1.66)	0.860
Lightness	$T_0 - T_2$	0.13 (0.02–0.25)	0.14 (0.02–0.26)	0.008 (−0.11–0.12)	0.885	1.05 (0.57–1.94)	0.870
Chroma	$T_0 - T_1$	0.03 (−0.05–0.11)	0.01 (−0.07–0.09)	−0.017 (−0.09–0.06)	0.668	0.87 (0.51–1.49)	0.608
Chroma	$T_1 - T_2$	0.07 (−0.01–0.15)	0.08 (0.004–0.16)	0.017 (−0.06–0.09)	0.648	1.16 (0.68–1.98)	0.587
Chroma	$T_0 - T_2$	0.10 (0.01–0.19)	0.10 (0.01–0.19)	0.000 (−0.7–0.07)	1.000	0.97 (0.56–1.69)	0.911
L^*	$T_0 - T_1$	0.34 (−0.27–0.94)	0.40 (−0.20–1.00)	0.066 (−0.41–0.54)	0.786	1.04 (0.65–1.66)	0.879
L^*	$T_1 - T_2$	0.03 (−0.65–0.70)	−0.004 (−0.68–0.67)	−0.033 (−0.51–0.44)	0.889	0.83 (0.52–1.33)	0.436
L^*	$T_0 - T_2$	0.37 (−0.001–0.73)	0.40 (0.03–0.77)	0.032 (−0.37–0.43)	0.873	0.92 (0.57–1.47)	0.726
C^*_{ab}	$T_0 - T_1$	0.19 (−0.43–0.81)	0.18 (−0.44–0.80)	−0.008 (−0.48–0.47)	0.972	1.06 (0.66–1.69)	0.809
C^*_{ab}	$T_1 - T_2$	0.42 (−0.13–0.96)	0.29 (−0.26–0.83)	−0.129 (−0.55–0.29)	0.543	0.85 (0.53–1.36)	0.498
C^*_{ab}	$T_0 - T_2$	0.61 (0.19–1.03)	0.47 (0.05–0.89)	−0.138 (−0.51–0.23)	0.464	0.78 (0.49–1.25)	0.302
ΔE	$T_0 - T_1$	2.10 (1.50–2.69)	2.46 (1.86–3.05)	0.360 (−0.16–0.89)	0.176	1.43 (0.88–2.33)	0.154
ΔE	$T_1 - T_2$	2.15 (1.64–2.66)	2.35 (1.84–2.86)	0.197 (−0.33–0.72)	0.460	1.23 (0.77–1.97)	0.392
ΔE	$T_0 - T_2$	1.80 (1.39–2.22)	1.86 (1.45–2.28)	0.062 (−0.37–0.49)	0.777	1.11 (0.68–1.81)	0.688
d(OM1)	$T_0 - T_1$	0.38 (−0.46–1.22)	0.42 (−0.41–1.26)	0.043 (−0.56–0.65)	0.889	1.01 (0.63–1.61)	0.979
d(OM1)	$T_1 - T_2$	0.32 (−0.48–1.12)	0.21 (−0.59–1.01)	−0.11 (−0.66–0.44)	0.691	0.92 (0.58–1.47)	0.739
d(OM1)	$T_0 - T_2$	0.70 (0.22–1.18)	0.63 (0.15–1.11)	−0.068 (−0.55–0.41)	0.781	0.96 (0.60–1.54)	0.882
2D system							
L^*	$T_0 - T_1$	0.31 (−0.17–0.80)	0.30 (−0.19–0.78)	−0.016 (−0.35–0.32)	0.926	1.01 (0.63–1.60)	0.975
L^*	$T_1 - T_2$	0.06 (−0.37–0.50)	0.05 (−0.39–0.49)	−0.012 (−0.31–0.29)	0.936	0.91 (0.57–1.46)	0.704
L^*	$T_0 - T_2$	0.38 (−0.03–0.78)	0.33 (−0.06–0.75)	−0.028 (−0.31–0.26)	0.847	0.93 (0.58–1.48)	0.748
C^*_{ab}	$T_0 - T_1$	0.23 (−0.29–0.75)	0.17 (−0.35–0.69)	−0.053 (−0.36–0.26)	0.738	0.84 (0.53–1.33)	0.449
C^*_{ab}	$T_1 - T_2$	0.20 (−0.25–0.66)	0.17 (−0.28–0.62)	−0.034 (−0.31–0.24)	0.805	0.90 (0.56–1.44)	0.668
C^*_{ab}	$T_0 - T_2$	0.43 (0.05–0.82)	0.34 (−0.04–0.73)	−0.087 (−0.33–0.15)	0.471	0.77 (0.49–1.23)	0.279
ΔE	$T_0 - T_1$	1.63 (1.17–2.10)	1.74 (1.28–2.21)	0.111 (−0.26–0.48)	0.552	1.33 (0.83–2.14)	0.239
ΔE	$T_1 - T_2$	1.45 (1.03–1.87)	1.65 (1.22–2.07)	0.199 (−0.16–0.56)	0.271	1.32 (0.82–2.13)	0.260
ΔE	$T_0 - T_2$	1.61 (1.24–1.97)	1.39 (1.03–1.76)	−0.214 (−0.51–0.08)	0.155	0.80 (0.49–1.28)	0.346

Nevertheless, there are some limitations concerning the electronical measurement methods, including light condition, calibration of the measurement device, reproducibility of the measurements, and visual threshold discussed in the literature [32]. The spectrophotometer Shade Inspector™ was used in our study, because of its good results regarding reproducibility of lightness and chroma found in pilot studies [15, 33]. Other studies, investigating dental color measuring devices did show reliable results as well [34–38].

The Shade Inspector™ is calibrated with a factory-provided selection of industrially fabricated color reference scale (VITAPAN® Classical and VITA 3D-Master®). These color scales originating of different batches were read in and the measurements averaged. Therefore, variations in measurements due to the calibration process are conceivably [39]. The study of Kohlmeyer and Scheller evaluating VITAPAN® Classical color scale samples, revealed that the individual color scale samples failed to invariably correspond to the respective primary color [40]. In addition, unequivocal findings

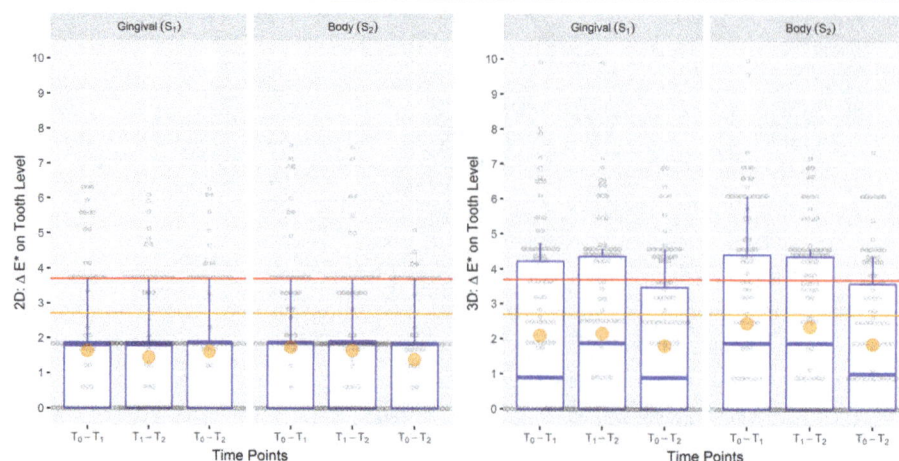

Fig. 6 a, b Box plots showing the distribution of ΔE for the 2D-system (**a**; left) and the 3D-system (**b**; right) on tooth level. Orange circle: mean; bold line: median; box: interquartile range (between 25 and 75%); whiskers: range between 12.5 and 87.5%; grey dots figure the 120 observations; red line: clinically important difference at 3.7 units or 2.7 units

were reported on color consistency alongst shade guides from the same manufacturer [41, 42]. One in vitro study found that repeatability and accuracy of a dental color measuring instrument (ShadeScan) was influenced by shade guide systems used for testing [43]. In our study, the complete clinical procedure was performed by an experienced orthodontist under standardized conditions (color neutral such as same room, same dental unit and same light conditions by dental unit lamp, patient was covered by a drape, tooth surfaces were always saliva-wet). The electronical measurements were performed by a calibrated examiner [15] in a pilot study. The tooth color measuring device itself operates independently of light on the principle of spectral photometry. However, in a study, evaluating the effect of different illuminants (natural daylight, dental unit lamp, and daylight lamp), the matching repeatability of 2 intraoral spectrophotometers was not completely satisfactory for clinical practice [44]. Therefore, our measurements were taken under standardized conditions as described before. Thus, we do not assume relevant effects by the surrounding light conditions.

Our study has methodological strengths. Notably, two measurements (2D, 3D) at each time point were used, thereby reducing problems due to regression to the mean, which is here the tendency of tooth segment's colors at the extremes to have less extreme values on subsequent measurements [30]. To reduce the influence of extreme values at the first measurement, it is common to discard the first of three blood pressure measurements of the same examination [45] or to measure the periodontium by the Florida probe thrice given disagreement in first two measurements. Importantly for interpreting of the analysis of change as done herein, the second measurement was performed by the 3D-system,

which was considered as the primary outcome. Moreover, we used mixed models as a shrinkage approach and "a way of discounting observed variation that accounts for regression to the mean" [31]. Second, the 2D-system measured at quarter points for the second shade designation number. As the 3D-system did not cover the space of the most frequent 2D shades, the 2D-system added essential information, although limited by the regression to the mean. Third, tooth type as a potentially substantial confounder can only be considered in multilevel analysis. Further, it is not possible to address confounding due to tooth type by the study design. Thus, tooth type cannot be subject of randomizing in a MB study; analysis restricted to the subject level can be misleading. Fourth, we presented not only the original codes of the 2D- and 3D-system but also the transformed values based on the CIE system. As B2 > B1 > B4 > B3 on the L^* scale [16], the shade designation numbers of the original 2D codes cannot be well interpreted. Finally, we used not only ΔE to estimate the treatment effect but also the measure d(0 M1) to allow for purer or lighter changes. In terms of L^*, ΔE does not differentiate a lighter change from a darker change given the same ΔE; in terms of C^*_{ab}, ΔE does not differentiate a purer change from a stronger change. The 3D shade 0 M1 as the new origin of the coordinate system enables us to differentiate lighter/purer changes from darker/stronger changes. 0 M1 as the new origin of the 3D-system is justified for its lightest *lightness* and its purest *chroma*, including the purest red (a^*) and the purest yellow (b^*). For the 2D- system, no shade has these properties [16].

Unfortunately, there was no sample size calculation for this study. However, we accounted for subject and tooth level to increase statistical power. Moreover, other

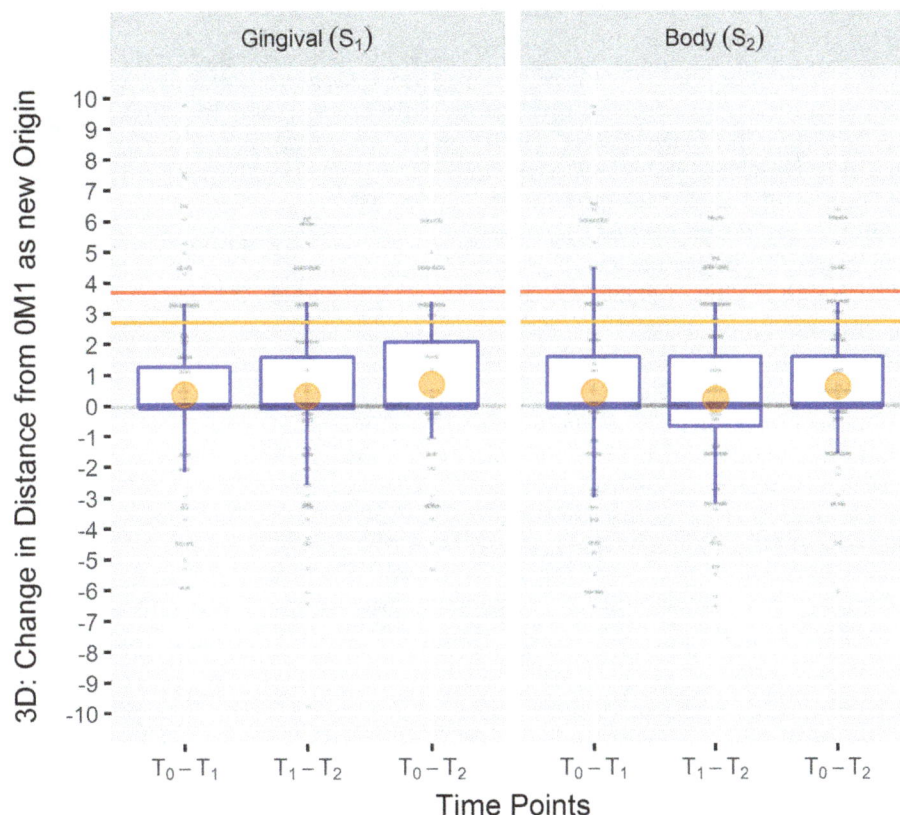

Fig. 7 Box plots showing the distribution of the change in distance from 0 M1 for the 3D system on tooth level. Orange circle: mean; bold line: median; box: interquartile range (between 25 and 75 - 50% of the values); whiskers: range between the 12.5 and 87.5% (75% of the values); grey dots figure the 120 observations; change > 0 indicates darker or stronger colors; change <0 indicates lighter or purer colors; red line: clinically important difference at 3.7 units or 2.7 units

studies included similar numbers of participants [10, 46]. Besides this limitation, it was not sensitive to adjust for baseline values [47–49], because segments could not be randomized to treatment groups. Therefore, we compared the difference in change from baseline between segments [28, 50, 51].

Discussion of results

Confidence intervals for the treatment effect for both color systems indicated no clinically important differences between body and gingival segments. Further, changes from baseline to 3 months after MBA treatment $(T_0 - T_2)$ were at worst 2.3 units for 3D- system and 2.0 units for 2D-system, respectively, which are less than the threshold of 2.7 units for a clinical meaningful difference.

Previous studies [4, 14] have shown that the enamel color variables are affected by orthodontic bonding and debonding procedures due to tooth cleaning [52], enamel conditioning procedures (etching) [53], and enamel scratches [54]. Other effects, such as staining of enamel and resin material used for the bonding brackets, may

also induce color change of teeth during orthodontic treatment. These color change may be the result of demineralization [55], or direct food dye [12, 56]. The staining of the resin material is associated with the color instability of the polymer [57].

Several experimental studies [3, 4, 12–14, 58] investigated the impact of the bonding process on tooth color. Three studies [3, 12, 14] investigating color change after bonding of extracted teeth have not found any indication of a significant influence of the bonding process on tooth color. In another experimental study [13] assessing color changes in bracket areas, significant differences in ΔE were found. Despite the significance of the results, the authors did not consider the color changes visually perceivable for the majority of examiners. *Eliades* et al. [4] reached similar conclusions when examining the influence of different bonding materials. Furthermore, enamel color alterations might also derive from the irreversible penetration of resin into the enamel surface [4]. Moderate evidence exits that shorter resin tags penetration produces less change in enamel color following clean-up procedure and polishing [58]. Self-etching primers produce less resin penetration and these systems produce less iatrogenic color change in enamel following orthodontic treatment [58]. In our study 35%-phosphoric acid was used.

The results of a prospective clinical trial conducted by *Karamouzos* et al. [10] showed significant changes of tooth color (2.1 to 3.6 ΔE units) after orthodontic treatment. The value for the parameter *lightness* (L*) decreased, whereas the values for the parameters a* (value for green-red) and b* (value for blue-yellow) increased. These changes indicated a decrease in tooth *lightness* as well as a change in *hue*, which may be perceptible if a threshold of 1.2 is assumed [26]. In our study, however, we did not find ΔE values greater than 2.7 units, which are considered clinically relevant [26]. Nevertheless, our results are in accordance to a recently published review by *Chen* that there is no strong evidence that orthodontic treatment with fixed appliances alters the original color of enamel [8].

Conclusion
Within the limitation of this study the MBA treatment can be seen as a safe method with respect to tooth color.

Funding
The study was not funded.

Informed consent
Informed consent was obtained from all individual participants and parents included in the study.

Explanation of any issues relating to journal policies
No issues.

Authors' contributions
AR Contributed to data acquisition, design, analysis and interpretation, writing of manuscript. CS Contributed to statistical analysis and interpretation, writing statistical part of manuscript. AT Contributed to data acquisition. AF Critically revised the manuscript. AW Contributed to design, analysis and interpretation, writing of manuscript. All authors gave final approval and agree to be accountable for all aspects of the work. All authors have read and approved the manuscript.

Consent for publication
The authors confirm that the content of the manuscript has not been published or submitted for publication elsewhere.

Competing interests
The authors declare that they have no competing interests.

Author details
[1]Department of Orthodontics and Department of Dental Propaedeutics/Community Dentistry, Dental School, University Medicine, Walther-Rathenau Straße 42a, 17475 Greifswald, Germany. [2]Department of Prosthetic Dentistry, Gerodontology and Biomaterials, University of Greifswald, Fleischmannstraße 42, 17475 Greifswald, Germany. [3]Private Dental Office, Bahnhofstraße 4, 18581 Putbus, Germany. [4]Department of Orthodontics, Dental School, University Medicine, Franz-Josef-Strauß-Allee 11, 93053 Regensburg, Germany. [5]Department of Restorative Dentistry, Periodontology, Endodontology, Preventive and Pediatric Dentistry, Dental School, University Medicine, Walther-Rathenau Straße 42a, 17475 Greifswald, Germany.

References
1. Watts A, Addy M. Tooth discolouration and staining: a review of the literature. Br Dent J. 2001;190:309–16. https://doi.org/10.1038/sj.bdj.4800959a.
2. Burrows S. A review of the safety of tooth bleaching. SADJ. 2010;65(6):8–13.
3. Wriedt S, Keller S, Wehrbein H. The effect of debonding and/or bleaching on enamel color - an in-vitro study. J Orofac Orthop. 2008;69:169–76. https://doi.org/10.1007/s00056-008-0737-2.
4. Eliades T, Kakaboura A, Eliades G, Bradley TG. Comparison of enamel colour changes associated with orthodontic bonding using two different adhesives. Eur J Orthod. 2001;23:85–90.
5. Silverstone LM, Saxton CA, Dogon IL, Fejerskov O. Variation in the pattern of acid etching of human dental enamel examined by scanning electron microscopy. Caries Res. 1975;9:373–87.
6. Baumann DF, Brauchli L, van Waes H. The influence of dental loupes on the quality of adhesive removal in orthodontic debonding. J Orofac Orthop. 2011;72:125–32. https://doi.org/10.1007/s00056-011-0010-y.
7. Ogaard B, Fjeld M. The enamel surface and bonding in orthodontics. Semin Orthod. 2010;16:37–48.
8. Chen Q, Zheng X, Chen W, Ni Z, Zhou Y. Influence of orthodontic treatment with fixed appliances on enamel color: a systematic review. BMC Oral Health. 2015;15:31. https://doi.org/10.1186/s12903-015-0014-x.
9. Janiszewska-Olszowska J, Szatkiewicz T, Tomkowski R, Tandecka K, Grocholewicz K. Effect of orthodontic debonding and adhesive removal on the enamel - current knowledge and future perspectives - a systematic review. Med Sci Monit. 2014;20:1991–2001. https://doi.org/10.12659/MSM.890912.
10. Karamouzos A, Athanasiou AE, Papadopoulos MA, Kolokithas G. Tooth-color assessment after orthodontic treatment: a prospective clinical trial. Am J Orthod Dentofac Orthop. 2010;138(537):e531–8; discussion 537–539. https://doi.org/10.1016/j.ajodo.2010.03.026.
11. Boncuk Y, Cehreli ZC, Polat-Ozsoy O. Effects of different orthodontic adhesives and resin removal techniques on enamel color alteration. Angle Orthod. 2014;84:634–41. https://doi.org/10.2319/060613-433.1.
12. Trakyali G, Ozdemir FI, Arun T. Enamel colour changes at debonding and after finishing procedures using five different adhesives. Eur J Orthod. 2009;31:397–401. https://doi.org/10.1093/ejo/cjp023.
13. Jahanbin A, Ameri H, Khaleghimoghaddam R. Effect of adhesive types on enamel discolouration around orthodontic brackets. Aust Orthod J. 2009;25:19–23.
14. Hintz JK, Bradley TG, Eliades T. Enamel colour changes following whitening with 10 per cent carbamide peroxide: a comparison of orthodontically-bonded/debonded and untreated teeth. Eur J Orthod. 2001;23:411–5.
15. Ratzmann A, Klinke T, Schwahn C, Treichel A, Gedrange T. Reproducibility of electronic tooth colour measurements. Biomed Tech (Berl). 2008;53:259–63. https://doi.org/10.1515/BMT.2008.036.
16. Park JH, Lee YK, Lim BS. Influence of illuminants on the color distribution of shade guides. J Prosthet Dent. 2006;96:402–11. https://doi.org/10.1016/j.prosdent.2006.10.007.
17. Paravina RD. Performance assessment of dental shade guides. J Dent. 2009; 37(Suppl 1):e15–20. https://doi.org/10.1016/j.jdent.2009.02.005.
18. Vita Z. Dental Shade Guides. In J Am Dent Assc. 2002;133:366–7.
19. Cook RJ, Farewell VT. Multiplicity considerations in the design and analysis of clinical trials. J R Stat Soc Ser. 1996;159:93–110. https://doi.org/10.2307/2983471.
20. ICH E9 Expert Working Group. Statistical principles for clinical trials: ICH harmonized tripartite guideline. Stat Med. 1999;18:1905–42.
21. Ahn JS, Lee YK. Color distribution of a shade guide in the value, chroma, and hue scale. J Prosthet Dent. 2008;100:18–28. https://doi.org/10.1016/S0022-3913(08)60129-8.

22. Paravina RD, Powers JM, Fay RM. Color comparison of two shade guides. Int J Prosthodont. 2002;15:73–8.

23. Wasserstein RL, Assoc AS. ASA statement on statistical significance and P-values. Am Stat. 2016;70:131–3. https://doi.org/10.1080/00031305.2016.1154108.

24. Greenland S, Senn SJ, Rothman KJ, Carlin JB, Poole C, Goodman SN, Altman DG. Statistical tests, P values, confidence intervals, and power: a guide to misinterpretations. Eur J Epidemiol. 2016;31:337–50. https://doi.org/10.1007/s10654-016-0149-3.

25. Rabe-Hesketh S, Skrondal A. Multilevel and longitudinal modeling using Stata. 3rd ed. College Station: Stata Press; 2012.

26. Paravina RD, Ghinea R, Herrera LJ, Bona AD, Igiel C, Linninger M, Sakai M, Takahashi H, Tashkandi E, Perez MM. Color difference thresholds in dentistry. J Esthet Restor Dent. 2015;27(Suppl 1):S1–9. https://doi.org/10.1111/jerd.12149.

27. Kenward MG, Roger JH. Small sample inference for fixed effects from restricted maximum likelihood. Biometrics. 1997;53:983–97.

28. Harrell FE Jr. With applications to linear models, logistic and ordinal regression, and survival analysis. In: Regression modeling strategies. 2nd ed. Heidelberg: Springer; 2015. https://doi.org/10.1007/978-3-319-19425-7.

29. Wickham H. Elegant graphics for data analysis. New York: Springer; 2009.

30. Fletcher RH, Fletcher SW, Fletcher GS. Clinical epidemiology: the essentials. 5th ed. Philadelphia: Lippincott Williams & Wilkins; 2014.

31. Harrell FE, Jr., Slaughter JE. Biostatistics for biomedical research. Harell FE ed. pp. 1- 11-22-11: biostat.mc.vanderbilt.edu; 2017. http://www.fharrell.com/. Accessed 25 May 2018.

32. Chu SJ, Trushkowsky RD, Paravina RD. Dental color matching instruments and systems. Review of clinical and research aspects. J Dent 2010;38 Suppl 2:e2–16; doi: https://doi.org/10.1016/j.jdent.2010.07.001.

33. Ratzmann A, Treichel A, Langforth G, Gedrange T, Welk A. Experimental investigations into visual and electronic tooth color measurement. Biomed Tech (Berl). 2011;56:115–22. https://doi.org/10.1515/BMT.2011.008.

34. Ishikawa-Nagai S, Ishibashi K, Tsuruta O, Weber HP. Reproducibility of tooth color gradation using a computer color-matching technique applied to ceramic restorations. J Prosthet Dent. 2005;93:129–37.

35. Da Silva JD, Park SE, Weber HP, Ishikawa-Nagai S. Clinical performance of a newly developed spectrophotometric system on tooth color reproduction. J Prosthet Dent. 2008;99:361–8. https://doi.org/10.1016/S0022-3913(08)60083-9.

36. Dozic A, Kleverlaan CJ, El-Zohairy A, Feilzer AJ, Khashayar G. Performance of five commercially available tooth color-measuring devices. J Prosthodont. 2007;16:93–100. https://doi.org/10.1111/j.1532-849X.2007.00163.x.

37. Kim-Pusateri S, Brewer JD, Davis EL, Wee AG. Reliability and accuracy of four dental shade-matching devices. J Prosthet Dent. 2009;101:193–9. https://doi.org/10.1016/S0022-3913(09)60028-7.

38. Olms C, Setz JM. The repeatability of digital shade measurement--a clinical study. Clin Oral Investig. 2013;17:1161–6. https://doi.org/10.1007/s00784-012-0796-z.

39. Hugo B, Witzel T, Klaiber B. Comparison of in vivo visual and computer-aided tooth shade determination. Clin Oral Investig. 2005;9:244–50. https://doi.org/10.1007/s00784-005-0014-3.

40. Kohlmeyer B, Scheller H. Computerised tooth color determination with measuring device "digital shade guide". Dtsch Zahnarztl Z. 2002;57:172–5.

41. Cal E, Sonugelen M, Guneri P, Kesercioglu A, Kose T. Application of a digital technique in evaluating the reliability of shade guides. J Oral Rehabil. 2004;31:483–91.

42. Tashkandi E. Consistency in color parameters of a commonly used shade guide. Saudi Dent J. 2010;22:7–11. https://doi.org/10.1016/j.sdentj.2009.12.002.

43. Kim-Pusateri S, Brewer JD, Dunford RG, Wee AG. In vitro model to evaluate reliability and accuracy of a dental shade-matching instrument. J Prosthet Dent. 2007;98:353–8. https://doi.org/10.1016/S0022-3913(07)60119-X.

44. Sarafianou A, Kamposiora P, Papavasiliou G, Goula H. Matching repeatability and interdevice agreement of 2 intraoral spectrophotometers. J Prosthet Dent. 2012;107:178–85. https://doi.org/10.1016/S0022-3913(12)60053-5.

45. Friedman LM, Furberg CD, DL DM, Reboussin DM, granger CB. Fundamentals of Clinical Trials. 5th ed. Heidelberg: Springer; 2015.

46. Hammad SM, El Banna M, El Zayat I, Mohsen MA. Effect of resin infiltration on white spot lesions after debonding orthodontic brackets. Am J Dent. 2012;25:3–8.

47. Cologne JB. Re: "when is baseline adjustment useful in analyses of change? An example with education and cognitive change". Am J Epidemiol. 2006;164:1138–9. https://doi.org/10.1093/aje/kwj359.

48. Chen JT, Weuve J, Glymour M, Rehkopf D. Quantifying survivor bias in lifecourse epidemiologic studies. Am J Epidemiol. 2006;163:S69.

49. Glymour MM, Weuve J, Berkman LF, Kawachi I, Robins JM. When is baseline adjustment useful in analyses of change? An example with education and cognitive change. Am J Epidemiol. 2005;162:267–78. https://doi.org/10.1093/Aje/Kwi187.

50. Senn S. Change from baseline and analysis of covariance revisited. Stat Med. 2006;25:4334–44. https://doi.org/10.1002/sim.2682.

51. Harrell FE, Jr.: Statistical Errors in the Medical Literature. 2017; http://www.fharrell.com/post/errmed/#change. Accessed 16 April 2018.

52. Thompson RE, Way DC. Enamel loss due to prophylaxis and multiple bonding/debonding of orthodontic attachments. Am J Orthod. 1981;79:282–95.

53. van Waes H, Matter T, Krejci I. Three-dimensional measurement of enamel loss caused by bonding and debonding of orthodontic brackets. Am J Orthod Dentofac Orthop. 1997;112:666–9.

54. Sandison RM. Tooth surface appearance after debonding. Br J Orthod. 1981;8:199–201.

55. Ogaard B, Rolla G, Arends J. Orthodontic appliances and enamel demineralization. Part 1. Lesion development. Am J Orthod Dentofac Orthop. 1988;94:68–73.

56. Eliades T, Gioka C, Heim M, Eliades G, Makou M. Color stability of orthodontic adhesive resins. Angle Orthod. 2004;74:391–3. https://doi.org/10.1043/0003-3219(2004)074<0391:CSOOAR>2.0.CO;2.

57. Faltermeier A, Rosentritt M, Reicheneder C, Behr M. Discolouration of orthodontic adhesives caused by food dyes and ultraviolet light. Eur J Orthod. 2008;30:89–93. https://doi.org/10.1093/ejo/cjm058.

58. Zaher AR, Abdalla EM, Abdel Motie MA, Rehman NA, Kassem H, Athanasiou AE. Enamel colour changes after debonding using various bonding systems. J Orthod. 2012;39:82–8. https://doi.org/10.1179/1465312512Z.0000000009.

29

Evaluating the biomechanical effects of implant diameter in case of facial trauma to an edentulous atrophic mandible: a 3D finite element analysis

Aysa Ayali[*] 🆔 and Kani Bilginaylar

Abstract

Background: Rehabilitation using an implant supported overdenture with two implants inserted in the interforaminal region is the easiest and currently accepted treatment modality to increase prosthetic stabilization and patient satisfaction in edentulous patients. The insertion of implants to the weakend mandibular bone decreases the strength of the bone and may lead to fractures either during or after implant placement. The aim of this three dimensional finite element analysis (3D FEA) study was to evaluate the biomechanical effects of implant diameter in case of facial trauma (2000 N) to an edentulous atrophic mandible with two implant supported overdenture.

Methods: Three 3D FEA models were simulated; Model 1 (M1) is edentulous atrophic mandible, Model 2 (M2), 3.5x11.5 mm implants were inserted into lateral incisors area of same edentulous atrophic mandible, Model 3 (M3), 4.3x11.5 mm implants were inserted into lateral incisors area of same edentulous atrophic mandible.

Results: In M1 and M2 highest stress levels were observed in condylar neck, whereas highest stress values in M3 were calculated in symphyseal area.

Conclusions: To reduce the risk of bone fracture and to preserve biomechanical behavior of the atrophic mandible from frontal traumatic loads, implants should be inserted monocortically into spongious bone of lateral incisors area.

Keywords: Mandible, Fracture, Dental implant, Overdenture, Finite element analysis

Background

Although dental implant placement has become a usual treatment in recent years, the treatment of patients with atrophic mandible is still challenging. In the moderately or severely resorbed edentulous mandible, rehabilitation using an implant supported overdenture with two implants inserted in the interforaminal region is the easiest treatment modality to increase prosthetic stabilization and patient satisfaction [1, 2]. Such surgical procedures are anticipated, however, complications can be seen such as infection, improper placement, neurosensory injury, bleeding and mandible fracture which has a reported occurrence rate of 0.2%. The rate of incidence seems to be low, but it leads to overwhelming outcomes such as malunion, non-union,

paresthesia, osteomyelitis and prolonged functional and nutritional disturbances [3]. On the other hand, the mandible is the most common broken bone by cause of facial injuries with the ratio of 23–97% [4]. The insertion of implants to the weakend mandibular bone decreases the strength of the bone and may lead to fractures either during or after implant placement [5]. Numerous case reports of fractured athrophic mandible secondary to implant insertion were reported in the literature [3, 6–8].

The principal areas of mandibular fracture are located in the condylar neck, the body or the angle and the symphysis of the mandible. The biomechanical behaviour of the mandible is important to know to understand the mechanism of fractures and to optimize treatment scenarios [9]. Clinically, the pattern of mandible fracture is related to various causes such as intensity and direction of the force, location of the impact point, position of the

---
* Correspondence: aysaayali@hotmail.com
Department of Oral and Maxillofacial Surgery, Near East University, Faculty of Dentistry, Near East Boulevard, Nicosia Cyprus, 99138 Mersin 10, Turkey

mandible at the time of injury, biomechanical properties of the mandible, overlying soft tissue, and the presence of teeth [10]. Although many studies have been reported that focused on these topics, declarations relating to the impacts of implant number, diameter, design, and length on the weakening of the atrophic edontulous mandible are rare and not depend on biomechanical evidence.

The Finite Elemet Analysis (FEA) has now become widely accepted and non-invasive tool that provides valuable results to estimate different parameters of the complex biomechanical behaviour of mandible [11–13].

The aim of this three dimensional finite element analysis (3D FEA) study was to evaluate the biomechanical effects of implant diameter in case of facial trauma to an edentulous atrophic mandible with two implant supported overdenture.

Methods

The three-dimensional models that were used in the current study were prepared with the help of single software to standardize all of the parameters of the models. Models were divided into three groups (Fig 1):

1. Model 1 (M1): Edentulous atrophic mandible (control model) (Fig 1a).
2. Model 2(M2): 3.5 × 11.5 mm Nobel Replace implants (Nobel Biocare USA, Yorba Linda, CA) were placed in the areas of both lateral incisors at a distance of 7 mm from the central point of the arch with the same vertical height level and Locator® attachments (Zest Anchors LLC, CA, USA) were used to connect implants to overdenture prosthesis (Fig 1b).
3. Model 3(M3): 4.3 × 11.5 mm Nobel Replace implants (Nobel Biocare USA, Yorba Linda, CA) were placed in the areas of both lateral incisors at a

distance of 7 mm from the central point of the arch with the same vertical height level and Locator® attachments (Zest Anchors LLC, CA, USA) were used to connect implants to overdenture prosthesis (Fig 1c).

The data obtained from the Visible Human Project® (U.S. National Library of Medicine, Bethesda, MD, USA) were modified with the use of VRMESH (VirtualGrid Inc, Bellevue City, WA, USA) and Rhinoceros 4.0 (McNeel North America, Seattle, WA, USA) software to establish a 3D mandible FEA model to simulate clinical situation of edentulous atrophic mandible.

Mechanical properties of the materials that were simulated were taken from the literature [14–16] and are presented in Table 1. For standardization, the same overdentures were used by assuming that the material properties were the same for both the base part and artificial teeth. The implant-bone interface was considered to be static. The contact area of the overdenture and mucosa was assumed to be frictionless. ALGOR FEMPRO SOFTWARE (ALGOR Inc. Pittsburgh, PA, USA) was used to mesh final models with 3D parabolic tetrahedral solid elements with surface to surface contact. And then a refined mesh was performed in the mandible model to reproduce the compound stress formation observed in bone and implants. Total numbers of nodes and elements are listed in Table 2. Same software was also used to perform static analysis of the models.

The mandibular condyles were fixed in all degrees of freedom. There are several muscles take place to close or elevate the mandible (Fig 1d). These muscles are masseter, temporal, medial and lateral pterygoid muscles. These muscles were modelled with no resistance during compression. Muscle tension stiffness values were reported previously in the literature: masseter muscle (16.35 N/mm), medial pterygoid muscle (15 N/mm), lateral pterygoid muscle (12 N/mm), anterior temporal muscle (14 N/mm) and posterior temporal muscle (13 N/mm) [10]. Traumatic force of 2000 N was applied perpendicularly to the frontal region on a 1 cm diameter circular area (Fig 1d). In previous FEA studies, force

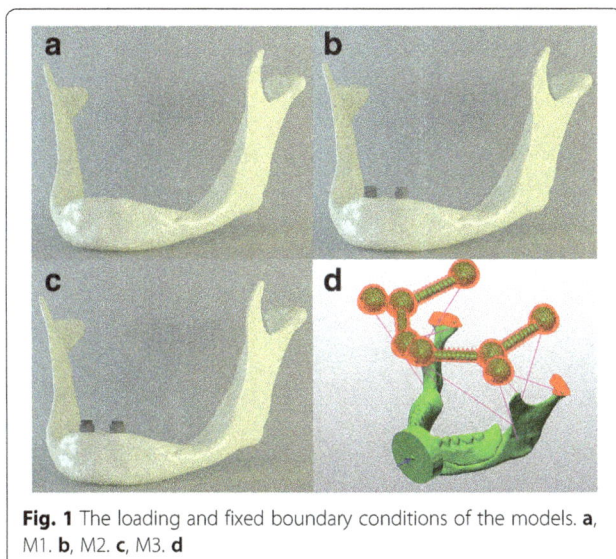

Fig. 1 The loading and fixed boundary conditions of the models. **a**, M1. **b**, M2. **c**, M3. **d**

Table 1 Mechanical properties of the materials

Material	Young's Modulus (MPa)*	Poisson's ration
Cortical Bone	13,700	0.3
Cancellous Bone	1,370	0.3
Titanium alloy	110,000	0.35
PMMA*	3,000	0.35
Mucosa	680	0.45

*Abbreviations: *MPa* Megapascal, *PMMA* Polymethyl methacrylate

Table 2 Total numbers of nodes and elements

Models	Nodes	Elements
Model 1	150440	691104
Model 2	282843	1339942
Model 3	280872	1319489

magnitude of 2000 N was used as a representative of a punch [10, 17].

After performing the FEA, maximum (Pmax) and minimum (Pmin) principle and Von Mises (VM) stresses were evaluated numerically and color coded.

Results

Von mises stresses in M1, M2 and M3 models

The highest calculated values of Von Mises stresses in M1 (979.261 N/mm^2) and M2 (1454.74 N/mm^2) have been identified in the condylar area, whereas the highest value in M3 (3866 N/mm^2) was observed in symphyseal area (Fig 2).

The evaluation of Von Mises stress patterns in the titanium implants of M3 showed that the stresses distributed all along the buccal surface of the implants, whereas in M2 high stresses were concentrated around the implant neck region (Fig 3).

Pmax stresses in M1, M2 and M3 models

The highest Pmax stress values in M1 (1112.74 N/mm^2) and M2 (2047.92 N/mm^2) were located in condylar area, whereas the highest value in M3 (2560.68 N/mm2) was observed in symphyseal area (Fig 4).

Pmin stresses in M1, M2 and M3 models

The highest Pmin stress values were isolated in symphyseal area in all models.−1203.38 N/mm^2,−1811.51 N/mm^2 and−4125.3 N/mm^2, respectively (Fig 5).

Discussion

Patients that have atrophic edentulous mandibles suffer from psychosocial and functional problems related to their dentures. Insufficient stability and reduced retention of a lower denture because of a poor load–bearing capacity of the mandibular bone and remaining soft tissues hamper proper prosthodontic rehabilitation of these patients [7]. The insertion of two endosseous implants in the interforaminal region of an atrophic edentulous mandible is currently accepted and a widespread treatment option for improving retention and stability of a mandibular overdenture [5, 7, 18, 19].

Mandible fracture caused by endosseous implants was first reported by Albrektsson [20]. The ratio of a physician encountering a fractured atrophic mandible with dental implants has increased with the increase in use of dental implants [14]. Despite improvements in surgical fixation instruments, because of decreased vascularization, limited bone quality and quantity and absence of teeth in a patient with a fractured atrophic mandible, current procedures of fracture immobilization continues to be difficult and have been shown to be insufficient. Furthermore, fracture treatment is often complicated due to the poor health status and complex medical problems of older patients [21]. Clinicians involved in dental implant rehabilitation should realize that prevention is the best treatment for implant related mandibular fracture. That requires selection of patient, careful surgical technique, and postoperative care. Although such complications are rare, it is needed to be discussed preoperatively since the treatment of mandible fractures related to implants is complicated [3].

The aim of this tree-dimensional finite element analysis study was to evaluate the biomechanical behaviour of an atrophic mandible with two endoessous implants in response to traumatic force, based on differences in implant width. Additionally, this study will lead to find best insertion point of implants and selection of

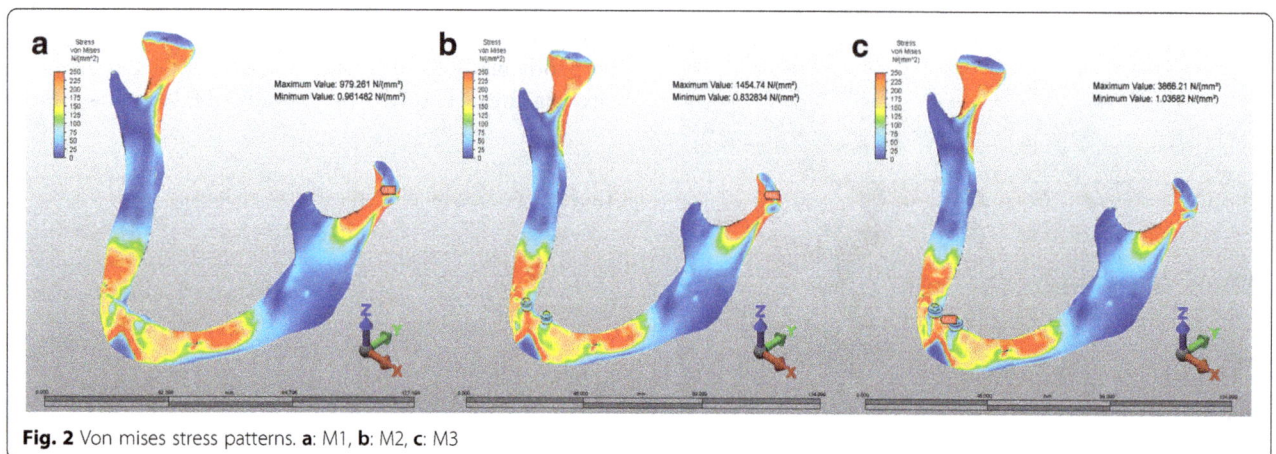

Fig. 2 Von mises stress patterns. **a**: M1, **b**: M2, **c**: M3

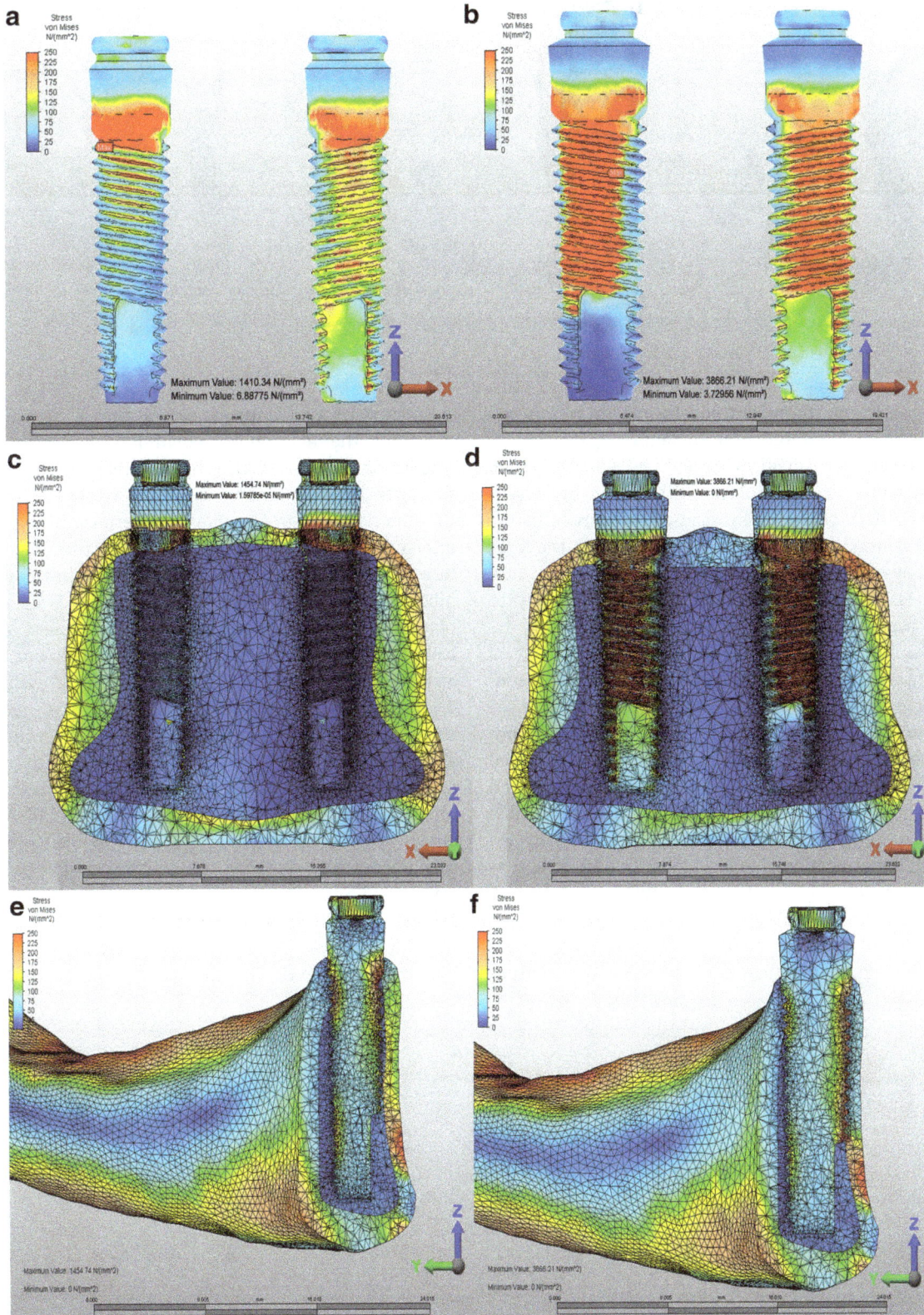

Fig. 3 Von mises stress patterns of titanium implants. **a**: M2, **b**: M3, **c**: M2 frontal plane, **d**: M3 frontal plane, **e**: M2 sagittal plane, **f**: M3 sagittal plane

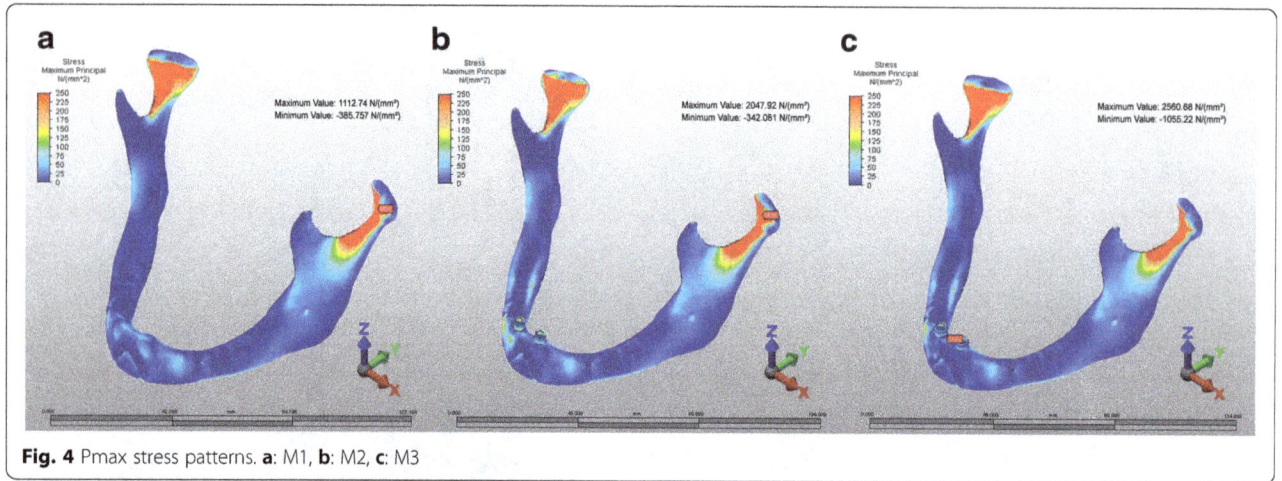

Fig. 4 Pmax stress patterns. **a**: M1, **b**: M2, **c**: M3

implant's diameter, to prevent edentulous atrophic mandible fractures related to dental implants.

FEA is regarded as an adequate and convenient method for investigating stress and strain distribution by investigating the effect of the biomechanical properties of the bone and dental implants. It is difficult to assess the force distribution on jaws and dental implants due to the heterogeneous structure of the bones and the inability to simulate the effects of the muscles and soft tissues on the bones [14, 22, 23]. However, with the improvement of FEA software, dental implants and effects of soft tissues and muscles of the human jaws have demonstrated in the present study compatible with those of clinical situations. In the literature recent studies compared FEA analysis of mandible fracture with actual clinical cases and reported FEA to be an accurate, non-invasive, and repeatable method for studying the biomechanical behaviour of human mandibles under mechanical loads. Therefore, in ethical considerations FEA reduces the need for animal and cadaveric studies [9, 16, 22].

It was stated in the McGill (2002) and York (2009) Consensus Statements that a mandibular overdenture supported by two implants is the first choice of treatment for the mandibular edentulous patient [18, 19]. According to Kan et al. [14] placement of implants in the lateral incisor area is a better treatment modality than insertion in the canine area because of increase in inter-implant distance increases the fracture risk with in terms of frontal plane trauma. Previous clinical and biomechanical studies have reported that, long implant placement results in more stress to the implant and surrounding bone than short implant placement in the atrophic mandibles [5, 8, 14, 24]. In the present study 3.5 mm and 4.3 mm implant diameters have been used since these types of implants are widely regarded as standard diameter implants. Implants with narrow diametes of 3.0 to 3.25 mm are well documented only for single-tooth, non-load-bearing regions [25]. A meta-analysis study showed that narrower implants had significantly lower survival rates compared with wider implants [26]. Moreover, most authors advice at least 1 mm residual bone present to the adjacent to the implant surface [25]. Therefore, narrower and wider implant diameters were not used in the current study.

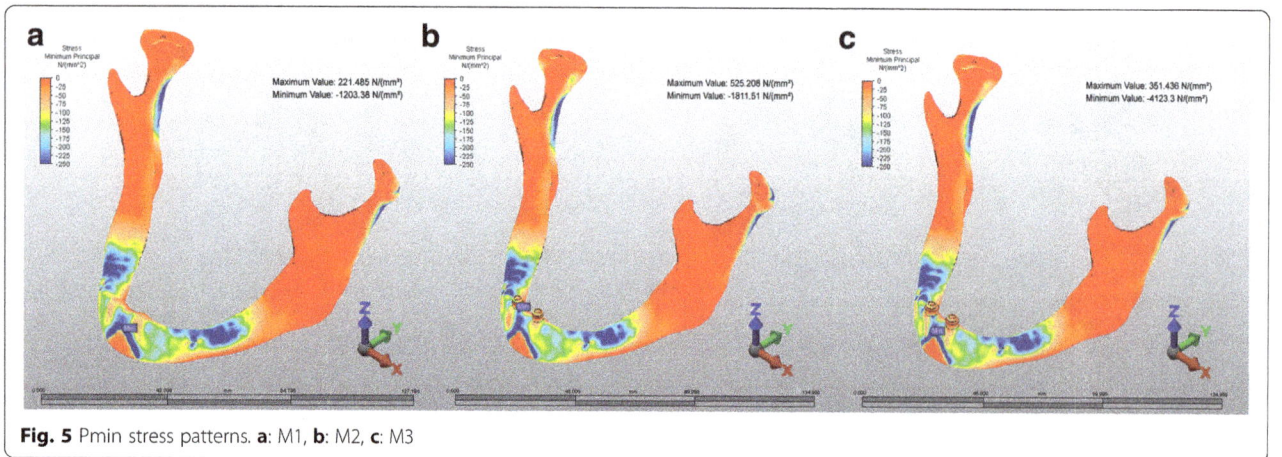

Fig. 5 Pmin stress patterns. **a**: M1, **b**: M2, **c**: M3

For all these reasons, two monocortically inserted implants into lateral incisor areas of an atrophic mandible were simulated in the present study.

Previous FEA studies showed that the impact in the symphysis region of a dentate or edentulous mandible produced highest stress values in both the condylar neck areas which were similar with M1 model of current study [9, 16]. The highest calculated values of Von Mises stresses and Pmax stresses have been identified in the condylar area in M1 and M2, whereas the highest value in M3 was observed in symphyseal area. This could be because, there was spongious bone that may provide a homogenous stress distribution all around the implants in M2, whereas in M3 there wasn't any spongious bone between implants and cortical bone on buccal side of implants. In M2, implants tend to tilt backwards in spongious bone and mandible moves to posteroinferior direction. Therefore, stresses accumulate at condylar neck areas. But in M3, because of absence of spongious bone on buccal side, implants are not able to move like in M2, therefore cortical bone transfers stresses directly to implants that makes the mandible to move only to posterior direction. That makes the stresses to distribute at the contact point of the implants to the bone (symphyseal area). Moreover in M2 high stress levels have been observed in implant neck area which is surrounded by only cortical bone. All these results showed that higher stress levels occur where implants directly come in contact with cortical bone. No experimental data can be found directly relevant to present study in the previous literatures to compare these results. Therefore, further studies in this area are needed.

Conclusions

In conclusion, according to present study, to reduce the risk of bone fracture and to preserve biomechanical behavior of the atrophic mandible from frontal traumatic loads, implants should be inserted into lateral incisors area and into spongious bone monocortically.

Abbreviations
3D: Three dimensional; FEA: Finite element analysis; Fig: Figure; M1: Model 1; M2: Model 2; M3: Model 3; MPa: Megapascal; N: Newton; N/mm: Newton/milimeter; N/mm^2: Newton/milimeter square; Pmax: Maximum principle; Pmin: Minimum principle; PMMA: Polymethyl methacrylate; VM: Von mises

Acknowledgement
Not applicable.

Funding
This work was supported by the Near East University Scientific Research Project (SAG-2016-2-005).

Authors' contributions
AA and KB participated to the conception and design of the work, to the acquisition of data, wrote the paper, participated in the analysis and interpretation of data and reviewed the manuscript. All the authors read and approved the final manuscript.

Competing interests
The authors declare that they have no competing interests.

Consent for publication
Not applicable.

References
1. de Souza Batista VE, de Souza Batista FR, Vechiato-Filho AJ, Lemos CA de A, Pellizzer EP, Verri FR. Rehabilitation With Mandibular Implant-Retained Complete Overdenture Using the Association of Two Retention Systems. J Craniofac Surg. 2016;27:e620–2.
2. Karbach J, Hartmann S, Jahn-Eimermacher A, Wagner W. Oral Health-Related Quality of Life in Edentulous Patients with Two- vs Four-Locator-Retained Mandibular Overdentures: A Prospective, Randomized, Crossover Study. Int J Oral Maxillofac Implants. 2015;30:1143–8.
3. Almasri M, El-Hakim M. Fracture of the anterior segment of the atrophic mandible related to dental implants. Int J Oral Maxillofac Surg. 2012;41:646–9.
4. Coskunses FM, Kocyigit ID, Atil F, Tekin U, Suer BT, Tuz HH, et al. Finite-Element Analysis of a New Designed Miniplate which is Used via Intraoral Approach to the Mandible Angle Fracture: Comparison of the Different Fixation Techniques. J Craniofac Surg. 2015;26:e445–8.
5. Torsiglieri T, Raith S, Rau A, Deppe H, Hölzle F, Steiner T. Stability of edentulous, atrophic mandibles after insertion of different dental implants. A biomechanical study. J Craniomaxillofac Surg. 2015;43:616–23.
6. Meijer HJA, Raghoebar GM, Visser A. Mandibular Fracture Caused by Peri-Implant Bone Loss: Report of a Case. J Periodontol. 2003;74:1067–70.
7. Raghoebar GM, Stellingsma K, Batenburg RH, Vissink A. Etiology and management of mandibular fractures associated with endosteal implants in the atrophic mandible. Oral Surg Oral Med Oral Pathol Oral Radiol Endod. 2000;89:553–9.
8. Oh W, Roumanas ED, Beumer J. Mandibular fracture in conjunction with bicortical penetration, using wide-diameter endosseous dental implants. J Prosthodont. 2010;19:625–9.
9. Gallas Torreira M, Fernandez JR. A three-dimensional computer model of the human mandible in two simulated standard trauma situations. J Craniomaxillofac Surg. 2004;32:303–7.
10. Antic S, Vukicevic AM, Milasinovic M, Saveljic I, Jovicic G, Filipovic N, et al. Impact of the lower third molar presence and position on the fragility of mandibular angle and condyle: A Three-dimensional finite element study. J Craniomaxillofac Surg. 2015;43:870–8.
11. Vollmer D, Meyer U, Joos U, Vègh A, Piffkò J. Experimental and finite element study of a human mandible. J Cranio-Maxillofac Surg. 2000;28:91–6.
12. Kilinç Y, Erkmen E, Kurt A. Biomechanical Evaluation of Different Fixation Methods for Mandibular Anterior Segmental Osteotomy Using Finite Element Analysis, Part One: Superior Repositioning Surgery. J Craniofac Surg. 2016;27:32–5.
13. Li Q, Ren S, Ge C, Sun H, Lu H, Duan Y, et al. Effect of jaw opening on the stress pattern in a normal human articular disc: finite element analysis based on MRI images. Head Face Med. 2014;10:24.
14. Kan B, Coskunses FM, Mutlu I, Ugur L, Meral DG. Effects of inter-implant distance and implant length on the response to frontal traumatic force of two anterior implants in an atrophic mandible: three-dimensional finite element analysis. Int J Oral Maxillofac Surg. 2015;44:908–13.
15. Ozan O, Ramoglu S. Effect of Implant Height Differences on Different Attachment Types and Peri-Implant Bone in Mandibular Two-Implant Overdentures: 3D Finite Element Study. J Oral Implantol. 2015;41:e50–9.
16. Santos LS de M, Rossi AC, Freire AR, Matoso RI, Caria PHF, Prado FB. Finite-element analysis of 3 situations of trauma in the human edentulous mandible. J Oral Maxillofac Surg. 2015;73:683–91.
17. Takada H, Abe S, Tamatsu Y, Mitarashi S, Saka H, Ide Y. Three-dimensional bone microstructures of the mandibular angle using micro-CT and finite element analysis: relationship between partially impacted mandibular third molars and angle fractures. Dent Traumatol. 2006;22:18–24.
18. Thomason JM, Feine J, Exley C, Moynihan P, Müller F, Naert I, et al. Mandibular two implant-supported overdentures as the first choice standard of care for edentulous patients–the York Consensus Statement. Br Dent J. 2009;207:185–6.
19. Thomason JM, Kelly SAM, Bendkowski A, Ellis JS. Two implant retained overdentures–a review of the literature supporting the McGill and York consensus statements. J Dent. 2012;40:22–34.

20. Albrektsson T. A multicenter report on osseointegrated oral implants. J Prosthet Dent. 1988;60:75–84.

21. Flores-Hidalgo A, Altay MA, Atencio IC, Manlove AE, Schneider KM, Baur DA, et al. Management of fractures of the atrophic mandible: a case series. Oral Surg Oral Med Oral Pathol Oral Radiol. 2015;119:619–27.

22. Trivedi S. Finite element analysis: A boon to dentistry. J oral Biol craniofacial Res. 2014;4:200–3.

23. Tsouknidas A, Lympoudi E, Michalakis K, Giannopoulos D, Michailidis N, Pissiotis A, et al. Influence of Alveolar Bone Loss and Different Alloys on the Biomechanical Behavior of Internal-and External-Connection Implants: A Three-Dimensional Finite Element Analysis. Int J Oral Maxillofac Implants. 2015;30:e30–42.

24. Steiner T, Torsiglieri T, Rau A, Möhlhenrich SC, Eichhorn S, Grohmann I, et al. Impairment of an atrophic mandible by preparation of the implant cavity: a biomechanical study. Br J Oral Maxillofac Surg. 2016;54:619–24.

25. Klein MO, Schiegnitz E, Al-Nawas B. Systematic review on success of narrow-diameter dental implants. Int J Oral Maxillofac Implants. 2014;29(Suppl):43–54.

26. Ortega-Oller I, Suárez F, Galindo-Moreno P, Torrecillas-Martínez L, Monje A, Catena A, et al. The influence of implant diameter on its survival: a meta-analysis based on prospective clinical trials. J Periodontol. 2014;85:569–80.

30

Vestibulo-Oral inclination of maxillary and mandibular canines and bicuspids - a CBCT investigation

Jan Hourfar[1], Dirk Bister[2], Jörg A. Lisson[3], Christine Goldbecher[4] and Björn Ludwig[3,5*]

Abstract

Background: The aim of this retrospective study was to measure tooth and crowns axes of canines, first and second bicuspids of orthodontically untreated subjects with near normal occlusion to: 1. Define norms and reveal potential gender differences and 2. Discuss implications of the findings for orthodontics.

Methods: The CBCT-datasets of 167 patients, 56 males (mean age 28.63 years ± 11.99 years) and 111 females (mean age 29.72 years ± 11.47 years) were used. Tooth- and crown axes were measured for right and left sides. Normal distribution was evaluated with the Kolmogorov-Smirnov-test. For gender comparison independent t-Tests and for comparison of right and left sides a paired t-Test were used for normally distributed data. For data not following normal distribution for gender comparison the Mann-Whitney-U-Test was used and for data comparing the two sides the Wilcoxon signed rank test was applied.
The level of statistical significance was set at $p \leq 0.05$.

Results: Measurement of tooth axes revealed buccal inclination for both genders with maximum values for maxillary and mandibular canines. Statistical significant differences were only found for maxillary canines ($P = 0.025$) and lower second bicuspids ($P = 0.016$) respectively. Values for crown axes revealed oral inclination for both genders with maximum values for maxillary first bicuspids and in the mandible for first and second bicuspids. No statistical significant differences were found between the genders apart from asymmetry for crown axes for the upper first bicuspids for males ($P = 0.006$) and females ($P < 0.001$).

Conclusions: Our study reveals that irrespective of gender, oral inclination of the crowns of canines and premolars is the norm. The values of the most commonly used bracket prescriptions coincide with the average values found in our investigation. For esthetic reasons modifications of torque values can be considered.

Keywords: Cone beam computed tomography, Tooth axis, Crown axis, Vestibulo-oral inclination, Torque

Background

Orthodontics aims at achieving good functional occlusion and dental aesthetics [1, 2]. A fundamental aspect to achieving good aesthetics and function is the predictable three-dimensional positioning of teeth. To accomplish this, contemporary orthodontics mostly relies on using pre-adjusted standard edgewise fixed appliances that are available with a range of different bracket prescriptions and slot sizes. By using these different prescriptions different torque values are applied.

Although not the sole determinant [3] of smile aesthetics, the vestibulo-oral inclination of the canines and bicuspids, particularly in the upper jaw [4], play an important role for the smile aesthetics. Approximately 90 % of people show either the maxillary first and second premolar when smiling [5] and the vestibulo-oral inclination of the maxillary canines and bicuspids can influence the width of the buccal corridor [4–6]. The buccal corridor is defined as the space between the facial surfaces of the posterior teeth and the corners of the lips when smiling [7]. Whether smaller or wider buccal corridors are preferable

---
* Correspondence: bludwig@kieferorthopaedie-mosel.de
[3]Department of Orthodontics, University of Saarland, Homburg/Saar, Germany
[5]Private Practice, Am Bahnhof 54, 56841 Traben-Trarbach, Germany
Full list of author information is available at the end of the article

has been debated before [8] and there is some evidence suggesting gender differences [9].

Some authors recommend to give upper canines and bicuspids buccal crown torque to improve aesthetics [5]. However a number of commonly used bracket prescriptions apply negative torque to canines and bicuspids, causing oral inclination. A recent study by Xu et al., [4] however, investigating three dimensional digital models revealed a broad range of esthetic acceptability for vestibulo-oral inclinations of the maxillary canines and premolars. Vestibulo-oral inclination of crowns can be measured on study models or with Cone Beam Computed Tomography (CBCT) images. Only the latter are able to measure tooth axis and crown inclination with precision [10–12], because CBCT images show the roots as well as adjacent dentofacial structures undistorted in a 1:1 ratio [13]. Conventional two dimensional radiographs do not allow for precise measurements of buccolingual inclination of teeth [14].

The aim of this retrospective study was to measure vestibulo-oral inclination of roots and crowns of canines, first and second bicuspids in both jaws of orthodontically untreated subjects to:

1. Define norms and reveal possible gender differences and
2. Discuss implications for orthodontic treatment.

Methods
Definition of abbreviations can be found in Table 1.

Patients and radiographic material
Anonymized, relevant CBCT images that had been taken between 2009 and 2012 were analyzed; the images were sourced from a practice that specializes in orthodontics and oral surgery.

Inclusion criteria were:

– Justification for the radiographs and written consent were available.
– The indications for imaging included: diagnosis of intraosseus and dental pathologies and both pre-operative risk assessment and surgical planning for various interventions, complying with the "as low as reasonably achievable" (ALARA) principle [15].

CBCT-scans
The CBCT scans used in this study were all taken with the same equipment: Veraviewpocs 3D®, (J. Morita Corp., Osaka, Japan). Images were acquired with the following settings: 5 mA, 80 kV, pixel size: 0.125 mm × 0.125 mm; voxel size was 0.125 mm³. All CBCT images provided a slice thicknesses of 0.25 mm. Patients were positioned according to the manufacturer's instructions.

Patient selection and inclusion criteria
CBCT datasets of a total of 1007 patients were available. Only datasets with field of view (FOV) including complete dentition of both jaws without artifacts and only patients of Caucasian origin without history of previous orthodontic treatment were included. Further inclusion criteria included presence of fully erupted teeth that exhibited neither prosthetic restorations/fillings or dental caries. Only patients with near normal occlusion (NNO) were included. NNO was verified using available plaster models.

Measurements on CBCT datasets
Software
All measurements were performed using DICOM imaging software (OsiriX®, Version 2.0.1, 64 Bit, Pixmeo, Bernex, Switzerland) for MacOS® (Apple Inc., Cupertino, Ca, USA). The software features 3 split windows for coronal, sagittal and axial view. After screening of the respective 3D-data sets, orthoradial adjustments to the x-, y- and z-plane level were made to enable reproducible

Table 1 Abbreviations

Abbreviation	Type	Definition
mrp	RPL	Median reference plane, aligned parallel to the dental arch of the split axial view.
ap	RP	apex. Most apical point of the root.
cej	RP	cemento-enamel-junction
i	RP	cusp tip
cf	RP	Central fossa. Deepest occlusal notch between cusps in bicuspids
FA	RP	FA-Point according to Andrews
α	AM	Tooth axis: Angle between long axis of the tooth (i-ap and cf-ap respectively) and midsagittal plane (msp).
β	AM	Crown axis: Angle between long axis of the tooth (i-ap and cf-ap respectively) and tangent through FA-point (constructed using parallel shift of the connective line between cej and i).

RPL reference plane, RP reference point, AM angular measurement (degrees)

three-dimensional measurements. The validity and accuracy of measurements performed with Osirix® software have been demonstrated by various previous studies [16–22].

Dental measurements

The dental measurements consisted of 1. crown and 2. tooth axis. These two different measurements were performed using a median reference plane and a set of radiographic reference points and lines (Fig. 1, Table 1). The exact protocol for the measurement of crown axes and tooth axes are described in detail below. Tooth and crown axes were measured for canines, first bicuspids, and second bicuspids in both jaws. A section through each tooth measured it at its widest occlusal vestibulo-oral distance and was adjusted on the axial and sagittal split window respectively. All angular measurements were undertaken on the coronal split window of the imaging software using the built in angle measuring tool. Negative values indicate oral inclination of crown or root respectively whereas positive values indicate vestibular inclination of crown or root respectively. Mandibular and maxillary measurements were undertaken in the same way.

1. Crown axis
   The crown axis (i.e. the vestibulo-oral inclination of the crown) was defined and measured as the angle between the median reference plane ("mrp") and the line through the FA-point according to Andrews [23]. As described by Smith et al. [24] a parallel shift of the connective line between the clearly defined reference points "cej" (cemento-enamel-junction) and "i" (cusp tip) for was used to construct the line through FA.

2. Tooth axis
   The tooth axis (i.e. the vestibulo-oral inclination of the root) was measured as the angle between the median reference plane ("mrp") and a line passing through the cusp tip ("i") of the canines (or "cf" of the bicuspids) and the apical reference point ("ap"). In case of root apex dilaceration, the middle third of the root was used as the apical reference point, similar to conventional cephalometry.

Data collection and statistical analysis

All data were collated on an Excel® spreadsheet (Microsoft Corp., Redmond, Washington, USA). Statistical analyses were carried with SPSS® for Windows, version 22.0 (IBM Corp., Armonk, New York, USA). Normal distribution

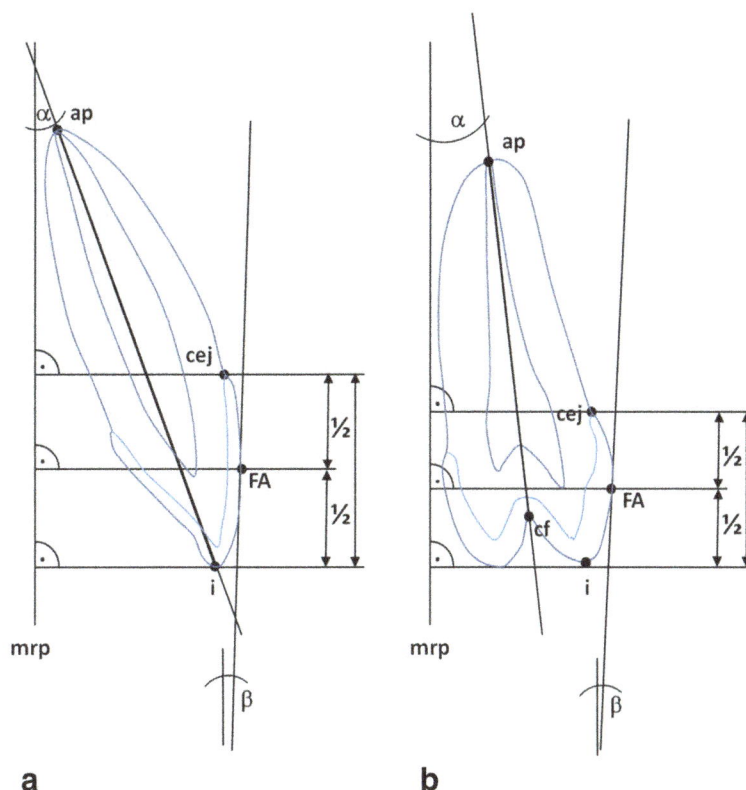

Fig. 1 Measurement of crown and tooth axes. Measurements were undertaken using different reference points as defined in Table 1. Left upper canine (**a**) and left bicuspid (**b**) are shown here. Negative values (-) indicate oral inclination of crown or root whereas positive (+) values indicate vestibular inclination

was evaluated with the Kolmogorov-Smirnov-test. For gender comparison independent t-Tests and for comparison of right and left sides a paired t-Test were used for normally distributed data. For data not following normal distribution for gender comparison the Mann-Whitney-U-Test was used and for data comparing the two sides the Wilcoxon signed rank test was applied. Descriptive statistics (Medians and Interquartile Ranges (IQR)) are presented for data not following normal distribution whereas descriptive statistics (Means and Standard Deviations (SD)) are presented for normally distributed data.

For intra-examiner reliability the same operator repeated all measurements for 50 randomly selected cases 3 months after the initial measurements and the coefficient of variation (COV) was calculated. The COV was mean 0.13 (range: 0.03–0.34) for males and mean 0.17 (range: 0.03–0.72) for females. No statistical difference ($P = 0.554$) was found between the COVs. The level of statistical significance was set at $p \leq 0.05$.

Results

Sample demographics

A total of 167 patients, 56 males (mean age 28.63 years ± 11.99 years) and 111 females (mean age 29.72 years ± 11.47 years) fulfilled the criteria for inclusion. No statistically significant difference ($P = 0.569$) was found between age of both genders.

CBCT-measurements

Descriptive values of the CBCT measurements and results of the statistical analysis are presented in Tables 2, 3, 4 and 5. Mean and median values for tooth axes presented buccal inclination for males and females with maximum values for maxillary and mandibular canines. Statistical significant gender differences were only found in maxillary canines ($P = 0.025$) and lower second bicuspids ($P = 0.016$) respectively (Tables 2 and 3). Conversely, mean and median values for crown axes revealed oral inclination for both genders with maximum values for maxillary first bicuspids and in the mandible for first

and second bicuspids. No statistical significant differences were found between the genders. Interestingly there was statistically significant asymmetry for crown inclinations for the upper first bicuspids for males ($P = 0.006$) and females ($P < 0.001$) (Tables 4, 5).

Discussion

The aim of our study was to define norms for vestibulo-oral inclination of teeth for an untreated Caucasian population, to investigate gender differences and to discuss possible implications of the findings for orthodontic treatment.

The results of our study referring the tooth axes were consistent with those of another CBCT study using similar methodology [13]; although neither crown axes nor gender differences were investigated by that group. The only difference were the lower second bicuspids, which showed vestibular inclination. Our study investigated only Caucasian patients whereas the sample assessed by Tong et al. [13] was comprised of 6 ethnicities: Hispanic, Black, White, Asian and Middle Eastern; Caucasian white patients constituted their smallest group and the differences between the ethnicities were not investigated.

In our study two comparisons between genders referring to tooth axes reached the level of statistical significance; these differences were likely to be spurious however. There was no difference between right and left that reached level of significance.

Crown axes did not exhibit statistically significant differences ($P > 0.05$) between male and female subjects and demonstrated oral inclination. It is interesting to note that a number of widely used prescriptions of commercially available bracket systems have negative torque values for canines and bicuspids: negative torque values (-7) can be found for maxillary canines (Andrews and MBT prescriptions) as well as for maxillary bicuspids (Roth, MBT, and Andrews prescriptions) [25]. Except for maxillary first bicuspids, the results of our study for crown axes of maxillary canines and second bicuspids resemble the torque values of the aforementioned prescriptions (Tables 2, 3). Interestingly our study showed asymmetry of the upper first premolar torque values

Table 2 Tooth axes (in degrees) - *males*

Tooth	Mean, R	SD, R	Mean, L	SD, L	Avg (R, L)	SD, avg (R, L)	Mean diff (R-L)	P value (R vs L)	P value (M vs F)
U3	+12.62	6.96	+12.19	7.66	+12.40	7.28	0.43	0.668	0.025*
U4	+3.36	6.67	+3.99	6.17	+3.67	6.41	−0.64	0.636	0.237
U5	+4.33	7.14	+3.83	5.78	+4.09	6.48	0.50	0.374	0.190
L3	+17.41	7.44	+18.88	8.02	+18.15	7.73	−1.47	0.336	0.114
L4	(+5.24)	(7.79)	(+3.14)	(7.87)	(+3.40)	(7.84)	(2.10)	0.056	0.526
L5	(+6.20)	(7.23)	(+4.36)	(8.23)	(+5.58)	(8.24)	(1.84)	0.149	0.016*

*$P \leq 0.05$; not normally distributed data in brackets
R right, *L* left, *Avg* average, *diff* difference, *M* male, *F* female, *U* upper, *L* lower; 3, canine; 4, first bicuspid; 5, second bicuspid

Table 3 Tooth axes (in degrees) - *females*

Tooth	Mean, R	SD, R	Mean, L	SD, L	Avg (R, L)	SD, avg (R, L)	Mean diff (R-L)	P value (R vs L)	P value (M vs F)
U3	+14.96	6.89	+14.47	8.19	+14.71	7.55	0.48	0.293	0.025*
U4	(+3.10)	(7.50)	(+2.58)	(7.12)	(+2.63)	(8.00)	(0.52)	0.387	0.237
U5	+2.61	7.48	+3.41	6.43	+2.99	6.99	−0.80	0.147	0.190
L3	+20.33	7.33	+19.32	8.77	+19.83	8.07	1.01	0.098	0.114
L4	+4.22	5.67	+3.56	5.47	+3.89	5.56	0.67	0.283	0.526
L5	+8.55	7.20	+7.16	6.44	+7.85	6.84	1.39	0.212	0.016*

*$P \leq 0.05$; not normally distributed data in brackets
R right, L left, Avg average, *diff* difference, M male, F female, U upper, L lower; 3, canine; 4, first bicuspid; 5, second bicuspid

between right and left hand sides for both males and females indicating asymmetry of approximately three degrees (−8.66 and −11.74 for males and −8.48 and −11.80 for females). This has to our knowledge not previously been described.

One factor contributing to an attractive or esthetic smile is the size of the buccal corridor [7] and numerous papers have been published on this [6, 9, 26–32] and the literature is inconclusive. In a systematic review, Janson et al. [33] pointed out that the influence of the buccal corridor on a smile was thought more important if digitally modified patient photographs were used for evaluation, rather than natural images; however a broader smile was preferred by most authors [5, 34]. Another study found smaller buccal corridors for male subjects and larger buccal corridors for female subjects aesthetically more pleasing [9], suggesting a gender difference.

Our study supports the notion that oral inclination of the maxillary bicuspids is the norm; approximately −7.5° for first and −10° for second bicuspids. An earlier investigation speculated that application of buccal crown torque to canines and posterior teeth might alleviate pronounced buccal corridors and enhance esthetics [5]. If application of buccal crown torque is desired, applying more positive values will subsequently move the roots of the teeth palatal potentially reducing the risk of developing vestibular bony dehiscence or recession [35].

A recent study found that orthodontists prefer ranges of 0° to −7° of vestibulo-oral inclination for the canines and −3° to −11° for the bicuspids esthetically pleasing.

For laypersons the values were +3 to −10° for the canines and +5 to −11° of inclination for bicuspids [4]. Our investigation appears to confirm that orthodontists prefer naturally occurring inclinations of teeth, in contrast to the lay population.

Indiscriminate treatment of patients with a pre-adjusted standardized straight wire fixed appliances, using commercially available brackets and archwires is not consistent with individualized treatment. However torque prescriptions 'programmed' in bracket systems usually not fully expressed. This can be due to a variety of factors such as: inaccuracies of bracket positioning, differences in tooth morphology between individuals, because of torque loss (the 'play' between the archwire and slot) or the properties of the orthodontic materials themselves [36, 37]. Our study confirms that the torque values used in most commercially available bracket prescriptions are found in the untreated population.

The need for individualized treatment of the patient may be particularly interesting when considering extractions: One CBCT study demonstrated that non-extraction treatment increased the buccal crown torque of the upper bicuspids but that extraction treatment lead to lingual crown torque of upper canines [11].

Aesthetic considerations aside, the functional occlusion must not be neglected. Applying buccal crown torque to maxillary canines and bicuspids for esthetic reasons might interfere with functional occlusal contacts: canine guidance might be lost and for maxillary bicuspids the palatal cusps can interfere during lateral excursion and our study

Table 4 Crown axes (in degrees) - *males*

Tooth	Mean, R	SD, R	Mean, L	SD, L	Avg (R,L)	SD, avg (R,L)	Mean diff (R-L)	P value (R vs L)	P value (M vs F)
U3	−6.23	6.01	−6.98	5.89	−6.61	5.92	0.74	0.426	0.358
U4	−8.66	7.40	−11.74	6.97	−10.12	7.32	3.08	0.006**	0.944
U5	−7.17	6.73	−7.80	5.95	−7.48	6.48	0.63	0.069	0.668
L3	(−0.37)	(5.22)	(−0.03)	(5.70)	(−0.36)	(5.79)	(−0.34)	0.981	0.345
L4	−11.35	8.25	−12.47	9.37	−13.08	8.77	1.12	0.540	0.743
L5	−13.53	8.50	−10.54	7.83	−12.98	8.23	−2.99	0.149	0.734

**$P \leq 0.01$; not normally distributed data in brackets
R right, L left, Avg average, *diff* difference, M male, F female, U upper, L lower; 3, canine; 4, first bicuspid; 5, second bicuspid

Table 5 Crown axes (in degrees) - *females*

Tooth	Mean, R	SD, R	Mean, L	SD, L	Avg (R,L)	SD, avg (R,L)	Mean diff (R-L)	P value (R vs L)	P value (M vs F)
U3	−7.08	7.19	−6.76	7.02	−7.43	6.72	−0.32	0.075	0.358
U4	−8.48	6.24	−11.80	6.08	−10.06	6.36	3.32	<0.001***	0.944
U5	−7.79	7.48	−7.97	6.30	−7.91	6.83	0.18	0.898	0.668
L3	(−0.65)	(4.81)	(−1.55)	(8.15)	(−1.00)	(5.94)	(0.91)	0.104	0.345
L4	−11.67	7.06	−11.53	8.28	−12.69	7.69	−0.14	0.309	0.743
L5	−12.18	8.04	−12.54	7.94	−13.40	8.03	0.35	0.369	0.734

***$P \leq 0.001$; not normally distributed data in brackets
R right, L left, Avg average, diff difference, M male, F female, U upper, L lower; 3, canine; 4, first bicuspid; 5, second bicuspid

appears to suggest that orally inclined teeth are the norm for the untreated population. Although not part of this investigation we can speculate that a mutually balanced and protected occlusion may well be the norm. It has been recommended that post-treatment occlusion should be subjected to dynamic evaluation as well as the commonly used static assessment of the occlusion [38]; particularly with regard to desired postorthodontic treatment outcome: the majority of the referring dentists rank canine guidance as most important feature of the occlusion [39].

Conclusions

- Our study revealed that irrespective of gender, oral inclination of canine and premolars crowns were the norm for the Caucasian white population investigated.
- The torque values of most commonly used bracket prescriptions coincide with the average values found in our investigation.
- There was an asymmetry in upper first premolar torque for both males and females that has not previously been reported.

Acknowledgements
Not applicable.

Funding
None.

Authors' contributions
JH conceived the project, performed the measurements, gathered and processed i.e. created the material presented (tables, electronic images, references, etc.) and drafted the manuscript. DB translated and critically revised the manuscript. JAL helped in conceiving this project and critically revised the manuscript. CG helped selecting the material and took part in the acquisition of data. BL had the idea for this project and reviewed every step of the process. All authors read and approved the final manuscript.

Competing interests
The authors declare that they have no competing interests.

Author details
[1]Department of Orthodontics, University of Heidelberg, Heidelberg, Germany. [2]Department of Orthodontics, Guy's and St Thomas' NHS Foundation Trust and King's College London Dental Institute, London, UK. [3]Department of Orthodontics, University of Saarland, Homburg/Saar, Germany. [4]Private Practice, Halle/Saale, Germany. [5]Private Practice, Am Bahnhof 54, 56841 Traben-Trarbach, Germany.

References
1. Peck S, Peck L. Selected aspects of the art and science of facial esthetics. Semin Orthod. 1995;1:105–26.
2. Shaw WC, Rees G, Dawe M, Charles CR. The influence of dentofacial appearance on the social attractiveness of young adults. Am J Orthod. 1985;87:21–6.
3. Gill D, Naini FB. Orthodontics: Principles and Practice. 1. edn: Chichester, West Sussex, UK: Wiley-Blackwell; 2011.
4. Xu H, Han X, Wang Y, Shu R, Jing Y, Tian Y, Andrews WA, Andrews LF, Bai D. Effect of buccolingual inclinations of maxillary canines and premolars on perceived smile attractiveness. Am J Orthod Dentofacial Orthop. 2015;147:182–9.
5. Zachrisson BU. Making the premolar extraction smile full and radiant. World J Orthod. 2002;3:260–5.
6. Moore T, Southard KA, Casko JS, Qian F, Southard TE. Buccal corridors and smile esthetics. Am J Orthod Dentofacial Orthop. 2005;127:208–13.
7. Frush JP, Fischer RD. The dynesthetic interpretation of the dentogenic concept. J Prosthet Dent. 1958;8:558–81.
8. Martin AJ, Buschang PH, Boley JC, Taylor RW, McKinney TW. The impact of buccal corridors on smile attractiveness. Eur J Orthod. 2007;29:530–7.
9. Oshagh M, Zarif NH, Bahramnia F. Evaluation of the effect of buccal corridor size on smile attractiveness. Eur J Esthet Dent. 2010;5:370–80.
10. Tong H, Enciso R, Van Elslande D, Major PW, Sameshima GT. A new method to measure mesiodistal angulation and faciolingual inclination of each whole tooth with volumetric cone-beam computed tomography images. Am J Orthod Dentofacial Orthop. 2012;142:133–43.
11. Chen G, Qin YF, Xu TM. Tip and torque changes in maxillary buccal segment after orthodontic treatment: a three-dimensional study. Zhonghua Kou Qiang Yi Xue Za Zhi. 2010;45:650–4.
12. Shewinvanakitkul W, Hans MG, Narendran S, Martin Palomo J. Measuring buccolingual inclination of mandibular canines and first molars using CBCT. Orthod Craniofac Res. 2011;14:168–74.
13. Tong H, Kwon D, Shi J, Sakai N, Enciso R, Sameshima GT. Mesiodistal angulation and faciolingual inclination of each whole tooth in 3-dimensional space in patients with near-normal occlusion. Am J Orthod Dentofacial Orthop. 2012;141:604–17.
14. Garcia-Figueroa MA, Raboud DW, Lam EW, Heo G, Major PW. Effect of buccolingual root angulation on the mesiodistal angulation shown on panoramic radiographs. Am J Orthod Dentofacial Orthop. 2008;134:93–9.
15. IRCP. Radiation and your patient - A Guide for Medical Practitioners. ICRP Supporting Guidance 2. Available at: http://www.icrp.org/publication.asp?id=ICRP%20Supporting%20Guidance%202. Accessed 29 Nov 2014. Ann IRCP 2001, 31.
16. Albert S, Cristofari JP, Cox A, Bensimon JL, Guedon C, Barry B. Mandibular reconstruction with fibula free flap. Experience of virtual reconstruction using Osirix(R), a free and open source software for medical imagery. Ann Chir Plast Esthet. 2011;56:494–503.

17. Fortin M, Battie MC. Quantitative Paraspinal Muscle Measurements: Inter-Software Reliability and Agreement Using OsiriX and ImageJ. Phys Ther. 2012.

18. Jalbert F, Paoli JR. Osirix: free and open-source software for medical imagery. Rev Stomatol Chir Maxillofac. 2008;109:53–5.

19. Melissano G, Bertoglio L, Civelli V, Amato AC, Coppi G, Civilini E, alori G, De Cobelli F, Del Maschio A, Chiesa R. Demonstration of the Adamkiewicz artery by multidetector computed tomography angiography analysed with the open-source software OsiriX. Eur J Vasc Endovasc Surg. 2009;37:395–400.

20. Sierra-Martinez E, Cienfuegos-Monroy R, Fernandez-Sobrino G. OsiriX, a useful tool for processing tomographic images in patients with facial fracture. Cir Cir. 2009;77:95–9.

21. Wang YC, Liu YC, Hsieh TC, Lee ST, Li ML. Aneurysmal subarachnoid hemorrhage diagnosis with computed tomographic angiography and OsiriX. Acta Neurochir (Wien). 2010;152:263–9. discussion 269.

22. Yamauchi T, Yamazaki M, Okawa A, Furuya T, Hayashi K, Sakuma T, Takahashi H, Yanagawa N, Koda M. Efficacy and reliability of highly functional open source DICOM software (OsiriX) in spine surgery. J Clin Neurosci. 2010;17:756–9.

23. Andrews LF. The six keys to normal occlusion. Am J Orthod. 1972;62:296–309.

24. Smith RN, Brook AH, Karmo M. The relationship between the mid-point and most-prominent point on the labial curve of upper anterior teeth. Open Dent J. 2009;3:167–72.

25. American Orthodontics (AO) Corporation, Sheboygan, WI, USA. AO product Catalog. Available at: http://www.americanortho.com/catalog/index.html#p=16. Accessed 24 Jun 2015.

26. Roden-Johnson D, Gallerano R, English J. The effects of buccal corridor spaces and arch form on smile esthetics. Am J Orthod Dentofacial Orthop. 2005;127:343–50.

27. Zange SE, Ramos AL, Cuoghi OA, de Mendonça MR, Suguino R. Perceptions of laypersons and orthodontists regarding the buccal corridor in long- and short-face individuals. Angle Orthod. 2010;81:86–90.

28. Valiathan A, Gandhi S. Buccal corridor spaces, arch form, and smile esthetics. Am J Orthod Dentofacial Orthop. 2005;128(5):557.

29. Yang IH, Nahm DS, Baek SH. Which hard and soft tissue factors relate with the amount of buccal corridor space during smiling? Angle Orthod. 2008;78:5–11.

30. Krishnan V, Daniel ST, Lazar D, Asok A. Characterization of posed smile by using visual analog scale, smile arc, buccal corridor measures, and modified smile index. Am J Orthod Dentofacial Orthop. 2008;133:515–23.

31. Ioi H, Kang S, Shimomura T, Kim SS, Park SB, Son WS, Takahashi I. Effects of buccal corridors on smile esthetics in Japanese and Korean orthodontists and orthodontic patients. Am J Orthod Dentofacial Orthop. 2012;142:459–65.

32. Parekh SM, Fields HW, Beck M, Rosenstiel S. Attractiveness of variations in the smile arc and buccal corridor space as judged by orthodontists and laymen. Angle Orthod. 2006;76:557–63.

33. Janson G, Branco NC, Fernandes TM, Sathler R, Garib D, Lauris JR. Influence of orthodontic treatment, midline position, buccal corridor and smile arc on smile attractiveness. Angle Orthod. 2011;81:153–61.

34. Zachrisson BU. Maxillary expansion: long-term stability and smile esthetics. World J Orthod. 2001;2:266–72.

35. Northway WM. Gingival recession–can orthodontics be a cure? Angle Orthod. 2013;83:1093–101.

36. Miethke RR, Melsen B. Effect of variation in tooth morphology and bracket position on first and third order correction with preadjusted appliances. Am J Orthod Dentofacial Orthop. 1999;116:329–35.

37. Gioka C, Eliades T. Materials-induced variation in the torque expression of preadjusted appliances. Am J Orthod Dentofacial Orthop. 2004;125:323–8.

38. Akhoundi MS, Hashem A, Noroozi H. Comparison of occlusal balance contacts in patients treated with standard edgewise and preadjusted straight-wire appliances. World J Orthod. 2009;10:216–9.

39. Hall JF, Sohn W, McNamara JA. Why do dentists refer to specific orthodontists? Angle Orthod. 2009;79:5–11.

31

Vertical bone regeneration using rhBMP-2 and VEGF

Lara Schorn[1], Christoph Sproll[1][*] (iD), Michelle Ommerborn[2], Christian Naujoks[1], Norbert R. Kübler[1] and Rita Depprich[1]

Abstract

Background: Sufficient vertical and lateral bone supply and a competent osteogenic healing process are prerequisities for the successful osseointegration of dental implants in the alveolar bone. Several techniques including autologous bone grafts and guided bone regeneration are applied to improve quality and quantity of bone at the implantation site. Depending on the amount of lacking bone one- or two-stage procedures are required. Vertical bone augmentation has proven to be a challenge particularly in terms of bone volume stability. This study focuses on the three dimensional vertical bone generation in a one stage procedure in vivo. Therefore, a collagenous disc-shaped scaffold (ICBM = Insoluble Collagenous Bone Matrix) containing rhBMP-2 (Bone Morphogenetic Protein-2) and/or VEGF (Vascular Endothelial Growth Factor) was applied around the coronal part of a dental implant during insertion. RhBMP-2 and VEGF released directly at the implantation site were assumed to induce the generation of new vertical bone around the implant.

Methods: One hundred eight titanium implants were inserted into the mandible and the tibia of 12 mini pigs. Four experimental groups were formed: Control group, ICBM, ICBM + BMP-2, and ICBM + BMP-2 + VEGF. After 1, 4 and 12 weeks the animals were sacrificed and bone generation was investigated histologically and histomorphometrically.

Results: After 12 weeks the combination of ICBM + rhBMP2 + VEGF showed significantly more bone volume density (BVD%), a higher vertical bone gain (VBG) and more vertical bone gain around the implant (PVBG) in comparison to the control group.

Conclusion: By using collagenous disc-shaped matrices in combination with rhBMP-2 and VEGF vertical bone can be generated in a one stage procedure without donor site morbidity. The results of the presenting study suggest that the combination of rhBMP-2 and VEGF applied locally by using a collagenous carrier improves vertical bone generation in vivo. Further research is needed to establish whether this technique is applicable in clinical routines.

Keywords: Vertical bone regeneration, Cytokines, rhBMP-2, VEGF, Tissue engineering

Background

Successful osseointegration of dental implants depends on implant stability, quality and quantity of alveolar bone [1], and bone-to-implant contact [2]. Lower quality or quantity of residual bone can be caused by trauma, systemic or local illnesses or local atrophic processes [3] eventually resulting in the need for bone augmentation. Various studies showed that vertical bone regeneration in particular remains a challenge [4–7]. At posterior

---
* Correspondence: christoph.sproll@med.uni-duesseldorf.de
[1]Department of Oral-, Maxillo- and Plastic Facial Surgery, Heinrich-Heine-University Duesseldorf, Moorenstr. 5, 40225 Duesseldorf, Germany
Full list of author information is available at the end of the article

regions of the upper jaw a sinus floor augmentation procedure is suitable to regain bone height whereas in the lower jaw there is no such option [8]. In cases where the remaining bone is still 5–8 mm in height mini implants can be an option nowadays but sometimes there even is not sufficient bone for the use of those [9, 10].

Several augmentative techniques and materials have been described for bone regeneration. Autogenous, allogenic, xenogenic or alloplastic onlay or inlay bone grafts can be used for horizontal or vertical bone regeneration. Autogenous bone is the most commonly used and current gold standard [11–14], especially in combination with the tent pole technique (were the periosteum is tented up for bone to grow underneath) [15, 16]. A recent meta-analysis reviewed the use of grafting materials for alveolar ridge augmentation in combination with implant placement. Troeltzsch et al. showed that in terms of vertical bone augmentation autogenous bone blocks harvested from the iliac crest and the calvarium seem to be the only ones capable of gaining larger bone volumes [17]. The main disadvantages of bone grafts are donor site morbidity, limited supply, and possible postoperative complications [18]. When it comes to quality of life after surgery, patients' discomfort appears to be significantly higher when autogenous bone grafts (especially iliac crest grafts) are used in comparison to other augmentative techniques or materials [6, 17, 19–23]. Bone grafts often cause insufficient bone consolidation and sometimes are limited in size (e.g. space at implantation site is limited due to obligatory gingival coverage) [8]. Screws or other fixation devices might be necessary to keep the graft in place [7]. Furthermore, when used without a membrane technique, there might be fibrous encapsulation of the graft and as a consequence no sufficient bone-to-implant contact [8, 24].

A different approach is guided bone regeneration (GBR) which makes use of occlusive membranes preventing soft tissue ingrowth into the bone thereby allowing osteogenic cells originating from the adjacent bone to immigrate the restoration site [13, 25]. In addition, there are combinations of bone substitutes and membrane techniques [26]. Small volume vertical defects can be augmented by particulate grafting materials. If no skeletal scaffold is available, the combination with titanium meshes seems to be most beneficial for three-dimensional stability [17]. GBR has led to promising results in the past [8, 27–29]: there is unlimited supply and no need of a donor site. Nevertheless, membranes tend to collapse leaving the problem of bone volume stability. Non resorbable membranes or titanium meshes have to be removed in a second surgery. As in any other surgical procedure, infections, tissue inflammation and wound dehiscence have been reported as complications [8, 27].

Distraction osteogenesis is another option for vertical bone gain [13, 30]. Advantages of distraction osteogenesis are soft tissue expansion simultaneously with bone growth and again no donor site morbidity compared to the harvest of autogenous bone [8, 31]. Disadvantages are the long duration of the treatment, high relapse rates and possible post-operative complications such as early, delayed or completely absent bone consolidation, nerve injury and infection [32]. A minimum of bone height and stability is necessary for device application which usually precludes the use of this technique in the severely atrophic jaw [8]. Furthermore, several surgical procedures are required for installation and removal of the distraction device, and at least implant insertion [8, 33].

All of the above mentioned options for bone augmentation are technically highly demanding and depend on good manual skills of the surgical staff [34]. Depending on the augmentation techniques several months are required for bone consolidation and additional surgery might be necessary to finally insert the implant and/or remove the non resorbable materials/devices. Postoperative complications (e.g. infection, wound dehiscence, nerve injury, bleeding) or insufficient bone formation might occur [9]. GBR, onlay grafts and alveolar ridge distraction seem to deliver stable results of bone regeneration after up to 5 years but overall there is very little reliable data to show whether those approaches are successful over time (>10 years) [9, 35].

Since bone tissue engineering holds the promise to provide an alternative to all these above described techniques, research on this topic has become increasingly popular over the last years. Along with mesenchymal and embryonal stem cells, cytokines and growth factors blaze a trail to bone augmentation [36]. The BMPs constitute a family of proteins with the ability to initiate osteoblastic differentiation [37] and have proven to enhance osteoinductive characteristics of bone graft substitutes (e.g. in combination with autogenous bone blocks or collagenous sponges) [38–43]. rhBMP-2 in particular has shown the highest osteoinductive potential of the BMP family [44]. VEGF–A promotes angiogenesis by proliferation and migration of endothelial cells and regulates vasculogenesis [45, 46]. Furthermore, it influences osteoblastic differentiation and plays an important role in early and late enchondral ossification due to resorption of cartilage and promotion of angiogenesis [47]. It has proven to be important for craniofacial and mandibular ossification in particular [48]. By combining VEGF and rhBMP-2 angiogenesis and blood supply can be increased and formation of new bone can be enhanced [44].

The aim of this study was to generate vertical bone growth with the help of a disc-shaped collagenous scaffold containing rhBMP-2 and VEGF placed around the coronal part of the implant during insertion. The following advantages were postulated:

1. Sufficient volume stability and adequate bone consolidation are ensured by application of rhBMP-2 and VEGF directly on implantation site.
2. No membranes, screws or titan meshes are necessary to hold the augmentative materials in place or prevent soft tissue from ingrowth.
3. In comparison to other studies and techniques no consecutive surgery is necessary in order to remove foreign materials [49, 50].
4. The implant can be set directly at its ideal position. Simultaneously, the implant is able to integrate into

the residual bone and new vertical bone can grow at its top. Therefore, it can be used even where mini-implants are no option.

Moreover, this study was designed to verify whether rhBMP-2 and VEGF work synergistically in order to promote vertical bone growth. Former in vitro and in vivo studies suggested a positive effect on bone growth by using the combination of VEGF and rhBMP-2 [44, 48, 51] but it has not been tested for vertical bone augmentation in vivo yet.

Methods
Implants and scaffolds
The dental implants used were 11 mm in length and 3.5 mm in diameter (Nobel Replace Straight NP, Nobel Biocare, Goeteborg, Sweden). A disc–shaped scaffold of insoluble collagenous bone matrix (ICBM, 10 mm of diameter in total, inner diameter 3.5 mm, 5 mm of height and with a volume of 345 mm^3) was designed to exactly fit the coronal part of the implant whilst lying above the local bone. 138 µg rhBMP-2 (provided by Prof. Dr. W. Sebald, Wuerzburg, Germany) and 18.4 µg VEGF (Recombinant Human VEGF165 #293-VE-050, R&D Systems Europe, Ltd., Abington, United Kingdom) were applied onto the ICBM-Carrier.

Animal study
Twelve mini pigs (average body weight 66 kg of both genders) were treated in this study. They were kept according to official standards. The usage of mini pigs has been approved by the Animal Ethics Committee of the University of Duesseldorf.

For all surgical procedures animals underwent general anaesthesia. Preoperatively the animals were sedated by the use of 10 mg/kgKG Ketamin (Ketavet®, Pfizer, Karlsruhe, Germany) and 5 mg/kgKG Azaperon (Stresnil®, Janssen-Cilag, Neuss, Germany). General anaesthesia was induced by Thiopental (Thiopental inresa®, Inresa Arzneimittel GmbH, Freiburg, Germany), followed by endotracheal intubation. Endotracheal anaesthesia was performed by using Isofluran for induction and maintenance. In addition, for intraoperative pain management 0.5 ml Piritramid (Dipidolor®, Janssen-Cilag, Neuss, Germany) and Arti-cainhydrochloride (Ultracain® DS, 1:200.000, Aventis, Frankfurt, Germany) were used. For dental extraction, the oral cavity was cleaned by antiseptic mouthwash (Hexoral®, Pfizer, Karlsruhe, Germany), gingival margins were cut and relieving incisions were made. The mucoperiosteal flap was raised and the two premolars and the first molar teeth were removed. Bone ridges were flattened, plastic reconstruction of the extraction site and subsequent saliva proof wound closure was performed (Vicryl® 2/0, Ethicon GmbH, Norderstedt, Germany).

After 3 months 108 dental implants were inserted into the mandible (72 implants) and the tibia (36 implants) of the 12 mini pigs. All surgery was performed under sterile conditions in a veterinary operating theatre. The intraorally, gingival margins were cut, relieving incisions were made and a mucoperiosteal flap was elevated. Three implants on each side of the mandible were inserted according to manufacturer's instructions. They were implanted overlapping the residing bone by 5 mm. Depending on the experimental group the implant was either allowed to heal by itself (group 1), covered with ICBM (group 2), covered with ICBM containing rhBMP-2 (group 3), or covered by ICBM containing rhBMP-2 and VEGF (group 4). The periosteum was incised allowing the mucoperiosteal flap to tensionless cover the implanted area. Saliva-proof wound closure was performed by interrupted sutures using Vicryl 2.0. At the tibia, bone was exposed over a distance of 10 cm by atraumatic preparation towards the bone after incision of the skin and the subcutaneous tissue. The periosteum was incised and implants were inserted following manufacturer's instructions according to test groups. A multi-layered wound closure was performed by interrupted sutures using Vicryl 2.0.

During surgery and for 3 days postoperatively the mini pigs received oral antibiotic coverage (Amoxicillin 10 mg/kg body weight, Duphamox LA®, Fort Dodge, Wuerselen, Germany) and decongestant medication (Carproven p.o. 4.4 mg/kg body weight, Rimadyl®, Pfizer, Karlsruhe, Germany). 4 of the animals were euthanized by pentobarbital overdosing (Eutha 77® ad us. vet, Essex Pharma, Muenchen, Germany) after 2, 4 and 12 weeks, respectively. Afterwards, tibial and mandibular block specimens were harvested.

Histological and histomorphometric preparation
Specimens were fixed in 4% formaldehyde, dehydrated, embedded in Technovit® 7200 VLC (Heraeus Kulzer GmbH, Wehrheim, Germany), and polymerized. Utilizing the cutting-grinding technique according to Donath, longitudinal sections were grounded to about 20–40 µm for conventional microscopy (EXACT-Apparatebau, Norderstedt, Germany). Samples were stained according to manufacturer's protocols with Masson-Trichrom-Goldner and toluidine blue. To examine, evaluate, and photograph the specimens light microscopes (Leica DM 5000B, Leica Microsystems, Wetzlar, Germay, and Olympus BX50, Olympus, Hamburg, Germany) equipped with a microscopic high resolution camera (Leica DFC 40020C, Leica Wetzlar, Germany) were used. With the help of image measuring software (Cell D®, Soft Imaging System, Muenster, Germany and Leica Application-Suite LA5 V3.7 Leica Microsystems Imaging Solutions Ltd., 2003, Wetzlar, Germany) four main measurements were performed: Bone-to implant-contact % (BIC%) was

measured by manually marking the areas in which bone was attached to the surface of the implant using 40-fold magnification. The result was then divided by the measured length of the implant including windings and multiplied by 100. Bone-volume-density % (BVD%) was measured marking a distinct $2mm^2$ area, one side of the cube touching the residing bone and one side touching the implant. Within the cube the measurement software (colour coded and manually adjusted beforehand) detected the percentage of newly generated young bone. Furthermore, the length of the defect and the most coronal bone-implant-contact were measured. Using those two parameters, the amount of newly generated periimplant vertical bone (periimplant vertical bone gain = PVBG) could be calculated. Moreover, by dividing the measured most coronal bone formation by the length of the defect, vertical bone gain (VBG) in total was calculated.

Statistical analysis

Seventy seven implants were used for evaluation (51 Mandible, 26 Tibia). Twenty seven implants were separated for a different study. Four specimens were lost during preparation process. A Kolmogorov-Smirnov-Test was used to detect normal distribution of values. A linear regression analysis was executed to detect dependencies. $P < 0.05$ was set for a significant divergence, whereas $p > 0,01$ was considered to be highly significant. Calculations were performed by the use of SPSS

21 for Windows (SPSS Inc., Chicago, IL, USA) and with the help of Dr. Wolfgang Kaisers (CBiBs, Heinrich-Heine-University Duesseldorf, Deutschland).

Results

Light microscopic examinations of the control group and the ICBM group showed no or very little new bone formation after 2 weeks (Fig. 1). Around implants covered by ICBM + BMP-2 and ICBM + BMP-2 + VEGF islands of osteoid could be found within the area of the ICBM-scaffold. After 4 weeks in all groups new bone was formed. In the ICBM + BMP-2 + VEGF group new bone grew circumferentially around the implant presenting trabecular bone and primary bone marrow. After 12 weeks of healing all groups presented trabecular bone formation and primary bone marrow. Areas of dense lamellar bone showed around implants with ICBM + BMP-2 + VEGF (Fig. 2).

Slight bone-to implant-contact (Fig. 3) was noticeable in all groups after 2 weeks (Table 1). ICBM and ICBM + BMP-2 + VEGF covered implants showed the highest mean values (ICBM 34.4% (±8.9%), ICBM + BMP-2 + VEGF 30.2% (±11.7%)). The other two groups showed less bone-to implant-contact. In terms of bone-volume density the ICBM group started off with the highest value of 10.3% (±7.9%) whereas there was no BVD measurable in the control group. Vertical bone gain (VBG) showed to be almost the same in ICBM + BMP-2 (45% (±40%)) and ICBM + BMP-2+ VEGF (46% (±54%)). In the ICBM

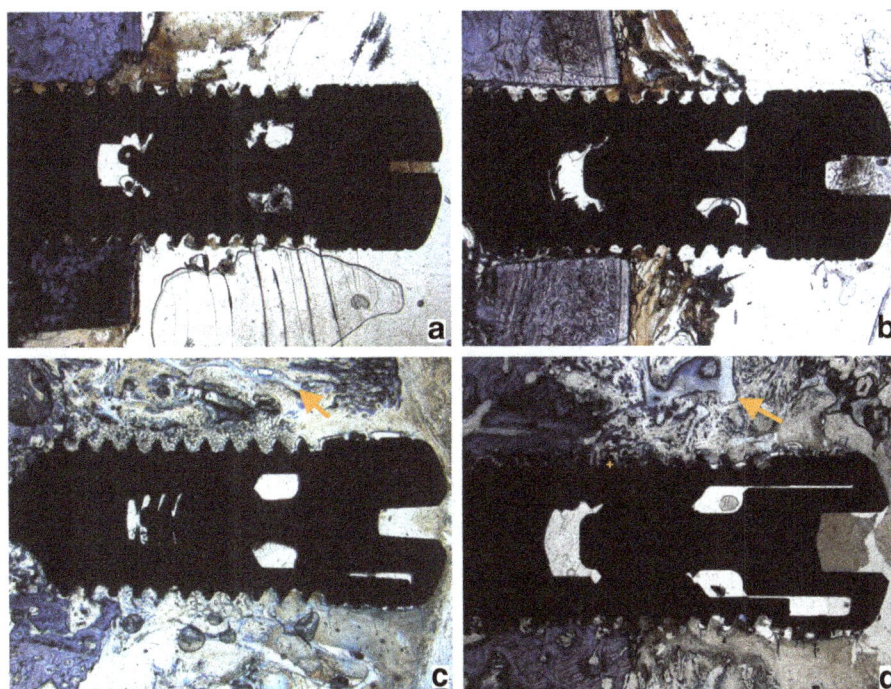

Fig. 1 Histological results after 2 weeks: **a** Implant by itself, **b** Implant with ICBM-Carrier, **c** Implant with ICBM-Carrier and rhBMP-2, **d** Implant with ICBM, rhBMP-2 and VEGF, + indicates new bone formation around the windings of the implant, → indicates islands of newly formed osteoid matrix

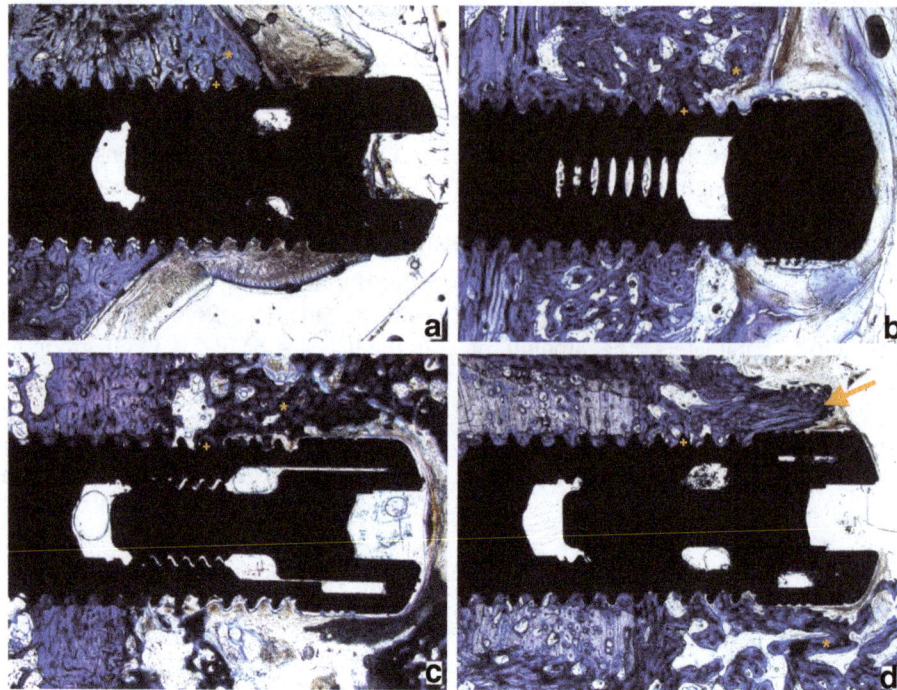

Fig. 2 Histological results after 12 weeks: **a** Implant by itself, **b** Implant with ICBM-Carrier, **c** Implant with ICBM-Carrier and rhBMP-2, **d** Implant with ICBM, rhBMP-2 and VEGF, + indicates new bone formation around the winding of the implant, * indicates newly formed trabeculae of woven bone, → indicates lamellar bone

group an average of (17% (±8%)) was calculated. There was no VBG measurable in specimens containing only the implant. In terms of periimplant vertical bone ICBM + BMP-2 reached 3.1 mm (±3.1 mm) and ICBM + BMP-2 + VEGF came to 3.1 mm (±3 mm) after 2 weeks. Upon 4 weeks of the healing mean BIC percentages varied from 38.9% (±10.37%) in the ICBM group to 49.3% (±19.7%) in the ICBM + BMP-2 + VEGF group. BVD percentages varied even more. The average BVD (Fig. 4) regarding the implant on its own was

15.8% (±22.57%). A measured negative value (below zero) equalled bone resorption. ICBM + BMP-2 + VEGF came to 61.3% (±14.5). Vertical bone gain (Fig. 5) shows a similar distribution. Mean VBG in the control group was measured 24% (±29%), whereas ICBM + BMP-2 + VEGF group averages measured ICBM + BMP-2 + VEGF 91% (±40%). Periimplant vertical bone gain (Fig. 6) sums up to 1.34 mm (±2.3 mm) in the control group, to 4.34 mm (±4.5 mm) in the ICBM-group, 4 mm (±3.1 mm) in the ICBM + BMP-2

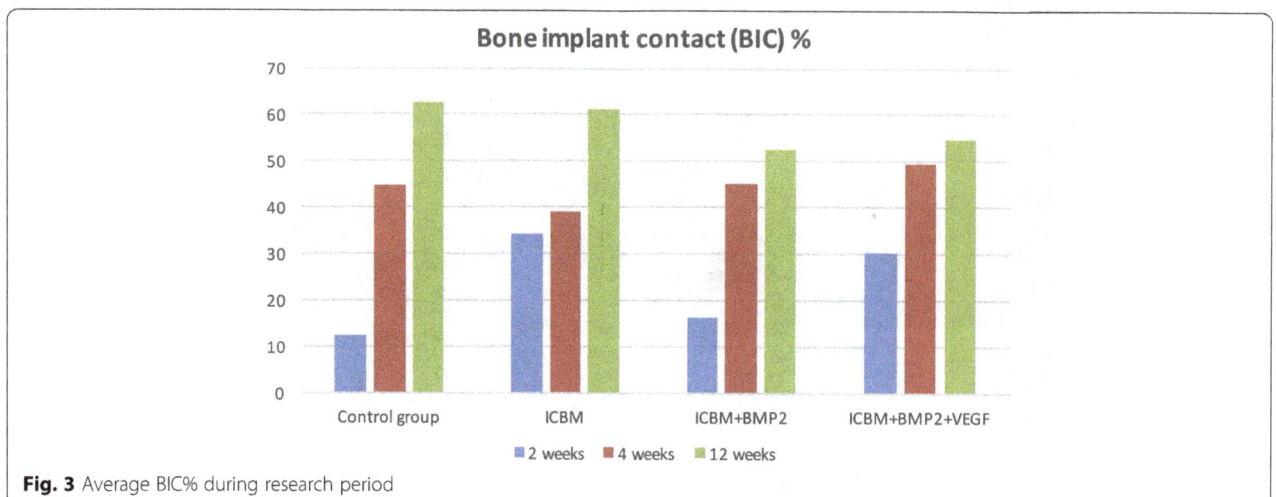

Fig. 3 Average BIC% during research period

Table 1 Summary of measured mean values for Bone-implant-contact, Bone-volume-density, Vertical-bone-gain and periimplant-vertical-bone gain

	Control group	ICBM	ICBM + BMP-2	ICBM + BMP-2 + VEGF
BIC%				
2 weeks	12.5	34.4	16.3	30.2
4 weeks	44.6	38.9	45	49.3
12 weeks	62.7	61.3	52.7	54.7
BVD%				
2 weeks	0	10.3	3	6.1
4 weeks	15.8	31.4	33.1	61.3
12 weeks	27.5	55.8	46.1	65
VBG%				
2 weeks	0	17	45	48
4 weeks	24	64	53	91
12 weeks	48	42	84	94
PVBG (mm)				
2 weeks	0	1.1	3.1	3.1
4 weeks	1.3	4.3	4	7.6
12 weeks	2.1	3.1	5.7	5.8

group and 7.6 mm (±3.01 mm) in the ICBM + BMP-2 + VEGF group. After 12 weeks mean BIC percentages for control and ICBM groups were almost equal accounting for 62.7%, (±15.1%) for the implant alone and 61.3% (±16.2%) for ICBM. ICBM + BMP-2 and ICBM + BMP-2 + VEGF stayed behind. Implants covered by ICBM + BMP-2 + VEGF showed the highest percentages (65% (±20.5%)).

The lowest values were found in the control group (27.5% (±47.6%)). Vertical bone gain (VBG) in specimens containing only the implant added up to 48% (±83%). Those implants being covered by ICBM + BMP-2 + VEGF

added up to 94% (±54%). In terms of vertical bone gain around the implant (PVBG) ICBM + BMP-2 (5.8 mm (±3.2 mm)) and ICBM + BMP-2 + VEGF (5.6 mm (±3.8 mm)) groups showed similar values after 12 weeks and the control group displayed (2.1 mm (±3.6 mm)) of gained bone height (Table 1). Statistically significant differences could be seen in vertical bone gain between control and ICBM + BMP-2 + VEGF groups ($p = 0.0158$). Highly significant differences were detected in bone-volume density ($p = 0.0011$) and in periimplant vertical bone gain ($p = 0.0018$) between the control and the ICBM + BMP-2 + VEGF group.

With the intention of using as few animals as possible, implants were inserted into the tibia and into the lower jaw. Although bone recovery differs and the exposure to bacteria in the oral cavity is missing, the tibia equals the lower jaw best in terms of bone size and volume. Furthermore, oral hygiene cannot be managed in mini-pigs, resulting in an increased loss of implants. Overall, implants inserted into the tibia showed higher values than implants inserted into the lower jaw but in order to get a reliable statistical outcome results could not be analysed separately (Table 2).

Discussion

All individual parts of this study were subject of former research studies. RhBMP-2 has proven to enhance bone regeneration adjacent to dental implants [52]. VEGF is known to induce angiogenesis [45, 46, 53]. Bai et al. [54] and Lin et al. [55] tested the combination of rhBMP-2 and VEGF, which seems to accelerate bone healing. Different carrier materials [2, 5, 34, 56, 57] have been examined but the ultimate carrier is yet to be found. ICBM itself has shown bone regenerative capacity in combination with embryonal stem cells [58, 59]. A combination of all of those materials in vivo, however, has never been described before.

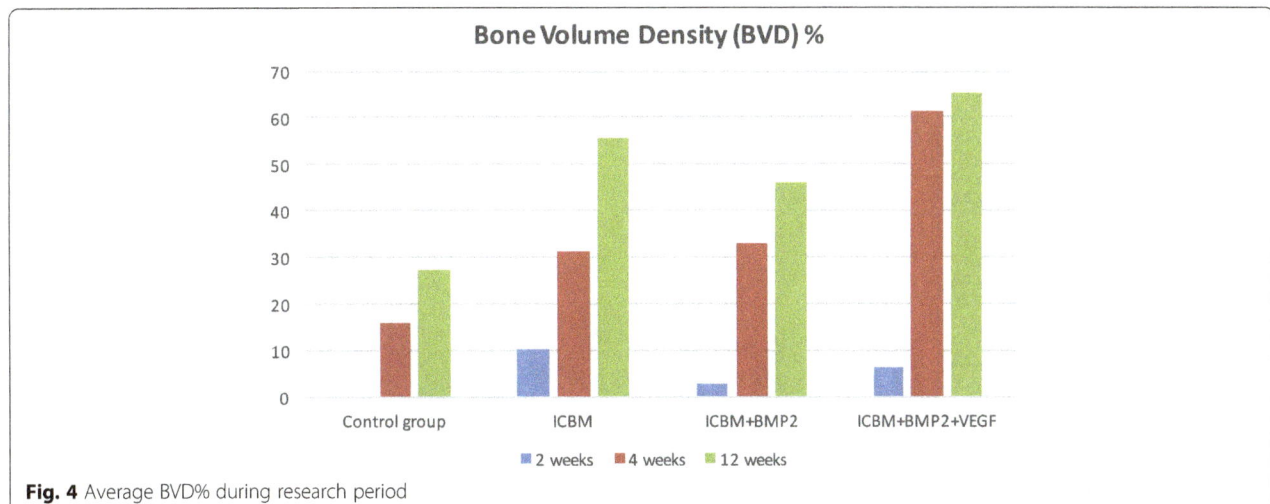

Fig. 4 Average BVD% during research period

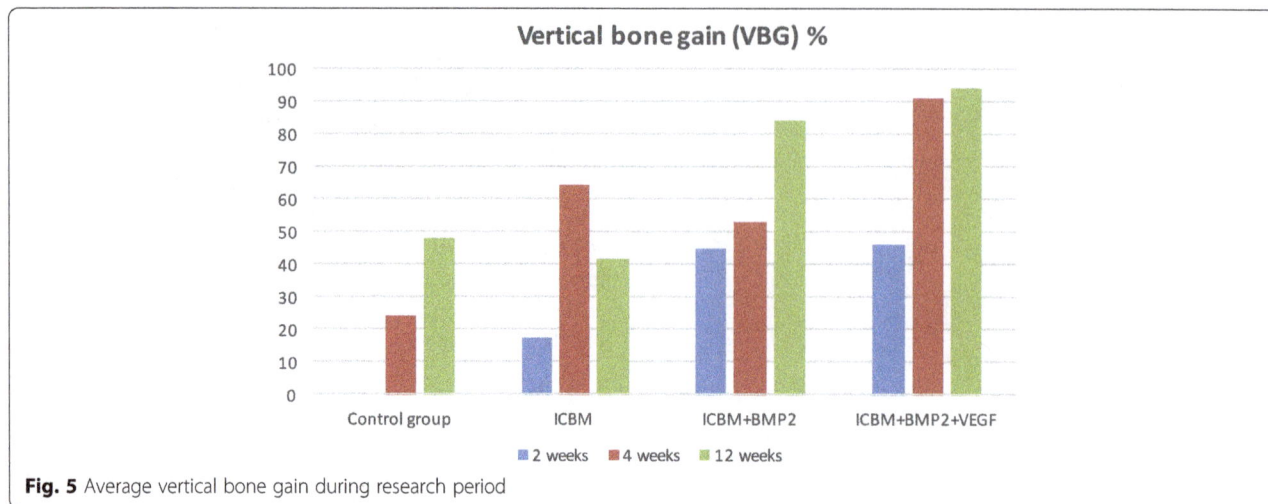

Fig. 5 Average vertical bone gain during research period

The surface of dental implants is decisive for chemotaxis and cell activation [60]. Sand-blasted and acid etched surfaces are particularly useful for reliable osseointegration of dental implants [6, 61, 62]. Titan implants with sand-blasted and acid etched surfaces were used as control group in this study. During the 12 week-period of this study linear bone growth could be detected. To release cytokines at implantation site, a carrier system is needed [63]. Ideally, the carrier emits cytokines continuously over a longer period and simultaneously serves as a stable scaffold for immigrating cells. Giesenhagen harvested disc-shaped autogenous bone blocks of the chin and placed them around the coronal part of the implant. He found them to be particularly helpful in regeneration of three-dimensional vertical bone defects [64]. Carrel et al. 3D printed a tricalciumphosphate and hydroxyapatite scaffold to enhance three - dimensional bone augmentation [57]. The meta-analysis by Troeltzsch et al. indicated that bone blocks significantly enhanced horizontal augmentation in comparison to particulate materials. In terms of vertical augmentation beneficial results depended on the origin of the bone block material [17]. In this study disc-shaped collagenous scaffolds (ICBM carrier) were used fitting precisely around the coronal part of the implants. Results showed that the ICBM alone seems to accelerate periimplant bone regeneration. After 2 weeks, implants covered with ICBM reached higher values in every measurement in comparison to the control group. After 12 weeks, apart from BVD which was higher than in the control group (BVD Control group after 2 weeks 27.5% and BVD ICBM-after 2 weeks 55.8%), no or little difference could be seen. This might be due to collagenous structures of the ICBM acting as a scaffold for osteoblasts to migrate and generate new bone. Over time reabsorbing processes around the implant take place. Therefore, ICBM alone only seems to provide an advantage in vertical bone growth during the first 4 weeks of implantation.

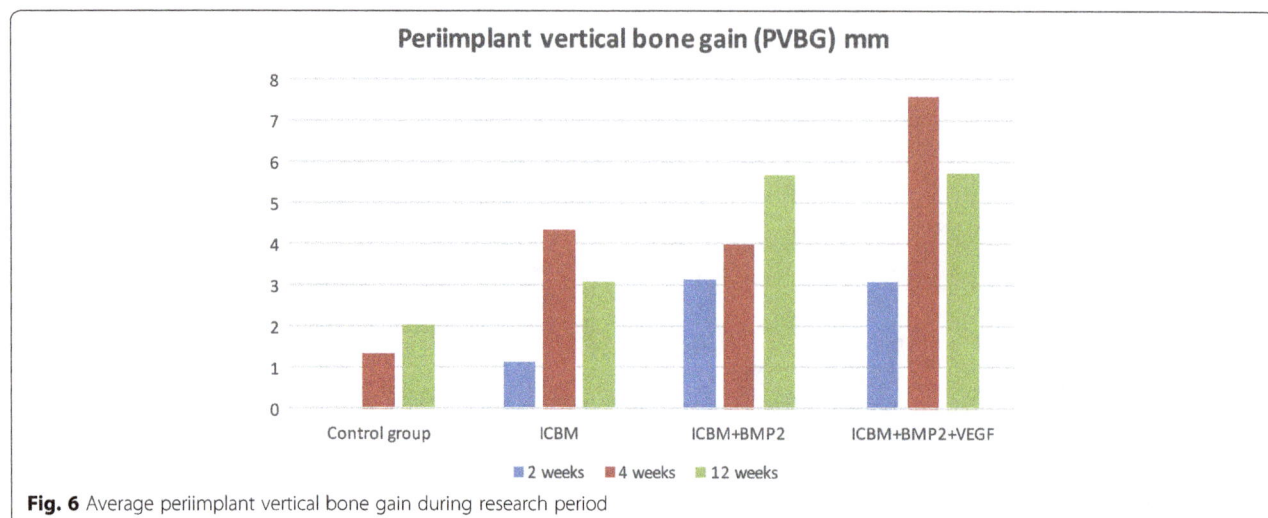

Fig. 6 Average periimplant vertical bone gain during research period

Table 2 Summary of mean values for Bone-implant-contact, Bone-volume-density, Vertical-bone-gain and periimplant-vertical-bone gain divided into mandible and tibia

	Control Group		ICBM-Carrier		ICBM + BMP-2		ICBM + BMP-2 + VEGF	
	Mandible	Tibia	Mandible	Tibia	Mandible	Tibia	Mandible	Tibia
BIC%								
2 weeks	no data	12.5	no data	34.4	18.4	14.1	42	10.7
4 weeks	44.6	no data	39.6	37.4	40.3	73.3	43.8	60.4
12 weeks	68.1	51.8	43.3	70.3	49.1	57.2	49.4	65.2
BVD%								
2 weeks	no data	0	no data	10.3	5.9	0	9.7	0
4 weeks	15.8	no data	13.5	67.1	1.1	68.6	58.5	66.9
12 weeks	0	82.4	2.1	82.7	42.9	50	59.7	75.6
VBG%								
2 weeks	no data	0	no data	17.3	40	35.1	46.1	44.9
4 weeks	24	no data	30.1	137.2	41.8	117.5	66.1	139.8
12 weeks	0	143.4	0.6	62.6	38.4	141	66.8	148.8
PVBG (mm)								
2 weeks	no data	0	no data	1.1	4.4	1.9	3.2	3.1
4 weeks	1.3	no data	2.5	8	3.5	6.7	5.9	10.9
12 weeks	0	6.2	0.1	4.9	3.1	9	5	7.2

Recombinant rhBMP-2 enhances bone regeneration [2, 65, 66]. RhBMP-2 initiates differentiation of embryonal stem cells into chondroblasts, osteoblasts or adipocytes. While lower concentrations of rhBMP-2 are assumed to boost initial chondrification higher concentrations are supposed to enhance osteogenesis [67]. Over the entire examination period ICBM + BMP-2 showed lower BIC% values compared to the implant alone. However, measured values of VBG, PVBG and BVD were higher compared to the control group. A study of Jones et al. showed a similar outcome. RhBMP-2 induced periimplant bone regeneration showed a higher BIC%, more new bone formation and a better filling of the defect after 4 weeks but after 12 weeks no difference was detectable anymore [2]. This effect was thought to be due to negative feedback mechanisms of the rhBMP-2 signalling cascade putting a break on new bone formation. Nevertheless, given that case, VBG, PVBG and BVD would decrease as well. A different explanation could be a lack of angiogenesis to support rhBMP-2-accelerated bone growth. Matsubara et al. stated that bone formation can be delayed in order to ensure sufficient vascularization [68]. This could explain the reduced growth rate after 4 weeks. The carrier-complex itself might also be the reason for a reduced BIC in comparison to the control group. Directly around the implant concentrations of rhBMP-2 might have been lower than at the centre of the ring (approximately 2 mm away from implant surface). Three possible explanations might be: 1. more rhBMP-2 was available in these areas,

2. less rhBMP-2 was necessary for sufficient bone growth or 3. rhBMP-2 could be used more effectively. In a similar study Refaat et al. used ICBM-Carriers and rhBMP-2 for spinal fusion. They used much lower doses of rhBMP-2 (2 µg and 10 µg). RhBMP-2 was released by 100% within 20 days, irrespective of the dose provided [69]. If these results were to be transferred to this study, a positive effect of BMP2 would only be possible in the first 4 weeks after implantation.

Angiogenesis is crucial for bone formation. Local application of VEGF prolongs angiogenesis at defect sites and therefore reinforces osteogenesis [46, 47]. For craniofacial and mandibular bone in particular, sufficient amounts of VEGF are necessary for ossification [48]. Peng et al. examined the synergistic potential of rhBMP-2 and VEGF. Outcomes described a dependant relationship between these two [70]. Jiang et al. found increased bone generation combining VEGF and rhBMP-2 compared to only using one of them. Furthermore, they stated VEGF to be the determining factor of enhancement in bone formation in vitro [44]. The present in vivo study supports those findings. Measured results of ICBM + BMP-2 + VEGF were similar or higher compared to ICBM + BMP-2. Especially bone volume density and vertical bone gain were substantially higher after 4 and 12 weeks of the healing process compared to ICBM + BMP-2. There might even be a higher dependency of rhBMP-2 and VEGF than formerly thought. According to Matsubara et al. vascular endothelial cells and muscle cells are supposed to be the primary source of rhBMP-2 expression during osteogenesis. Results of their studies showed that mainly blood vessels release rhBMP-2 and mesenchymal stem cells synthesize VEGF [68]. In this study ICBM + BMP-2 + VEGF showed a rapid bone growth which wears off after 4 weeks in comparison to implants alone. These results indicate along with other studies [55] that prolonged artificial high levels of VEGF over the physiological period of 31 days do not improve bone healing. This might be due to decreasing VEGF and rhBMP-2 levels according to consumption over time. Kumar et al. solved this problem by using stem cells producing VEGF and rhBMP-2 [47]. To sum up, the combination of ICBM + BMP-2 + VEGF significantly outranks implants alone in terms of bone volume density, vertical bone gain and periimplant vertical bone gain. Only short term improvement of bone to implant contact could be seen.

This study being an animal study, the number of samples had to be held small. Therefore, values varied significantly. In order to get more reliable results further research has yet to follow.

Conclusion

Results of this study suggest that the combination of rhBMP-2 and VEGF applied locally by using a collagenous carrier enhances vertical bone generation around the implant in vivo. In defect areas high quality and quantity of bone could be detected in comparison to implants alone, implants covered with ICBM and implants covered with ICBM+ rhBMP-2. A one stage procedure and the use of a collagenous disc-shaped scaffold reduced the number of surgery to a minimum, eliminated donor site morbidity and maintained satisfactory volume stability as there was only little resorption over time.

Further investigations have yet to show how rhBMP-2 and VEGF can be used in a safe and predictable way in order to use them for bone regeneration in clinical routines.

Abbreviations
GBR: Guided bone regeneration; ICBM: Insoluble collagenous bone matrix; rhBMP-2: Recombinant human bone morphogenetic protein-2; VEGF: Vascular endothelial growth factor

Acknowledgements
The authors thank Prof. Sager and Mrs. Schrey for their support in carrying out the experimental animal studies, Dr. Kaisers for the help with data analysis and Dr. Berr for the help with laboratory work.

Funding
Implants were generously donated by Nobel Biocare, Goeteborg, Sweden rhBMP-2 was generously donated by Prof. Dr. W. Sebald, Wuerzburg, Germany.

Authors' contributions
NRK made substantial contributions to conception and study design; RD and CN performed surgery; LS performed the histological examination; RD, LS analyzed and interpreted the data; LS, CS and RD were major contributors in writing the manuscript. CN and MO were involved in revising the manuscript critically. All authors read and approved the final manuscript.

Authors' information
Not applicable.

Competing interests
The authors declare that they have no competing interests.

Consent for publication
Not applicable.

Ethics approval
The animal study has been approved by the Animal Ethics Committee of the University of Duesseldorf (G/90/2005).

Author details
[1]Department of Oral-, Maxillo- and Plastic Facial Surgery, Heinrich-Heine-University Duesseldorf, Moorenstr. 5, 40225 Duesseldorf, Germany. [2]Department of Operative and Preventive Dentistry and Endodontics, Heinrich-Heine-University Duesseldorf, Moorenstr. 5, Duesseldorf 40225, Germany.

References
1. Cochran DL, Schenk R, Buser D, Wozney JM, Jones AA. Recombinant human bone morphogenetic protein-2 stimulation of bone formation around endosseous dental implants. J Periodontol. 1999;70:139–50.
2. Jones AA, Buser D, Schenk R, Wozney J, Cochran DL. The effect of rhBMP-2 around endosseous implants with and without membranes in the canine model. J Periodontol. 2006;77:1184–93.
3. Clementini M, Morlupi A, Canullo L, Agrestini C, Barlattani A. Success rate of dental implants inserted in horizontal and vertical guided bone regenerated areas: a systematic review. Int J Oral Maxillofac Surg. 2012;41:847–52.
4. Daga D, Mehrotra D, Mohammad S, Singh G, Natu SM. Tentpole technique for bone regeneration in vertically deficient alveolar ridges: a review. J Oral Biol Craniofac Res. 2015;5:92–7.
5. Sigurdsson TJ, Nygaard L, Tatakis DN, Fu E, Turek TJ, Jin L, et al. Periodontal repair in dogs: evaluation of rhBMP-2 carriers. Int J Periodontics Restorative Dent. 1996;16:524–37.
6. Esposito M, Grusovin MG, Felice P, Karatzopoulos G, Worthington HV, Coulthard P. The efficacy of horizontal and vertical bone augmentation procedures for dental implants - a Cochrane systematic review. Eur J Oral Implantol. 2009;2:167–84.
7. Restoy-Lozano A, Dominguez-Mompell JL, Infante-Cossio P, Lara-Chao J, Espin-Galvez F, Lopez-Pizarro V. Reconstruction of mandibular vertical defects for dental implants with autogenous bone block grafts using a tunnel approach: clinical study of 50 cases. Int J Oral Maxillofac Surg. 2015;44:1416–22.
8. Zakhary IE, El-Mekkawi HA, Elsalanty ME. Alveolar ridge augmentation for implant fixation: status review. Oral Surg Oral med Oral Pathol Oral Radiol. 2012;114:S179–89.
9. Octavi CF, Genis BB, Rui F, Jung RE, Cosme GE, Eduard VC. Interventions for dental implant placement in atrophic edentulous mandibles: vertical bone augmentation and alternative treatments. A meta-analysis of randomized clinical trials. J Periodontol. 2016;87:1–23.
10. Nosouhian S, Rismanchian M, Sabzian R, Shadmehr E, Badrian H, Davoudi A. A mini-review on the effect of mini-implants on contemporary orthodontic science. J Int Oral Health. 2015;7:83–7.
11. Schuckert KH, Jopp S, Osadnik M. Modern bone regeneration instead of bone transplantation: a combination of recombinant human bone morphogenetic protein-2 and platelet-rich plasma for the vertical

augmentation of the maxillary bone-a single case report. Tissue Eng Part C Methods. 2010;16:1335–46.

12. Handschel J, Meyer U, Wiesmann HP. Embryonic stem cell use. In: Meyer U, Meyer T, Handschel J, Wiesmann HP, editors. Fundamentals of tissue engineering and regenerative medicine. Heidelberg: Springer-Verlag; 2009. p. 159–66.

13. Keestra JA, Barry O, Jong L, Wahl G. Long-term effects of vertical bone augmentation: a systematic review. J Appl Oral Sci. 2016;24:3–17.

14. Kahnberg KE, Nystrom E, Bartholdsson L. Combined use of bone grafts and Branemark fixtures in the treatment of severely resorbed maxillae. Int J Oral Maxillofac Implants. 1989;4:297–304.

15. Marx RE, Shellenberger T, Wimsatt J, Correa P. Severely resorbed mandible: predictable reconstruction with soft tissue matrix expansion (tent pole) grafts. J Oral Maxillofac Surg. 2002;60:878–88. discussion 888-879

16. Wannfors K, Johansson C, Donath K. Augmentation of the mandible via a "tent-pole" procedure and implant treatment in a patient with type III osteogenesis imperfecta: clinical and histologic considerations. Int J Oral Maxillofac Implants. 2009;24:1144–8.

17. Troeltzsch M, Troeltzsch M, Kauffmann P, Gruber R, Brockmeyer P, Moser N, et al. Clinical efficacy of grafting materials in alveolar ridge augmentation: a systematic review. J Craniomaxillofac Surg. 2016;44:1618–29.

18. Fahmy RA, Mahmoud N, Soliman S, Nouh SR, Cunningham L, El-Ghannam A. Acceleration of alveolar ridge augmentation using a low dose of recombinant human bone morphogenetic protein-2 loaded on a Resorbable bioactive ceramic. J Oral Maxillofac Surg. 2015;73:2257–72.

19. Felice P, Checchi V, Pistilli R, Scarano A, Pellegrino G, Esposito M. Bone augmentation versus 5-mm dental implants in posterior atrophic jaws. Four-month post-loading results from a randomised controlled clinical trial. Eur J Oral Implantol. 2009;2:267–81.

20. Felice P, Marchetti C, Piattelli A, Pellegrino G, Checchi V, Worthington H, et al. Vertical ridge augmentation of the atrophic posterior mandible with interpositional block grafts: bone from the iliac crest versus bovine anorganic bone. Eur J Oral Implantol. 2008;1:183–98.

21. Felice P, Pistilli R, Lizio G, Pellegrino G, Nisii A, Marchetti C. Inlay versus onlay iliac bone grafting in atrophic posterior mandible: a prospective controlled clinical trial for the comparison of two techniques. Clin Implant Dent Relat res. 2009;11(Suppl 1):e69–82.

22. Felice P, Scarano A, Pistilli R, Checchi L, Piattelli M, Pellegrino G, et al. A comparison of two techniques to augment maxillary sinuses using the lateral window approach: rigid synthetic resorbable barriers versus anorganic bovine bone. Five-month post-loading clinical and histological results of a pilot randomised controlled clinical trial. Eur J Oral Implantol. 2009;2:293–306.

23. Chiapasco M, Di Martino G, Anello T, Zaniboni M, Romeo E. Fresh frozen versus autogenous iliac bone for the rehabilitation of the extremely atrophic maxilla with onlay grafts and endosseous implants: preliminary results of a prospective comparative study. Clin Implant Dent Relat res. 2015;17(Suppl 1):e251–66.

24. Becker W, Clokie C, Sennerby L, Urist MR, Becker BE. Histologic findings after implantation and evaluation of different grafting materials and titanium micro screws into extraction sockets: case reports. J Periodontol. 1998;69:414–21.

25. Lang NP, Hammerle CH, Bragger U, Lehmann B, Nyman SR. Guided tissue regeneration in jawbone defects prior to implant placement. Clin Oral Implants res. 1994;5:92–7.

26. Rocchietta I, Fontana F, Simion M. Clinical outcomes of vertical bone augmentation to enable dental implant placement: a systematic review. J Clin Periodontol. 2008;35:203–15.

27. Buser D, Bragger U, Lang NP, Nyman S. Regeneration and enlargement of jaw bone using guided tissue regeneration. Clin Oral Implants res. 1990;1:22–32.

28. Gotfredsen K, Nimb L, Buser D, Hjorting-Hansen E. Evaluation of guided bone generation around implants placed into fresh extraction sockets: an experimental study in dogs. J Oral Maxillofac Surg. 1993;51:879–84. discussion 885-876

29. Penarrocha MA, Vina JA, Maestre L, Penarrocha-Oltra D. Bilateral vertical ridge augmentation with block grafts and guided bone regeneration in the posterior mandible: a case report. J Oral Implantol. 2012;38 Spec No:533-537.

30. Chin M. Distraction osteogenesis for dental implants. Atlas Oral Maxillofac Surg Clin North Am. 1999;7:41–63.

31. Rachmiel A, Srouji S, Peled M. Alveolar ridge augmentation by distraction osteogenesis. Int J Oral Maxillofac Surg. 2001;30:510–7.

32. Wolvius EB, Scholtemeijer M, Weijland M, Hop WC, van der Wal KG. Complications and relapse in alveolar distraction osteogenesis in partially dentulous patients. Int J Oral Maxillofac Surg. 2007;36:700–5.

33. Gaggl A, Schultes G, Karcher H. Distraction implants: a new operative technique for alveolar ridge augmentation. J Craniomaxillofac Surg. 1999;27:214–21.

34. Asa'ad F, Pagni G, Pilipchuk SP, Gianni AB, Giannobile WV, Rasperini G. 3D-printed scaffolds and biomaterials: review of alveolar bone augmentation and periodontal regeneration applications. Int J Dent. 2016;2016:1239842.

35. Roccuzzo M, Savoini M, Dalmasso P, Ramieri G. Long-term outcomes of implants placed after vertical alveolar ridge augmentation in partially edentulous patients: a 10-year prospective clinical study. Clin Oral Implants Res. 2016; doi:10.1111/clr.12941.

36. Amini AR, Laurencin CT, Nukavarapu SP. Bone tissue engineering: recent advances and challenges. Crit rev Biomed Eng. 2012;40:363–408.

37. Roelen BA, Dijke P. Controlling mesenchymal stem cell differentiation by TGFBeta family members. J Orthop Sci. 2003;8:740–8.

38. Depprich RA. Biomolecule use in tissue engineering. In: Meyer U, Meyer T, Handschel J, Wiesmann HP, editors. Fundamentals of tissue engineering and regenerative engineering. Heildelberg: Springer-Verlag; 2009. p. 121–36.

39. Jamjoom A, Cohen RE. Grafts for ridge preservation. J Funct Biomater. 2015;6:833–48.

40. Wallace SC, Pikos MA, Prasad H. De novo bone regeneration in human extraction sites using recombinant human bone morphogenetic protein-2/ACS: a clinical, histomorphometric, densitometric, and 3-dimensional cone-beam computerized tomographic scan evaluation. Implant Dent. 2014;23:132–7.

41. Wikesjo UM, Qahash M, Huang YH, Xiropaidis A, Polimeni G, Susin C. Bone morphogenetic proteins for periodontal and alveolar indications; biological observations - clinical implications. Orthod Craniofac Res. 2009;12:263–70.

42. Jovanovic SA, Hunt DR, Bernard GW, Spiekermann H, Wozney JM, Wikesjo UM. Bone reconstruction following implantation of rhBMP-2 and guided bone regeneration in canine alveolar ridge defects. Clin Oral Implants res. 2007;18:224–30.

43. Glowacki J. Demineralized bone and BMPs: basic science and clinical utility. J Oral Maxillofac Surg. 2015;73:S126–31.

44. Jiang J, Fan CY, Zeng BF. Experimental construction of BMP2 and VEGF Gene modified tissue engineering bone in vitro. Int J Mol Sci. 2011;12:1744–55.

45. Neufeld G, Cohen T, Gengrinovitch S, Poltorak Z. Vascular endothelial growth factor (VEGF) and its receptors. Faseb J. 1999;13:9–22.

46. Kleinheinz J, Wiesmann HP, Stratmann U, Joos U. Beeinflussung der Angiogenese und Osteogenese unter dem Einfluss von vascular endothelial growth factor (VEGF). Mund-Kiefer GesichtsCHir. 2002;6:175–82.

47. Kumar S, Wan C, Ramaswamy G, Clemens TL, Ponnazhagan S. Mesenchymal stem cells expressing osteogenic and angiogenic factors synergistically enhance bone formation in a mouse model of segmental bone defect. Mol Ther. 2010;18:1026–34.

48. Duan X, Bradbury SR, Olsen BR, Berendsen AD. VEGF stimulates intramembranous bone formation during craniofacial skeletal development. Matrix Biol. 2016;52-54:127–40.

49. Katanec D, Granic M, Majstorovic M, Trampus Z, Panduric DG. Use of recombinant human bone morphogenetic protein (rhBMP2) in bilateral alveolar ridge augmentation: case report. Coll Antropol. 2014;38:325–30.

50. Stimmelmayr M, Beuer F, Schlee M, Edelhoff D, Guth JF. Vertical ridge augmentation using the modified shell technique–a case series. Br J Oral Maxillofac Surg. 2014;52:945–50.

51. Du Z, Chen J, Yan F, Doan N, Ivanovski S, Xiao Y. Serum bone formation marker correlation with improved osseointegration in osteoporotic rats treated with simvastatin. Clin Oral Implants Res. 2013;24:422–7.

52. Matin K, Senpuku H, Hanada N, Ozawa H, Ejiri S. Bone regeneration by recombinant human bone morphogenetic protein-2 around immediate implants: a pilot study in rats. Int J Oral Maxillofac Implants. 2003;18:211–7.

53. Cross MJ, Dixelius J, Matsumoto T, Claesson-Welsh L. VEGF-receptor signal transduction. Trends Biochem Sci. 2003;28:488–94.

54. Bai Y, Li P, Yin G, Huang Z, Liao X, Chen X, et al. BMP-2, VEGF and bFGF synergistically promote the osteogenic differentiation of rat bone marrow-derived mesenchymal stem cells. Biotechnol Lett. 2013;35:301–8.

55. Lin Z, Wang JS, Lin L, Zhang J, Liu Y, Shuai M, et al. Effects of BMP2 and VEGF165 on the osteogenic differentiation of rat bone marrow-derived mesenchymal stem cells. Exp Ther Med. 2014;7:625–9.

56. Schliephake H. Application of bone growth factors–the potential of different carrier systems. Oral Maxillofac Surg. 2010;14:17–22.

57. Carrel JP, Wiskott A, Moussa M, Rieder P, Scherrer S, Durual S. A 3D printed TCP/HA structure as a new osteoconductive scaffold for vertical bone augmentation. Clin Oral Implants Res. 2016;27:55–62.

58. Kahle M, Wiesmann HP, Berr K, Depprich RA, Kubler NR, Naujoks C, et al. Embryonic stem cells induce ectopic bone formation in rats. Biomed Mater Eng. 2010;20:371–80.

59. Langenbach F, Naujoks C, Kersten-Thiele PV, Berr K, Depprich RA, Kubler NR, et al. Osteogenic differentiation influences stem cell migration out of scaffold-free microspheres. Tissue Eng Part A. 2012;16:759–66.

60. Jennissen H, Zumbrink T, Chatzinikolaidou M, Steppuhn J. Biocoating of implants with mediator molecules: surface enhancement of metals by treatment with Chromosulfuric acid-Biologisierung von Implantaten mit Biomolekülen: Oberflächenveredelung von Metallen durch Behandlung mit Chromschwefelsäure. Weinheim: Wiley-VCH Verlag GmbH; 1999.

61. Novaes AB Jr, Souza SL, de Oliveira PT, Souza AM. Histomorphometric analysis of the bone-implant contact obtained with 4 different implant surface treatments placed side by side in the dog mandible. Int J Oral Maxillofac Implants. 2002;17:377–83.

62. Rammelt S, Schulze E, Bernhardt R, Hanisch U, Scharnweber D, Worch H, et al. Coating of titanium implants with type-I collagen. J Orthop Res. 2004;22:1025–34.

63. Li RH, Wozney JM. Delivering on the promise of bone morphogenetic proteins. Trends Biotechnol. 2001;19:255–65.

64. Giesenhagen B. Die einzeitige vertikale Augmentation mit ringförmigen Knochentransplantaten. Z Zahnärztl Impl. 2008;24:129–32.

65. Huh JB, Kim SE, Kim HE, Kang SS, Choi KH, Jeong CM, et al. Effects of anodized implants coated with Escherichia Coli-derived rhBMP-2 in beagle dogs. Int J Oral Maxillofac Surg. 2012;41:1577–84.

66. Weng D, Poehling S, Pippig S, Bell M, Richter EJ, Zuhr O, et al. The effects of recombinant human growth/differentiation factor-5 (rhGDF-5) on bone regeneration around titanium dental implants in barrier membrane-protected defects: a pilot study in the mandible of beagle dogs. Int J Oral Maxillofac Implants. 2009;24:31–7.

67. Zur Nieden NI, Kempka G, Rancourt DE, HJ AHR. Induction of chondro-, osteo-and adipogenesis in embryonic stem cells by bone morphogenetic protein-2: effect of cofactors on differentiating lineages. BMC Dev Biol. 2005;5:1.

68. Matsubara H, Hogan DE, Morgan EF, Mortlock DP, Einhorn TA, Gerstenfeld LC. Vascular tissues are a primary source of BMP2 expression during bone formation induced by distraction osteogenesis. Bone. 2012;51:168–80.

69. Refaat M, Klineberg EO, Fong MC, Garcia TC, Leach JK, Haudenschild DR. Binding to COMP reduces the BMP2 dose for spinal fusion in a rat model. Spine (Phila Pa 1976). 2016;41:E829–36.

70. Peng H, Usas A, Olshanski A, Ho AM, Gearhart B, Cooper GM, et al. VEGF improves, whereas sFlt1 inhibits, BMP2-induced bone formation and bone healing through modulation of angiogenesis. J Bone Miner Res. 2005;20:2017–27.

32

Classification and characterization of class III malocclusion in Chinese individuals

Cai Li, Ying Cai, Sihui Chen and Fengshan Chen*

Abstract

Background: Class III malocclusion is a maxillofacial disorder that is characterised by a concave profile and can be attributed to both genetic inheritance and environmental factors. It is a clinical challenge due to our limited understanding of its aetiology. Revealing its prototypical diversity will contribute to our sequential exploration of the underlying aetiological information. The objective of this study was to characterize phenotypic variations of Class III malocclusion via a lateral cephalometric analysis in a community of Chinese individuals.

Method: One-hundred-and-forty-four individuals (58 males ≥18 and 86 females ≥16) with Class III malocclusion ranging from mild to severe were enrolled in this study. Principal component analysis and cluster analysis were performed using 61 lateral cephalometric measurements.

Results: Six principal components were discovered in the examined population and were responsible for 73.7 % of the variability. Four subtypes were revealed by cluster analysis. Subtype 1 included subjects with mild mandibular prognathism with a steep mandibular plane. Subjects in subtype 2 showed a combination of prognathic mandibular and retrusive maxillary with a flat or normal mandibular plane. Subtype 3 included individuals with purely severe mandibular prognathism and a normal mandibular plane. Individuals in subtype 4 had a mild maxillary deficiency and severe mandibular prognathism with the lowest mandibular plane angle.

Conclusion: The six principal components extracted among the 61 variables improve our knowledge of lateral cephalometric analysis for diagnoses. We successfully identified four Class III malocclusion subtypes, indicating that cluster analysis could supplement the classification of Class III malocclusion among a Chinese population and may assist in our on-going genetic study.

Keywords: Class III malocclusion, Mandibular prognathism, Subtypes, Multivariate, Principal component analysis, Cluster analysis

Background

Class III malocclusion has long been considered a complicated maxillofacial disorder that is characterised by a concave profile, which may exhibit mandibular protrusion, maxillary retrusion or a combination of both [1] as well as possible anatomic heterogeneity of this malocclusion. The prevalence of Class III malocclusion varies greatly both among and within populations, and the highest prevalence of 15.8 % has been observed in Southeast Asian populations in previous studies [2]. In recent years, it has been widely accepted that both genetic inheritance and environmental factors contribute to

Class III malocclusion [3, 4], and diversity loci and suspicious genes associated with Class III malocclusion have been identified using linkage analysis and association studies [4–10]. Although informative, the previous genetic studies have limitations, including modest sample sizes, the exclusion of environmental factors, the lack of a systematic estimation of genetic variants associated with the disease, and perhaps more importantly, limited phenotypes that cannot capture the complexities of Class III malocclusion [11]. Owing to the limited knowledge of the underlying aetiologies of this condition, it is still a challenge for dentists to diagnose and treat Class III malocclusion [12]. Distinguishing phenotypes that are related to different expressions of a genotype is an

* Correspondence: orthodboy@126.com
Department of Orthodontics, School & Hospital of Stomatology, Shanghai Engineering Research Centre of Tooth Restoration and Regeneration, Tongji University, Shanghai 200072, China

essential step in establishing the genetic contribution to Class III malocclusion.

Lateral cephalometric radiographs provide rich phenotypic data, which provide information about the cranial, facial bony and soft tissue structures. Cephalometric analysis is an economic and convenient accessory examination and plays a predominant role in approaching the definition of phenotypes among and within the Class III population [13, 14]. Recently, multivariate analyses such as discriminant analyses, principal component analyses (PCA) and cluster analyses have been used to distinguish the phenotypic variations of Class III malocclusion in several studies [11, 14–16]. PCA is a powerful method that is used to provide an overview of complex multivariate data [17]. In contrast, cluster analysis complements PCA organized variables to select homogeneous information such that the underlying phenotype may be identified. This method has also been applied to determine the subtypes of other diseases [18–20].

A large sample of patients with Class III malocclusion from the University of North Carolina was studied by Bui et al., including a wide age range from 5.9 to 56.3 years and racial diversity [14]. In this study, five clusters were identified to represent distinct subtypes via PCA and cluster analyses. Recently, Moreno Uribe et al. characterized Class III malocclusion phenotypes by using the same method with 63 cephalometric measures derived from 292 Caucasian adults. The PCA reduced 63 cephalometric variables into six principal components that explained 81 % of the variability within the samples, and the cluster analysis classified the individuals into five distinct subtypes, which differed from the findings of previous research [11].

Although a few previous studies have contributed to the characterization of Class III malocclusion, there is still uncertainty about whether Class III phenotypic classifications can be generalizable to other samples and populations. We may identify different phenotypic subgroups specific to the Chinese population. Our group has been engaged in genetic studies of Class III malocclusion and has obtained important findings [21–23]. In this study, we aimed to identify additional phenotypic variation within a large group of Chinese samples using methods similar to those of Moreno Uribe. These findings will facilitate clinical diagnoses and will enhance future genetic studies.

Methods

Study samples

We enrolled 144 subjects (58 males ≥18 and 86 females ≥16), with a clinical diagnosis of Class III malocclusion who were seeking orthodontic treatment at the Affiliated Stomatology Hospital of Tongji University from January 2014 to September 2015. The subjects ranged in age from 16 to 35 years, with a mean age of approximately 23 (22.61 ± 4.58) years. All participants were of Han Chinese ancestry and their conditions ranged from mild to severe phenotypes, and the patients all met at least two of the eligibility criteria (Table 1), including an ANB angle (Point A-Nasion-Point B) of the centric jaw relationship < 0.0°, an anterior crossbite, and a Wits appraisal greater than –2.0 mm [3, 4, 24]. Participants who had previous orthodontic treatments, congenital abnormalities (e.g., cleft lip and palate), severe facial trauma, or general physical disease (e.g., endocrine diseases) were excluded.

Cephalometric analysis

All the lateral cephalograms involved in our study were digital films. The exposures were made by a standardized technique with the patients' jaws in centric occlusion with an equipment of dental X-ray (Veraviewepocs X550, Kyoto, Japan). Captured images were saved as JPG files. The obtained digital radiographs were then standardized with a 10-mm ruler and imported into the NemoCeph NX software (version 6.0, Nemotec, Madrid, Spain). Cephalometric tracing and measurement were performed using the analysis software with a computer by an experienced orthodontist. Sixty-one cephalometric parameters digitized with 20 skeletal landmarks and 10 soft tissue landmarks were selected, which represented comprehensive craniofacial information, including information about the skeletal structure, teeth, soft tissue and their relationships to each other (Table 2). An additional file shows the data of the cephalometric analysis in more detail (see Additional file 1). A sample of 15 random lateral cephalograms were traced twice at least 2 weeks apart. The reliability of the landmark location (intraexaminer agreement) was assessed using intra-class correlation methods (ICC) [25]. The result showed that the intra-examiner reliability ranged from ICC = 85.21 % to ICC = 99.99 %, which is generally acceptable.

Statistical analysis

All measured values were adjusted with multiple linear regression to assess the possible effects of age and gender and eliminate the interaction of age and gender. It was necessary to systematically search for factors that

Table 1 Characteristics of the study group

	Inclusion Criteria	Exclusion Criteria
1	ANB ≤ 0°	History of orthodontic treatments
2	Overjet ≤ 0 at least edge-to-edge or anterior crossbite	Congenital abnormalities (e.g., cleft lip and palatee)
3	Wits ≤ −2°	Severe facial trauma
4		General physical disease (e.g., endocrine diseases)

Table 2 Cephamotric variables

Cranial Base		
	Condylion to Gnathion (Co-Gn)(mm)	IMPA (L1-MP) (°)
Saddle/Sella Angle (SN-Ar) (°)	**Intermaxillary**	L1-NB (°)
Anterior Cranial Base (SN) (mm)	Midface Length (Co-A) (mm)	L1-NB (mm)
Posterior Cranial Base (S-Ar) (mm)	ANB (°)	L1 Protrusion (L1-APg) (°)
Maxilla	Facial Plane to AB (NP-AB) (°)	L1 Protrusion (L1-APg) (mm)
SNA (°)	Post-Ant Face Height (S-Go/N-Me) (%)	FMIA (L1-FH) (°)
Convexity (NA-APg) (°)	Y-axis (N-S-Gn) (°)	Interincisal Angle (U1-L1) (°)
N to A through the Horizontal Plane (mm)	Maxillary-Mandibular Difference (mm)	UADH (U1-PP) (mm)
Na _|_ to A point (mm)	Wits Appraisal (AO-BO) (mm)	LADH (L1-MP) (mm)
Maxilla Length (Co-ANS) (mm)	Anterior Face Height (N-Me) (mm)	UPDH (U6-PP) (mm)
Mandible	Upper Face Height (N-ANS) (mm)	LPDH (L6 - MP) (mm)
SNB (°)	Inferior Facial Height (mm)	Overjet (mm)
Facial Angle (FH-NPg) (°)	Nasal Height (N-ANS/N-Me) (%)	Overbite (mm)
Gonial Angle (Ar-Go-Me)(°)	MP-SN (°)	**Soft Tissue**
Ramus Height (Ar-Go) (mm)	FMA (FH-MP) (°)	Upper Lip to E-Plane (mm)
Facial Taper (N-Gn-Go) (°)	GoGn-SN (°)	Lower Lip to E-Plane (mm)
Articular Angle (S-Ar-Go) (°)	Occlusal plane To SN (°)	Upper lip length (Sn-ULI)
N to B through Horizontal Plane (mm)	Occlusal Plane to FH (OP-PoOr) (°)	Lower lip length (LLS-Me')
N to Pg through Horizontal Plane (mm)	**Dental**	Facial angle (G'-Sn-Pog') (°)
Pg to Na Perpendicular (mm)	U1-SN (°)	Upper lip anterior (ULA-TVL) (°)
Mandibular Unit Length (Co-Gn) (mm)	U1-NA (°)	Lower lip anterior (LLA - TVL) (°)
Pg - NB (mm)	U1-NA (mm)	
Posterior Facial Height (Co-Go) (mm)	U1-FH (°)	

Boldface indicates six categories of the sixty-one cephalometric parameters

impacted the variables and to group these factors into homogeneous categories. Principal component analysis (PCA) was performed, and 61 principal component scores were then calculated one by one to eliminate interactions between variables. Components with a cumulative variance > 70 % were used in the following cluster analysis. Partitioning cluster analysis (CA) based on principal components (PCs) was applied to construct a

hierarchical structure in all of the Class III malocclusion individuals. We performed CA by the k-means method, which sorted participants into groups by maximizing differences and minimizing differences [26, 27]. The clustering algorithm was performed separately for a range of 3 to 6 clusters. A three-dimensional plot was produced using the R statistical program to implement the visualization of the cluster analysis results. The representative subject that was closest to the mean values of the cluster was chosen as the template. One-way analysis of variance (ANOVA) and the Wilcoxon signed rank test were performed to compare the commonly used variables among each cluster, with the aim of identifying major differences across groups. In this study, IBM SPSS 22.0 was used for all analyses, and the significant difference level was set as $p < 0.05$.

Results

PCA transformed the 61 selected variables into 61 independent components. The first 6 PCs contributed significantly to representing the relationship of the 61 variables chosen for cluster analysis, which accounted for 73.7 % of all variation (Fig. 1). The first principal component (PC 1) that contributed most of the variation (20.59 %) mainly consisted of vertical length measurements. The second principal component (PC 2), which explained 19.34 % of the variation, mainly referred to the vertical and sagittal positions of the mandible in relation to the cranial base. The third principal component (PC 3) represented the protrusion and inclination of the lower incisor and explained 12.17 % of the variation. Principal component 5 (PC 5) consisted mainly of parameters for the upper incisor and accounted for only 6.60 % of the variation. Components 4 and 6 were highly correlated with the Na _|_ to A point, APDI (NP-FH), Ao-Bo (Wits), overbite (mm), and the articular angle, which cannot be easily summarized anatomically. Table 3 summarizes the correlations of the identified principal components and the variables making the greatest contributions. An additional file shows the results of the PCA in more detail (see Additional file 2).

This group of 144 individuals with class III malocclusion were subjected to cluster analysis (CA) and were classified into 4 groups (Fig. 2; Table 4), which are both clinically meaningful and statistically acceptable based on the value of K-means in the classifier: Cluster 1 ($n = 48$) was a vertical type of Class III malocclusion that showed mild mandibular prognathism with a steep mandibular plane, and a labial inclination of the upper incisors. This group contained the largest number of observations. Cluster 2 ($n = 38$) represented individuals with moderate skeletal Class III malocclusion with a combination of a prognathic mandibular and a retrusive

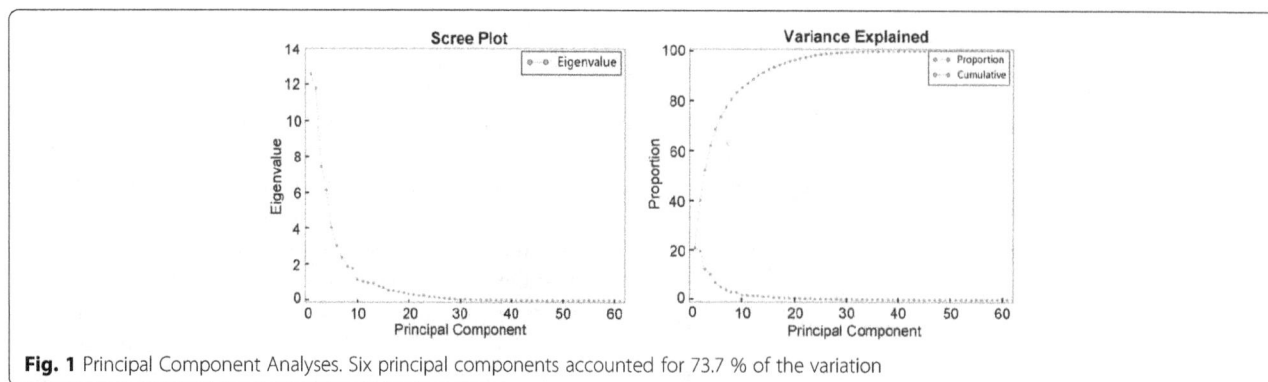

Fig. 1 Principal Component Analyses. Six principal components accounted for 73.7 % of the variation

maxilla and a flat or normal mandibular plane. Cluster 3 (n = 46) was centrally located, and the subjects with this type had severe mandibular prognathism, a normal mandibular plane, and the most serious lingual inclination of the lower incisors. Subjects in Cluster 4 had the most severe phenotype of skeletal Class III malocclusion, exhibiting maxillary deficiency and severe mandibular prognathism with the lowest mandibular plane angle and an obvious labial inclination of the upper incisors. Cluster 4 also had the fewest observations (n = 12). Figure 3 displays templates of each cluster. Table 5 presents the descriptive statistics of each subtype, including the means and standard deviations for the variables used in each cluster, and the p-values for the significance level of each cluster are shown in Table 6. The most significant difference was observed in the FH-MP variable among the four clusters, but no evident difference was found between each cluster for the SNB and Wits variables. An additional file shows the results of the CA in more detail (see Additional file 3).

Discussion

By the end of the nineteenth century, Angle had first classified malocclusions into three groups (Class I, Class II and Class III) based on the relationship of the first molars; shortly thereafter, it was recognized that this classification could not capture the breadth of clinical characteristics. Gradually, Class III malocclusion was extended to refer to the skeletal jaw relationship in a mesial position of the mandible to the maxilla [2]. Class III malocclusion was a mixture of various patterns of maxillofacial deformity rather than a homogenous group. Organization of the phenotypic heterogeneity into its underlying hierarchical structure is of great necessity and may contribute to both etiological and therapeutic studies. In this study, principal component analysis and cluster analysis were performed using luxury lateral cephalometric measurements, which is a method that is frequently applied in classifications, especially when there are numerous variables. Sixty-one morphological features were included in the study, which may permit a comprehensive evaluation.

Table 3 Summary of the principal components analysis

Principal component	1	2	3	4	5	6
Variance explained[a]	0.20586	0.19340	0.12168	0.10028	0.06596	0.04932
Cumulative variance[b]		0.39926	0.52094	0.62122	0.68718	0.73650
Variables[c]	Posterior Facial Height (Co-Go) (mm)	GoGn-SN (°)	LI-NB (°)	Na ⊥ to A point (mm)	UI-SN (°)	Wits Appraisal (AO-BO) (mm)
	Upper Face Height (N-ANS) (mm)	MP-SN (°)	LI-NB (mm)	Pg to Na Perpendicular (mm)	U1-FH (°)	Convexity (NA-APg) (°)
	Midface Length (Co-A) (mm)	Facial Taper (N-Gn-Go) (°)	L1 Protrusion (L1-APg) (mm)	Facial Angle (FH-NPg) (°)	U1-NA (°)	Overbite (mm)
	LPDH (L6-MP) (mm)	Gonial Angle (Ar-Go-Me) (°)	L1 Protrusion (L1-APg) (°)	N to B through the horizontal plane (mm)	U1-NA (mm)	Facial angle (G' - Sn - Pog') (°)
	LADH (LI-MP) (mm)	Post-Ant Face Height (S-Go/N-Me) (%)	FMIA (L1-FH) (°)	N to A through the horizontal plane (mm)	Occlusal plane to FH (OP-PoOr) (°)	Articular Angle (S-Ar-Go) (°)

[a]represents the variance explained by each principal component in PCA
[b]shows the cumulative variance explained by each added PC sequentially
[c]displays the variables contributing the most in each PC

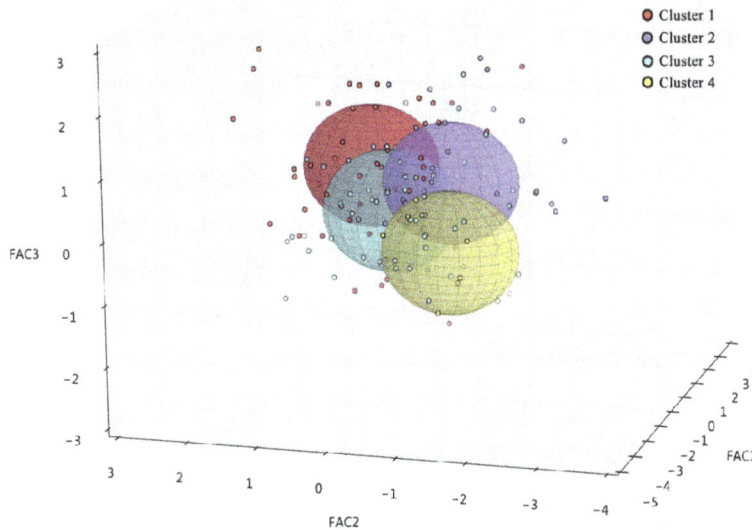

Fig. 2 Cluster analysis results of Class III malocclusion. A 3-D spherical image representing the four identified clusters. Each cluster is traced by a unique colour

In the principal component analysis, six PCs were identified from the 61 variables among the 144 participants, which were responsible for 73.7 % of the variation. Additionally, the variables in the first three PCs explained more than half (52.09 %) of the variation. PC 1 and PC 2 consisted mainly of vertical and sagittal parameters that defined the relationship of the mandible to the cranial base, whereas PC 3 characterized the protrusion and inclination of the lower incisors. This result almost corresponds to the earlier studies by Moreno Uribe and Bui [11, 14]. Interestingly, the ANB angle (Point A-Nasion-Point B) and the SNA and SNB angles were not captured in our study, whereas these variables existed for PC 1 in the PCA performed by Moreno Uribe and Bui. Perhaps the individuals who were recruited to our study had only mild and moderate cases of class III malocclusion, and the number of severe patients may have been relatively small. Moreover, some parameters, such as facial taper, the articular angle, and the facial angle, acted as vital parts of the principal components, thus indicating their important role as measurements of Class III malocclusion. PCA was applied to reduce the interaction among the variables on which CA was performed to eliminate noisy variables that may corrupt the cluster structure [28].

Although the existence of Class III malocclusion subtypes is recognized by researchers, a few subgroups were identified among Class III malocclusion patients, three of which are defined by a long face, an average face or postural Class III [16]. Because there is a variation in the determination of the number of clusters, subjective factors could not be completely avoided in the CA. In previous studies, the patterns of five and seven clusters were proposed following a cluster analysis of more detailed cephalometric measurements [11, 14, 15]. In this research, the clustering algorithm was performed separately for a range of 3 to 6 clusters. According to our results, the model with three clusters was too simple to summarize the clinical variations, whereas in the models that included five or six clusters, one of the clusters contained fewer than five cases. Thus, we determined the existence of four subtypes of Chinese individuals based on CA.

Compared with the previous studies conducted by Moreno Uribe and Bui, who captured 5 clusters by CA [11], the subtype of severe Class III malocclusion with a retrusive maxilla and a high angle was not observed in our study, which may have been due to the moderate sample size. In addition, the proportion of people in each subtype differed from their results. A study related to the dento-facial profile of the Polish population found specific characteristics compared with other European

Table 4 Summary of the clusters

Cluster	Frequency (%)	Standard Deviation[a]	Nearest Clusters	Distance
1	48(33.3 %)	0.63	3	1.89
2	38(26.4 %)	0.58	3	2.05
3	46(31.9 %)	0.46	1	1.89
4	12(8.3 %)	0.67	3	2.54
Total	144			

[a]indicates the average distance between subjects within each cluster

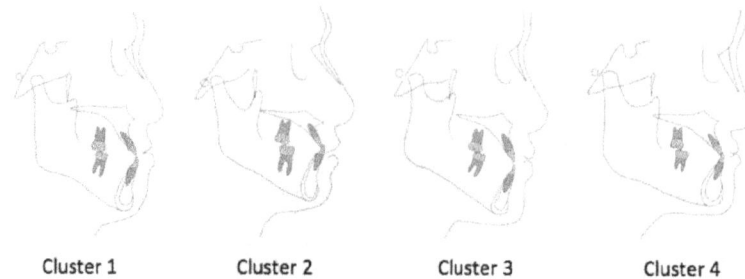

Fig. 3 Cluster templates. The cephalometric trace of the templates in each cluster as described in the results

populations. This may indicate that nationality should be considered when diagnosing facial structures [29]. Although the previous studies helped us expand the threshold of the types of Class III malocclusion, a systemic analysis to validate a practical classification system is necessary and should be the first step toward a comprehensive and accurate understanding of heterogeneity owing to ethnicity and large samples. The subjects of this study were Chinese adults and post-pubertal individuals who were not included in previous studies, which is a supplement to further systematic reviews.

In this study, a description of phenotypes based on a Chinese population was more detailed than in previous studies and was achieved by comparing the means of some commonly used measurements, such as the SNA angle, SNB angle, ANB angle, FH-MP angle, Wits and incisor angulation. The FH-MP angle rather than the ANB or SNB was the dominant classifier. Depending on the results of the PCA, this may suggest that the growth patterns rather than severity are involved in genotypes. Meanwhile, the lingual inclination of incisors in severe Class III malocclusion was significantly different from that of mild cases, which reminded orthodontists of the limitations of inclining incisors during the camouflage treatment [30]. In addition, differences in the Wits

appraisal, which is usually measured to predict whether the Class III patient is a poor or good grower, were also observed to be less significant when compared among clusters, indicating that Wits might be a confusing and ambiguous measurement for assessing Class III conditions.

When discussing these results, we must consider some limitations. It is regrettable that there was a lack of family history data, which are important for the assessment of disease progression and may be closely linked to certain subtypes. In Class III malocclusion patients, diagnosis and treatment are not only influenced by severity, the jaw discrepancy, the incisor inclination, and the mandibular plane but also by factors such as age and family history, which were not included in this study. Compared with the research conducted by Moreno Uribe a few years ago in Caucasian Class III samples [11], there is a necessity to enlarge our working sample size to approach a more clinically impeccable classification system. As auxiliary examinations have increased in recent years, Cone beam CT (CBCT) identifies three-dimensional landmarks of the maxillofacial region [31, 32]. A larger sample size, including informative data extracted from CBCT, will assist in the development of a more sophisticated classification system and a more accurate understanding of the genetic aetiology. As stated previously, the cephalograms were taken in centric occlusion in this study. We found 3 patients who have an antero-posterior shift in centric relation and centric occlusion. In these 3 cases, the cephalograms were taken

Table 5 Means and standard deviations of variables in each cluster

Variables	Cluster 1	Cluster 2	Cluster 3	Cluster 4
Frequency	48	38	46	12
Proportions	(33.33 %)	(26.39 %)	(31.94 %)	(8.33 %)
Age	21.29 ± 3.85	24.21 ± 5.03	21.87 ± 4.38	25.67 ± 4.10
Sex(m/f)	22/26	18/20	15/31	3/9
SNA(°)	81.50 ± 3.57	80.08 ± 2.78	82.95 ± 3.28	79.95 ± 3.72
SNB(°)	83.70 ± 4.06	83.08 ± 3.12	84.40 ± 3.83	85.01 ± 4.38
ANB(°)	−2.20 ± 2.07	−3.02 ± 1.98	−1.46 ± 1.72	−5.06 ± 1.77
Wits(°)	−7.56 ± 4.02	−7.48 ± 3.66	−7.77 ± 3.40	−5.98 ± 3.42
FH-MP(°)	30.95 ± 5.49	24.16 ± 5.32	26.82 ± 5.01	18.23 ± 3.98
UI-SN (°)	118.25 ± 6.07	108.85 ± 5.94	112. 80 ± 4.85	119.69 ± 8.29
LI-MP (°)	84.00 ± 8.35	88.47 ± 8.31	82.12 ± 7.96	88.19 ± 3.90

Table 6 P-values of two-way cluster comparisons

	1–2	1–3	1–4	2–3	2–4	3–4
SNA(°)	0.048[*]	0.035[*]	0.147	<0.001[*]	0.908	0.006[*]
SNB(°)	0.450	0.370	0.287	0.112	0.126	0.623
ANB (°)	0.053	0.061	<0.001[*]	<0.001[*]	0.002[*]	<0.001[*]
Wits (°)	0.926	0.777	0.186	0.721	0.219	0.135
FH-MP(°)	<0.001[*]	<0.001[*]	<0.001[*]	0.021[*]	0.001[*]	<0.001[*]
UI-SN (°)	<0.001[*]	<0.001[*]	0.450	0.003[*]	<0.001[*]	<0.001[*]
LI-MP (°)	0.011[*]	0.255	0.105	<0.001[*]	0.916	0.020[*]

[*]P-values < 0.05

in both centric occlusion and centric relation. Comparing the results of the cepholametric measurement, we found little difference between centric occlusion and centric relation of the three cases. That wouldn't cause significant influence on the final results. While among a larger sample size, it is appropriate that the cephalograms be taken in centric relation in those cases during the further studies.

Our ultimate goal is to describe the variants of Class III malocclusion and identify the genetic basis of the disease. The replication of genetic variant studies in Class III malocclusion and many other complex diseases is rare [33]. For example, what we previously identified in a large Class III malocclusion pedigree was inconsistent with the loci identified in other studies [4–10]. Considering all of these limitations, disease heterogeneity may be a difficult factor. A novel taxonomy via cluster analysis might facilitate genetic research. Additionally, clinical relevance should be investigated across subgroups in therapy after the completion of approximately 2-year-long treatment procedures in longitudinal studies. The integration of therapies related to craniofacial phenotypes would eventually lead to improved and distinct treatment schedules.

Conclusions

Cluster analysis produced four clusters of Class III malocclusion, which represented characteristics of maxillary or mandibular discrepancy, corresponding to short or long faces, the inclination of the incisors and severity. With PCA, six PCs were extracted from the 61 variables among 144 participants, which were responsible for 73.7 % of the variation. Our study provided much more detailed information relative to previous studies by applying ANOVA and the Wilcoxon signed rank test to the variables in each cluster.

Abbreviation

CA: Cluster analysis; PC: Principal component; PCA: Principal component analysis

Acknowledgments

The authors would like to thank the Affiliated Stomatology Hospital of Tongji University for help in providing excellent samples.

Funding

This work was supported by the National Natural Science Foundation of China (No. 81371129).

Authors' contributions

CL carried out the cephalometric measurements and drafted the manuscript. YC and SC participated in the design of the study and the statistical analysis. FC conceived of the study and contributed to its design. All authors read and approved the final manuscript.

Competing interests

The authors declare that they have no competing interests.

Consent for publication

Not applicable.

References

1. Chang HP, Tseng YC, Chang HF. Treatment of mandibular prognathism. J Formos Med Assoc. 2006;105(10):781–90.
2. Ngan P, Moon W. Evolution of Class III treatment in orthodontics. Am J Orthod Dentofacial Orthop. 2015;148(1):22–36.
3. Cruz RM, Krieger H, Ferreira R, Mah J, Hartsfield Jr J, Oliveira S. Major gene and multifactorial inheritance of mandibular prognathism. Am J Med Genet A. 2008;146(1):71–7.
4. Yamaguchi T, Park SB, Narita A, Maki K, Inoue I. Genome-wide linkage analysis of mandibular prognathism in Korean and Japanese patients. J Dent Res. 2005;84(3):255–59.
5. Frazier-Bowers S, Rincon-Rodriguez R, Zhou J, Alexander K, Lange E. Evidence of linkage in a Hispanic cohort with a Class III dentofacial phenotype. J Dent Res. 2009;88(1):56–60.
6. Jang JY, Park EK, Ryoo HM, Shin HI, Kim TH, Jang JS, Park HS, Choi JY, Kwon TG. Polymorphisms in the Matrilin-1 gene and risk of mandibular prognathism in Koreans. J Dent Res. 2010;89(11):1203–07.
7. Perillo L, Monsurrò A, Bonci E, Torella A, Mutarelli M, Nigro V. Genetic Association of ARHGAP21 Gene Variant with Mandibular Prognathism. J Dent Res. 2015;94(4):569–76.
8. da Fontoura CSG, Miller SF, Wehby GL, Amendt BA, Holton NE, Southard TE, Allareddy V, Moreno Uribe LM. Candidate gene analyses of skeletal variation in malocclusion. J Dent Res. 2015;94(7):913–20.
9. Tassopoulou-Fishell M, Deeley K, Harvey EM, Sciote J, Vieira AR. Genetic variation in myosin 1H contributes to mandibular prognathism. Am J Orthod Dentofac Orthop. 2012;141(1):51–9.
10. He S, Hartsfield Jr JK, Guo Y, Cao Y, Wang S, Chen S. Association between CYP19A1 genotype and pubertal sagittal jaw growth. Am J Orthod Dentofac Orthop. 2012;142(5):662–70.
11. Moreno Uribe LM, Vela KC, Kummet C, Dawson DV, Southard TE. Phenotypic diversity in white adults with moderate to severe Class III malocclusion. Am J Orthod Dentofac Orthop. 2013;144(1):32–42.
12. Sugawara J, Mitani H. Facial growth of skeletal class III malocclusion and the effects, limitations, and long-term dentofacial adaptations to chincap therapy. Seminars in Orthodontics. 1997;3(4):244–54.
13. Mouakeh M. Cephalometric evaluation of craniofacial pattern of Syrian children with Class III malocclusion. Am J Orthod Dentofac Orthop. 2001; 119(6):640–49.
14. Bui C, King T, Proffit W, Frazier-Bowers S. Phenotypic characterization of Class III patients: a necessary background for genetic analysis. Angle Orthod. 2006;76(4):564–69.
15. Hong SX, Yi CK. A classification and characterization of skeletal class III on etio-pathogenic basis. Int J Oral Maxillofac Surg. 2001;30(4):264–71.
16. Abu Alhaija ES, Richardson A. Growth prediction in Class III patients using cluster and discriminant function analysis. Eur J Orthod. 2003; 25(6):599–608.
17. Bro R, Smilde AK. Principal component analysis. Anal Methods. 2014;6(9): 2812–31.
18. Burgel PR, Paillasseur JL, Caillaud D, Tillie-Leblond I, Chanez P, Escamillae R, Court-Fortune I, Perez T, Carre P, Roche N. Clinical COPD phenotypes: a novel approach using principal component and cluster analyses. Eur Respir J. 2010;36(3):531–39.
19. Burgel P-R, Paillasseur J-L, Peene B, Dusser D, Roche N, Coolen J, Troosters T, Decramer M, Janssens W. Two distinct chronic obstructive pulmonary disease (COPD) phenotypes are associated with high risk of mortality. PLoS One. 2012;7(12):e51048.
20. Chen CZ, Wang LY, Ou CY, Lee CH, Lin CC, Hsiue TR. Using cluster analysis to identify phenotypes and validation of mortality in men with COPD. Lung. 2014;192(6):889–96.
21. Li Q, Li X, Zhang F, Chen F. The identification of a novel locus for mandibular prognathism in the Han Chinese population. J Dent Res. 2011;90(1):53 7.

22. Li Q, Zhang F, Li X, Chen F. Genome scan for locus involved in mandibular prognathism in pedigrees from China. PLoS One. 2010;5(9):e12678.

23. Chen F, Li Q, Gu M, Li X, Yu J, Zhang Y-B. Identification of a Mutation in FGF23 Involved in Mandibular Prognathism. Sci Rep. 2015;5:11250.

24. Alexander AEZ, McNamara Jr JA, Franchi L, Baccetti T. Semilongitudinal cephalometric study of craniofacial growth in untreated Class III malocclusion. Am J Orthod Dentofac Orthop. 2009;135(6):700. e1-00. e14.

25. Shrout PE, Fleiss JL. Intraclass correlations: uses in assessing rater reliability. Psychol Bull. 1979;86(2):420.

26. Vogt W, Nagel D. Cluster analysis in diagnosis. Clin Chem. 1992;38(2):182–98.

27. Chen L, Lin Z-X, Lin G-S, Zhou C-F, Chen Y-P, Wang X-F, Zheng Z-Q. Classification of microvascular patterns via cluster analysis reveals their prognostic significance in glioblastoma. Hum Pathol. 2015;46(1):120–28.

28. Ben-Hur A, Guyon I. Detecting stable clusters using principal component analysis. Functional Genomics: Methods and Protocols. 2003. p. 159–82. http://citeseerx.ist.psu.edu/viewdoc/download?doi=10.1.1.155.5532&rep=rep1&type=pdf.

29. Jolanta EL, Stephen W, Aneta W, Bartłomiej WL. The Polish face in profile: a cephalometric baseline study. Head Face Med. 2015;11:5.

30. Hall-Scott J. The maxillary-mandibular planes angle (MM o) bisector: A new reference plane for anteroposterior measurement of the dental bases. Am J Orthod Dentofac Orthop. 1994;105(6):583–91.

31. Hodges RJ, Atchison KA, White SC. Impact of cone-beam computed tomography on orthodontic diagnosis and treatment planning. Am J Orthod Dentofac Orthop. 2013;143(5):665–74.

32. Merrett SJ, Drage NA, Durning P. Cone beam computed tomography: a useful tool in orthodontic diagnosis and treatment planning. J Orthod. 2009;36(3):202–10.

33. Munafò MR. Replication validity of genetic association studies of smoking behavior: What can meta-analytic techniques offer? Nicotine Tob Res. 2004;6(2):381–82.

33

Effect of DACH1 on proliferation and invasion of laryngeal squamous cell carcinoma

Jiarui Zhang, Xiuxia Ren, Bo Wang, Jing Cao, Linli Tian* and Ming Liu*

Abstract

Background: To investigate the effect of DACH1 over-expression on proliferation and invasion of laryngeal squamous cell carcinoma (LSCC).

Methods: The 120 cases of LSCC tumors and 114 adjacent non-neoplastic tissues were collected to detect the expression of DACH1 by immunohistochemistry. The changes of DACH1 expression from each group were assessed and correlated to the clinical parameters of the patients. Plasmid-DACH1 was transfected into Hep-2 cells to up-regulate the expression of DACH1C. Real-time PCR, Western blot, CCK8 and transwell assay were used to verify the cell proliferation and invasion after plasmid-DACH1 transfection.

Results: The results indicated that DACH1 was downregulated in LSCC tissues as compared to corresponding adjacent non-neoplastic tissues. Decreased expression of DACH1 was found in the tumors upraglottic tumor, lymph node metastases, T3–4 stage and advanced clinical stage. In Hep-2 cells, transfection with plasmid-DACH1 could suppress cell proliferation, invasion and induce G1 phase extension in cell cycle.

Conclusions: DACH1 may act as a tumor suppressor gene and could be a potential target for therapeutic intervention of LSCC.

Keywords: LSCC, DACH1, Proliferation, Invasion

Background

One of the most common head and neck cancers is laryngeal cancer, which is also the third most common otolaryngological cancer [1]. The majority of laryngeal cancers are laryngeal squamous cell carcinomas (LSCC). Despite improvements in diagnostic and therapeutic modalities, there has been no significant improvement in laryngeal cancer survival over the past 20 years [2, 3]. Therefore, new diagnostic and therapeutic targets for LSCC are urgently needed.

The dachshund (DAC) gene was first elucidated in drosophila and isolated as a dominant suppressor of mutation ellipse. DACH1, as a homologous gene in humans, associates with the Retinal Determination Gene Network (RDGN), which includes DAC/DACH, eya/Eya, so/Six, ey and toy [4, 5]. DACH1 is a tumor suppressor gene in many cancers such as colorectal, oral and breast cancers [6–8]. Among the mammals, the expressions of DACH1 target genes could be through DNA-binding transcription factors and DNA-sequence specific binding to Forkhead binding sites [9]. DACH1 was reported to be related to epithelial-mesenchymal transition (EMT): E-cadherin and γ-catrnin that belong to the epithelial protein are down-regulated, while N-cadherin and vimentin that belong to mesenchymal protein are up-regulated [6]. DACH1 can negatively regulate TGF-β and Wnt pathways, repress SNAI1 and CXCL5 signaling [4, 7, 8, 10]. The acetylated carboxyl terminus of DACH1 binds to P53 and enhances its tumor suppressor function in breast cancer [11]. The methylation of DACH1 also promotes the motility and invasion of tumors [8]. Although DACH1 has been studied in many cancers, its role in LSCC remains unknown. Therefore, we examined the in vivo and in vitro relationship between DACH1

* Correspondence: tianlinli78@163.com; liuming002@outlook.com
Department of Otorhinolaryngology, Head and Neck Surgery, Second
Affiliated Hospital, Harbin Medical University, Harbin 150081, China

expression and LSCC to determine if DACH1 had any anticancer effects in LSCC.

Methods
Patients and samples
A total of 120 cases of LSCC tumors and 114 adjacent non-neoplastic tissues were collected from the Department of Pathology in the Second Affiliated Hospital of Harbin Medical University. The LSCC patients were treated by surgery from 2014 to 2016, and no patient received any anticancer treatment before surgery. All patients had no prior history of other cancer and precursor lesions. The fresh tissues were immediately fixed in buffered formalin. We analyzed gender, age, smoking, drinking, T classification, lymph node metastases, primary location and histopathological differentiation, which were obtained from patient records. Smoking and alcohol consumption were calculated according to [12].

Cell culture and transfection
The human LSCC cell line Hep-2 was purchased from The Cell Bank of Chinese Academy of Science (Shanghai, China). Plasmid-DACH1 was constructed by Origene. Hep-2 cells were cultured in DMEM (Hyclone) supplemented with 10% fetal bovine serum (NQBB) and incubated at 37under humidified atmosphere containing 5% CO_2. DACH1 plasmid with GFP as a reporter gene was transfected into Hep-2 cells with Lipofectamine 2000 (Invitrogen) according to the manufacturer's instructions. Hep-2 cells were plated onto 6-well plates (2.5×10^5 cell/well) for a day till they reached 80–85% confluency. The plasmid and Lipofectamine 2000 were each diluted in 250 uL of serum-free OPTI-MEM (Gibco BRL) and incubated for 5 min at room temperature. The diluted plasmid and Lipofectamine 2000 were combined at a 1:2 ratio (3 μg of plasmid with 6 uL of Lipofectamine 2000), mixed gently and incubated for 20 min at room temperature. A total of 500 uL of the mixture was added to each well in a final volume of 2 mL per well. Then the cells were analyzed by Real-time PCR and Western blot.

Real-time PCR and Western blotting
Total RNA was isolated using Trizol reagent (Invitrogen) according to the manufacturer's instructions. About 500 ng of total RNA was used to synthesize cDNA according to the manufacturer's manual (TOYOBO FSQ-301). The primer sequences of DACH1 were designed and synthesized by Invitrogen: Forward primer was 5′-TGCC GCATTCTGTCCCT-3′ and Reverse primer was 5′-G AGTCTGCTCCATGTTGGTTATT-3′. After reverse transcription at 37 °C for 15 min, 50 °C for 5 min and 98 °C for 5 min, Real-time PCR was performed using SYBR-Green Master Mix (TOYOBO QPK-201). Reaction con

ditions were 95 °C for 60 s, 40 cycles at 95 °C for 15 s, 56 °C for 15 s, and 72 °C for 45 s. Data calculated from the Ct values were normalized to the expression of human β-actin gene, and $2^{-\triangle\triangle Ct}$ was used to calculate the expression of DACH1. Each sample was run in triplicate.

Untreated Hep-2 cells and GFP-plasmid groups were collected and analyzed by western blot to assess the expression of DACH1. Total protein was extracted from each group. Anti-DACH1 antibody was purchased from Origene. The membrane with anti-DACH1 (diluted 1:5000 in TBST) was incubated overnight at 4 °C, followed by incubation with the secondary antibody for 1 h at room temperature. β-actin was used as a loading control. The signal intensities were determined using Image J program.

Cell proliferation and invasion assays
Black Hep-2 cells were used as controls for cells transfected with DACH1 plasmid. Cells were plated in 96-well plates at a density of 5×10^3 cells per well. To measure cell proliferation at 24 h, 48 h, 72 h, 10 uL CCK8 reagent was added to cells according to the manufacturer's protocol, and incubated at 37 °C for 2 h. The absorbance at 450 nm was measured using a micro-well plate reader. Each group had five replicate wells. The percentage rate of cell growth was calculated using the following formula: (mean absorbance of the treatment group/mean absorbance of the control group) × 100.

The invasion ability between plasmid-DACH1 levels and black Hep-2 cells was compared using 24-well Boyden chambers (8 mm pore size) coated with matrigel (BD). A total of 2×10^4 cells in 200 uL serum-free media were resuspended in the upper chambers. The lower chamber contained 600 uL of medium containing 10% fetal bovine serum to serve as a chemoattractant. Cells were incubated for 36 h at 37 °C, then cells in the upper chambers were mechanically removed. The cells that had migrated to the lower chambers were fixed in crystal violet for 10–30 min, and five random fields were observed and counted under microscope at × 200 magnification. The experiments were repeated at least three times.

Cell cycle analysis
After transfecting with plasmid-DACH1 for 72 h, the cells were washed twice with cold PBS and fixed in 75% ethanol for 24 h. Then the cells were stained as per the manufacturer's instructions (BD), and cell cycle was analyzed by flow cytometry.

Immunohistochemistry
The samples were embedded in paraffin and incised into thin sections (4um). Then the sections were dewaxed with xylene and different doses alcohol, and washed

three times with distilled water. Antigen retrieval was performed with repair solution according to the manufacturer's instructions. Slices were infiltrated with 3% H_2O_2, put into humidors for 10 min, and washed three times with PBS. Rabbit anti-DACH1 (OriGene) was added and the slices were incubated overnight at 4 °C. Slices were rinsed five times with PBS for five minutes each time, incubated with secondary antibody for 30 min at room temperature, and then washed three times with PBS. The slides were stained with a drop of 3,3-di-aminobenzidine (DAB) and counterstained with hematoxylin for three minutes, dehydrated by alcohol, and sealed by neutral gum. Positive cells showed a brownish color and negative cells were blue.

DACH1 scores

The DACH1 IHC staining results were evaluated by three independent pathologists. DACH1 expression was observed in the nucleus of cells in five random fields. The staining intensity was evaluated based on a 4-point scale (0, no staining, 1, weak intensity, 2, moderate intensity, and 3, strong intensity). The positive cancer cells were also evaluated on a 5-point scale according to the fraction of stained cells (0, < 1%, 1, 1–10%, 2, 10–50%, 3, 50–80%, 4, 80–100%). The DACH1 expression was calculated as the percentage of positive cells in whole tumor cells. DACH1 low-expression based on the percentage of positive cells was lower than the mean value. The IHS was equal to the staining intensity multiplied by the fraction of stained cells.

Statistical analysis

The expression of DACH1 was analyzed by Chi-square test. Independent-sample t-test were used to compare the differences between the two groups. $P < 0.05$ was considered to be significant. All statistical calculations were expressed as mean ± SD using the SPSS statistical software. Graphpad Prism 5 was used to create the artworks.

Results

DACH1 expression is low in LSCC

IHC staining for DACH1 in 120 LSCC and 114 adjacent non-neoplastic mucosa paraffin specimens showed that the intensity and percentage of stained cells in the former samples were obviously lower than the latter. DACH1 was mainly found in the nucleus (Fig. 1), and its expression was associated with several clinical parameters, including smoking, drinking, T classification, lymph node metastases, primary location and clinical stage in LSCC paraffin specimens (Table 1). The low-expression was related to supraglottic tumors, T3–4 stage, and III-IV clinical stage. DACH1 had no significant difference with age, gender, and differentiation.

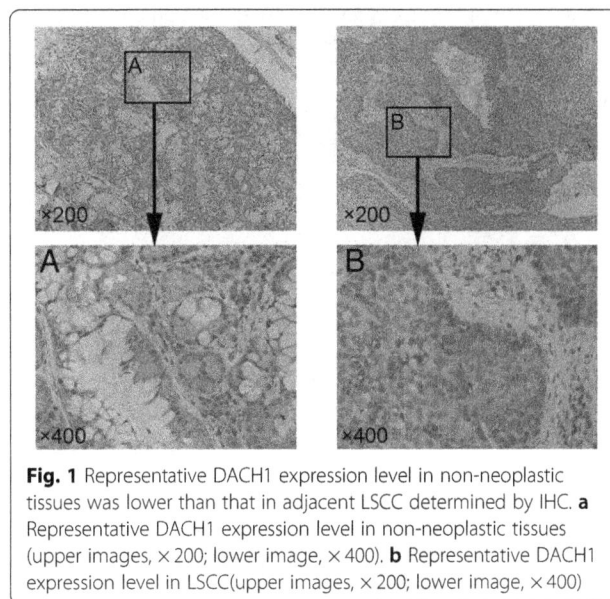

Fig. 1 Representative DACH1 expression level in non-neoplastic tissues was lower than that in adjacent LSCC determined by IHC. **a** Representative DACH1 expression level in non-neoplastic tissues (upper images, × 200; lower image, × 400). **b** Representative DACH1 expression level in LSCC(upper images, × 200; lower image, × 400)

DACH1 expression was up-regulated after DACH1 plasmid transfection in Hep-2 cells

Plasmid-DACH1 was transfected in Hep-2 cells to up-regulate the expression of DACH1 in order to further explore the functional roles of DACH1 in LSCC (Fig. 2). Real-time PCR and Western blot were used to verify the translational level after plasmid-DACH1 transfection, which showed that both mRNA (Fig. 3a) and protein (Fig. 3b) levels were higher in the plasmid-DACH1 transfected group than in the uninfected group. These results indicated that DACH1 was effectively expressed after plasmid-DACH1 transfection in Hep-2 cells.

Overexpression of DACH1 inhibited proliferation and invasion of Hep-2 cells

After transfecting plasmid-DACH1 in Hep-2 cells, we tested its influence on the proliferation and invasion of cells. As shown in Fig. 4a, proliferation of Hep-2 cells transfected with plasmid-DACH1 was effectively inhibited at 72 h. The growth curve was plotted according to OD values. Transwell assay suggested that the invasion of Hep-2 cells was significantly lower in the transfected group than in the control group (Fig. 4b, c and d). The results implied that DACH1 inhibited the proliferation and invasion of Hep-2 cells in vitro. Therefore, DACH1 may play a role in inducing the proliferation and invasion of LSCC.

Overexpression of DACH1 suppressed cell cycle

We detected cell cycle to study the antiproliferative mechanism of DACH1 and flow cytometry analysis indicated that up-regulation of DACH1 in Hep-2 cells could suppress cell cycle in G1 phase, as compared to the

Table 1 Relationship between DACH1 expression and clinicopathological characteristics in 120 LSCC patients

Clinicopathological characteristics	DACH1 <mean value%	expression ≥mean value%	p-value
N = 120	60 (50.0%)	60 (50.0%)	
Age (mean ± SD; years)			0.239
< 61 ± 8.11	38 (31.7%)	44 (36.7%)	
≥ 61 ± 8.11	22 (18.3%)	16 (13.3%)	
Gender			0.194
Male	32 (26.7%)	39 (32.5%)	
Female	28 (23.3%)	21 (17.5%)	
T classification			0.002
T_1-T_2	49 (40.8%)	33 (27.5%)	
T_3-T_4	11 (9.2%)	27 (22.5%)	
Lymph node metastases			0.010
Yes	40 (33.3%)	52 (43.3%)	
No	20 (16.7%)	8 (6.7%)	
Primary location			0.006
Supraglottic	41 (34.2%)	26 (21.7%)	
Glottic	19 (15.8%)	34 (28.3%)	
Differentiation			0.099
G1	23 (19.2%)	32 (26.7%)	
G2-G3	37 (30.8%)	28 (23.3%)	
Clinical stage			0.016
I-II	29 (24.2%)	42 (35.0%)	
III-IV	31 (2ss5.8%)	18 (15.0%)	
Smoking			0.002
Never	4 (3.3%)	17 (14.2%)	
Ever	56 (46.7%)	43 (35.8%)	
Drinking			0.039
Never	11 (9.2%)	21 (17.5%)	
Ever	49 (40.8%)	39 (32.5%)	

uninfected group, the G1 phase of the plasmid-DACH1 transfected group was markedly prolonged (Fig. 5).

Discussion

LSCC accounts for a vast proportion of head and neck cancers. In 2011, LSCC accounted for approximately 0.7% of all new cancer diagnoses and about 0.6% of all cancer-related deaths [13]. Metastasis is one of the main reasons for poor prognosis. Studies have shown that EMT may contact with tumor invasion and metastasis [14]. DACH1 could repress EMT by repressing gene transcription in the nucleus and translation in the cytoplasm [15].

DACH1 has been identified in several human cancers as a novel tumor suppressor gene [16–18]. Our study showed that DACH1 was significantly down-regulated in LSCC as compared to non-neoplastic tissues. In addition, it was found that lower expression of DACH1 was closely correlated with supraglottic tumor, lymph node metastases, T3–4 stage and advanced clinical stage. Considering the association of these clinicopathological parameters with the poor prognosis of patients with LSCC, these results imply that DACH1 may play a role in the progression and influence the prognosis in LSCC. To explore the effect of the overexpression of DACH1on the metastasis and progression of LSCC, we examined the alterations in cell growth and behavior following DACH1overexpression in the Hep-2 cells. Elevated expression of DACH1 suppressed proliferation, induced cell cycle arrest.

in the G1 phase, and suppressed cell invasion in the Hep-2 cells. Taken together, these results suggest that DACH1 is a tumor-suppressor in the growth and progression of LSCC. These results were similar to previous studies on the expression of DACH1 in esophageal cancer, hepatocellular carcinoma and colorectal cancer [10, 18, 19]. Smoking and alcohol consumption were risk factors of laryngeal carcinoma, and DACH1 increased the risk of laryngeal carcinoma which is consistent with other study [12].

Patients with relatively low DACH1 expression showed lower 5-year overall survival among lung adenocarcinoma, endometrial cancer and luminal breast cancer [4, 17, 20]. DACH1 may be a prognosis gene in LSCC.

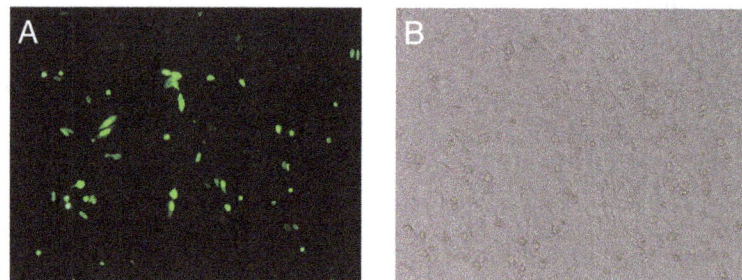

Fig. 2 (**a**) GFP plasmid-DACH1 expression in Hep-2 cells after 72 h. **b** No GFP expression in black Hep-2 cells. Fluorescence microscope images (× 200)

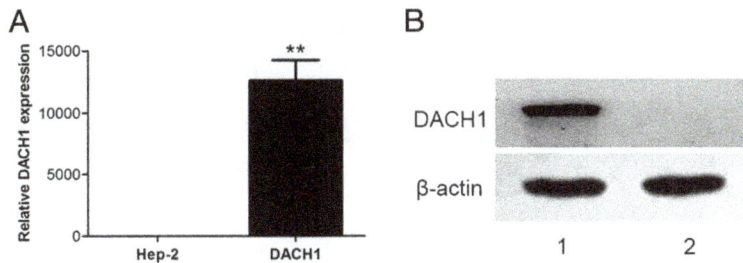

Fig. 3 The expression level of DACH1 in two groups. **a** Real-time PCR analysis showed that DACH1 expression was significantly up-regulated after plasmid-DACH1 transfection, $P < 0.05$. **b** Western blot showed the protein level of DACH1 in transfected Hep-2 cells(1), and control Hep-2 cells (2)

However, DACH1 is up-regulated in myeloid leukemia via interaction with HOXA9 and overexpression in ovarian cancer with poor prognosis as promotion sensitivity gene [21, 22]. So, in order to examine how DACH1 suppresses LSCC, we transfected plasmid-DACH1 in Hep-2 cells, and used RT-PCR and Western blot assays to verify its successful expression. The results showed that over-expression of DACH1 suppressed Hep-2 cell growth and invasion, which was in agreement with previous studies that showed that low-expression of DACH1 promoted the activation of MMP-2 and MMP-9 through TGF-β signaling to promote invasion in gastric cancer [23] and high-expression of DACH1 blocked Wnt pathway to suppress viability and invasion in hepatocellular carcinoma [24]. DACH1 was found to be the less frequent methylation in oral carcinoma cell lines as the negative regulator of Wnt pathway [8]. Furthermore, we found that over-expression of DACH1 suppressed

the G1 phase to prolong cell cycle. These results indicated that DACH1 may act as an anti-tumor gene in Hep-2 cells. The underlying mechanism needs further investigation.

MiRNA-194 and miRNA-217 are known to target DACH1 in pancreatic ductal adenocarcinoma and breast cancer, respectively. They could block the expression of DACH1, and promote the development of tumors [25, 26]. However, the relationship between these miRNAs and DACH1 in LSCC remains unknown and needs to be examined. Increasing DACH1 expression is reported to bind to AP-1 and NF-kB sites to suppress IL-8 in cellular migration, and its carboxyl terminus binds to TCERG1 FF2 domain to repress transcription through DNA binding and YB-1C-terminus and DNA Binding Domain (DBD) to inhibit the development of breast cancer [15, 27, 28]. In our study, DACH1 suppressed the function of Hep-2 cells. DACH1 blocked both FOXM1

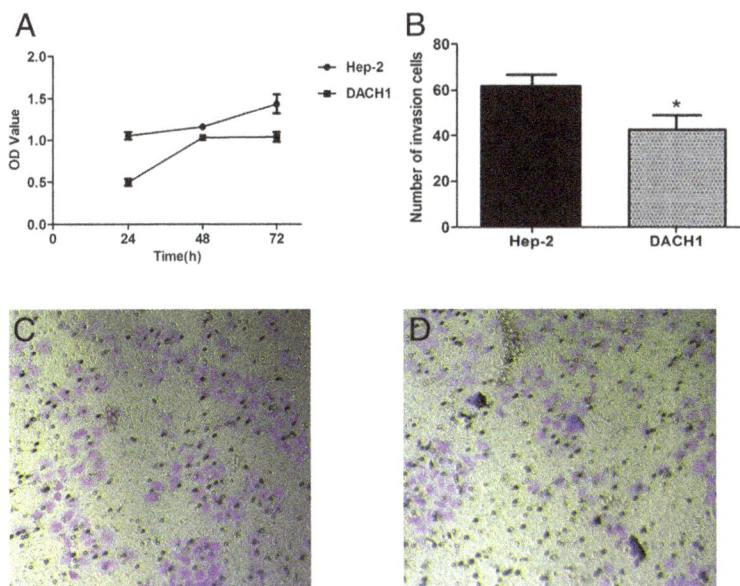

Fig. 4 DACH1 inhibited proliferation and invasion of Hep-2 cells. **a** After plasmid-DACH1 transfection, the OD of the transfected group had no obvious increase as compared to the infected group at 72 h, $P < 0.05$. **b** After 72 h transfection, the number of invasive cells in each group. **c** The number of invasive cells in the black Hep-2 cells group. **d** The plasmid-DACH1 group, $P < 0.05$

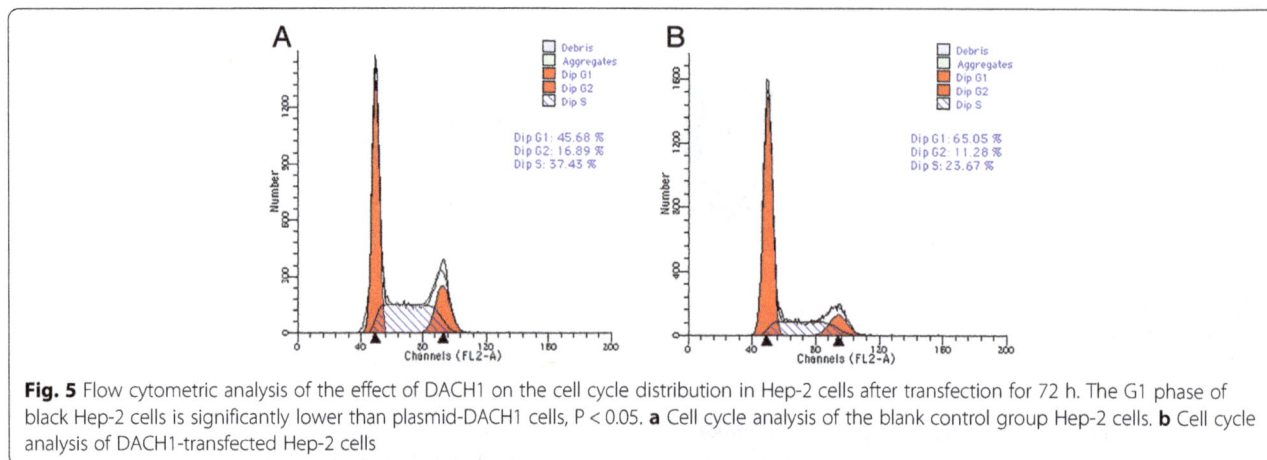

Fig. 5 Flow cytometric analysis of the effect of DACH1 on the cell cycle distribution in Hep-2 cells after transfection for 72 h. The G1 phase of black Hep-2 cells is significantly lower than plasmid-DACH1 cells, P < 0.05. **a** Cell cycle analysis of the blank control group Hep-2 cells. **b** Cell cycle analysis of DACH1-transfected Hep-2 cells

and FOXC2 to inhibit cell invasion, migration and cell cycle [5, 9]. C-Jun, as a component of AP-1 transcription factor complex, is inhibited by DACH1 to repress DNA synthesis and Cyclin D1 [29–31]. TIC or CSC is a stem cell that facilitates tumor initiation, however, re-expression of DACH1 decreased the tumor and mammosphere formation, reduced the CD44high/CD24low proportion in BTIC, and repressed the expression of Sox2, Oct4, Nanog, KLF4 and c-Myc [5, 32]. More recently, through Artificial Neural Networks (ANNs), DACH1 was shown as the biomarker that binds to ERa, and PELP1 is the target gene of DACH1 in ERa signaling [20, 33].

DACH1 is highly expressed in the nuclei, and is a new suppressor gene located on chromosome 13q22 [6]. DACH1 contains two domains: DachBOX-N and DachBOX-C, the former associates with SKI/SNO proteins (DS), and binds to HDAC3 and SIX6; while the latter binds to UBC9 [34]. DACH1 can block cell cycle progression and synergistic action with p53 protein and repress CXCL5 through protein-protein association in lung cancer and NSCLC [4, 35]. In vitro studies have shown that DACH1 negatively regulates colorectal cancer via Wnt pathway and malignant peripheral nerve sheath tumors through RAS signaling [19, 36]. Furthermore, DACH1 binds Smad4 and NCoR to repress TGF-β signaling [37], enhances chemosensitivity by inducing the expression of P21 [18], and regulates hormone levels in breast and prostate cancers [33, 38]. DACH1 responsive element (DRE) competes with FOXA-responsive element for binding sites, hence DACH1 attenuates FOX signaling [9, 28]. CCK8 and transwell assays showed that DACH1 inhibited cell proliferation and invasion in vitro, and its expression is lower in stage III-IV than in stage I-II. Therefore, DACH1 can inhibit cell invasion and metastasis, and loss of its function can facilitate the development of oncogenes.

DACH1 is thought to be an effective therapeutic target to suppress the invasion and growth of many tumors [39, 40]. Although surgery and radiation are the main treatments, the sequential treatment is not yet perfected and tumor cell recurrence cannot be controlled. Our study showed lower DACH1 in LSCC tissues than in normal tissues. Although over-expression of DACH1 suppressed cell proliferation and invasion, the underlying mechanisms need further study.

Conclusion

In summary, this is the first report on the significance of DACH1 in LSCC. The expression of DACH1 was lower in LSCC than in adjacent normal tissues, and decreased expression of DACH1 was found in the tumors upraglottic tumor, lymph node metastases, T3–4 stage and advanced clinical stage. Positive regulation of DACH1 could suppress proliferation and invasion, and induce apoptosis of Hep-2 cells. Therefore, DACH1 may be a new therapeutic target to improve the prognosis of LSCC.

Abbreviations
DAC: Dachshund; EMT: Epithelial-mesenchymal transition; LSCC: laryngeal squamous cell carcinoma; RDGN: Retinal Determination Gene Network

Funding
The research was supported by Linli Tian's grant from the national science foundation of china (81402234), Ming Liu's grants from the national science foundation of china (81241085, 81372902), and Linli Tian's grant from postdoctoral scientific research developmental fund (LBH-Q16157).

Authors' contributions
The authors had roles in study design, data collection and analysis, decision to publish, or preparation of the manuscript. All authors read and approved the final manuscript.

Authors' information
Linli Tian is a professor of ENT at the Harbin Medical University, who serves at the second affiliated hospital from 2003 to now. She specializes in working with the laryngopharyngeal diseases.

Consent for publication

All patients have consent to publish. The authors all consent for publition.

Competing interests

The authors declare that they have no competing interests.

References

1. Chu EA, Kim YJ. Laryngeal cancer: diagnosis and preoperative work-up. Otolaryngol Clin N Am. 2008;41:673–95. https://doi.org/10.1016/j.otc.2008.01.016.
2. Ellis L, Coleman MP, Rachet B. The impact of life tables adjusted for smoking on the socio-economic difference in net survival for laryngeal and lung cancer. Br J Cancer. 2014;111:195–202. https://doi.org/10.1038/bjc.2014.217.
3. Connor KL, Pattle S, Kerr GR, et al. Treatment, comorbidity and survival in stage III laryngeal cancer. Head Neck. 2015;37:698–706. https://doi.org/10.1002/hed.23653.
4. Han N, Yuan X, Wu H, et al. DACH1 inhibits lung adenocarcinoma invasion and tumor growth by repressing CXCL5 signaling. Oncotarget. 2015;6:5877–88. https://doi.org/10.18632/oncotarget.3463.
5. Liu Y, Han N, Zhou S, et al. The DACH/EYA/SIX gene network and its role in tumor initiation and progression. Int J Cancer. 2016;138:1067–75. https://doi.org/10.1002/ijc.29560.
6. Wang P. Suppression of DACH1 promotes migration and invasion of colorectal cancer via activating TGF-β-mediated epithelial-mesenchymal transition. Biochem Biophys Res Commun. 2015;460:314–9. https://doi.org/10.1016/j.bbrc.2015.03.032.
7. Zhao F, Wang M, Li S, et al. DACH1 inhibits SNAI1-mediated epithelial-mesenchymal transition and represses breast carcinoma metastasis. Oncogenesis. 2015;4:e143. https://doi.org/10.1038/oncsis.2015.3.
8. Jarosław P, Joanna S, Magdalena KP, et al. The negative regulators of Wnt pathway—DACH1, DKK1, and WIF1 are methylated in oral and oropharyngeal cancer and WIF1 methylation predicts shorter survival. Tumour Biol. 2015;36:2855–61. https://doi.org/10.1007/s13277-014-2913-x.
9. Zhou J, Wang C, Wang Z, et al. Attenuation of Forkhead signaling by the retinal determination factor DACH1. Proc Natl Acad Sci U S A. 2010;107:6864–9. https://doi.org/10.1073/pnas.1002746107.
10. Wu L, Herman JG, Brock MV, et al. Silencing DACH1 promotes esophageal Cancer growth by inhibiting TGF-β signaling. PLoS One. 2014;9:e95509. https://doi.org/10.1371/journal.pone.0095509.
11. Chen K, Wu K, Gormley M, et al. Acetylation of the cell-fate factor dachshund determines p53 binding and signaling modules in breast Cancer. Oncotarget. 2013;4:923–35. https://doi.org/10.18632/oncotarget.1094.
12. Hui HF, Pan H, Wang BQ, et al. Association between UGT1A1 polymorphism and risk of laryngeal squamous cell carcinoma. Int J Environ Res Public Health. 2016;13. https://doi.org/10.3390/ijerph13010112.
13. Siegel R, Ward E, Brawley O, et al. Cancer statistics, 2011: the impact of eliminating socioeconomic and racial disparities on pre-mature cancer deaths. CA-Cancer J Clin. 2011;61:212–36. https://doi.org/10.3322/caac.20121.
14. Sun R, Qin C, Jiang B, et al. Down-regulation of MALAT1 inhibits cervical cancer cell invasion and metastasis by inhibition of epithelial-mesenchymal transition. Mol BioSyst. 2016;12:952–62. https://doi.org/10.1039/c5mb00685f.
15. Wu K, Chen K, Wang C, et al. Cell fate factor DACH1 represses YB-1-mediated oncogenic transcription and translation. Cancer Res. 2015;74:829–39. https://doi.org/10.1158/0008-5472.CAN-13-2466.
16. Zhu J, Wu C, Li H, et al. DACH1 inhibits the proliferation and invasion of lung adenocarcinoma through the downregulation of peroxiredoxin 3. Tumour Biol. 2016;37:9781–8. https://doi.org/10.1007/s13277-016-4811-x.
17. Nan FF, Lü QT, Zhou J, et al. Altered expression of DACH1 and cyclin D1 in endometrial cancer. Cancer Biol Ther. 2009;8:1534–9.
18. Zhu HB, Wu HM, Yan WJ, et al. Epigenetic silencing of DACH1 induces loss of transforming growth factor β1 antiproliferative response in human hepatocelluar carcinoma. Hepatology. 2013;58:2012–22. https://doi.org/10.1002/hep.26587.
19. Yan WJ, Wu KM, Herman JG, et al. Epigenetic regulation of DACH1, a novel Wnt signaling component in colorectal cancer. Epigenetics. 2013;8:1373–83. https://doi.org/10.4161/epi.26781.
20. Powe DG, Dhondalay GKR, Lemetre C, et al. DACH1: its role as a classifier of long term good prognosis in luminal breast Cancer. PLoS One. 2014;9: e84428. https://doi.org/10.1371/journal.pone.0084428.
21. Lee JW, Kim HS, Hwang J, et al. Regulatiion of HOXA9 activity by predominant expression of DACH1 against C/EBPα and GATA-1 in myeloid leukemia with MLL-AF9. Biochem Biophys Res Commun. 2012;426:299–305. https://doi.org/10.1016/j.bbrc.2012.08.048.
22. Liang F, Lü Q, Sun S, et al. Increased expression of dachshund homolog 1 in ovarian cancer as a predictor for poor outcome. Int J Gynecol Cancer. 2012; 22:386–93. https://doi.org/10.1097/IGC.0b013e31824311e6.
23. Yan WJ, Wu KM, Herman JG, et al. Epigenetic silencing of DACH1 induces the invasion and metastasis of gastric cancer by activating TGF-β signalling. J Cell Mol Med. 2014;18:2499–511. https://doi.org/10.1111/jcmm.12325.
24. Liu Y, Zhou R, Yuan X, et al. DACH1 is a novel predictive and prognostic biomarker in hepatocellular carcinoma as a negative regulator of Wnt/ β-catenin signaling. Oncotarget. 2015;6:8621–34. https://doi.org/10.18632/oncotarget.3281.
25. Zhang J, Zhao CY, Zhang SH, et al. Upregulation of miR-194 contributes to tumor growth and progression in pancreatic ductal adenocarcinoma. Oncol Rep. 2014;31:1157–64. https://doi.org/10.3892/or.2013.2960.
26. Zhang Q, Yuan YH, Cui JC, et al. MiR-217 promotes tumor Proloferation in breast Cancer via targeting DACH1. J Cancer. 2015;6:184–91. https://doi.org/10.7150/jca.10822.
27. Wu KM, Katiyar S, Li A, et al. Dachshund inhibits oncogene-induced breast cancer cellular migration and invasion through suppression of interleukin-8. PNAS. 2008;105:6924–9. https://doi.org/10.1073/pnas.0802085105.
28. Zhou J, Liu Y, Zhang W, et al. Transcription elongation regulator 1 is a co-integrator of the cell fate determination factor dachshund homolog 1. J Biol Chem. 2010;285:40342–50. https://doi.org/10.1074/jbc.M110.156141.
29. Wu KM, Li AP, Rao M, et al. DACH1 is a cell fate determination factor that inhibits cyclin D1 and breast tumor growth. Mol Cell Biol. 2006;26:7116–29. https://doi.org/10.1128/MCB.00268-06.
30. Wu KM, Liu MR, Li AP, et al. Cell fate determination factor DACH1 inhibits c-Jun–induced contact-independent growth. Mol Biol Cell. 2007;18:755–67. https://doi.org/10.1091/mbc.E06-09-0793.
31. Chu Q, Han N, Yuan X, et al. DACH1 inhibits cyclin D1 expression, cellular proliferation and tumor growth of renal cancer cells. J Hematol Oncol. 2014; 7:73. https://doi.org/10.1186/s13045-014-0073-5.
32. Wu K, Jiao X, Li Z, et al. Cell fate determination factor dachshund reprograms breast Cancer stem cell function. J Biol Chem. 2011;286:2132–42. https://doi.org/10.1074/jbc.M110.148395.
33. Popov VM, Zhou J, Shirley LA, et al. The cell fate determination factor DACH1 is expressed in estrogen receptor-alpha-positive breast cancer and represses estrogen receptor-alpha signaling. Cancer Res. 2009;69:5752–60. https://doi.org/10.1158/0008-5472.CAN-08-3992.
34. Popov VM, Wu K, Zhou J, et al. The dachshund gene in development and hormone-responsive tumorigenesis. Trends Endocrinol Metab. 2010;21:41–9. https://doi.org/10.1016/j.tem.2009.08.002.
35. Chen K, Wu K, Cai S, et al. Dachshund binds p53 to block the growth of lung adenocarcinoma cells. Cancer Res. 2013;73:3262–74. https://doi.org/10.1158/0008-5472.CAN-12-3191.
36. Miller SJ, Lan ZD, Hardiman A, et al. Inhibition of eyes absent homolog 4 expression induces malignant peripheral nerve sheath tumor necrosis. Oncogene. 2010;29:368–79. https://doi.org/10.1038/onc.2009.360.
37. Wu K, Yang Y, Wang C, et al. DACH1 inhibits transforming growth factor-β signaling through binding Smad4. J Biol Chem. 2003;278:51673–84. https://doi.org/10.1074/jbc.M310021200.
38. Wu K, Katiyar S, Witkiewicz A, et al. The cell fate determination factor dachshund inhibits androgen receptor signaling and prostate cancer cellular growth. Cancer Res. 2009;69:3347–55. https://doi.org/10.1158/0008-5472.CAN-08-3821.
39. Zhang L, Wang CQ, Liu F, et al. Effects of human dachshund homolog 1 on the proliferation, migration, and adhesion of squamous cell carcinoma of the tongue. Oral Surg Oral Med Oral Pathol Oral Radiol. 2016;121:58–66. https://doi.org/10.1016/j.oooo.2015.08.021.
40. Chen K, Wu K, Jiao X, et al. The endogenous cell-fate factor dachshund restrains prostate epithelial cell migration via repression of cytokine secretion via a CXCL signaling module. Cancer Res. 2015;75:1992–2004. https://doi.org/10.1158/0008-5472.CAN-14-0611.

34

Three dimensional evaluation of soft tissue after orthognathic surgery

Junho Jung, Chi-Heun Lee, Jung-Woo Lee and Byung-Joon Choi[*]

Abstract

Background: To evaluate the nasolabial soft tissue change three-dimensionally after orthognathic surgery, using a structured light scanner.

Methods: Thirty-two malocclusion patients, who underwent orthognathic surgery, were evaluated. CBCT and 3D facial scans were obtained before surgery and 3 months after surgery. The 3D changes in the 26 landmarks, and the relative ratio of the soft tissue movement to the bony movement, were evaluated.

Results: In the Le Fort I advancement patients, the nasal tip moved 17% forward, compared to the maxillary bony movement, but the nasal prominence decreased 15%. The alar width increased 4 mm after the advancement, and the width decreased 4.7 mm after Le Fort I setback. The relative ratio of the soft tissue movement to the bony movement after bilateral sagittal split osteotomy was about 66% at the Li point in the anteroposterior direction, and it was 21% in the Le Fort I advancement and 14% in Le Fort I setback at the Ls point.

Conclusion: Alar cinch suturing may not be sufficient to overcome the effect of the maxilla advancement compressing the nasal complex. Alar width widening was prevented in Le Fort I setback. However, it is uncertain that the alar cinch suturing was solely responsible. The soft tissue around the mandible tends to accompany the bony movement more than the maxillary area. In addition, structured light scanning system proved to be a useful tool to evaluate the nasolabial soft tissue.

Keywords: Orthognathic surgery, Structured light-based scanners, 3D measurement, Nasolabial soft tissue

Background

Orthognathic surgery restores not only the occlusal function, but also aesthetics by improving facial harmony. Needless to say, improving soft tissue esthetics is of the ultimate treatment goal. According to skeletal movements from orthognathic surgery, there are consistent nasolabial soft tissue changes. Consequently, various attempts have tried to establish a correlation between the hard and soft tissue changes [1–4].

Conventional two-dimensional (2D) lateral cephalogram is used to predict and evaluate surgical outcomes before and after surgery. Although these methods are convenient and have economic advantages, due to the limitation of its midsagittal projection and the projection angle and distance, the information of soft tissue changes and the accuracy is lacking and unsatisfactory [5]. Moreover, since various soft tissue closure techniques, including the alar cinch suture and the "V-Y" lip mucosal closure, control the nasal base and upper lip [6–8], 2D imaging methods may not be adequate to evaluate the nasolabial tissue.

In recent years, 3D imaging has gained popularity to overcome the limitations of 2D analysis. Cone beam computed tomography (CBCT) provides sufficient information about skeletal structures, and is used to measure soft tissue changes [9]. Moreover, it is frequently applied in dentistry. However, owing to its low resolution and lack of data of skin texture and color, the accuracy of the evaluation for facial soft tissues is not guaranteed [10]. Therefore, noncontact optical scanning methods such as Laser surface scanning and light emitting diode (LED) white light scanning, were introduced as 3D imaging tools [11]. The LED white light scanning has advantages of innocuousness to the human eyes and immediacy to acquire data, making the scanning method suitable for long-term studies and for a larger population of patients [12].

* Correspondence: sjnb2@khu.ac.kr
Department of Oral and Maxillofacial Surgery, School of Dentistry, Kyung Hee University, 26, Kyungheedae-ro, Dongdaemun-gu, 02447 Seoul, Republic of Korea

This study was undertaken to assess and describe the nasolabial soft tissue changes three-dimensionally, after bilateral sagittal split osteotomy (BSSRO) or Le Fort I osteotomy with BSSRO, using structured light system-one of the LED white light scanning system. In addition, this study also investigated the effect of the alar base cinch suture following Le Fort I osteotomy, by measuring nasal soft tissue.

Methods

Subjects

The patients enrolled for this study included 32 malocclusion cases (17 men, 15 women; mean age, 23.8 ± 3.60 years; range, 17–33 years) who had undergone BSSRO or/and Le Fort I advancement or setback osteotomy, between 2010 and 2016, in the department of oral and maxillofacial surgery at Kyung Hee university Medical Center (Table 1). The patients were divided into 3 groups: BSSRO only (9 patients; mean age, 23.2 ± 3.5; range, 19–31), Le Fort I advancement (13 patients; mean age, 24.0 ± 3.4; range, 17–31), and Le Fort I setback (10 patients; mean age, 24.1 ± 4.1; range, 19–33). All subjects underwent pre- and post-operative orthodontic treatment. In each case, the surgical procedure consisted of BSSRO only, or Le Fort I osteotomy with BSSRO and rigid fixation. After Le Fort I osteotomy and rigid fixation with four L-type titanium plates, alar cinch suture was applied to prevent widening of the nose for all patients. A hole was made at the anterior nasal spine through lateral to lateral by a 1.6 Ø drill. The suture (2/0 non-absorbable (Ethibond)) was passed through the perinasal musculature and fibroadipose tissue at the right alar base from a lateral to medial, the needle then passed through the hole in the nasal spine. The tissue at the left alar base was grasped by the same suture, and the needle then passed through the hole again. A knot of the suture was made at the alar base. The mandible was set back with BSSRO, and the proximal segment fixed with one 4-hole plate and screws. A surgical wafer was placed for 5–6 weeks postoperatively, and inter-arch elastics were used in order to stabilize the inter-maxillary relationship with the surgical wafer. This study was approved by the Ethics Committee at the Kyung Hee University Dental Hospital (KHD IRB 1603–4).

Patients who underwent superior or inferior positioning of the maxilla and previous nasal surgery and have any craniofacial anomalies and a history of trauma were excluded in this study.

Data acquisition

3D facial image scans using a LED white light scanning system (Morpheus 3D, Morpheus Co., Ltd., Seoul, Korea) were acquired preoperatively and at 3 months postoperative (scan time: 0.8 s, 33 frame rate: 15 frames/s, data accuracy: ±0.2 mm). Each patient was instructed to relax their lips and set the head in a natural position, while the images were taken. Afterwards, three images from three different views were reconstructed into one 3D image by a merging process.

CBCT scans were acquired preoperatively and at 3 months postoperative, using the Alphard 3030 Dental CT system (Asahi Roentgen Ind. Co., Ltd., Kyoto, Japan) with the following imaging protocol: 80 kVp, 5 mA, 17 s, and 15.4 cm × 15.4 cm field of view. All patients were seated upright with maximum intercuspation, and the Frankfort horizontal (FH) plane of the patient was maintained parallel to the floor during scanning. Voxels were isotropic, each of 0.3 mm width. The CBCT data were exported into the DICOM format, and OnDemand 3D (CyberMed Inc., Seoul, Korea) was used to measure the movement of the maxilla and mandible by superimposition of the data. The actual movement of B-point was measured after BSSRO; both A-point and B-point were measured after Le Fort I osteotomy.

Landmarks and coordinate system

To evaluate the nasolabial soft tissue changes after surgery, 26 landmarks were set on the 3D image along the lip border, and around the lip and the nostrils (Figs. 1a, 2, Table 2). [12] The landmark values were recorded with a

Table 1 Details of the subjects

Group	Mean age	Gender (M/F)	Diagnosis	Ethnicity
Le Fort I Advancement & BSSRO	24.0 ± 3.4	9/4	Class I malocclusion: 1	Korean
			Class II malocclusion: 2	
			Class III malocclusion: 10	
Le Fort I Setback & BSSRO	24.1 ± 4.1	4/6	Class I malocclusion: 3	Korean
			Class II malocclusion: 2	
			Class III malocclusion: 5	
BSSRO	23.2 ± 3.5	4/5	Class I malocclusion: 0	Korean
			Class II malocclusion: 0	
			Class III malocclusion: 9	

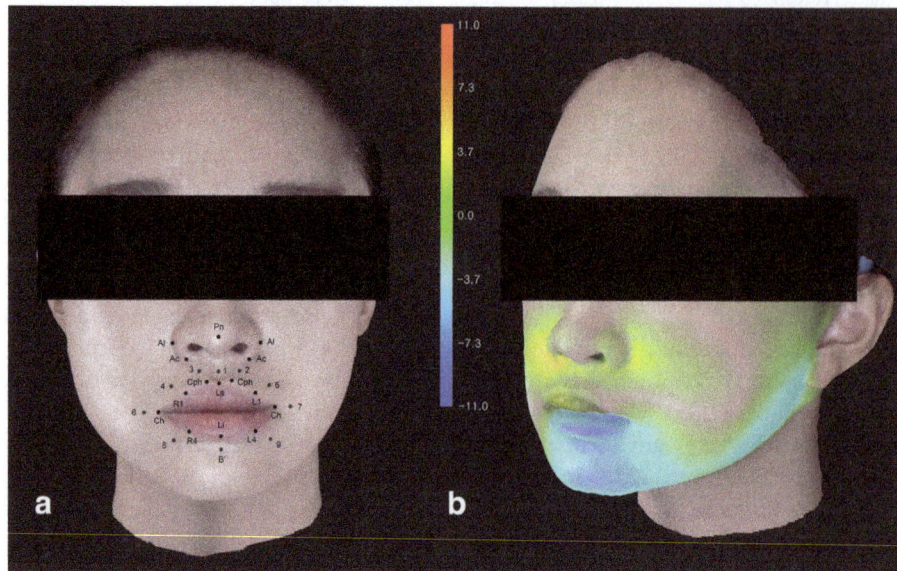

Fig. 1 (**a**) Three-dimensionally reconstructed facial image and twenty-six landmarks around the nasolabial tissue. (**b**) A superimposed color map image of facial soft tissue change after orthognathic surgery

3D Cartesian coordinate system. The left (x-axis), front (z-axis) and above (y-axis) of a patient were defined as positive values; the reference planes were set as below [13]:

The horizontal reference plane (x-axis): the ala-tragus plane was rotated 7.5 degree upward on the axis connecting both tragi, and translated until soft tissue nasion.

The sagittal reference plane (y-axis): the plane perpendicular to the horizontal plane and passing the soft tissue nasion.

The coronal reference plane (z-axis): the plane perpendicular to the other reference planes and passing the soft tissue nasion.

Superimposition of pre-and post-operative image data was performed by reference points including left and right exocanthion, endocanthion, N′, and wide face of forehead using 3D Image Overlay [13]. The differences were evaluated by superimposed 3D image with one coordinate system.

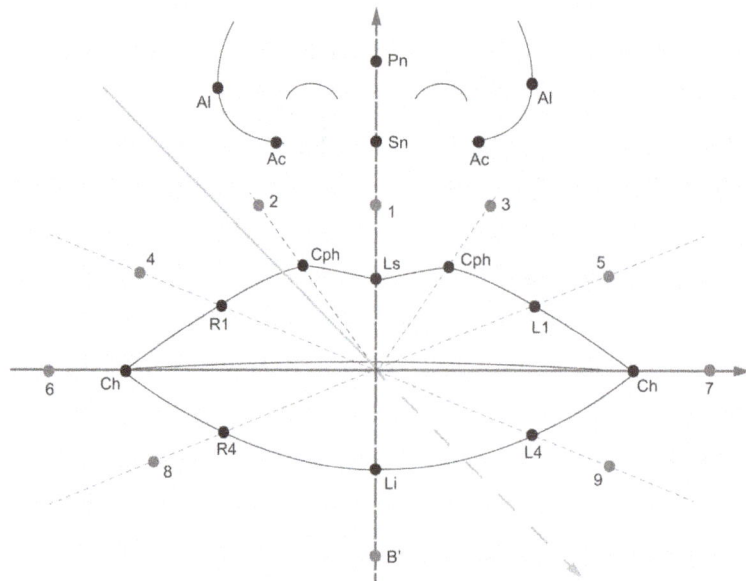

Fig. 2 Twenty-six landmarks around the nasolabial tissue [12]

Table 2 Definitions of the landmarks

Region	Landmarks	Description
Along the lips	Cph (L), Cph (R)	The highest point of the Cupid's bow (left, right)
	Ls	The lowest point of the middle area of the Cupid's bow
	Ch (L), Ch(R)	The most lateral point of vermilion border (left, right)
	Li	The lowest point of vermilion border
	L1, L4, R1, R4	Midpoints of curved vermilion border
Around the lips	1–9 B′	Perioral points which are counterparts of each point along the lip border, being apart by the same distance Soft tissue B point
Around the nostril	Al (L), Al (R)	Most lateral point of the alar contour (left, right)
	Pn	Most anterior point of the nose
	Sn	Midpoint of the nasolabial angle at the columellar base
	Ac (L), Ac (R)	Labial insertion of each alar base

Statistical analysis

Two weeks after the first measurement, re-evaluation was performed by the same investigator, and both values were compared using the Pearson correlation analysis. The coefficient was above 0.98 at the 95% confidence level. Thus, the mean of the two values was used for the statistical analysis. The Shapiro-Wilk test was used to confirm the Normality of the data distribution. The paired Student t-test analyzed the data, and α-level was set to 0.05.

Results

The amount of movement at point A was about 2.4 mm ($\pm$1.4) after the Le Fort I advancement, and the relative ratio of the soft tissue movement to the bony movement are shown in Table 3 and Fig. 3. Unplanned superoinferior movements of the maxilla was not observed during the measurement. The alar width increased approximately 4 mm after surgery, which was statistically significant. In addition, a significant forward movement

Table 3 The relative ratio of soft tissue movement to bony movement in the anteroposterior direction and three-dimensional changes of perioral soft tissue after Le Fort I advancement & BSSRO

Landmarks	Soft tissue/bony movement (%)	X-axis			Y-axis			Z-axis		
		mean	SD	P-value	Mean	SD	P-value	Mean	SD	P-value
Cph (L)	22%	−0.21	0.54	0.19	0.36	1.54	0.42	0.53	1.72	0.07
Cph (R)	31%	0.19	0.54	0.24	0.29	1.09	0.35	0.73	1.52	*0.02
Ls	21%	−0.07	0.17	0.16	2.85	8.55	0.25	0.51	1.87	*0.00
Lip (L1)	14%	0.11	1.16	0.73	0.46	1.39	0.26	0.34	1.80	*0.00
Lip (R1)	32%	−0.01	0.91	0.98	1.01	2.57	0.19	0.77	1.53	*0.00
Ch (L)	35%	0.63	1.05	0.05	0.94	1.88	0.10	−1.72	3.17	0.29
Ch (R)	47%	1.24	5.77	0.45	0.80	2.88	0.34	−2.35	3.20	0.11
1	40%	0.04	0.25	0.57	−0.11	0.87	0.67	−0.96	1.46	*0.04
2	39%	0.29	0.61	0.11	0.31	0.55	0.07	−0.93	37.24	0.39
3	34%	0.39	0.51	*0.02	−0.09	0.88	0.71	−0.82	1.44	0.62
4	26%	0.18	0.82	0.45	−0.02	0.88	0.95	−0.63	1.61	0.18
5	20%	0.08	0.83	0.74	0.14	0.93	0.59	−0.49	1.87	0.37
Al (L)	31%	1.23	0.80	*0.00	0.02	0.36	0.88	0.74	0.09	*0.01
Al (R)	33%	2.89	5.51	*0.04	0.14	0.47	0.29	0.78	1.06	*0.02
Ac (L)	18%	−5.17	13.75	0.20	−1.87	12.03	0.59	0.44	7.85	0.84
Ac (R)	29%	1.66	10.43	0.13	−3.82	15.25	0.38	0.70	5.70	0.67
Sn	115%	0.04	1.72	0.93	−2.05	11.91	0.52	−2.74	4.03	*0.03
Pn	18%	−0.04	0.37	0.72	0.02	0.22	0.71	0.43	0.43	*0.00

SD standard deviation
Asterisks indicate statistical significance between the values of pre- and post-operative measurement ($P < 0.05$)s

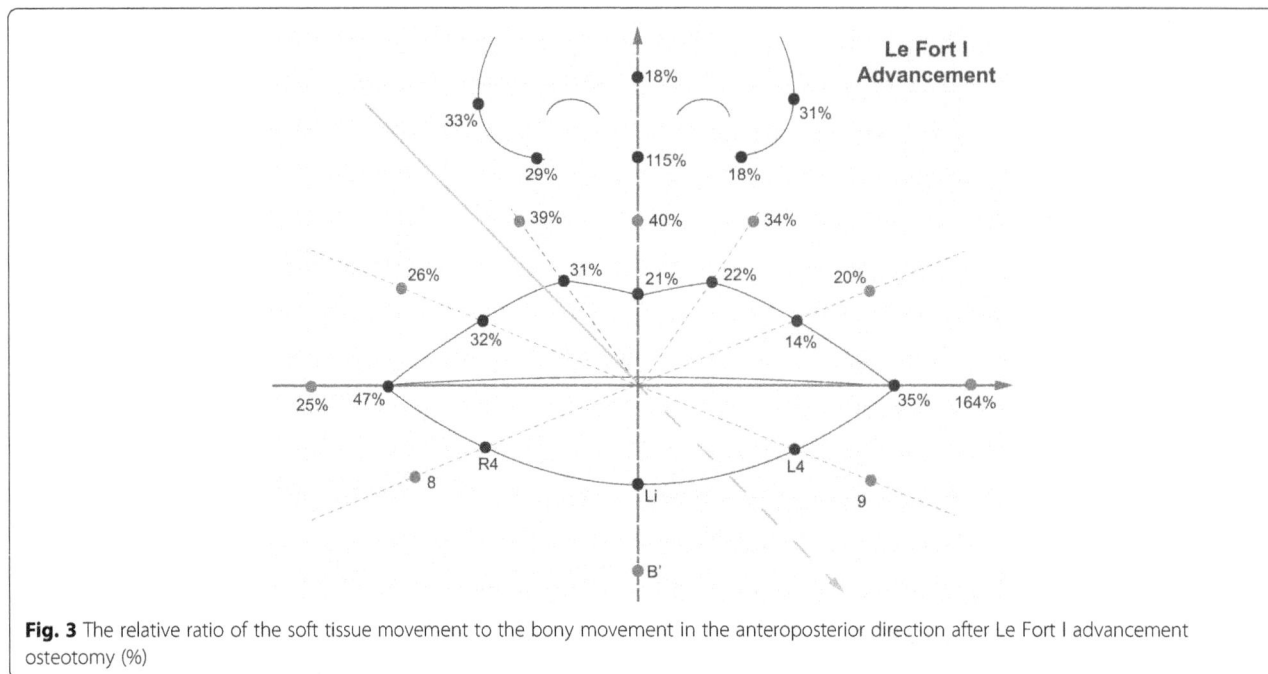

Fig. 3 The relative ratio of the soft tissue movement to the bony movement in the anteroposterior direction after Le Fort I advancement osteotomy (%)

of almost all upper lip landmarks was observed due to the maxilla advancement ($P < 0.05$). In the upper lip, the percentage of the soft tissue movement compared to the bony movement was 14–31%. In the nasal area, the ratio was 18–48%, which was higher than the lip area. However, the nasal tip movement was the least among the nasal areas.

After the Le Fort I setback osteotomy, on an average, point A moved posteriorly by about 2.1 mm (±1.0). Unplanned superoinferior movements of the maxilla was not observed during the measurement. Also, postoperatively the alar width decreased about 4.7 mm (Table 4, Fig. 4). In the upper lip area, the soft tissue movement was 3–52% compared to the bony movement, and it was 15% at the nasal tip. However, the proportion was 63–84% at the alar and alar base areas.

The amount of setback movement after BSSRO was measured as the mean value of 6.6 mm (±2.8) at point B by CBCT (Table 5). The Li and soft tissue B point movement was 4.3 and 4.85 mm, respectively. The relative ratio of soft tissue movement to bony movement was about 66% and 73% in the anteroposterior direction at the landmarks.

Discussion

Le Fort I osteotomy has the potential to alter the mid-facial region. However, despite precise planning and surgery, it is difficult to predict soft tissue changes. Hence, this study aimed to demonstrate the 3D change in postoperative nasolabial soft tissue, in order to optimize surgical outcomes and patient satisfaction. Especially, undesirable effects such as widening of the alar

base or alteration of the nasal tip projection [3, 14–16] were measured.

2D techniques have been broadly used until recent years. However, due to their limitations, the measurements might be somewhat biased [14]. Therefore, various methods, including laser scanners, stereophotogrammetry, and structured light systems, have recently been introduced for 3D soft tissue assessment. The accuracy of the structured light system used in this study compares the direct anthropometric measurements, and 3D facial scan values were less than 1 mm [17, 18]. Moreover, as the face of the subject was simultaneously scanned from multiple angles in less than 1 s, we expect more reliable collections of 3D datasets. The facial scanning device used in study is now available more than 10 countries in America, Europe and Asia. The cost for the procedure is less than the one for CBCT taking in our clinic.

In our study, the nasolabial soft tissue changes were compared with the actual movement of point A measured in CBCT. The average movement of the nasal tip was about 17% compared to the maxillary bony movement. However, the nasal prominence (measured from the alar groove to the tip) decreased by about 15% of the total maxillary advancement. In other words, although the actual nasal tip moved forward, the nasal prominence itself decreased as the piriform aperture compressed the nasal complex, and it widened and became obtuse. According to the tripod theory, the widened alar may pull the nasal tip back, despite an increase in relative nasal tip position to the face, so that intrinsic nasal tip projection decreased while the extrinsic nasal projection increased [19–21].

Table 4 The relative ratio of soft tissue movement to bony movement in the anteroposterior direction and three-dimensional changes of perioral soft tissue after Le Fort I setback & BSSRO

Landmarks	Soft tissue/bony movement (%)	X-axis			Y-axis			Z-axis		
		mean	SD	P-value	Mean	SD	P-value	Mean	SD	P-value
Cph (L)	25%	− 0.32	0.56	0.13	0.39	1.26	0.38	−0.52	0.92	0.13
Cph (R)	19%	0.33	0.44	0.06	7.23	20.66	0.32	−0.41	0.93	0.23
Ls	14%	0.09	0.41	0.52	0.27	1.29	0.55	−0.29	0.95	0.39
Lip (L1)	3%	−0.06	0.38	0.65	0.26	0.85	0.38	−0.06	0.88	0.84
Lip (R1)	16%	−0.54	1.74	0.38	0.21	0.64	0.36	−0.33	0.62	0.15
Ch (L)	22%	0.02	0.62	0.94	0.48	1.45	0.35	0.96	2.72	0.32
Ch (R)	40%	−0.52	1.02	0.17	−7.08	21.63	0.36	1.69	3.13	0.14
1	52%	0.02	0.10	0.51	−0.45	0.39	*0.01	−1.10	0.65	*0.00
2	40%	0.37	0.37	*0.02	−6.79	18.91	0.31	−0.83	0.65	*0.01
3	43%	−0.49	0.38	*0.01	−0.51	0.58	*0.03	−0.90	0.72	*0.01
4	38%	0.43	0.58	0.06	−0.19	0.41	0.19	−0.80	1.01	*0.04
5	31%	−0.28	0.40	0.07	−0.12	0.15	*0.04	−0.64	0.73	*0.03
Al (L)	63%	−1.26	1.29	*0.01	−1.92	5.47	0.32	−1.32	0.93	*0.00
Al (R)	77%	−3.42	13.50	0.47	−0.06	0.11	0.15	−1.62	2.22	0.06
Ac (L)	74%	−1.26	1.29	*0.01	−1.92	5.47	0.32	−1.32	0.93	*0.00
Ac (R)	84%	−3.42	13.50	0.47	−0.06	0.11	0.15	−1.62	2.22	0.06
Sn	29%	−0.09	0.12	0.06	−2.72	9.20	0.40	−0.62	1.31	0.20
Pn	15%	−0.03	0.05	0.13	0.01	0.04	0.69	−0.32	0.41	*0.04

SD standard deviation

Asterisks indicate statistical significance between the values of pre- and post-operative measurement ($P < 0.05$)

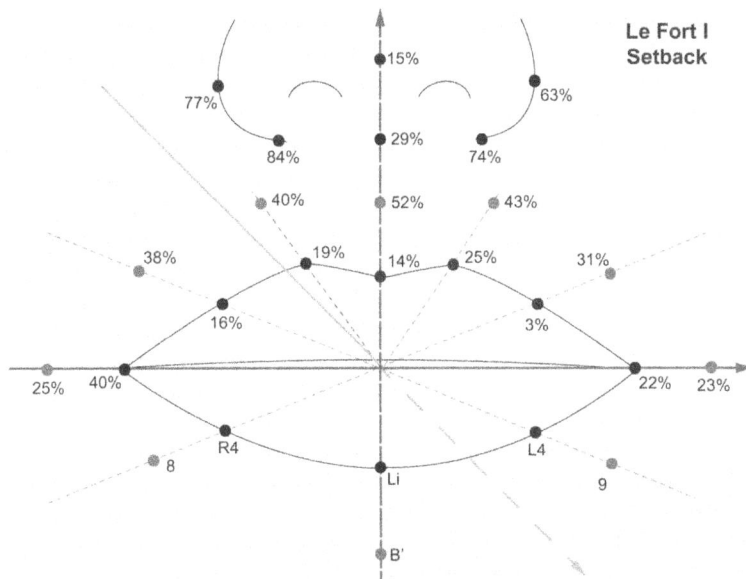

Fig. 4 The relative ratio of the soft tissue movement to the bony movement in the anteroposterior direction after Le Fort I setback osteotomy (%)

Table 5 The relative ratio of soft tissue movement to bony movement in the anteroposterior direction and three-dimensional changes of perioral soft tissue after BSSRO

Landmarks	Soft tissue/bony movement (%)	X-axis			Y-axis			Z-axis		
		mean	SD	P-value	Mean	SD	P-value	Mean	SD	P-value
Ch (L)	37%	0.45	0.60	0.09	0.26	1.27	0.60	−0.18	0.88	0.60
Ch (R)	25%	−0.04	1.19	0.94	−0.33	0.54	0.16	−0.62	0.91	0.13
L4	57%	1.16	1.71	0.12	−13.89	3.94	0.39	−3.77	1.67	*0.00
R4	52%	3.32	11.19	0.46	11.60	3.14	0.37	−3.44	1.05	*0.00
Li	66%	−0.26	0.82	0.44	11.48	3.11	0.37	−4.35	1.25	*0.03
6	114%	−1.17	1.64	0.11	1.08	1.07	*0.04	−7.50	2.14	0.39
7	11%	0.51	1.68	0.45	0.82	2.06	0.44	0.73	0.74	*0.04
8	55%	−1.26	2.15	0.17	16.70	45.04	0.37	3.61	1.30	*0.00
9	309%	1.08	1.47	0.10	−0.12	1.36	0.82	20.39	44.57	0.27
B′	73%	−0.54	0.69	0.08	−0.91	1.33	0.12	4.82	2.13	*0.00

SD standard deviation

Asterisks indicate statistical significance between the values of pre- and post-operative measurement ($P < 0.05$)

In this study, despite alar cinch suturing, the alar width resulted in an increase of 4 mm after Le Fort I advancement. However, in case of Le Fort I setback, the width decreased by about 4.7 mm. Therefore, we surmise that the effect of the maxilla advancement compressing the nasal complex exceeds the effect of the cinch suturing. Although alar width widening was prevented in Le Fort I setback, it is uncertain that the alar cinch suturing was solely responsible, because the backward movement of the supporting bony structure may also have effects to prevent the widening.

The relative ratio of the soft tissue movement to the bony movement after BSSRO was only about 66% at the Li point, and 73% at B′ point. In Le Fort I advancement, the ratio was 21% at the Ls point, and 14% in the Le Fort I setback. These results indicate that considering the labial tissue, more soft tissue movements occur around the mandible than the maxillary area. A similar tendency was observed in other studies. Biak and Kim reported that the proportion of soft tissue changes to hard tissue changes at the Ls point was 34% in Le Fort I advancement, and 81% at Li point in BSSRO [22]. Soncul and Bamber also presented 49% of the proportion at Upper vermillion in Le Fort I advancement, and 71% at the Lower vermillion in BSSRO [23].

Previous studies describe that nasolabial soft tissue change following Le Fort I osteotomy occurs inconsistently, indicating that hard-to-soft tissue prediction is a difficult task. Nasal tip movement has been reported in 30–60% of the total maxillary advancement, and the columellar base was known to be advanced more than the nasal tip, after the anterior movement of the maxilla [24–26]. However, reports of this finding are also inconsistent [6]. The alar width increased along the maxillary advancement, but with wide ranges. [27–29] Van Loon et al. presented no difference in the alar width after Le Fort I advancement, between patients who had underwent an alar cinch and those who had not [30]. Howley et al. also compared a group of patients who underwent an alar cinch suture with a control group, and concluded that the alar base width eventually increased 6 months after the surgery [31]. These results are in accordance with this study, which implicates that it is hard to control the alar width despite the alar cinch suture after the maxillary advancement osteotomy.

We observed a wide variety of soft tissue response to the bony movement in this study, and this result could originate due to soft adaptation process after surgery. Although this study helps us predict the outcomes of orthognathic surgery, a large sample number is required to increase reliability and confirm the factors that influence the nasolabial soft tissue changes after orthognathic surgery. However, a structured light system such as a 3D imaging method to measure facial soft tissues, provides useful and accurate information conveniently. Hence, this system can serve as a worthwhile tool in dentistry. In addition, there are other factors to observe soft tissue response after orthognathic surgery, such as lip thickness, volume and tonicity, which were not evaluated in this study. It should be evaluated for a future study to better understand soft tissue response.

Conclusions

Alar cinch suturing does not appear sufficient to overcome the effect of the maxilla advancement compressing the nasal complex. The nasal complex became obtuse and the alar width increased. Alar width widening was prevented in Le Fort I setback. However, it is uncertain that the alar cinch suturing was solely responsible. The soft tissue around the mandible tends to accompany the bony movement more than the maxillary area. In addition, structured light scanning system proved to be a useful tool to evaluate the nasolabial soft tissue.

Abbreviations
2D: Two-dimensional; 3D: Three dimensional; BSSRO: Bilateral sagittal split osteotomy; CBCT: Cone beam computed tomography; LED: Light emitting diode

Authors' contributions
B-JC conceived the study design and treated the patients. JJ wrote the manuscript, and JJ and C-HL carried out the measurement of the outcomes. JJ and JWL interpreted the data and edited the manuscript. All authors read and approved the final manuscript.

Consent for publication
Not applicable.

Competing interests
The authors declare, that they have no competing interests.

References
1. Chew MT, Sandham A, Wong HB. Evaluation of the linearity of soft- to hard-tissue movement after orthognathic surgery. Am J Orthod Dentofac Orthop. 2008;134:665–70.
2. Olate S, Zaror C, Blythe JN, Mommaerts MY. A systematic review of soft-to hard tissue ratios in orthognathic surgery. Part III: double jaw surgery procedures. J Craniomaxillofac Surg. 2016;44:1599–606.
3. Bailey LJ, Collie FM, White RP Jr. Long-term soft tissue changes after orthognathic surgery. Int J Adult Orthodon Orthognath Surg. 1996;11:7–18.
4. McFarlane RB, Frydman WL, McCabe SB, Mamandras AM. Identification of nasal morphologic features that indicate susceptibility to nasal tip deflection with the LeFort I osteotomy. Am J Orthod Dentofac Orthop. 1995;107:259–67.
5. Lane C, Harrell W, Jr. Completing the 3-dimensional picture. Am J Orthod Dentofac Orthop 2008;133:612–620.
6. Muradin MS, Rosenberg AJ, van der Bilt A, Stoelinga PJ, Koole R. The influence of a Le fort I impaction and advancement osteotomy on smile using a modified alar cinch suture and V-Y closure: a prospective study. Int J Oral Maxillofac Surg. 2012;41:547–52.
7. Mustafa K, Shehzana F, Bhat HH. Assessment of alar flare and efficacy of alar cinch suture in the Management of Alar Flare Following Le Fort 1 superior repositioning: a comparative study. J Maxillofac Oral Surg. 2016;15:528–34.
8. Muradin MS, Seubring K, Stoelinga PJ, vd Bilt A, Koole R, Rosenberg AJ. A prospective study on the effect of modified alar cinch sutures and V-Y closure versus simple closing sutures on nasolabial changes after Le fort I intrusion and advancement osteotomies. J Oral Maxillofac Surg. 2011;69:870–6.
9. Gorgulu S, Gokce SM, Olmez H, Sagdic D, Ors F. Nasal cavity volume changes after rapid maxillary expansion in adolescents evaluated with 3-dimensional simulation and modeling programs. Am J Orthod Dentofac Orthop. 2011;140:633–40.
10. Miracle AC, Mukherji SK. Conebeam CT of the head and neck, part 1: physical principles. AJNR Am J Neuroradiol. 2009;30:1088–95.
11. Kau CH, Richmond S, Incrapera A, English J, Xia JJ. Three-dimensional surface acquisition systems for the study of facial morphology and their application to maxillofacial surgery. Int J Med Robot. 2007;3:97–110.
12. Ahn HW, Chang YJ, Kim KA, Joo SH, Park YG, Park KH. Measurement of three-dimensional perioral soft tissue changes in dentoalveolar protrusion patients after orthodontic treatment using a structured light scanner. Angle Orthod. 2014;84:795–802.
13. Lee WJLK, Yu HS, Baik HS. Lip and perioral soft tissue changes after bracket bonding using 3-D laser scanner. Korean J Orthod. 2011;41:411–22.
14. Vasudavan S, Jayaratne YS, Padwa BL. Nasolabial soft tissue changes after Le fort I advancement. J Oral Maxillofac Surg. 2012;70:e270–7.
15. Kim YI, Park SB, Son WS, Hwang DS. Midfacial soft-tissue changes after advancement of maxilla with Le fort I osteotomy and mandibular setback surgery: comparison of conventional and high Le fort I osteotomies by superimposition of cone-beam computed tomography volumes. J Oral Maxillofac Surg. 2011;69:e225–33.
16. Altug-Atac AT, Bolatoglu H, Memikoglu UT. Facial soft tissue profile following bimaxillary orthognathic surgery. Angle Orthod. 2008;78:50–7.
17. Ma L, Xu T, Lin J. Validation of a three-dimensional facial scanning system based on structured light techniques. Comput Methods Prog Biomed. 2009;94:290–8.
18. Kim SH, Jung WY, Seo YJ, Kim KA, Park KH, Park YG. Accuracy and precision of integumental linear dimensions in a three-dimensional facial imaging system. Korean J Orthod. 2015;45:105–12.
19. Sheen JH. Secondary rhinoplasty. Plast Reconstr Surg. 1975;56:137–45.
20. Sheen JH. Spreader graft: a method of reconstructing the roof of the middle nasal vault following rhinoplasty. Plast Reconstr Surg. 1984;73:230–9.
21. Metzler P, Geiger EJ, Chang CC, Sirisoontorn I, Steinbacher DM. Assessment of three-dimensional nasolabial response to Le fort I advancement. J Plast Reconstr Aesthet Surg. 2014;67:756–63.
22. Baik HS, Kim SY. Facial soft-tissue changes in skeletal class III orthognathic surgery patients analyzed with 3-dimensional laser scanning. Am J Orthod Dentofac Orthop. 2010;138:167–78.
23. Soncul M, Bamber MA. Evaluation of facial soft tissue changes with optical surface scan after surgical correction of class III deformities. J Oral Maxillofac Surg. 2004;62:1331–40.
24. Freihofer HP, Jr. Changes in nasal profile after maxillary advancement in cleft and non-cleft patients. J Maxillofac Surg 1977;5:20–27.
25. Mansour S, Burstone C, Legan H. An evaluation of soft-tissue changes resulting from Le fort I maxillary surgery. Am J Orthod. 1983;84:37–47.
26. Bundgaard M, Melsen B, Terp S. Changes during and following total maxillary osteotomy (le fort I procedure): a cephalometric study. Eur J Orthod. 1986;8:21–9.
27. Schendel SA, Williamson LW. Muscle reorientation following superior repositioning of the maxilla. J Oral Maxillofac Surg. 1983;41:235–40.
28. Carlotti AE Jr, Aschaffenburg PH, Schendel SA. Facial changes associated with surgical advancement of the lip and maxilla. J Oral Maxillofac Surg. 1986;44:593–6.
29. Honrado CP, Lee S, Bloomquist DS, Larrabee WF Jr. Quantitative assessment of nasal changes after maxillomandibular surgery using a 3-dimensional digital imaging system. Arch Facial Plast Surg. 2006;8:26–35.
30. van Loon B, Verhamme L, Xi T, de Koning MJ, Berge SJ, Maal TJ. Three-dimensional evaluation of the alar cinch suture after Le fort I osteotomy. Int J Oral Maxillofac Surg. 2016;45:1309–14.
31. Howley C, Ali N, Lee R, Cox S. Use of the alar base cinch suture in Le fort I osteotomy: is it effective? Br J Oral Maxillofac Surg. 2011;49:127–30.

Permissions

List of Contributors

Michael Vaiman
Department of Otolaryngology, Head and Neck Surgery, Assaf Harofe Medical Center, Affiliated to Sackler Faculty of Medicine, Tel Aviv University, Zerifin, Israel
33 Shapiro Street, Bat Yam 59561, Israel

Paul Gottlieb and Inessa Bekerman
Department of Radiology, Assaf Harofe Medical Center, Affiliated to Sackler Faculty of Medicine, Tel Aviv University, Zerifin, Israel

Ozkan Ozgul
Department of Oral and Maxillofacial Surgery, Faculty of Medicine, Ufuk University, Ankara, Turkey

Fatma Senses, Umut Tekin, Ismail Doruk Kocyigit and Fethi Atil
Department of Oral and Maxillofacial Surgery, Faculty of Dentistry, Kırıkkale University, Kırıkkale, Turkey

Nilay Er
Department of Oral and Maxillofacial Surgery, Faculty of Dentistry, Trakya University, Edirne Turkey

Hakan Hıfzı Tuz
Department of Oral and Maxillofacial Surgery, Faculty of Dentistry, Hacettepe University, Ankara, Turkey

Alper Alkan
Department of Oral and Maxillofacial Surgery, Faculty of Dentistry, Erciyes University, Kayseri, , Turkey

Sareh Said Yekta-Michael and Jamal M Stein
Department of Conservative Dentistry, Periodontology and Preventive Dentistry, Aachen University, Aachen, North Rhine-Westphalia, Germany

Sareh Said Yekta-Michael and Ernst Marioth-Wirtz
Interdisciplinary Center for Clinical Research, RWTH Aachen University, Aachen, North Rhine-Westphalia, Germany

Markus Kaup, Christoph Heinrich Dammann and Till Dammaschke
Department of Operative Dentistry, Westphalian Wilhelms-University, Albert-Schweitzer-Campus 1, building W 30, 48149 Münster, Germany

Edgar Schäfer
Central Interdisciplinary Ambulance in the School of Dentistry, Albert-Schweitzer-Campus 1, building W 30, 48149 Münster, Germany

Casiano Del Angel-Mosqueda, Ada Pricila López-Lozano, Ricardo Emmanuel Romero-Zavaleta, Carlos Eduardo Medina-De la Garza and Myriam Angélica De la Garza-Ramos
Unidad de Odontología Integral y Especialidades, Centro de Investigación y Desarrollo en Ciencias de la Salud, Universidad Autónoma de Nuevo León, Monterrey, Nuevo León, México

Casiano Del Angel-Mosqueda, Yolanda Gutiérrez-Puente and Ada Pricila López-Lozano
Instituto de Biotecnología, Facultad de Ciencias Biológicas, Universidad Autónoma de Nuevo León, San Nicolás de los Garza, Nuevo León, México

Yolanda Gutiérrez-Puente
Departamento de Química, Facultad de Ciencias Biológicas, Universidad Autónoma de Nuevo León, San Nicolás de los Garza, Nuevo León, México

Ada Pricila López-Lozano and Myriam Angélica De la Garza-Ramos
Facultad de Odontología, Universidad Autónoma de Nuevo León, Monterrey, Nuevo León, México

Andrés Mendiola-Jiménez, Carlos Eduardo Medina-De la Garza and Marcela Márquez-M
Facultad de Medicina, Universidad Autónoma de Nuevo León, Monterrey, Nuevo León, México

Marcela Márquez-M
Department of Oncology-Pathology, CCK, Karolinska Institutet, Stockholm, Sweden

Chrisanthi Karapantzou
ENT-Department, University of Göttingen Medical Center, Göttingen, Germany

Dirk Dressler
Department of Neurology, University of Hannover Medical Center, Hannover, Germany

Saskia Rohrbach
Department of Audiology and Phoniatrics, University of Berlin Medical Center, Berlin, Germany

Rainer Laskawi
HNO-Klinik Universitätsmedizin Göttingen, Robert-Koch-Str. 40, 37075 Göttingen, Germany

T. Roberts, L. Stephen, T. di Pasquale, A. Nasereldin, M. Chetty and S. Shaik
Faculty of Dentistry, University of the Western Cape, Private Bag X08, Mitchell's Plain, 7785 Cape Town, South Africa

C. Scott and P. Beighton
Faculty of Health Sciences, University of Cape Town, Observatory, 7925 Cape Town, South Africa

L. Lewandowski
Duke Global Health Institute, Pediatric Rheumatology, Global Health, Duke University Medical Center, Durham, USA

Benoît Imholz and Paolo Scolozzi
Department of Surgery, Service of Maxillofacial and Oral Surgery, University Hospital and Faculty of Medicine, Geneva, Switzerland

Thomas Schouman
Hôpital Pitié-Salpêtrière, Service de Chirurgie Maxillofaciale et Stomatologie, UPMC Université Paris, Paris, France

Philippe Rouch
Arts et Métiers ParisTech, LBM, 151, Boulevard de l'hôpital, Paris, France

Jean Fasel
Department of Anatomy, Faculty of Medicine -University of Geneva, Geneva, Switzerland

Delphine Courvoisier
CRC and Division of Clinical Epidemiology, Department of Health and Community Medicine, University of Geneva and University Hospitals of Geneva, Geneva, Switzerland

Michael Vaiman
Department of Otolaryngology – Head and Neck Surgery, Assaf Harofe
Medical Center, Affiliated to Sackler Faculty of Medicine, Tel Aviv University
Zerifin, Israel

Judith Luckman
Department of Radiology, Neuroradiology section, Beilinson campus, Rabin medical center, Holon, Israel

Tal Sigal and Inessa Bekerman
Department of Radiology, Assaf Harofe Medical Center, Affiliated to Sackler Faculty of Medicine, Tel Aviv University, Zerifin, Israel

Maisa O Al-Sebaei
Department of Oral and Maxillofacial Surgery, King AbdulAziz University, Faculty of Dentistry, PO Box 80209, Jeddah 21589, Kingdom of Saudi Arabia

Sihui Chen, Ying Cai and Fengshan Chen
Department of Orthodontics, Laboratory of Oral Biomedical Science and Translational Medicine, School of Stomatology, Tongji University, Middle Yanchang Road 399, Shanghai, P. R. China

Katharina Storck, Johannes Hauber, Anna-Maria Buchberger, Rainer Staudenmaier and Murat Bas
Department of Otorhinolaryngology, Klinikum Rechts der Isar, Technische Universität München, Ismaningerstrasse 22, 81675 Muenchen, Germany

Kornelia Kreiser
Department of Diagnostic and Interventional Neuroradiology, Klinikum Rechts der Isar, Technische Universität München, Ismaningerstrasse 22, 81675 Muenchen, Germany

Kilian Kreutzer
Department of Maxillofacial Surgery, Universitaetsklinikum Eppendorf, Martinistraße 52, 20246 Hamburg, Germany

Jörg Neunzehn and Hans-Peter Wiesmann
Technische Universität Dresden, Institute of Material Science, Chair for Biomaterials, Budapester Strasse 27, D-01069 Dresden, Germany

Thomas Szuwart
Department of Cranio-Maxillofacial Surgery, University Hospital of Muenster, Research Group Vascular Biology of Oral Structures (VABOS), Waldeyerstr 30, Muenster 48149, Germany

Ikenna Onwuekwe, Birinus Ezeala-Adikaibe and Oluchi Ekenze
Neurology Unit, Department of Medicine, University of Nigeria Teaching Hospital, Ituku-Ozalla, Enugu, Nigeria

Tonia Onyeka
Department of Anaesthesia/Pain and Palliative Care Unit, University of Nigeria Teaching Hospital, Ituku-Ozalla, PMB 01129 Enugu, Nigeria

Emmanuel Aguwa
Department of Community Medicine, University of Nigeria Teaching Hospital, Ituku-Ozalla, Enugu, Nigeria

Elias Onuora
Department of Anaesthesia, University of Nigeria Teaching Hospital, Ituku-Ozalla, Enugu, Nigeria

Florian Bauer, Steffen Koerdt, Niklas Rommel, Klaus-Dietrich Wolff, Marco R. Kesting and Jochen Weitz
Department of Oral and Maxillofacial Surgery at the Klinikum rechts der Isar, Technische Universität München, Ismaningerstrasse 22, 81675 Munich, Germany

Shabahang Mohammadi, Mohammad Mohseni, Masoumeh Eslami and Hessein Arabzadeh
Ear Nose Throat (ENT) and Head and Neck Surgery Research Center, Hazrat Rasoul Akram Hospital, Iran University of Medical Sciences, Sattarkhan St, Tehran, Iran

Morteza Eslami
Medical student of Iran University of Medical Sciences, ENT Department of Firouzgar Hospital, Vali Asr Street, Tehran, Iran

Se-Ho Lim, Moon-Key Kim and Sang-Hoon Kang
Department of Oral and Maxillofacial Surgery, National Health Insurance Service Ilsan Hospital, Goyang, Republic of Korea

Moon-Key Kim and Sang-Hoon Kang
Department of Oral and Maxillofacial Surgery, College of Dentistry, Yonsei University, Seoul, Republic of Korea

Julio Cifuentes, Alfredo Gantz, Ariel Barrera and Nicolas Yanine
Department of Oral and Maxillofacial Surgery, Clinica Alemana, Av Vitacura 5951, Vitacura, Santiago, Chile

Christian Teuber
Department of Oral and Maxillofacial Surgery, Pontificia Universidad Católica de Chile, Av Libertador Bernardo O'Higgins 340, Santiago, Chile

Gholamreza Danesh
Department of Orthodontics, Faculty of Health, University Witten/Herdecke, Alfred-Herrhausen-Strasse 44, 58455 Witten, Germany

Carsten Lippold
Department of Orthodontics, Universitätsklinikum Münster, Albert-Schweitzer-Campus 1, Gebäude W30, Waldeyerstraße 30, 48149 Münster, Germany

B. Lee, C. Flores-Mir and M. O. Lagravère
Department of Dentistry, University of Alberta, Edmonton, Canada

M. O. Lagravère
Department of Medicine and Dentistry, School of Dentistry, University of Alberta, 5524 Edmonton Clinic Health Academy, 11405-87 Ave, Edmonton T6G 1C9, Canada

Marc A. Polacco, Andrew M. Pintea, Benoit J. Gosselin and Joseph A. Paydarfar
Department of Otolaryngology, Dartmouth-Hitchcock Medical Center, Lebanon, NH, USA

Marc A. Polacco
Dartmouth-Hitchcock Medical Center, One Medical Center Drive, Lebanon, NH 03766, USA

Xiaoxian Chen and Jie Zhong
Department of Pediatric Dentistry, First clinical Division, Peking University School and Hospital of Stomatology, Beijing, China

Xinggang Liu
Department of Prosthodontics, Beijing Stomatological Hospital&School of Stomatology, Capital Medical University, 4 Tian Tan Xi Li, Beijing 100050, People's Republic of China

W. H. Arnold, Ch. Gröger and E. A. Naumova
Department of Biological and Material Sciences in Dentistry, School of Dentistry, Witten/Herdecke University, Witten, Germany

M. Bizhang
Department of Preventive and Operative Dentistry, School of Dentistry, Witten/Herdecke University, Witten, Germany

Marwa Mohammed Ali, Nadia Khalifa and Mohammed Nasser Alhajj
Department of Oral Rehabilitation, Faculty of Dentistry, University of Khartoum, Khartoum, Sudan

Nadia Khalifa
Department of Preventive and Restorative Dentistry, Faculty of Dental Medicine, University of Sharjah, Sharjah, United Arab Emirates

Mohammed Nasser Alhajj
Department of Prosthodontics, Faculty of Dentistry, Thamar University, Dhamar, Yemen

Michele Tepedino, Francesco Masedu and Claudio Chimenti
Department of Biotechnological and Applied Clinical Sciences, University of L'Aquila, Viale S.Salvatore, Edificio Delta 6, 67100 L'Aquila, Italy

Beatriz Vera-Sirera and Leopoldo Forner-Navarro
Department of Stomatology, Faculty of Medicine and Dentistry, University of Valencia, Valencia, Comunidad Valenciana, Spain

Luis Rubio-Martínez
Molecular Pathology Unit, Department of Pathology, La Fe University Hospital, University of Valencia, Valencia, Comunidad Valenciana, Spain

Francisco Vera-Sempere
Department of Pathology, Faculty of Medicine and Dentistry, La Fe University Hospital, University of Valencia, Torre A, 2° planta, Avda. Fernando Abril Martorell 106, 46026 Valencia, Comunidad Valenciana, Spain

Marcel Hanisch, Leopold F. Fröhlich and Johannes Kleinheinz
Department of Cranio-Maxillofacial Surgery, University Hospital Münster, Albert-Schweitzer-Campus 1, Gebäude W 30, Münster D-48149, Germany

Xu-Dong Yang, Su-Feng Zhao, Qian Zhang, Yu-Xin Wang, Wei Li, Xiao-Wei Hong and Qin-Gang Hu
Department of Oral and Maxillofacial Surgery, Nanjing Stomatological Hospital, Medical School of Nanjing University, No. 30 Zhong Yang Rd, Nanjing 210008, People's Republic of China

Anja Ratzmann
Department of Orthodontics and Department of Dental Propaedeutics/Community Dentistry, Dental School, University Medicine, Walther-Rathenau Straße 42a, 17475 Greifswald, Germany

Christan Schwahn
Department of Prosthetic Dentistry, Gerodontology and Biomaterials, University of Greifswald, Fleischmannstraße 42, 17475 Greifswald, Germany

Anja Treichel
Private Dental Office, Bahnhofstraße 4, 18581 Putbus, Germany

Andreas Faltermeier
Department of Orthodontics, Dental School, University Medicine, Franz-Josef-Strauß-Allee 11, 93053 Regensburg, Germany

Alexander Welk
Department of Restorative Dentistry, Periodontology, Endodontology, Preventive and Pediatric Dentistry, Dental School, University Medicine, Walther-Rathenau Straße 42a, 17475 Greifswald, Germany

Aysa Ayali and Kani Bilginaylar
Department of Oral and Maxillofacial Surgery, Near East University, Faculty of Dentistry, Near East Boulevard, Nicosia Cyprus, 99138 Mersin 10, Turkey

Jan Hourfar
Department of Orthodontics, University of Heidelberg, Heidelberg, Germany

Dirk Bister
Department of Orthodontics, Guy's and St Thomas' NHS Foundation Trust and King's College London Dental Institute, London, UK

Jörg A. Lisson and Björn Ludwig
Department of Orthodontics, University of Saarland, Homburg/Saar, Germany

Christine Goldbecher
Private Practice, Halle/Saale, Germany

Björn Ludwig
Private Practice, Am Bahnhof 54, 56841 Traben-Trarbach, Germany

Lara Schorn, Christoph Sproll, Christian Naujoks, Norbert R. Kübler and Rita Depprich
Department of Oral-, Maxillo- and Plastic Facial Surgery, Heinrich-Heine-University Duesseldorf, Moorenstr. 5, 40225 Duesseldorf, Germany

Michelle Ommerborn
Department of Operative and Preventive Dentistry and Endodontics, Heinrich-Heine-University Duesseldorf, Moorenstr. 5, Duesseldorf 40225, Germany

Cai Li, Ying Cai, Sihui Chen and Fengshan Chen
Department of Orthodontics, School and Hospital of Stomatology, Shanghai Engineering Research Centre of Tooth Restoration and Regeneration, Tongji University, Shanghai 200072, China

Jiarui Zhang, Xiuxia Ren, Bo Wang, Jing Cao, Linli Tian and Ming Liu
Department of Otorhinolaryngology, Head and Neck Surgery, Second Affiliated Hospital, Harbin Medical University, Harbin 150081, China

Junho Jung, Chi-Heun Lee, Jung-Woo Lee and Byung-Joon Choi
Department of Oral and Maxillofacial Surgery, School of Dentistry, Kyung Hee University, 26, Kyungheedae-ro, Dongdaemun-gu, 02447 Seoul, Republic of Korea

Index

www.ingramcontent.com/pod-product-compliance
Lightning Source LLC
Chambersburg PA
CBHW080458200326
41458CB00012B/4017